Clinical Radiation Oncology

Clinical Radiation Oncology

Editor: Andra Quinn

FOSTER ACADEMICS

www.fosteracademics.com

www.fosteracademics.com

FOSTER ACADEMICS

Cataloging-in-Publication Data

Clinical radiation oncology / edited by Andra Quinn.
p. cm.
Includes bibliographical references and index.
ISBN 978-1-63242-948-3
1. Cancer--Radiotherapy. 2. Radiotherapy. 3. Oncology. I. Quinn, Andra.
RC271.R3 C55 2020
616.994 064 2--dc23

Foster Academics,
118-35 Queens Blvd., Suite 400,
Forest Hills, NY 11375, USA

ISBN 978-1-63242-948-3 (Hardback)

Contents

Preface

The purpose of the book is to provide a glimpse into the dynamics and to present opinions and studies of some of the scientists engaged in the development of new ideas in the field from very different standpoints. This book will prove useful to students and researchers owing to its high content quality.

Radiation oncology is a field of medical specialization which involves the use of radiation for the treatment of cancer, and the management of pain and other symptoms. It can be applied to treat varied cancers and may be used alone or in conjunction with chemotherapy, surgery and other treatments. Radiation therapy generally works on cancerous tumors owing to its ability to control cell growth. Ionizing radiation damages the DNA of cancerous tissue thus leading to cellular death. The objective of radiotherapy depends on the location, stage and type of the tumor, and accordingly it may be called adjuvant, curative, neoadjuvant therapeutic or palliative. The field of radiation oncology has undergone significant advancements resulting in higher cure rates, improved quality of life and fewer side effects. New imaging technologies of tumors specifically allow radiation beams to be directed at the cancer, thereby limiting damage to adjacent organs. This book is a compilation of chapters that discuss the most vital concepts and emerging trends in the field of radiation oncology. It aims to shed light on some of the unexplored aspects and the recent researches in this field. This book, with its detailed analyses and data, will prove immensely beneficial to professionals and students involved in this area at various levels.

At the end, I would like to appreciate all the efforts made by the authors in completing their chapters professionally. I express my deepest gratitude to all of them for contributing to this book by sharing their valuable works. A special thanks to my family and friends for their constant support in this journey.

Editor

1

A patient-specific three-dimensional couplant pad for ultrasound image-guided radiation therapy

Heejung Kim[1,2], Ah Ram Chang[2], Sungwoo Cho[3] and Sung-Joon Ye[4,5,6*]

Abstract

Background: A wide application of ultrasound for radiation therapy has been hindered by a few issues such as skin and target deformations due to probe pressure, optical tracking disabilities caused by irregular surfaces and inter-user variations. The purpose of this study was to overcome these barriers by using a patient-specific three-dimensional (3D) couplant pad (CP).

Methods: A patient skin mold was designed using a skin contour of simulation CT images and fabricated by a 3D printer. A CP was then casted by pouring gelatin solution into a container accommodating the mold. To validate the use of the CP in positioning accuracy and imaging quality, phantom tests were carried out in our ultrasound-based localization system and then daily ultrasound images of four patients were acquired with and without the CP before treatment.

Results: In the phantom study, the use of CP increased a contrast-to-noise ratio from 2.4 to 4.0. The positioning accuracies in the US scans with and without the CP were less than 1 mm in all directions. In the patient study, the use of CP decreased the centroid offset of the target volume after target position alignment from 4.4 mm to 2.9 mm. One patient with a small volume of target showed a substantial increase in the inter-fractional target contour agreement (from 0.07 (poor agreement) to 0.31 (fair agreement) in Kappa values) by using the CP.

Conclusions: Our patient-specific 3D CP based on a 3D mold printing technique not only maintained the tracking accuracy but also reduced the inter-user variation, as well as that could potentially improve detectability of optical markers and target visibility for ultrasound image-guided radiotherapy.

Keywords: 3D couplant, Ultrasound, IGRT, 3D printing

Background

Ultrasound (US) can provide a superior soft tissue contrast and a high-spatial resolution (i.e. in the sub-millimeter range) [1]. In addition, US needs no extra radiation exposure for imaging, which potentially allows a daily image guidance over the course of radiation therapy (RT). One of the most widely used US applications in RT is a B-mode acquisition and tracking system (BAT; Nomos, Cranberry Township, PA, USA), which was first introduced in the 1990s. The most up-to-date US imaging system for IGRT is Clarity® (Elekta Ltd., Montréal, Québec, Canada). The advantage of this system over the conventional BAT system is that it eliminates inter-modality discrepancy by installing US devices in both a CT simulation room and a treatment room.

However, there have been a few issues in ultrasound image-guided radiation therapy (US IGRT). First, its main difference with the diagnostic US is the optical position-tracking system. Since the optical tracking system fixed on the ceiling should detect the reflective marker attached on the probe in the same coordinates as in the treatment room, the tracking range of the optical tracking system is limited by such geometry [2, 3]. In addition, the probe rotation is limited due to the marker position. Since the markers should be facing

* Correspondence: sye@snu.ac.kr
[4]Department of Transdisciplinary Studies, Seoul National University, Seoul, Korea
[5]Advanced Institutes of Convergence Technology, Seoul National University, Suwon, Korea
Full list of author information is available at the end of the article

toward the camera, irregularities and steep slopes of patient's skin hinder detectability of optical markers. Second, to improve the image quality of US, the air gap between the probe and the patient's skin must be removed. For this, during the US scan the pressure should be applied to the probe, which may deform the scanning region and distort images. As a result, target positional discrepancies in US images between the simulation and the treatment might be a concern [1, 4–7]. In order to minimize the probe pressure when the target lies underneath the skin or under an irregular surface, copious US gel and careful probe movement must be applied [8]. Third, the pressure manually applied to the US probe significantly varies depending on the users and thus influences the image quality of US. Such inter-personal variation has been an issue in US IGRT systems [7]. Moreover, US imaging involves the manual movement of a probe device over potentially irregular patient surfaces, which can be an another source of inter-personal variation. Therefore, achieving consistent and reproducible US scanning requires adequate user experience and training [4, 5]. Since an RT course consists of multiple fractions scheduled over 7–8 weeks, it is difficult even for a skilled user to maintain scanning consistency over the entire treatment period [9]. Forth, B-mode US is inherently limited by the dead zone artifact that occurs around the imaging region near the probe, depending on the probe frequency [10]. In order to avoid the acoustic noise near the transducer and to bring the lesion into the focal zone (geometric focus) of probe and out of the dead zone, a sufficient thickness of US coupling gel above the patient's skin has to be used especially for the superficial targets [11].

Conventionally, US gel, nipple pads and gel pads have been used as a coupling material. However, for irregular surfaces, the viscosity of US gel is too low. Nipple pads can be applied, but are limited to the breast nipple. Alternatively, gel pads (pad-type acoustic coupling materials) are commercially available with high prices. To facilitate US scanning on irregular surfaces, coupling pads of various materials have been investigated [12–17]. However, due to their very low viscosity, these pads require additional gels in some cases to remove air gap between the probe and patient skin surface. With their standard size, fixed thickness and shape, they are not flexible enough to fit over the scanning area of skin surface for each patient. To overcome the aforementioned problems in US IGRT, this study developed a patient-specific 3D couplant pad (CP) with an aid of 3D printing technology. We optimized the design and composition of the pad to facilitate its use in US IGRT. Finally, we investigated the feasibility of our CP and its clinical application through phantom and patient studies.

Methods

Equipment for IGRT

In this study, the US system used for IGRT was Clarity® 3.1 (Elekta Ltd., Montréal, Québec, Canada). Its main difference from the diagnostic US is the optical position-tracking system that consists of a ceiling-mounted optical camera system and eight infrared reflecting markers attached to the probe. This optical tracking system with the probe was calibrated with respect to the room reference coordinate by using the specific US calibration phantom (provided by the manufacturer). During the US scanning, it detects the marker position to determine the target location. The CT simulation scanner and the LINAC system used in this study were Philips Brilliance Big Bore 16-slice CT-simulator (Philips Healthcare, Cleveland, OH, USA) and Elekta Infinity™ (Elekta AB, Stockholm, Sweden), respectively.

Couplant pad (CP)

A couplant material should have appropriate acoustic properties to avoid image artifacts. An acoustic property (e.g., speed of sound) can be computed by measuring a signal trigger time to signal response time with the distance to a specific target. However, Clarity US probe acts as both a transmitter and receiver. It does not only have a functionality in clinical mode to measure the signal trigger and response time, but also it does not support any kind of hydrophone connection to be synchronized to Clarity transducer. According to the literatures [18, 19], the water-based gel has the desired ultrasonic transmission properties. Gelatin has been known to have a speed of sound from 1500 m/s to 1600 m/s and its density of 1 g/cm^3 with low attenuation (0.05 dB/cm*MHz). Thus, in this study, gelatin was selected for the CP material.

The CP making process was as follows: (1) the MIM® (MIM Software Inc., Cleveland, OH, USA) software was used to contour the skin and the treatment target on the CT images and to export the contour as a dicom file; (2) the dicom file of the patient skin contour was imported into the 3D Slicer (BWH and 3D Slicer contributors) software, which was used to make a skin surface model using the SlicerRT module and to convert it to the STL file format for 3D printing [20, 21]; (3) by using a 3D printer (CubePro®, Cubify, 3DSYSTEMS, Rock Hill, SC, USA), the patient skin mold for the area to be scanned by US was made using PLA (Polylactic acid); (4) the edible gelatin powder was mixed with hot water and 83% ethanol as a preservative with the ratio of 1:5:0.5; (5) the patient skin mold was fixed in the container; (6) the gelatin solution was poured into the container and put into the refrigerator for 2 h for solidifying; (7) finally the CP was separated from the container and the patient skin mold. The minimum depth of the CP should be 1 cm or more in order to bring the target into the focal zone.

According to the literature, oil can be used as a low viscosity coupling agent substitute for ultrasound gel [22]. To achieve a better contact between the phantom and the CP, baby oil was used. After spreading oil (mineral or vegetable) inside the CP or on the patient skin, the CP was put on the patient. At first US scan, skin markings were done at the CP edges. The CP was positioned by the skin marks and then the US scan was performed. All US scans for all patients were acquired by all three users.

Phantom study

Prior to the clinical implementation of CP, an in-house phantom was fabricated with a mixture of gelatin and agarose and a CP was fabricated with gelatin only for the phantom study. The mixture of gelatin and agarose was used as a soft tissue and a piece of a commercial gel pad (Aquaflex, Parker Laboratories, INC., Fairfield, NJ, USA) was inserted into the phantom as a target. Figure 1 shows the in-house phantom images acquired using CT and US with and without the CP. US scanning was performed in four different sweeping directions on the CP. Target volume and image contrast were evaluated by contouring volumes of interest (one target and four spheres with 1 cm diameter 2 cm away from target) on CT and US images.

To validate the positioning accuracy of the US-based localization with and without the CP, the Clarity Calibration Phantom (Elekta Ltd., Montréal, Québec, Canada) was used. It was scanned using the simulation CT to be used as a reference. Applying 20 different combination of intentional table shifts (ranged from 1 mm to 30 mm) from the reference location (0, 0, 0) in the left-right (LR), the anterior-posterior (AP) and the inferior-superior (IS) directions, CBCT and US images with and without the CP were acquired.

Patient study

Among the subjects eligible for US IGRT, four patients were selected in this study to evaluate the effectiveness of the developed CP. The four patients participated in the study after the institutional review board (IRB) approval (IRB number 2014–11-029). Patient 1 had a metastatic inguinal lymph node under an irregular surface. Patient 2 also had a metastatic inguinal lymph node at the depth of about 2 cm from the skin. Patient 3 had a tonsil cancer. Due to the surface curvature of this patient's head and neck, the probe movement had a difficulty; the probe marker was not detectable by the shoulder. Patient 4 had a soft tissue sarcoma on the shoulder placed at the shallow depth underneath the irregular surface and thus it was difficult to apply pressure with the probe. The curved probe was used for patients 1 and 3 and the linear probe was used for patients 2 and 4.

For all patients, the US scanning was performed at every treatment day before the treatment and the x-ray image acquisition was performed minimum once a week and maximum twice a week before the treatment by using the CBCT. For four patients (patient 1–4), the simulation CT image, US images with and without the

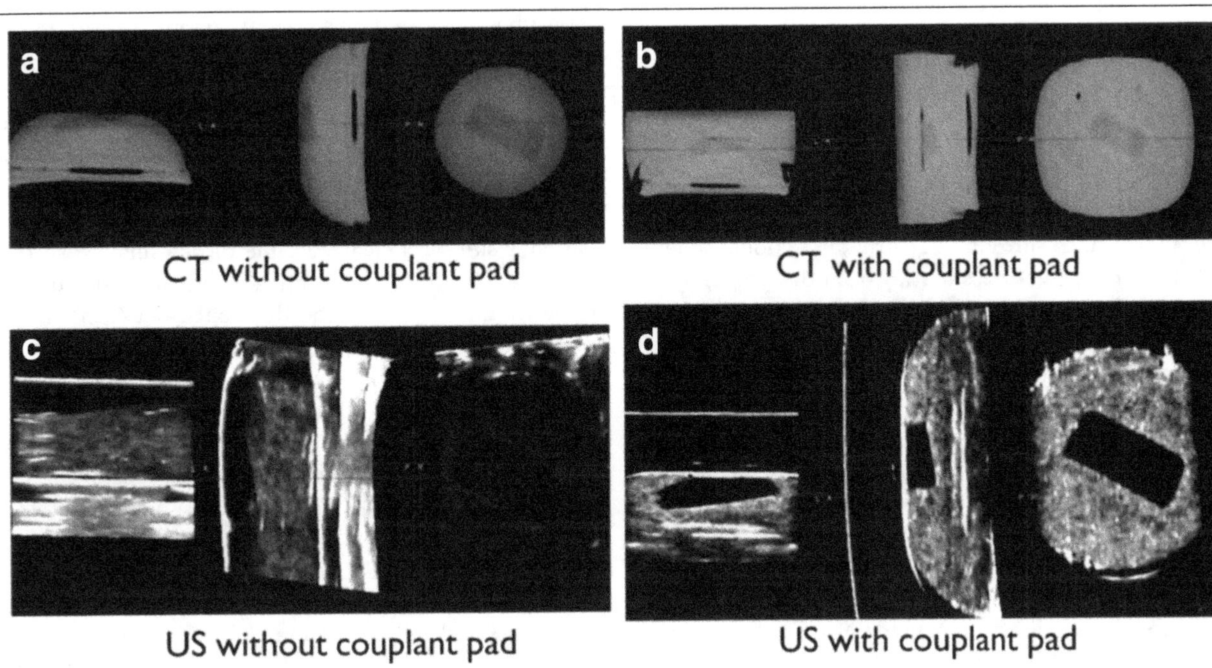

Fig. 1 In-house phantom images: **a** The simulation CT image acquired without couplant pad (CP). **b** The simulation CT acquired with CP. **c** The US image acquired without CP. **d** The US image acquired with CP

CP and CBCT images were acquired. Due to the patient's inevitable condition such as a deterioration of general condition and a low CBC (complete blood count) level that is not available to treat and due to the patient's treatment refusal, total 324 US images and 16 CBCT images were acquired in 21, 18, 6 and 9 fractions for patient 1, 2, 3 and 4. The US scanning time except of image registration process and patient setup was evaluated.

Data analysis and statistics

US images of four patients (patient 1–4) were acquired before the treatment by three different users (one physicist, two therapists) in both conditions with and without applying the CP. The first US image (taken at the first treatment day) for each patient was used as a reference and all US images were registered to it. The target volume (GTV) was contoured on the US images. The volume of the target and the target centroid shift were calculated. The contrast-to-noise ratio (CNR) was calculated an area inside and 3 mm outside the target volume in the US images. The variations in the volume of the target due to the deformation of the target depending on the US scanning conditions were also evaluated. Each target volume difference (%) was calculated by dividing a difference between the target volumes in the first US image and each US image by the target volumes in the first US image. Inter-user variation in US scanning was evaluated by analyzing the centroid shift of the target. The CERR (Computational Environment for Radiotherapy Research) software was used in order to evaluate the level of agreement among the target contours in terms of kappa values calculated using the Fleiss' eq. [23–25]. Using the SPSS software, a linear mixed model was calculated to investigate the developed CP in terms of image contrast and inter-user variation.

Results

Phantom study result

The target and surrounding structures (four spheres with 1 cm diameter at 2 cm away from the target) of the in-house phantom were delineated. Compared with the target volume (5.9 ml) in the CT image as a reference, it was not changed (less than 0.1 ml) by the probe sweeping direction in the US image with the CP, while it was varied by up to 1.6 ml in the US image without the CP because the target of the in-house phantom was located superficially. In addition, by using the CP, the CNR on the US image was increased from 2.4 to 4.0, comparing with the CNR (2.8) on the CT image.

Table 1 shows the Clarity Calibration Phantom test result for the localization accuracy of US scanning with and without the CP, comparing with CBCT. The US positioning errors were less than 0.6 mm in all directions, regardless of applying the CP. This result indicates that the Clarity® US image guidance system used in this study had no systematic error for target localization. Compared to CBCT as a ground truth, the US tracking for localization was accurate within 0.6 mm, even when using the CP: 0.1 ± 0.3 mm, 0.1 ± 0.2 mm and – 0.3 ± 0.7 mm for the US without the CP and 0.0 ± 0.2 mm, 0.2 ± 0.3 mm and – 0.6 ± 0.4 mm for the US with the CP in LR, AP and IS direction. For a reference, our couch and CBCT positioning accuracy are maintained to be within 1 mm by our monthly QA based on TG 142 report and the manufacturer engineer's periodic maintenance.

Table 1 Accuracy of US image-based localization with and without couplant pad (CP), comparing with CBCT: positioning errors from phantom test with intentional 3-dimensional table shifts (ranged from 1 mm to 30 mm in each direction)

	LR (mm)	AP (mm)	IS (mm)
CBCT	0.3 ± 0.3	0.5 ± 0.4	0.6 ± 0.5
US without CP	0.4 ± 0.2	0.6 ± 0.4	0.3 ± 0.3
US with CP	0.3 ± 0.2	0.5 ± 0.3	0.2 ± 0.1

Abbreviations: *LR* Left-Right, *AP* Anterior-Posterior, *IS* Inferior-Superior, *CBCT* Cone-Beam Computed Tomography, *US* Ultrasound, *CP* Couplant Pad

Patient study result

As shown in Fig. 2, the patient-specific CP for each patient was fabricated using the 3D printed-patient skin mold. Overall, by the use of the CP, the US hand-held probe could be easily swept on the flat side of the CP. In all patients, when the CP was not applied, a large amount of US coupling gel was needed in order to minimize the probe pressure due to the target being located at a shallow depth from the skin. For patient 4, the irregularity of patient's skin was excessive, so that the US scan could not cover the whole target region and the dark shadow due to the air was shown around the target. However, when the CP was applied, there was no difficulty for scanning and no need of a large amount of gel. Moreover, the patient's skin was clearly visible on US images, so that it was easier to fuse the images and to delineate the target. Figure 3 shows the difference between the US scans without and with the CP for all patients relative to their simulation CT images. Individually, for patient 1, the skin deformation due to the pressure from the hand-held probe was removed. For patient 2, the image contrast was improved and the edges of the target were clearly visible. For patient 3, the area between neck and shoulder with high curvature was filled by the CP so that the US scanning area between probe and CP became flat. Thus, the long target volume was scanned completely within the US optical tracking range. For patient 4, the shoulder surface was scanned without any artifact and deformation. In addition, the small superficial target near the shoulder became observable.

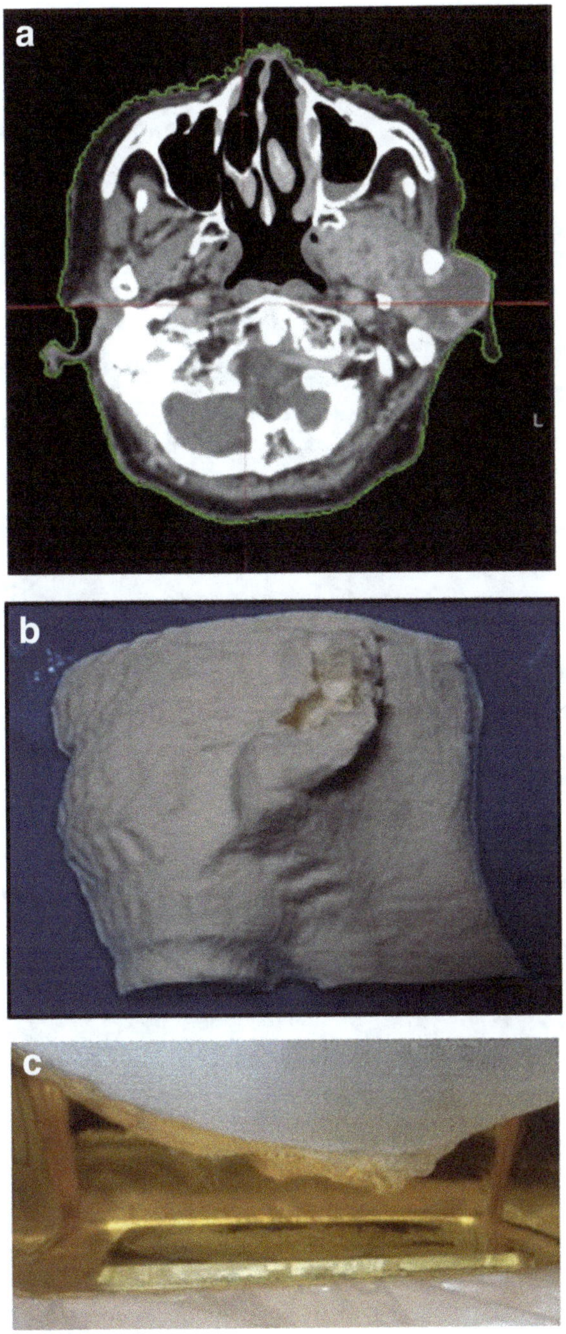

Fig. 2 Example of the process for fabricating a patient-specific 3D couplant pad (CP). **a** The patient skin contour is extracted from the simulation CT images. **b** The patient skin mold is fabricated by 3D printer. **c** A CP is casted by pouring gelatin solution into a container accommodating the mold

Except of image registration process and patient setup, the average US scanning time was 1 min 19 s for US without the CP and 1 min 24 s. For patient 1 and 2, it was less than 1 min 10 s on average regardless of the use of the CP. For patient 3 (large scanning area and large CP), US scanning without the CP took 56 s, but it increased to 1 min 39 s due to setting up the CP. However, for patient 4 (severely curved surface but small CP), it took 3 min 10 s without the CP and decreased to 2 min 20 s due to the use of CP.

The centroid shift of target in US images without the CP was − 0.7 ± 2.1 mm in LR and − 0.4 ± 4.2 mm in IS, but 2.1 ± 2.8 mm in AP. However, in US images with the CP it was less than 1 mm in all directions; 0.1 ± 1.7 mm in LR, 0.7 ± 1.7 mm in AP, − 0.6 ± 3.3 mm in IS. As shown in Fig. 4 (a), the 3D vector magnitude of the centroid shift decreased from 4.4 ± 3.9 mm (4.1 mm Median) to 2.9 ± 3.0 mm (2.1 mm Median). This effect of using CP on the centroid shift of target was statistically significant in LR, AP and 3D vector magnitude with p-values less than 0.001 for the linear mixed model. As listed in Table 2, the difference among the three different users in the mean and 1 SD values of the centroid offset of target was decreased due to the use of CP. Depending on the user's skills (e.g., probe pressure and scanning area coverage), the centroid offset was significantly different when the US scan was performed without the CP ($p < 0.05$ in all directions).

The image contrast between the target and the surrounding tissue were compared in terms of the CNR. Only for the patient 2 (small target on shoulder), the CNR was significantly increased from 3.7 ± 1.0 to 4.1 ± 1.1 with p-value less than 0.05. Contrary to the phantom study result, overall CNR had no statistically significant increase in the image contrast when applying the CP. It was 3.4 ± 1.5 for US without CP and 3.4 ± 1.3 for US with CP.

The target volume contouring variation among the different users were evaluated. As shown in Fig. 4 (b), the target volume contouring variation was decreased from 11.0% ± 10.2% to 5.5% ± 4.4% due to the use of CP ($p = 0.001$). The agreement of inter-fractional target contours on the registered US images was evaluated in terms of kappa values. For patient 1, 2 and 3, all kappa values were over 0.61 (good agreement) regardless of the use of CP. For the patient 4, the target volume was very small (about 0.2 ml) and the US scanning without the CP was very difficult because the target was placed under shoulder (steep and curved surface). The kappa values in US images without the CP were less than 0.07 (poor agreement); however, the kappa value was increased into over 0.31 (fair agreement) due to the use of CP.

The patient setup errors of US image-based localization with and without the CP were compared with CBCT which is a current gold standard method. As shown in Table 3, the average differences between CBCT and US localizations were less than 2 mm in all directions. In US without the CP, the maximum difference was − 1.9 mm

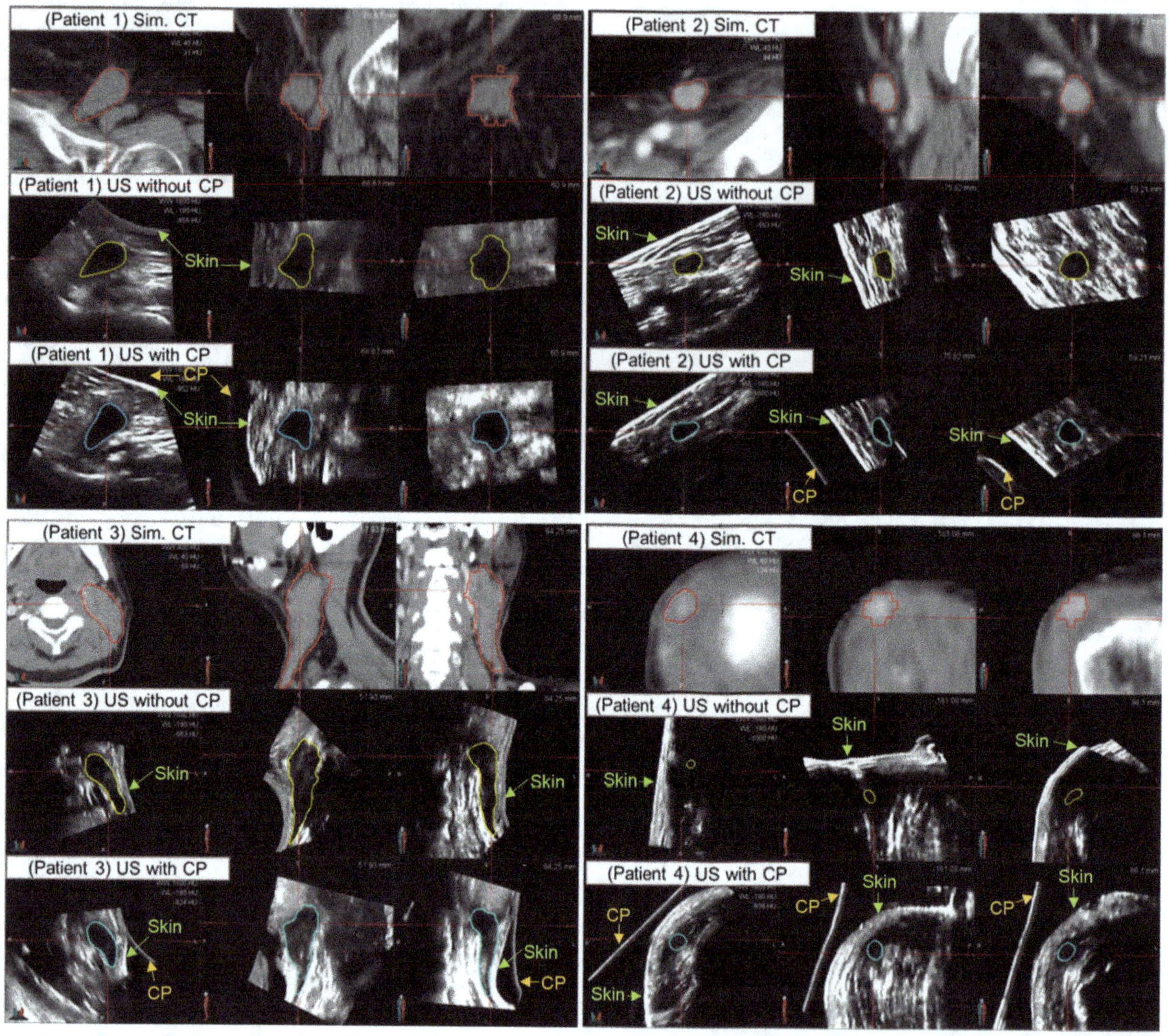

Fig. 3 US image acquisitions without and with using CP relative to the simulation CT image for four patients. The targets (GTV) were delineated on each images

on average in AP direction. When using the CP, it decreased by 1.1 mm. The 3D error magnitude decreased by 0.5 mm.

Discussion

Since the Clarity US system used in this study can use US images as reference images for image registration, no inter-modality effects were present and the scanning direction effects were negligible (less than 0.1 cc). In this study, the CP was made of gelatin, a homogeneous colloid gel that is produced from animal collagen. The collagen was combined with a sufficient amount of water so that the density of the CP ranged from 1004 kg/m^3–1024 kg/m^3, which is similar to that of water. Thus, the speed of sound in the CP (1500 m/s – 1600 m/s) may be similar to that in tissue (1520 m/s - 1650 m/s) [19, 26]. The gelatin was easy to use, cost-effective, homogeneous, and exhibited low acoustic attenuation. These highly desirable properties make gelatin an ideal material for a CP to be used during US scanning. To remove the air between the CP and the patient surface, conventional US gel has a higher viscosity than water or oil and did not sufficiently remove the air. The mineral oil yielded a clear interface and did not make air bubbles.

Ultrasound imaging noise is caused by excess gain or low gain [27]. This issue can be resolved by decreasing or increasing the overall gain. However, excessive gain can result in false echoes or oversaturation. To resolve low gain artifacts, applying more acoustic coupling material can help to increase the far gain and the overall gain. For these reasons, CNR for image contrast in the phantom test of this study was increased from 2.4 to 4.0

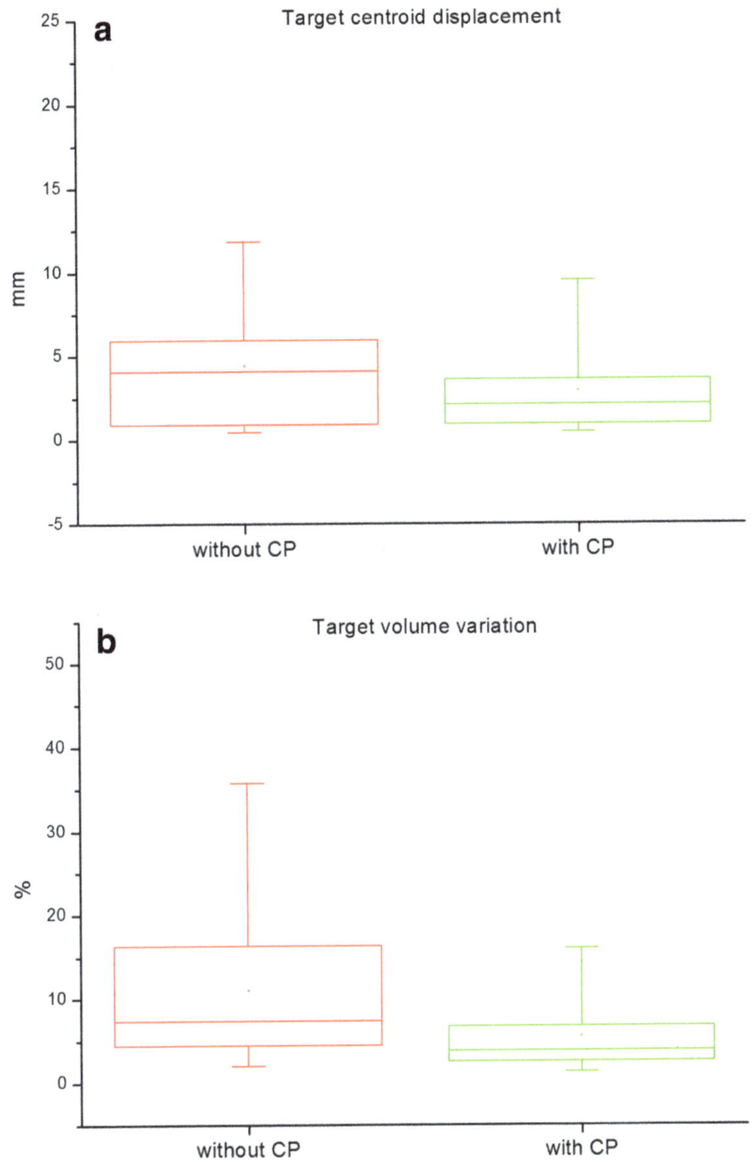

Fig. 4 Box-and-whisker charts for the results of (**a**) target centroid displacement and (**b**) target volume variation. The box is determined by the 25th and 75th percentiles and the whiskers are determined by the 5th and 95th percentiles. In the box, the line and small box represent the median and mean values

due to the use of the CP. Unlike the phantom study result, it was not significantly different in the patient study result when applying the CP. Only for the patient 2 who had a small target on shoulder, the CNR was increased from 3.7 to 4.1 ($p < 0.05$). An increase in noise in a target can be a possible reason of this different result for the CNR because the inside of target is very homogeneous in the phantom but heterogeneous in the patients.

The patient-specific 3D CP developed in this study can solve many problems that have been raised regarding the use of the Clarity® US system for IGRT. The specific contour of patient's skin above the target was used to make the mold for the CP. Theoretically, since the CP has a flat surface on the side where the probe can move with a constant pressure, the marker is always detectable without a dead angle. As in patient 3, the long and highly curved target volume between neck and shoulder was scanned without any difficulty to detect the reflective markers by filling the scanning area with the CP to become a flat surface. With the CP, the gel is used only for the probe surface. As experienced in the cases of patient 3 and patient 4, the flat surface of the CP faced to the US probe can potentially reduce the scanning time and remove the dependence on sweeping directions and multi-path artifact. In this study, the time required to perform a US scan with the CP decreased from 3 min

Table 2 Centroid offset of target after target position alignment: Analysis of the correlation of the centroid offset among the three different users by using the linear mixed model

	User 1	User 2	User 3	*p*-value
Without CP				
LR (mm)	− 0.7 ± 2.2	−0.2 ± 2.1	− 1.2 ± 2.0	0.005
AP (mm)	2.1 ± 2.8	1.5 ± 2.3	2.6 ± 3.2	0.002
IS (mm)	0.2 ± 4.7	0.5 ± 3.9	− 1.8 ± 3.5	< 0.001
3D (mm)	4.5 ± 4.4	3.9 ± 3.5	4.8 ± 3.8	0.020
		With CP		
LR (mm)	− 0.0 ± 1.4	0.3 ± 1.7	0.1 ± 1.8	0.081
AP (mm)	0.5 ± 1.4	0.7 ± 1.5	0.8 ± 2.2	0.582
IS (mm)	−1.0 ± 3.2	− 0.6 ± 3.2	− 0.4 ± 3.5	0.194
3D (mm)	2.7 ± 2.9	2.8 ± 2.9	3.3 ± 3.2	0.133

Abbreviations: *LR* Left-Right, *AP* Anterior-Posterior, *IS* Inferior-Superior, *3D* the amplitude of three-dimensional vector, *CP* Couplant Pad

10 s to 2 min 20 s due to the use of CP for the patient 4. For other patients, it was within 2 min, which is similar to CBCT. As shown in the case of patient 4, the inherent depth of the CP provided an additional benefit of removing dead-zone artifacts. Moreover, the contrast of US images was improved for patient 2 and inter-user variation in daily US scanning was mitigated in all patients. The CP developed in this study was conveniently fabricated with a lower cost (about 20 oz. and $4 per CP) than the commercial gel pad (about 5 oz. and $10 per price), requiring only 3 h from the extraction of patient's skin contours to the generation of the final CP. When a target volume is changed due to a patient's weight loss or tumor shrinkage, a planning CT can be re-acquired according to a radiation oncologist's decision and the CP also can be re-fabricated. In this study, there was no patient who needs the re-planning CT scan during entire treatment procedure.

The US localization accuracy comparing to CBCT has been studied but most studies were about prostate [28–34]. According to the literature which compared the setup errors between CBCT and Clarity transabdominal US, it resulted in the best agreement in LR direction and the largest discrepancy in US toward posterior due to the shift by 2.8 mm in AP direction [32]. According to Wong's breast US study, the skin displacement due to probe pressure was 3.0 mm compared to CT [35]. The results of US without CP versus CBCT in this study showed the maximum discrepancy (1.9 mm) in AP direction. Although this discrepancy was reduced to 1.3 mm due to the use of the CP, US is experimental up to the present and the patient setup verification using a standard methods (e.g. CBCT) should be performed additionally at least weekly. In addition, as shown in the result of the phantom test in this study, the US localization accuracy was not impaired even with the CP. Unfortunately, no literature exists on the topic of US CPs for US-IGRT. We could not compare our findings to other studies.

Table 3 Comparison of patient setup errors between CBCT and US image-based localization with and without couplant pad (CP)

	CBCT vs. US without CP	CBCT vs. US with CP
LR (mm)	− 0.3 ± 2.3	0.3 ± 1.9
AP (mm)	−1.9 ± 1.8	−0.8 ± 1.6
IS (mm)	0.8 ± 1.4	1.3 ± 1.2
3D (mm)	3.4 ± 1.4	2.9 ± 1.2

Abbreviations: *LR* Left-Right, *AP* Anterior-Posterior, *IS* Inferior-Superior, *3D* the amplitude of three-dimensional vector, *CBCT* Cone-Beam Computed Tomography, *US* Ultrasound, *CP* Couplant Pad

This study has some limitations. This findings were based on total 324 images from only four patients and thus additional images from more patients will be required to determine an appropriate PTV margin for our US IGRT. In this study, the 1st treatment US image was used as a reference US image for the image registration. Since the CP was generated from the simulation CT image, the CP was not available for a simulation US scan during a simulation CT scan. If the re-simulation CT and simulation US images using the CP are acquired at the same time before the treatment, the simulation US image can be used as a reference US image for the entire course of treatments. Alternatively, a 3D scanner can be used to make a patient-specific CP before the simulation CT/US.

Unlike the CBCT, the US does not provide an entire body or skin images. In this study, the skin marks for the CP edges were necessary to setup the CP on the patient surface. In addition, it could be difficult to place and fix the CP on the patient surface in a case like a breast which it slides off the skin. The supporting device for the CP can be helpful to immobilize the CP position and it is under development.

There is a limitation of the CP's lifespan. Once made, it should be put in a separate container and be stored in a refrigerator so that it can be used for up to 2 weeks safely without deformation. As long as the time that the CP is exposed to an air increase, the water consisting of the CP decrease and the CP can shrink. In addition, the ethanol is used as a conservative for fabricating the CP; nevertheless, when the CP is left at the room temperature or it is used more than 3 weeks, it can get moldy. Thus, the gelatin-based CP fabricated by our method in this study should be stored in an airtight container at a low temperature and it is proper to use within 2 weeks. If a sterilized separate space for a CP fabrication, a 3D printer, and a refrigerator for a CP storage are prepared, it will be practical to use it in an RT department for many patients. A new CP material for fabricating once and using it during entire treatment courses will be developed in our further study.

Conclusions

The patient-specific 3D CP based on the 3D mold printing technique not only maintained the tracking accuracy but also reduced the inter-user variation. This is a promising strategy that could potentially improve detectability of optical markers and target visibility. With taking advantage of non-ionizing radiation, ultrasound technology with this CP could potentially be used for a broader variety of radiotherapy targets.

Abbreviations

3D: 3-dimensional; AP: Anterior-Posterior; CNR: Contrast-to-noise ratio; CP: Couplant pad; CT: Computed tomography; IS: Inferior-Superior; LR: Left-Right; RT: Radiation therapy; SD: Standard deviation; US IGRT: Ultrasound image-guided radiation therapy; US: Ultrasound

Authors' contributions

HJK designed the study, acquired and interpreted the data, and wrote the manuscript. ARJ contributed to the data collection for patient study and involved in drafting the manuscript. SWC performed the 3D printing of patient skin mold. SJY contributed to the overall experimental design and involved in revising the manuscript critically. All authors have given final approval of the version to be published.

Competing interests

The authors declare that they have no competing interests.

Author details

[1]Department of Biomedical Engineering, Seoul National University, Seoul, Korea. [2]Department of Radiation Oncology, Soonchunhyang University Hospital, Seoul, Korea. [3]Department of Surgery, Soonchunhyang University Hospital, Seoul, Korea. [4]Department of Transdisciplinary Studies, Seoul National University, Seoul, Korea. [5]Advanced Institutes of Convergence Technology, Seoul National University, Suwon, Korea. [6]Biomedical Research Institute, Seoul National University Hospital, Seoul, Korea.

References

1. Enke KA C, Saw CB, Zhen W, Thompson RB, Raman NV. Inter-Observer Variation in Prostate Localization Utilizing BAT. Int J Radiat Oncol Biol Phys. 2002;54(2):269.
2. Robinson D, Liu D, Steciw S, Field C, Daly H, Saibishkumar EP, Fallone G. An evaluation of the Clarity 3D ultrasound system for prostate localization. J Appl Clin Med Phys. 2012;13:100–12.
3. Lachaine M, Falco T. Intrafractional prostate motion management with the clarity autoscan system. *Med Phys Int.* 2013;1:72–80.
4. Fiandra C, Guarneri A, Munoz F, Moretto F, Filippi AR, Levis M, Ragona R, Ricardi U. Impact of the observers' experience on daily prostate localization accuracy in ultrasound-based IGRT with the Clarity platform. *J Appl Clin Med Phys.* 2014;15:4795.
5. Fuss M, Cavanaugh SX, Fuss C, Cheek DA, Salter BJ. Daily stereotactic ultrasound prostate targeting: inter-user variability. *Technol Cancer Res Treat.* 2003;2:161–70.
6. Langen KM, Pouliot J, Anezinos C, Aubin M, Gottschalk AR, Hsu IC, Lowther D, Liu YM, Shinohara K, Verhey LJ, et al. Evaluation of ultrasound-based prostate localization for image-guided radiotherapy. *Int J Radiat Oncol Biol Phys.* 2003;57:635–44.
7. Serago CF, Chungbin SJ, Buskirk SJ, Ezzell GA, Collie AC, Vora SA. Initial experience with ultrasound localization for positioning prostate cancer patients for external beam radiotherapy. *Int J Radiat Oncol Biol Phys.* 2002; 53:1130–8.
8. Fargier-Voiron M, Presles B, Pommier P, Rit S, Munoz A, Liebgott H, Sarrut D, Biston M-C. Impact of probe pressure variability on prostate localization for ultrasound-based image-guided radiotherapy. *Radiother Oncol.* 2014;111:132–7.
9. Molloy JA, Chan G, Markovic A, McNeeley S, Pfeiffer D, Salter B, Tome WA. Quality assurance of U.S.-guided external beam radiotherapy for prostate cancer: report of AAPM Task Group 154. *Med Phys.* 2011;38:857–71.
10. Goodsitt MM, Carson PL, Witt S, Hykes DL, Kofler JM Jr. Real-time B-mode ultrasound quality control test procedures. Report of AAPM Ultrasound Task Group No. 1. *Med Phys.* 1998;25:1385–406.
11. American College of Radiology. Acr practice parameter for the performance of a breast ultrasound examination, Amended 2014 (Resolution 39). Reston: ACR (American College of Radiology); 2014.
12. Klucinec B. The effectiveness of the aquaflex gel pad in the transmission of acoustic energy. *J Athl Train.* 1996;31:313–7.
13. Tsui BCH, Tsui J. A flexible gel pad as an effective medium for scanning irregular surface anatomy. Can J Anesth. 2011;59:226–7.
14. Yasukawa K, Kunisue T, Tsuta K, Shikinami Y, Kondo T. P6C-9 An Ultrasound Phantom with Long-Term Stability Using a New Biomimic Soft Gel Material. In: Ultrasonics Symposium, 2007 IEEE; 2007. p. 2501–2.
15. Biller DS, Myer W. Ultrasound scanning of superficial structures using an ultrasound standoff pad. Vet Radiol. 1988;29:138–42.
16. Claes HP, Reygaerts DO, Boven FA, Leemans J, De Boeck M, Geurts JM. An echo-free silicone elastomer block for ultrasonography. Radiology. 1984;150:596.
17. Yeh HC, Wolf BS. A simple portable water bath for superficial ultrasonography. Am J Roentgenol. 1978;130:275–8.
18. Amin VR. Tissue characterization by ultrasound: a study of tissue-mimicking materials and quantitative ultrasonics, Retrospective Theses and Dissertations: Iowa State University; 1992. http://lib.dr.iastate.edu/.
19. Madsen EL, Zagzebski JA, Banjavie RA, Jutila RE. Tissue mimicking materials for ultrasound phantoms. Med Phys. 1978;5:391–4.
20. Fedorov A, Beichel R, Kalpathy-Cramer J, Finet J, Fillion-Robin JC, Pujol S, Bauer C, Jennings D, Fennessy F, Sonka M, et al. 3D Slicer as an image computing platform for the Quantitative Imaging Network. Magn Reson Imaging. 2012;30:1323–41.
21. Pinter C, Lasso A, Wang A, Jaffray D, Fichtinger G. SlicerRT: radiation therapy research toolkit for 3D Slicer. Med Phys. 2012;39:6332–8.
22. Gorny KR, Hangiandreou NJ, Hesley GK, Felmlee JP. Evaluation of mineral oil as an acoustic coupling medium in clinical MRgFUS. Phys Med Biol. 2007;52:N13–9.
23. Deasy JO, Blanco AI, Clark VH. CERR: a computational environment for radiotherapy research. Med Phys. 2003;30:979–85.
24. Fleiss JL. Statistical methods for rates and proportions. 2nd ed. New York: Wiley. 1981. p. 38–46.
25. Landis JR, Koch GG. The measurement of observer agreement for categorical data. Biometrics. 1977;33:159–74.
26. Bude RO, Adler RS. An easily made, low-cost, tissue-like ultrasound phantom material. J Clin Ultrasound. 1995;23:271–3.
27. Mohler ER. Essentials of Vascular Laboratory Diagnosis. Hoboken: Wiley; 2008.
28. McNair HA, Mangar SA, Coffey J, Shoulders B, Hansen VN, Norman A, Staffurth J, Sohaib SA, Warrington AP, Dearnaley DP. A comparison of CT- and ultrasound-based imaging to localize the prostate for external beam radiotherapy. Int J Radiat Oncol Biol Phys. 2006;65:678–87.
29. Boda-Heggemann J, Kohler FM, Kupper B, Wolff D, Wertz H, Mai S, Hesser J, Lohr F, Wenz F. Accuracy of ultrasound-based (BAT) prostate-repositioning: a three-dimensional on-line fiducial-based assessment with cone-beam computed tomography. Int J Radiat Oncol Biol Phys. 2008;70:1247–55.

30. van der Meer S, Bloemen-van Gurp E, Hermans J, Voncken R, Heuvelmans D, Gubbels C, Fontanarosa D, Visser P, Lutgens L, van Gils F, Verhaegen F. Critical assessment of intramodality 3D ultrasound imaging for prostate IGRT compared to fiducial markers. Med Phys. 2013;40:071707.
31. Li M, Ballhausen H, Hegemann NS, Ganswindt U, Manapov F, Tritschler S, Roosen A, Gratzke C, Reiner M, Belka C. A comparative assessment of prostate positioning guided by three-dimensional ultrasound and cone beam CT. Radiat Oncol. 2015;10:82.
32. Fargier-Voiron M, Presles B, Pommier P, Munoz A, Rit S, Sarrut D, Biston MC. Ultrasound versus Cone-beam CT image-guided radiotherapy for prostate and post-prostatectomy pretreatment localization. Phys Med. 2015;31:997–1004.
33. Richter A, Polat B, Lawrenz I, Weick S, Sauer O, Flentje M, Mantel F. Initial results for patient setup verification using transperineal ultrasound and cone beam CT in external beam radiation therapy of prostate cancer. Radiat Oncol. 2016;11:147.
34. Li M, Ballhausen H, Hegemann NS, Reiner M, Tritschler S, Gratzke C, Manapov F, Corradini S, Ganswindt U, Belka C. Comparison of prostate positioning guided by three-dimensional transperineal ultrasound and cone beam CT. Strahlenther Onkol. 2017;193:221–8.
35. Wong P, Muanza T, Reynard E, Robert K, Barker J, Sultanem K. Use of three-dimensional ultrasound in the detection of breast tumor bed displacement during radiotherapy. Int J Radiat Oncol Biol Phys. 2011;79:39–45.

2

ONE SHOT - single shot radiotherapy for localized prostate cancer: study protocol of a single arm, multicenter phase I/II trial

Thomas Zilli[1,2*], Marta Scorsetti[3,4], Daniel Zwahlen[5], Ciro Franzese[4], Robert Förster[6], Niccolò Giaj-Levra[7], Nikolaos Koutsouvelis[1], Aurelie Bertaut[8], Michel Zimmermann[5], Giuseppe Roberto D'Agostino[4], Filippo Alongi[7,9], Matthias Guckenberger[6] and Raymond Miralbell[1,2]

Abstract

Background: Stereotactic body radiotherapy (SBRT) is an emerging treatment alternative for patients with localized prostate cancer. Promising results in terms of disease control and toxicity have been reported with 4 to 5 SBRT fractions. However, question of how far can the number of fractions with SBRT be reduced is a challenging research matter. As already explored by some authors in the context of brachytherapy, monotherapy appears to be feasible with an acceptable toxicity profile and a promising outcome. The aim of this multicenter phase I/II prospective trialis to demonstrate early evidence of safety and efficacy of a single-fraction SBRT approach for the treatment of localized disease.

Methods: Patients with low- and intermediate-risk localized prostate cancer without significant tumor in the transitional zone will be treated with a single SBRT fraction of 19 Gy to the whole prostate gland with urethra-sparing (17 Gy). Intrafractional motion will be monitored with intraprostatic electromagnetic transponders. The primary endpoint of the phase I part of the study will be safety as assessed by CTCAE 4.03 grading scale, while biochemical relapse-free survival will be the endpoint for the phase II. The secondary endpoints include acute and late toxicity, quality of life, progression-free survival, and prostate-cancer specific survival.

Discussion: This is the first multicenter phase I/II trial assessing the efficacy and safety of a single-dose SBRT treatment for patients with localized prostate cancer. If positive, results of ONE SHOT may help to design subsequent phase III trials exploring the role of SBRT monotherapy in the exclusive radiotherapy treatment of localized disease.

Keywords: Prostate cancer, Stereotactic body radiotherapy, Urethra-sparing, Single fraction, Quality of life, Electromagnetic transponders

Background

Total dose and dose per fraction play an important role in the curative treatment of prostate cancer with radiotherapy (RT). Modern image-guided external RT allows safe dose escalation for prostate cancer. Doses above 74 Gy with conventional fractionation (2 Gy/day) have been shown to be beneficial. There are strong radiobiological considerations that suggest that treatment with a small number of large fractions (hypofractionation) may increase the therapeutic ratio of RT for prostate cancer.

The "α/β" ratio (i.e., cell sensitivity/cell repair) is a key parameter of the cell-survival linear-quadratic (LQ) model that purportedly defines the sensitivity of each tissue (healthy or tumoral) to changes in treatment fractionation. Prostate cancer cells may have a low α/β ratio (i.e.,~ 1.5 Gy), lower than that of most tumors or even of the late-responding normal tissues surrounding the tumor, the rectum and the bladder (α/β ratio 3–5 Gy)

* Correspondence: Thomas.Zilli@hcuge.ch; Thomas.Zilli@unige.ch
[1]Radiation Oncology, Geneva University Hospital, CH-1211, 14 Geneva, Switzerland
[2]Faculty of Medicine, Geneva University, Geneva, Switzerland
Full list of author information is available at the end of the article

[1]. Thus, hypofractionation may increase the tumor cell killing effect with relatively less toxic effect on the surrounding late responding normal tissues compared to conventional fractionation. Several authors have reported their respective experiences with moderate hypofractionation (i.e., dose per fraction 2.5 Gy to 4 Gy) for prostate cancer confirming the equivalence in terms of disease control and tolerance compared to standard fractionated treatments [2–5].

Bio-mathematical models using large patient data sets have focused on external beam RT schedules using less than 4 Gy fractions. It deserves to be acknowledged that the LQ model may not be predictive of cell survival and isoeffects with doses per fraction above 3-4Gy. Indeed, the predictions of the LQ model at very high dose/fraction (extreme hypofractionation) may be somehow "ambivalent", either overestimated (less repair of sublethal damage thus a lower value for "β") or underestimated (increased indirect cell-death secondary to intravascular endothelial damage). Staring from this background, clinical research on extreme hypofractionation started some 15 years ago when stereotactic body RT (SBRT) technology appeared as a treatment option against localized prostate cancer competing with high-dose rate brachytherapy (HDR-BT).

Indeed, preliminary results on extreme hypofractionation with SBRT have been reported during the last few years mainly for low-risk patients in single-institution [6–8] or multi-institutional [9] series. Most frequently, 5 fractions of 7.25 Gy have been delivered for a total equivalent dose to the tumor of 90 Gy in 2 Gy/fraction (LQ model) and a success rate of > 90%, 5-year biochemical relapse-free (bRFS) survival rates [10]. Data published so far for prostate SBRT have shown, although with a limited follow-up, late grade 3 toxicity rates for rectal and genitourinary (GU) toxicity lying within a ≤ 3% range [8, 11, 12]. Although, caution is recommended to avoid passing a too optimistic message regarding the potential biological benefits of extreme hypofractionation for prostate cancer (i.e., more cure with less side effects), financial and logistical advantages can undoubtedly be foreseen. In fact, a drop from 40 or more treatments to 5 or less sessions may reduce the cost of external beam RT, will increase the availability of treatment slots in otherwise busy departments (important issue in countries with limited resources), and significantly improve patient's convenience.

The question of how far can the number of fractions with SBRT be reduced is an exciting research matter with an undoubtful goal, face the challenge of assessing the potential for cure of prostate cancer patients with a single and unique fraction of high dose irradiation similar to what is already undertaken with radiosurgery against brain, lung, and liver targets. Such type of effort has already been attempted with HDR-BT. Recently, Prada et al. [13] reported a relatively disappointing 66% 6-year bRFS survival though a very good tolerance after a single interstitial application of 19 Gy to the prostate. Reasons for this suboptimal result may be related, for instance, to a suboptimal dose-distribution with HDR-BT compared to SBRT. Hoskin et al. have recently published the results on 49 patients treated with a single fraction of HDR-BT to 19/20 Gy [14]. With 49 months median follow-up, the 4-year estimates of grade-3 GU and gastrointestinal (GI) toxicity was 2% and 0%, respectively, with no grade 4 events, while the 4-year bRFS was 94%. Similarly, Morton et al. confirmed with a median follow-up time of 20 months the good tolerance of a single 19 Gy single HDR-BT fraction in terms of toxicity and impact on quality of life (QoL) [15] and Krauss et al. reported a 3-year bRFS rate of 93% [16], similar to results observed by Hoskin et al. In conclusion, for the authors one single fraction HDR-BT is feasible, weakly toxic, and with promising preliminary results.

Although, the effects are mostly encouraging, only controlled studies are able to properly address the impact of single fraction SBRT in prostate cancer outcomes. Therefore, a phase I/II approach will be a properly controlled study to demonstrate early evidence of safety and efficacy of the intervention and substantiate further the role of a single-fraction SBRT approach. If positive, the results of ONE SHOT will help determine the design of subsequent phase III trials in the exclusive RT setting for the treatment of localized disease.

Methods/Design

This study was approved by the Ethics committee of the Geneva University Hospital (2017–01236) and is registered on clinicaltrials.gov (NCT03294889). This is a phase I/II, prospective, multicenter, single-arm study.

Phase I, safety evaluation

The main objective of the phase I trial is to determine if a single fraction SBRT, with a dose of 19 Gy, is safe and well tolerated by assessing the occurrence of Grade ≥ 3 acute adverse events (AE) during the first 3 months.

Phase II, efficacy evaluation

The main objective of the phase II trial is to determine if a single fraction SBRT, with a dose of 19 Gy, is an effective treatment option by assessing bRFS at 3 years.

Objectives

Primary endpoint of the phase I trial Grade ≥ 3GU and GI acute AE will be assessed during the first three months following the single fraction treatment. AEs will be assessed according to National Cancer Institute

Common Terminology Criteria for Adverse Events (NCI CTCAE) v4.03. Special attention will be given to diarrhea, fecal incontinence, proctitis, rectal hemorrhage, rectal pain, hematuria, urinary frequency, urinary urgency, urinary retention, urinary incontinence, and cystitis non-infective. Persistent AE will be defined as any persistent toxicity during the first 3 months post-treatment (follow-up milestones: 1 week, 6 weeks, and 12 weeks).

Primary endpoint of the phase II trial bRFS, from time of inclusion until biochemical progression (according to recommendations of the Radiation Therapy Oncology Group - American Society for Radiation Oncology (RTOG-ASTRO), the Phoenix Consensus Conference recommendations) [17]:

- A rise by 2 ng/ml or more above the nadir prostate specific antigen (PSA) confirmed by a second observation taken 3–4 weeks later, where the nadir PSA is defined as the lowest PSA value observed on study.

Secondary endpoints of the phase II trial

- Acute AE (during the first 3 months follow-up) according to CTCAE v4.03
- Late AE (after 3 months follow-up) according to CTCAE v4.03
- Progression free survival (PFS) defined as time from inclusion until one of the following events, whichever comes first:
- Biochemical progression
- Clinical progression defined as either local or regional recurrence of the disease or the appearance of distant metastases
- Death from any cause
- Start of another line of systemic anti-neoplastic therapy
- Clinical progression free-survival
- Local progression free-survival
- Time to further anti-cancer therapy defined as the time from inclusion to the start of any type of salvage treatment.
- Prostate cancer-specific survival (PCSS)
- Overall survival (OS)
- QoL evaluated using EPIC 26 (Expanded prostate cancer index composite) [18], IPSS (International Prostate Symptoms Score) [19], and IIEF-5 (International Index of Erectile Function) [20]

Inclusion criteria

- Written informed consent according to ICH/GCP regulations before registration and prior to any trial specific procedures
- Histologically confirmed adenocarcinoma of the prostate without small cell features
- Tumor clinical stage cT1c-2c, pN0 or cN0, M0, according to UICC TNM 2009
- Magnetic Resonance Imaging (MRI) staging must confirm American Joint Committee on Cancer (AJCC) stage T1, T2a, T2b, or T2c
- Gleason score at biopsy 3 + 3 or 3 + 4 (World Health Organization, WHO 2016 Grade Groups 1, 2)
- PSA ≤15 ng/ml
- Age 18–85 years at time of registration
- WHO performance status 0–1
- IPSS ≤10 (alpha blockers allowed)
- MRI-based volume estimation of prostate gland ≤70 cc
- Patient agrees not to father a child during trial treatment and during 6 months thereafter

Exclusion criteria

- Evidence of T3a, T3b, or T4 disease as assessed by MRI
- Positive lymph-nodes or metastatic disease from prostate cancer on imaging studies.
- Significant tumor on the transitional zone as assessed by MRI
- Previous or ongoing androgen deprivation therapy
- Impossibility to implant electromagnetic transponders into the prostate
- History of hematologic or primary solid tumor malignancy, unless in remission for at least 3 years from registration with the exception of curatively treated localized non-melanoma skin cancer
- Prior pelvic RT
- Previous surgery for prostate cancer
- Previous transurethral resection of the prostate (< 12 weeks before registration)
- Hip prosthesis
- Severe or active co-morbidity likely to impact on the advisability of SBRT
- Any other serious underlying medical, psychiatric, psychological, familial, or geographical condition, which in the judgment of the investigator may interfere with the planned staging, treatment and follow-up, affect patient compliance, or place the patient at high risk from treatment-related complications

Intervention

In this trial, patients with localized prostate cancer are registered to receive the following target SBRT dose:

- 19 Gy in a single fraction to the whole prostate gland ± proximal seminal vesicles
- 17 Gy in a single fraction to the urethra planning-risk volume (PRV)

Before the SBRT treatment, all patients will be implanted transrectally or transperineally under ultrasound guidance with three electromagnetic transponders, the *Calypso®* beacons (*Varian Medical Systems, Palo Alto, CA*). Patients will be simulated a minimum of 4 days after the implant and treated with an empty rectum and full bladder. To help with the contouring of the urethra a 12 *French Foley* non-radiopaque catheter will be inserted before the CT simulation and before irradiation. Rigid or deformable co-registration with multi-parametric MRI is to be used for contouring purposes.

The Clinical Tumor Volume (CTV) is defined as the prostate +/− the proximal 2/3 of the seminal vesicles (SV) based on the risk of SV involvement as determined by the *Roach* score using a cutoff threshold of 15% [21]. The planning target volume (PTV) is defined as the CTV plus 5 mm margins in all directions except for a 3 mm margin posteriorly towards the rectal wall. The urethra PRV is defined on CT images by contouring a 12 *French Foley* catheter with a 2 mm isotropic rim expansion. Organs at risk (OAR) are contoured according to RTOG guidelines [22] and include the bladder wall and the rectal wall (both defined as a 5-mm internal margin created from the external surface), the penile bulb [23], and the proximal femurs. All patients will be treated with megavoltage beams from a *TrueBeam®* linear accelerator (*Varian Medical Systems, Palo Alto, CA*) with nominal photon energies ≥6 MV, 6 degrees of freedom couch, and a *Calypso®* localization system. The irradiation technique is *RapidArc®* (*Varian Medical Systems, Palo Alto, CA*), a rotational technique using a flattening filter-free (FFF) modality with patients treated in an isocentric setting.

Dose prescription, recording and reporting As volumetric modulated arc therapy (VMAT) techniques are mandatory in this trial, the definition of volumes and the dose reporting shall be in accordance with the ICRU (*International Commission on Radiation Units and Measurements*) report 83. The dose variation in the PTV shall be assessed by the near-minimum dose (D98%) and near-maximum dose (D2%). The proposed treatment verification schedule is presented in Fig. 1 using a threshold limit for *Calypso®* of ±3 mm with geometric check limits

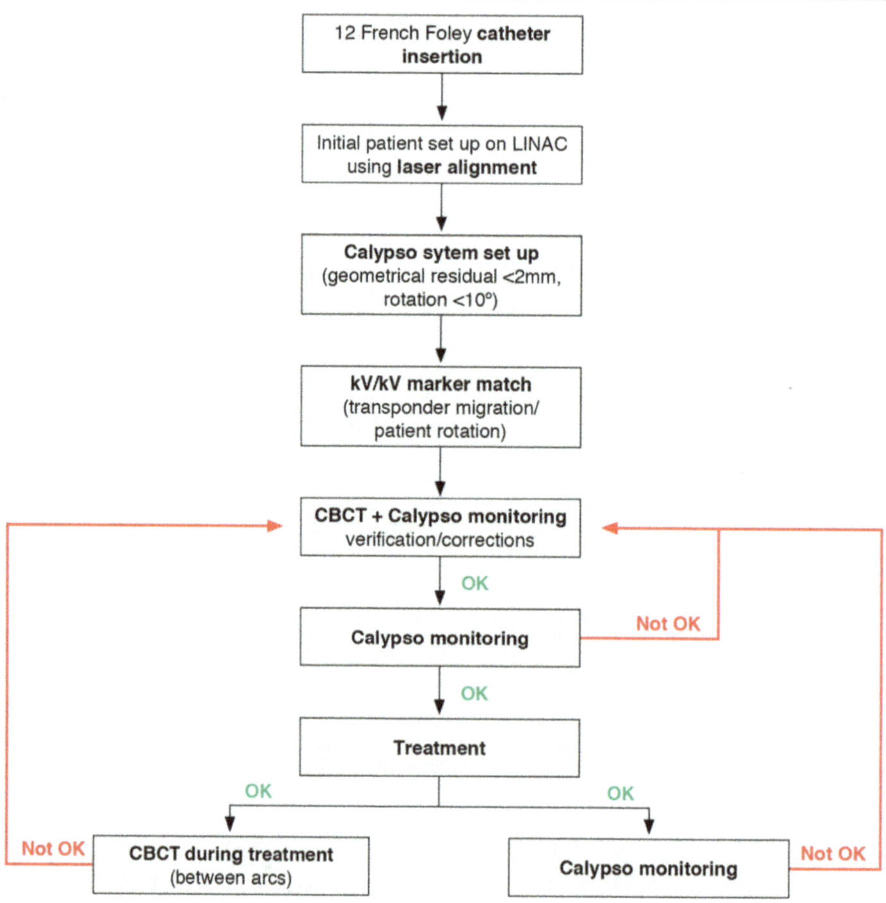

Fig. 1 Image-guided flowchart as per protocol

set to 2 mm (geometrical residual) and rotations of 10° (default values). Table 1 summarizes the dose constraints for the OAR [24].

Radiation Therapy Quality Assurance (RTQA) A RTQA program is based in Geneva and is an important asset of this multicentric trial. Electronic submission and assessment of target and OaR volumes, in addition to treatment plans as well, is a major step before any treatment can be validated and approved.

Follow-up

Patients are seen at day-5 after SBRT, at weeks 6 and 12, every 6 months for 2 years post treatment, and yearly up to 5 years of follow-up. A clinical update and a physical exam are conducted by recording any acute and/or late AE and the sequential PSA measurements. IPSS, IIEF-5, and QoL (EPIC-26 questionnaire) assessments are also performed. Radiological investigations including mpMRI, bone scan, choline-PET, and/or PSMA-PET will be repeated in case of progression, either biochemical or clinical.

Statistical analysis

Sample size

Phase I, safety evaluation

Only acute GU and/or GI grade 3 or higher toxicity will be considered for the safety evaluation. Three patients will be treated and evaluated for toxicity at 3 months. If the first 3 patients undergo any grade ≥ 3 toxicity or if 2 patients under go grade 4 toxicity, the trial will stop.

Otherwise, 3 additional patients will be recruited and treated. If 2/6 patients or fewer present with grade 3 AE, the trial will go on phase II and include 39 additional patients. Regarding these 6 patients, if one or more present with grade 4 toxicity, a meeting of the *Data Safety and Monitoring Board* (DSMB) will be carried on.

Phase II, efficacy evaluation

Based on published SBRT results on 5 fraction-trials and on one series of HDR-BT with 19 Gy single shot, a 3-yearsbRFS of 96% may be expected. Assuming this hypothesis and an expected dropout rate of 10%, 45 patients (including the 6 included in the phase I study) will allow evaluating 3-year bRFS with a 97.5% lower one-sided confidence interval and a width of the interval of 0.06 (upper bound = 90%).

Data analysis

Data description will be performed using the mean, standard deviation, median, and range for quantitative variables and the percentage for qualitative ones.

Phase I

Safety analyses shall be performed on the safety-evaluable population, defined as all subjects treated with the single shot SBRT. Toxicity and grade will be described at each follow-up visit according to the specificity of every

Table 1 Dose constraints

Structure	Standardized nomenclature	Dosimetric Parameter	Per Protocol	Acceptable Variation
PTV_19	PTV_19	D98% (Dnear min)	≥ 95% (i.e. 18 Gy)	
		D2% (Dnear max)	≤ 107% (ie. 20.3Gy)	D5% ≤ 107%, D2% ≤ 110%
Rectal_wall	Rectal_wall	V9.5Gy (50%)	< 40%	40–50%
		V15Gy (80%)	< 15%	15–20%
		V17Gy (90%) (NTD 68 Gy)	< 10%	< 15%
		V19Gy (100%) (NTD 83.6 Gy)	< 5%	< 10%
		V20Gy (105%) (NTD 92 Gy)	< 1 cc	
Bladder_wall	Bladder_wall	V9.5Gy (50%)	< 50%	50–60%
		V15Gy (80%)	< 20%	20–30%
		V17Gy (90%) (NTD 68 Gy)	< 15%	15–20%
		V19Gy (100%) (NTD 83.6 Gy)	< 10%	< 15%
		V20Gy (105%) (NTD 92 Gy)	< 1 cc	
Femurs (each)	Femur_Rt Femur_Lt	V14Gy (NTD 48 Gy)	< 5%	5–10%
Penile bulb	Penile_bulb	V14Gy (NTD 48 Gy)	< 5%	5–10%
Urethra PRV	Urethra_PRV	D98% (Dnear min)	≥ 95% (i.e. 16.2 Gy)	
		D5%	≤ 107% (i.e. 18.2 Gy)	
		D2% (Dnear max)	≤ 110% (i.e. 18.7 Gy)	

assessed endpoint, including the number and fraction of patients with at least one AE.

Phase II- statistical analysis of the primary endpoint

Efficacy analyses will be performed on an intention to treat basis (i.e., involving those patients following the major inclusion criteria and repeated one per protocol set). The primary endpoint is 3-years bRFS. bRFS, and its 97.5% one-sided confidence interval (CI), will be determined using the *Kaplan Meier* method. If the expected value of 96% isn't included in this interval, the efficacy of the experimental treatment will be questioned.

Phase II - statistical analysis of the secondary endpoints

Toxicity analyses will be performed. As for acute toxicity, late AE and grading will be reported at each follow up visit. Median survival time and its 95% bilateral confidence intervals (PFS, clinical PFS, local PFS, OS, and PCSS) will be determined using the *Kaplan Meier* method. The rate of survival will be given at 1, 2, 3, and 5 years. Univariate and multivariate *Cox* regression models will be fit to assess the effect of relevant baseline clinical and pathologic features on bRFS, PFS, and OS. Hazard ratio (HR) will be given with their 95% confidence intervals. Median follow-up will be estimated using the reverse *Kaplan Meier* method. QoL scores (EPIC, IPSS, IIEF-5) will be described at each clinical surveillance follow-up time by the mean, standard deviation, median, and range. Domain scores will be calculated only if sufficient items are completed in accordance with the relevant scoring manual. Mixt models will be used to characterize changes in QoL across time taken into account for confounding clinical and pathologic factors. All statistical analysis will be performed with SAS 9.4. *p*-values less than 5% will be considered as significant.

Discussion

Optimal management of localized low- or intermediate risk prostate cancer remains a challenging situation, with different treatment options available ranging from active surveillance to radical treatment [25]. Considering that patients under active surveillance have a greater risk of disease progression and metastases compared to definitive treatments [26], the choice of the more appropriate curative option is a crucial issue for clinicians.

SBRT represents a valid treatment option for these patients, combing a good toxicity profile, promising disease control rates, and limited impact on QoL. Recently reported, preliminary results of the Scandinavian phase III HYPO-RT-PC trial found in 1200 intermediate-risk prostate cancer patients similar biochemical control rates and toxicities results with extreme hypofractionation (42.7 Gy in seven fractions of 6.1 Gy over two and a half weeks) compared to standard fractionation 78 Gy [27]. However, the optimal SBRT fractionation schedule for curative treatment of patients with localized prostate cancer is, so far, unknown. Based on the promising results of HDR-BT monotherapy treatments [15, 28, 29], single-shot SBRT may represent an appealing treatment modality for prostate cancer patients.

To our knowledge, ONE SHOT is the first phase I/II trial assessing the efficacy and safety of a single-dose SBRT treatment for patients with localized prostate cancer in a multicenter setting. ONE SHOT proposes the same treatment technique under a strict RTQA protocol for all patients. By reducing significantly the beam-on time [30], our single shot linac-based FFF VMAT technique with intra-fractional control motion is expected to guarantee not only treatment reproducibility [31] but also minimize intra-fraction dose uncertainties [32]. Moreover, the implementation of patient-reported outcome using validated questionnaires will provide a reliable evaluation of the clinical impact of a single-dose SBRT by reporting a longitudinal follow-up on the long-term of radiation-induced side effects compared to physician-reported data.

While waiting for results of presently ongoing randomized phase III trials comparing SBRT with other fractionation or treatment, results of the ONE SHOT trial, if positive, may help to design subsequent studies exploring the role of SBRT monotherapy in the exclusive RT treatment of localized disease.

Abbreviations

AE: Adverse event; ASTRO: American Society for Radiation Oncology; bRFS: Biochemical relapse-free survival; CTV: Clinical target volume; DSMB: Data safety and monitoring board; EPIC 26: Expanded prostate cancer index composite; FFF: Flattening filter-free; HDR-BT: High-dose rate brachytherapy; ICRU: International Commission on Radiation Units and Measurements; IIEF-5: International Index of Erectile Function; IPSS: International Prostate Symptoms Score; LQ: Linear quadratic; mpMRI: Multi-parametric Magnetic Resonance Imaging; NCI CTCAE: National Cancer Institute Common Terminology Criteria for Adverse Events; OAR: Organs at risk; OS: Overall survival; PCSS: Prostate cancer-specific survival; PFS: Progression-free survival; PRV: Planning risk volume; PSA: Prostate specific antigen; PTV: Planning target volume; QoL: Quality of life; RT: Radiotherapy; RTOG: Radiation Therapy Oncology Group; RTQA: Radiation Therapy Quality Assessment; SBRT: Stereotactic body radiotherapy; SV: Seminal vesicles; VMAT: Volumetric modulated arc therapy; WHO: World Health Organization

Acknowledgements

Ms. Laurence Zulianello, PhD, Giovanna Dipasquale, MSc, Michel Rouzaud, MSc, *Geneva University Hospital, Geneva, Switzerland.*
MSc Stefano Tomatis and MSc Luca Cozzi, *Humanitas Cancer Center, Rozzano, IT.*
MSc Stephanie Tanadini-Lang, *University Hospital Zürich, Zürich, CH.*

Funding
This study is funded by a grant from the « *Fondation pour les recherches médicales et biologiques sur le cancer* » (Clinique de Carouge SA, Av. du Cardinal-Mermillod 1, 1227 Carouge GE, Forni Foundation, Switzerland). The granting bodies are not involved in data collection or analysis.

Authors' contributions
Study conception: *TZ, RM.* Initial Study design: *TZ, RM.* Revision of study design and protocol: *TZ, MS, DZ,* CF, *RF, NGL, NK, AB, MZ, GRD, FA, MG, RM* Study coordination: *TZ, NK, AB, RM.* Participating centers: *Geneva University Hospital, Geneva, CH; University Hospital Zürich, Zürich, CH; Kantonsspital Graubünden, Chur, CH; Humanitas Cancer Center, Rozzano, IT; Sacro Cuore Don-Calabria, Negrar, IT.* Drafting the manuscript: *TZ, MS, DZ,* CF, *NK, AB, GRD, FA, MG, RM.* All authors read and approved the final manuscript.

Competing interests
The authors declare that they have no competing interests.

Author details
[1]Radiation Oncology, Geneva University Hospital, CH-1211, 14 Geneva, Switzerland. [2]Faculty of Medicine, Geneva University, Geneva, Switzerland. [3]Radiation Oncology, Humanitas University, Rozzano, Milan, Italy. [4]Radiation Oncology, Humanitas Research Hospital and Cancer Center, Rozzano, Milan, Italy. [5]Radiation Oncology, Kantonsspital Graubünden, Chur, Switzerland. [6]Radiation Oncology, University Hospital Zürich, Zürich, Switzerland. [7]Radiation Oncology, Sacro Cuore Don-Calabria, Negrar, Italy. [8]Methodology and biostatistic unit, Centre Georges François Leclerc, Dijon, France. [9]Faculty of Medecine, University of Brescia, Brescia, Italy.

References

1. Miralbell R, Roberts SA, Zubizarreta E, Hendry JH. Dose-fractionation sensitivity of prostate cancer deduced from radiotherapy outcomes of 5,969 patients in seven international institutional datasets: alpha/beta = 1.4 (0.9-2. 2) gy. Int J Radiat Oncol Biol Phys. 2012;82:e17–24.
2. Aluwini S, Pos F, Schimmel E, van Lin E, Krol S, van der Toorn PP, et al. Hypofractionated versus conventionally fractionated radiotherapy for patients with prostate cancer (hypro): acute toxicity results from a randomised non-inferiority phase 3 trial. Lancet Oncol. 2015;16:274–83.
3. Arcangeli G, Saracino B, Arcangeli S, Gomellini S, Petrongari MG, Sanguineti G, et al. Moderate hypofractionation in high-risk, organ-confined prostate cancer: final results of a phase iii randomized trial. J Clin Oncol. 2017;35: 1891–7.
4. Dearnaley D, Syndikus I, Mossop H, Khoo V, Birtle A, Bloomfield D, et al. Conventional versus hypofractionated high-dose intensity-modulated radiotherapy for prostate cancer: 5-year outcomes of the randomised, non-inferiority, phase 3 chhip trial. Lancet Oncol. 2016;17:1047–60.
5. Lee WR, Dignam JJ, Amin MB, Bruner DW, Low D, Swanson GP, et al. Randomized phase iii noninferiority study comparing two radiotherapy fractionation schedules in patients with low-risk prostate cancer. J Clin Oncol. 2016;34:2325–32.
6. Fuller DB, Naitoh J, Mardirossian G. Virtual hdr cyberknife sbrt for localized prostatic carcinoma: 5-year disease-free survival and toxicity observations. Front Oncol. 2014;4:321.
7. Katz A, Kang J. Stereotactic body radiotherapy with or without external beam radiation as treatment for organ confined high-risk prostate carcinoma: a six year study. Radiat Oncol. 2014;9:1.
8. King CR, Brooks JD, Gill H, Presti JC Jr. Long-term outcomes from a prospective trial of stereotactic body radiotherapy for low-risk prostate cancer. Int J Radiat Oncol Biol Phys. 2012;82:877–82.
9. Hannan R, Tumati V, Xie XJ, Cho LC, Kavanagh BD, Brindle J, et al. Stereotactic body radiation therapy for low and intermediate risk prostate cancer-results from a multi-institutional clinical trial. Eur J Cancer. 2016;59:142–51.
10. King CR, Freeman D, Kaplan I, Fuller D, Bolzicco G, Collins S, et al. Stereotactic body radiotherapy for localized prostate cancer: pooled analysis from a multi-institutional consortium of prospective phase ii trials. Radiother Oncol. 2013;109:217–21.
11. Bolzicco G, Favretto MS, Scremin E, Tambone C, Tasca A, Guglielmi R. Image-guided stereotactic body radiation therapy for clinically localized prostate cancer: preliminary clinical results. Technol Cancer Res Treat. 2010;9:473–7.
12. Katz AJ, Santoro M, Ashley R, Diblasio F, Witten M. Stereotactic body radiotherapy for organ-confined prostate cancer. BMC Urol. 2010;10:1.
13. Prada PJ, Cardenal J, Blanco AG, Anchuelo J, Ferri M, Fernandez G, et al. High-dose-rate interstitial brachytherapy as monotherapy in one fraction for the treatment of favorable stage prostate cancer: toxicity and long-term biochemical results. Radiother Oncol. 2016;119:411–6.
14. Hoskin P, Rojas A, Ostler P, Hughes R, Alonzi R, Lowe G. Single-dose high-dose-rate brachytherapy compared to two and three fractions for locally advanced prostate cancer. Radiother Oncol. 2017;124:56–60.
15. Morton G, Chung HT, McGuffin M, Helou J, D'Alimonte L, Ravi A, et al. Prostate high dose-rate brachytherapy as monotherapy for low and intermediate risk prostate cancer: early toxicity and quality-of life results from a randomized phase ii clinical trial of one fraction of 19gy or two fractions of 13.5gy. Radiother Oncol. 2017;122:87–92.
16. Krauss DJ, Ye H, Martinez AA, Mitchell B, Sebastian E, Limbacher A, et al. Favorable preliminary outcomes for men with low- and intermediate-risk prostate cancer treated with 19-gy single-fraction high-dose-rate brachytherapy. Int J Radiat Oncol Biol Phys. 2017;97:98–106.
17. Roach M 3rd, Hanks G, Thames H Jr, Schellhammer P, Shipley WU, Sokol GH, et al. Defining biochemical failure following radiotherapy with or without hormonal therapy in men with clinically localized prostate cancer: recommendations of the rtog-astro phoenix consensus conference. Int J Radiat Oncol Biol Phys. 2006;65:965–74.
18. Szymanski KM, Wei JT, Dunn RL, Sanda MG. Development and validation of an abbreviated version of the expanded prostate cancer index composite instrument for measuring health-related quality of life among prostate cancer survivors. Urology. 2010;76:1245–50.
19. Barry MJ, Fowler FJ Jr, O'Leary MP, Bruskewitz RC, Holtgrewe HL, Mebust WK, et al. The american urological association symptom index for benign prostatic hyperplasia. The measurement committee of the american urological association. J Urol. 1992;148:1549–57. discussion 64
20. Rhoden EL, Teloken C, Sogari PR, Vargas Souto CA. The use of the simplified international index of erectile function (iief-5) as a diagnostic tool to study the prevalence of erectile dysfunction. Int J Impot Res. 2002;14:245–50.
21. Diaz A, Roach M 3rd, Marquez C, Coleman L, Pickett B, Wolfe JS, et al. Indications for and the significance of seminal vesicle irradiation during 3d conformal radiotherapy for localized prostate cancer. Int J Radiat Oncol Biol Phys. 1994;30:323–9.
22. Gay HA, Barthold HJ, O'Meara E, Bosch WR, El Naqa I, Al-Lozi R, et al. Pelvic normal tissue contouring guidelines for radiation therapy: a radiation therapy oncology group consensus panel atlas. Int J Radiat Oncol Biol Phys. 2012;83:e353–62.
23. Wallner KE, Merrick GS, Benson ML, Butler WM, Maki J, Tollenaar BG. Penile bulb imaging. Int J Radiat Oncol Biol Phys. 2002;53:928–33.
24. Dubouloz A, Rouzaud M, Tsvang L, Verbakel W, Bjorkqvist M, Linthout N, et al. Urethra-sparing stereotactic body radiotherapy for prostate cancer: how much can the rectal wall dose be reduced with or without an endorectal balloon? Radiat Oncol. 2018;13:114.
25. Mottet N, Bellmunt J, Bolla M, Briers E, Cumberbatch MG, De Santis M, et al. Eau-estro-siog guidelines on prostate cancer. Part 1: screening, diagnosis, and local treatment with curative intent. Eur Urol. 2017;71:618–29.
26. Hamdy FC, Donovan JL, Lane JA, Mason M, Metcalfe C, Holding P, et al. 10-year outcomes after monitoring, surgery, or radiotherapy for localized prostate cancer. N Engl J Med. 2016;375:1415–24.
27. Widmark A, Gunnlaugson A, Beckman L, Thellenberg-Karlsson C, Hoyer M, Lagerlund M. Oc-0599 ultrahypofrcationation for porstate cancer: outcome from the scandinavian phase 3 hypo-rt-pc trial. Radiother Oncol. 2018; 127(Suppl. 1):S314.

28. Gomez-Iturriaga A, Casquero F, Pijoan JI, Minguez P, Espinosa JM, Irasarri A, et al. Health-related-quality-of-life and toxicity after single fraction 19gy high-dose-rate prostate brachytherapy: phase ii trial. Radiother Oncol. 2018;126(2):278–82.
29. Hoskin P, Rojas A, Ostler P, Hughes R, Alonzi R, Lowe G, et al. High-dose-rate brachytherapy alone given as two or one fraction to patients for locally advanced prostate cancer: acute toxicity. Radiother Oncol. 2014;110:268–71.
30. D'Agostino G, Franzese C, De Rose F, Franceschini D, Comito T, Villa E, et al. High-quality linac-based stereotactic body radiation therapy with flattening filter free beams and volumetric modulated arc therapy for low-intermediate risk prostate cancer. A mono-institutional experience with 90 patients. Clin Oncol (R Coll Radiol). 2016;28:e173–e8.
31. Chen Z, Yang Z, Wang J, Hu W. Dosimetric impact of different bladder and rectum filling during prostate cancer radiotherapy. Radiat Oncol. 2016;11:103.
32. Reggiori G, Mancosu P, Tozzi A, Cantone MC, Castiglioni S, Lattuada P, et al. Cone beam ct pre- and post-daily treatment for assessing geometrical and dosimetric intrafraction variability during radiotherapy of prostate cancer. J Appl Clin Med Phys. 2010;12:3371.

3

Primary histiocytic sarcoma of the central nervous system: a case report with platelet derived growth factor receptor mutation and PD-L1/PD-L2 expression

Jackson M. May[1], Mark R. Waddle[1], Daniel H. Miller[1], William C. Stross[1], Tasneem A. Kaleem[1], Byron C. May[1], Robert C. Miller[1], Liuyan Jiang[3], Gerald W. Strong[1], Daniel M. Trifiletti[1], Kaisorn L. Chaichana[2], Ronald Reimer[2], Han W. Tun[4] and Jennifer L. Peterson[1,2*]

Abstract

Background: Histiocytic sarcoma (HS) is an aggressive malignant neoplasm. HS in the central nervous system is exceptionally rare and associated with a poor prognosis. This report documents a case of primary HS of the central nervous system with treatment including surgery, radiotherapy, and chemotherapy.

Case presentation: Our patient was a 47 year old female presenting with progressive ataxia, headaches, imbalance, nausea, vomiting, and diplopia. MRI showed a heterogeneously enhancing lesion approximately 2.9 × 3.0 × 2.3 cm centered upon the cerebellar vermis with mild surrounding vasogenic edema and abnormal enhancement of multiple cranial nerves. The patient underwent surgical debulking, which revealed histiocytic sarcoma with grossly purulent drainage. Staging revealed diffuse leptomeningeal involvement, primarily involving the brain and lower thoracic and lumbar spine. She underwent adjuvant radiotherapy to the brain and lower spine and was started on high dose methotrexate. However, she experienced progressive disease in the cervical and thoracic spine as well as pulmonary involvement. Genomic sequencing of her tumor showed a mutation in the platelet-derived growth factor receptor A (p.V0681) which could be targeted with Dasatinib. However, she did not tolerate Dasatinib and she succumbed to progressive disseminated disease eight months from original diagnosis. Our pathologic evaluation also revealed expression of PD-L1 and PD-L2 by tumor cells raising the potential therapeutic role for immune checkpoint inhibition.

Conclusions: This case provides an example of effective CNS control with resection and moderate doses of radiation therapy. A review of the literature confirms aggressive multidisciplinary treatment is the most effective treatment against this disease. In addition, genomic sequencing may play an important role in determining new therapeutic options. However, CNS histiocytic sarcoma remains an aggressive disease with a propensity for early widespread dissemination and few long term survivors.

Keywords: Histiocytic sarcoma, CNS, Radiation, Review

* Correspondence: peterson.jennifer2@mayo.edu
[1]Department of Radiation Oncology, Mayo Clinic, 4500 San Pablo Road South, Jacksonville, FL 32224, USA
[2]Department of Neurological Surgery, Mayo Clinic, Jacksonville, Florida, USA
Full list of author information is available at the end of the article

Background

Histiocytic sarcoma (HS) is an uncommon malignant neoplasm with morphological and immunophenotypic features of histiocytic tissue. HS presents most commonly with a mass involving soft tissues, gastrointestinal tract, and/or lymph nodes [16]. Primary histiocytic sarcoma of the central nervous system (CNS) is extremely rare and accounts for less than 1% of all lymphohematopoietic neoplasms [22]. A typical finding with CNS HS is the presence of an inflammatory infiltrate and the abundance of inflammatory cells can cause neoplastic cells to be overlooked and thus a misdiagnosis may occur [2]. Many previous cases are thought to be misdiagnosed due to lack of genetic markers, but the disease can now be recognized by its biological markers, such as positive expression of CD 163, CD 68, and lysozyme, which allow differentiation between CNS HS and other hematopoietic neoplasms [5], such as B-cell or T-cell non-Hodgkin's Lymphoma [16, 21]. While the optimal treatment for CNS HS is not well defined, surgery is the primary modality with radiotherapy and chemotherapy frequently used as adjuvant treatments. Overall, CNS HS carries a poor prognosis, but there have been reported cases of long term disease free survival in adults when multidisciplinary treatment of radiation therapy, chemotherapy, and surgery are applied [2, 11, 23]. Here, we present a case of primary CNS HS with leptomeningeal spread treated with tri-modality therapy and provide a review of the available literature for this aggressive disease.

Case presentation

Our patient was a 47 year old female with a history of ulcerative colitis, Sjogren's syndrome, migraines, and fibromyalgia who presented with a 6 month history of left lower extremity paresthesia followed by a 2 month history of progressive headaches, imbalance, ataxia, nausea, vomiting, and diplopia. Neurologic examination revealed severe gait ataxia requiring assistance to stand or walk and nystagmus with lateral gaze. MRI revealed a 3.0 cm heterogeneously enhancing mixed cystic and solid mass centered upon the cerebellar vermis with mild surrounding vasogenic edema and abnormal thickened enhancement of the bilateral vestibular nerves, left facial nerve, and right trigeminal nerve (Fig. 1).

The patient was promptly started on steroids, admitted to the hospital, and underwent a midline suboccipital craniotomy for debulking of the large intracerebellar tumor. Upon entering the cystic cavity, grossly purulent material without hemorrhage was noted. Gram stain and cultures were negative for infection. A subtotal resection was achieved and final pathology rendered the diagnosis of primary CNS histiocytic sarcoma (see Fig. 2). The H&E section (Fig. 2a and b) revealed sheets of large neoplastic cells with marked cytological atypia, brisk mitosis with occasional multilobated nuclei, and focal necrosis. Extensive immunohistochemical studies (Fig. 2c and d) showed the neoplastic cells positive for CD163, CD68, CD45, and Vimentin; negative for CD20, CD3, CD30, s-100, CD1a, CD21, CD23, pancytokeratin, MPO, CD61, CD123, GFAP, and BRAF. Further immunostains for PD-L1 with two different antibody clones (22C3 and 28–8) were also performed and showed more than 50% of the tumor cells were positive with membrane stain (Fig. 2e and f).

Post-operative MRI showed a midline posterior occipital craniotomy with subtotal resection of tumor and continued bilateral-enhancement along multiple cranial nerves, concerning for leptomeningeal spread (Fig. 3).

A staging PET scan was performed two weeks following surgery suggesting diffuse leptomeningeal spread. A complete spinal MRI confirmed diffuse leptomeningeal spread in the lower thoracic and lumbar spine as well as cauda equina involvement. Due to the convincing evidence on MRI, a CSF analysis was deferred. Standard lab work was within limits, including LDH (Fig. 4).

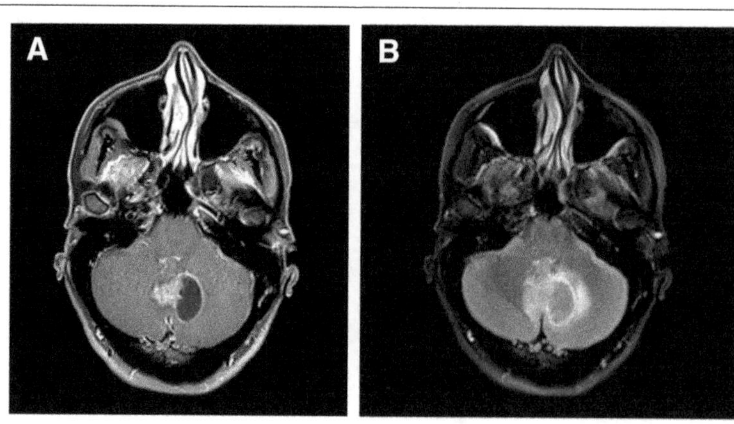

Fig. 1 a) Axial T1 Post Gadolinium Fat Saturation. **b**) T2 FLAIR Fat Saturation

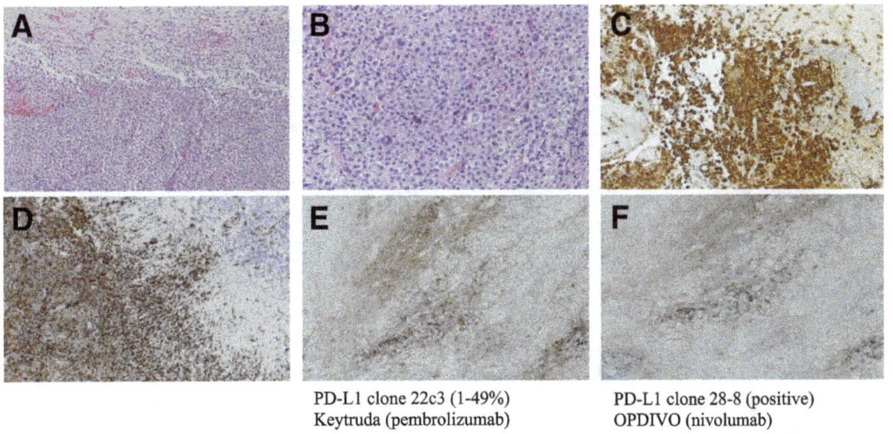

Fig. 2 Final Pathological Examination. The H&E section show the diffuse proliferation of neoplastic histiocytes invading normal brain parenchyma (**a** × 10, upper normal brain; bottom neoplastic histiocytes); the neoplastic histiocytes show marked cytological atypia with brisk mitosis (**b** × 20). Immunohistochemical studies show the histiocytes positive for CD 163 (**c** ×10), CD68 (**d** × 10), CD45 and vimentin; negative for CD20, CD3, CD30, s-100, CD1a, CD21, CD23, pancytokeratin, MPO, CD61, CD123, GFAP, and BRAF. The neoplastic histiocytes are also positive for PD-L1 with both clones (**e**× 10, 22C3 and **f**× 10, 28–8)

Three weeks following surgery, due to progressive lower back pain, she initiated radiation therapy including whole brain radiotherapy (30.6 Gy in 17 fractions) followed by a posterior fossa boost (5.4 Gy in 3 fractions) and a gross tumor boost (9 Gy in 5 fractions), for a total dose of 45 Gy in 25 fractions to gross disease with simultaneous radiation therapy to the lower thoracic and lumbar spine, receiving 40 Gy in 20 fractions, encompassing the areas of leptomeningeal disease in the spine and cauda equina. Full craniospinal radiotherapy was not performed to limit profound cytopenias that may have prevented further cytotoxic chemotherapy.

Interval follow up MRI showed a partial response with persistent posterior fossa disease but near complete resolution of previous leptomeningeal enhancement. Our plan was to initiate chemotherapy with a primary CNS lymphoma regimen with high CNS penetrating therapeutic agents including high-dose methotrexate, high-dose Ara-C, and thiotepa followed by high-dose chemotherapy with BCNU and thiotepa rescued by autologous stem cell transplantation. The patient was started on high dose intravenous methotrexate (HD-MTX) therapy, but received only one cycle secondary to patient intolerance.

A CT of the chest approximately two weeks after initiation of HD-MTX therapy for left sided rib pain showed new pulmonary nodules and a left sided pleural effusion, suspicious for metastatic disease. Thoracentesis revealed findings consistent with a malignant pleural effusion. The patient was initiated on cladribine (Leustatin).

Within two weeks after the completion of this infusion, the patient developed headaches, somnolence, fever, and nuchal rigidity. Malignant meningitis was suspected and the patient was started on IV antibiotics. Lumbar puncture was recommended but the patient declined. Her mental status significantly improved

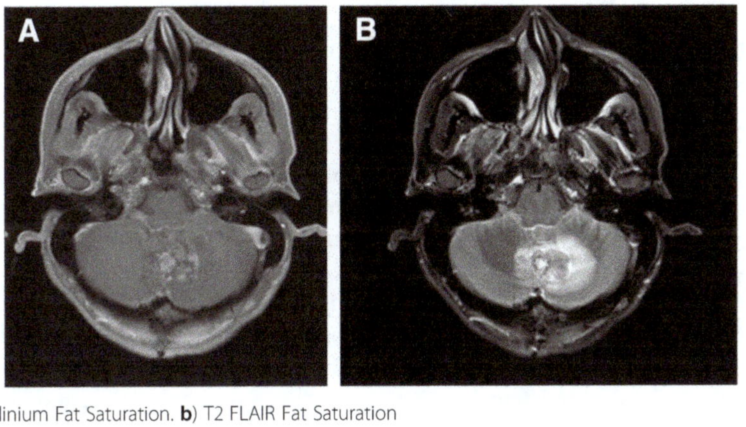

Fig. 3 **a**) Axial T1 Post Gadolinium Fat Saturation. **b**) T2 FLAIR Fat Saturation

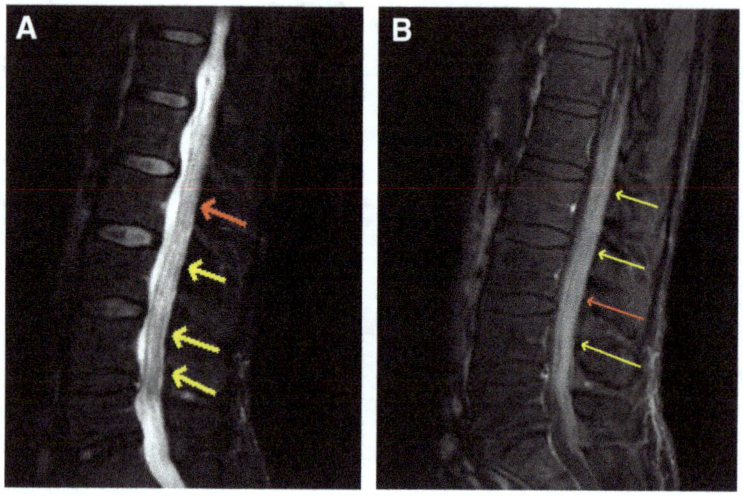

Fig. 4 a) Sagittal T2. **b**) Sagittal T1 Post Contrast

following antibiotic treatment. Brain MRI showed continued response of the cerebellar residual disease and no new intra-cranial lesions, but an MRI of the cervical spine showed new lesions consistent with metastatic disease in the untreated cervical spinal cord and thoracic vertebrae, including intramedullary involvement. She underwent further radiation therapy targeting C4-C6 and T1-T7 (20 Gy in 5 fractions). The patient rapidly showed improvement in symptoms.

Genomic sequencing of her tumor showed a novel mutation in the platelet-derived growth factor receptor A (p.V608I) and therefore, she was started on Dasatinib, a tyrosine kinase inhibitor (TKI) with known CNS penetration [24]. Unfortunately, this medication was poorly tolerated because of nausea, diarrhea, and acute pancreatitis so it was discontinued after one week.

The patient was readmitted to the hospital for continued decline in functional status, weakness, and failure to thrive. CT images of the chest, abdomen, and pelvis showed progressive bilateral pulmonary nodules. An MRI of the spine showed persistent but significantly improved leptomeningeal enhancement. Due to progression of symptoms, worsening systemic disease despite control of CNS disease, and limited systemic options available, the patient chose to enroll in hospice. The patient expired four weeks later, eight months after initial diagnosis.

Discussion

Histiocytic sarcoma of the CNS is an uncommon diagnosis with only about 30 total cases reported in the literature. The median age for diagnosis of HS is 46 years, which is equally distributed in males and females [20]. The prognosis for HS of the CNS is extremely poor with a median survival of 4.5 months, the longest recurrence free period reported being 42 months [6, 23].

This case was unique and merits discussion for several reasons. First, at the time of surgery, entry into the cerebellar lesion was associated with drainage of purulent material, which has been documented previously in only three other cases [1, 3, 26]. This was an unexpected finding at the time of surgery and no evidence of infection was identified. Second, this patient had extensive and symptomatic leptomeningeal disease with cranial nerve and spinal involvement by MRI. Leptomeningeal disease is relatively common in CNS HS, 10/31 (32%) documented cases had leptomeningeal involvement, which is associated with a poor quality of life and poor survival. In our case, this disease was treated aggressively with moderate dose radiation therapy, 45 Gy to the gross tumor in the cerebellum and 40 Gy to the leptomeningeal disease in the spine, which did achieve continued disease control, even 6 months after treatment. This raises the question as to whether patients with leptomeningeal spread would benefit from craniospinal radiotherapy. However, full craniospinal radiotherapy can induce profound cytopenias that could limit or delay the use of systemic therapy which has known benefit for histiocytic sarcoma. The other important aspect of this case is that we were able to obtain adequate amount of tissue from surgical resection of the brain tumor and performed genomic sequencing revealing a novel PDGFR mutation which is highly targetable with TKI's. There is very limited literature regarding genomic data in CNS histiocytic sarcoma. One additional case report describes a patient with CNS histiocytic sarcoma with genomic sequencing revealing BRAF V600E mutation. The patient experienced a

Table 1 Reported cases of Primary Histiocytic Sarcoma of the CNS and their characteristics

Author & Year	Age, Gender	Site(s)	Number of Lesions	Size (cm)	Primary Treatment	Outcome
[a]Gill-Samra et al. 2012 [14]	38 yr./F	Temporal	Multiple	5	Surgery+ WBRT: 45Gy in 25 fractions+ Chemotherapy	DOD 3 weeks after presentation
[a]Toshkezi et al. 2010 [29]	71 yr./F	Spine and leptomeninges	Solitary	2.5x 1x 1.1	Surgery+ RT: 44 Gy in 22 fractions	DOD 5 months after presentation
[a]Bell et al. 2012 [3]	62 yr./F	Cerebellum	Solitary	ND	Surgery	AWPD 24 months
[a]Bell et al. 2012 [12]	34 yr./M	Frontal	Solitary	2	Surgery	AWPD 10 months
[a] Devic et al., 2012 [10]	43 yr./F	Corpus callosum, Cerebellum, and Spine	Multiple	ND	Chemotherapy	DOD 10 months after presentation
[a]Wang et al., 2012 [31]	55 yr./F	Corpus callosum	Multiple	ND	Surgery+3D CRT: 16 Gy	DOD 4 months after presentation
[a]Torres et al., 1996 [28]	20 mo/M	Leptomeninges	Solitary	ND	Chemotherapy	DOD 3 months after presentation
[a] Cheuk et al., 2001 [9]	69 yr./F	Parietal	Solitary	1.5	Surgery+ WBRT+ Chemotherapy	DOD 8 months after presentation
[a] Cheuk et al., 2001 [9]	43 yr./M	Spine	Solitary	1.7	Surgery+ WBRT+ Chemotherapy	AWPD at 5 months
[a] Cheuk et al., 2001 [21]	11 yr./M	Cerebellum, occipital, and frontal	Multiple	.7–1	Surgery	DOD 4 months after presentation
[a] Sun et al., 2003 [26]	13 yr./M	Occipital and leptomeninges	ND	ND 1.1	Surgery	DOD 7 months after presentation
[a]Cao et al., 2007 [6]	53 yr./F	Cavernous sinus, relapsed to mediastinum	Solitary	3.1 × 2.9 × 2.2	Surgery+ RT 54 Gy	DOD 4 years after presentation
[a]Almefty et al., 2013 [1]	16 yr./M	Parietal	Solitary	3.5 × 4.4 × 4.0	Surgery+ IMRT: 60 Gy in 30 fractions	DOD 4 months after presentation
[a]Wu et al., 2013 [32]	50 yr./M	Parieto-occipital	Solitary	1.7	Surgery+ SRS: 30 Gy in 5 fractions	AWPD at 18 months
[a] Laviv et al., 2013 [19]	58 yr./M	Frontal	Solitary	6.5	Surgery	DOD 4 months after presentation
[a]Gomi et al.. 2012 [15]	17 mo/F	Cerebellum, dissemination to spine	Solitary	4.7 × 4.3 × 4.3	Surgery+ Chemotherapy	AWPD at 16 months
[a]Gentzler et al., 2011 [13]	52 yr./F	Parietal	Solitary	1.7	Palliative Care	Expired from lung cancer
[a] Perez-Ruiz et al., 2013 [23]	41 yr./F	Temporal and leptomeninges	Solitary	1.5 × 2	Surgery+ TMZ + IMRT: 61.2Gy	ANED 42 months
[a]Chalasani et al., 2013 [7]	44 yr./M	Corpus callosum	Multiple	3.5 and 2.6	Chemotherapy+ WBRT: 26 Gy + Boost to 46 Gy	DOD 27 weeks after presentation
[a]Idbaih et al., 2014 [17]	40 yr./M	Temporal	Solitary	ND	Chemotherapy	DOD 6 months after presentation
[a]Moulinger et al., 2014 [22]	63 yr./F	Pons	Multiple	ND	Chemotherapy	DOD 20 days after completion of treatment
[a] Bai et al., 2014 [2]	52 yr./M	Frontal	Solitary	ND	Surgery+ TMZ + IMRT: 54 Gy	ANED 16 months
[a]Foster et al., 2015 [11]	15 yr./F	Frontal	Solitary	5.8 × 4.7 × 4.0	Surgery+ TMZ + 3D CRT	ANED 23 months
[a] Chen et al.,	61 yr./M	Meckel's Cave	Solitary	1.5 × 1.1 ×	Radiotherapy 66Gy in 33	AWPD 31 months

Table 1 Reported cases of Primary Histiocytic Sarcoma of the CNS and their characteristics *(Continued)*

Author & Year	Age, Gender	Site(s)	Number of Lesions	Size (cm)	Primary Treatment	Outcome
2015 [8]				1.8	fractions + 1 cycle CVP + 2 cycles CHOP	
[a]Brown et al., 2015 [4]	23 yr./M	Cerebellopontine	Solitary	6	Chemotherapy+ IMRT	AWPD 60 months
[a]So et al., 2015 [25]	59 yr./M	Parietal, Corpus callosum, Frontal and Spine	Multiple	ND	Chemotherapy	DOD 8 months after presentation
Zanelli et al., 2017 [33]	45 yr./F	Leptomeninges	N/A	N/A	No therapy	DOD 2 months after presentation
[a] Ueno et al., 2016 [30]	65 yr./M	Frontal, parietal, spine, and leptomeninges	Multiple	ND	Radiotherapy	AWPD 11 months
Kim et al., 2017 [18]	16 yr./M	Corpus callosum, frontoparietal	Solitary	6.5 × 5.3	Surgery+ Chemotherapy+ Radiotherapy 60Gy	DOD 12 months after presentation
Marguet et al., 2018 [21]	67 yr./M	Periventricular, hypothalamic and sellar region, leptomeningeal involvement.	Multiple	2.1, 1.4	No therapy	DOD 7 months after presentation
Present case	47 yr/ F	Cerebellar vermis and leptomeninges	Multiple	3.0 × 2.9 × 2.3	Surgery + WBRT: 30.6 Gy + Boost to 45 Gy + Chemotherapy	DOD 8 months after presentation

ANED Alive and no evidence of disease, *AWPD* Alive with progressive disease, *DOD* Dead of disease, *ND* Not Determined, *PTV* Planning target volume, *WBRT* Whole Brain Radiation Therapy, *3D CRT* 3D Conformal Radiotherapy, *IMRT* Intensity modulated radiotherapy, *TMZ* Temozolomide, *CVP* Cyclophosphamide, vincristine, and prednisone, *CHOP* Cyclophosphamide, doxorubicin, vincristine, and prednisone
[a]Indicates patients from manuscript Zanelli et al., 2017 [33]

dramatic clinical and radiographic response with vemurafenib, though the response was not durable and the patient expired 6 months after initiation of treatment [17]. Our pathologic evaluation showed PD-L1 and PD-L2 expression by the tumor, which suggests that immunotherapy with checkpoint inhibitors should be explored. Using inhibitors to suppress PD-L1/PD-1 interaction has shown promising effects for treatment of various advanced cancers, but no literature is available for HS of the CNS [12]. Overexpression of PD-1 in an animal model has suggested antitumor immunity may be suppressed in histiocytic sarcoma, although this is yet to be shown in humans [27]. To the best of our knowledge, our case is the first report of PD-L1/PD-L2 expression in histiocytic sarcoma of the CNS.

A review of the literature for CNS HS was performed and the identified cases are shown in Table 1. Only three of thirty patients (10%) were alive with no evidence of disease at the time of publication, 16, 23, and 42 months after presentation [2, 11, 23]. Treatment for these cases consisted of surgery followed by concurrent chemoradiation with temozolomide and high dose focal radiation. In the two cases with radiation dose reported, the total dose given was 54 Gy and 61.4 Gy. This is consistent with the findings in our case that moderate doses of radiation are needed for local control.

The majority of cases in the literature received some form of surgery, radiation, and/or chemotherapy. The current standard treatment for CNS HS is surgery to achieve a maximal safe resection and for tissue diagnosis and relieving cerebral edema. An aggressive, multimodality approach is preferred with postoperative radiation therapy +/− chemotherapy, when the disease is unifocal. When the disease has become multifocal, further aggressive radiotherapy and combination chemotherapy is essential. Chemotherapeutics used previously include temozolomide (TMZ), cyclophosphamide, doxorubicin, vincristine and prednisone (CHOP), rituximab, ifosfamide, carboplatin, etoposide (ICE), methotrexate, and thalidomide. There are no documented cases in the literature of successful treatment of multifocal disease. Thus, HS is a very aggressive disease when found in the central nervous system which warrants aggressive treatment with multiple modalities. Despite limited long term survivals of this disease, there have been approximately 10% of cases with long term survival with aggressive treatment including surgery, dose escalated radiation therapy, and chemotherapy.

Conclusion

In this case we present a patient with a primary histiocytic sarcoma of the CNS, an extremely rare diagnosis with a poor prognosis. This patient was treated aggressively with surgery, radiation therapy, chemotherapy, and targeted therapy informed by genomic sequencing but ultimately expired of her progressive disease approximately 8 months after diagnosis. The genomic sequencing of the tumor tissue showed a novel PDGFR mutation, which could be targeted with TKI's. We showed expression of PD-L1 and PD-L2 by the tumor cells suggesting potential therapeutic role for immune checkpoint inhibitors. Our case demonstrates a durable response of CNS disease with radiation doses 40 Gy and above. Therefore, we recommend aggressive treatment with curative radiation doses to the CNS whenever appropriate and possible. Novel therapeutic agents such as TKI's and checkpoint inhibitors need to be explored.

Abbreviations

BCNU: Carmustine; CD: Cluster of differentiation; CHOP: Cyclophosphamide, Doxorubicin, Vincristine, and Prednisone; CNS: Central Nervous System; CSF: Cerebrospinal Fluid; CT: Computed Tomography; GFAP: Glial fibrillary acidic protein; Gy: Grey; H&E: Haemotoxylin and Eosin; HD-MTX: High Dose Methotrexate; HS: Histiocytic Sarcoma; ICE: Ifosfamide, Carboplatin, and Etoposide; IV: Intravenous; LDH: Lactate Dehydrogenase; MPO: Myeloperoxidase; MRI: Magnetic Resonance Imaging; PD-1: Programmed Cell Death Protein 1; PDGFR: Platelet Derived Growth Factor Receptor; PD-L1: Programmed Death-Ligand 1; PD-L2: Programmed Death Ligand-2; PET: Positron Emission Tomography; TKI: Tyrosine Kinase Inhibitor; TMZ: Temozolomide

Authors' contributions

JMM Collected patient data, composed manuscript, and produced final draft. MRW Assisted in composing drafts of manuscript. WCS Provided revisions for manuscript. TAK Provided edits for manuscript. DHM Assisted with manuscript composition. BCM Assisted with manuscript composition and provided recommendations to article. RCM Provided initial concept for research and revised manuscript. LJ Provided pathology report and excerpt regarding markers included in manuscript. GWS Collected patient's information including physician notes, procedure notes, and MRIs. DMT He revised and provided recommendations for the manuscript. KLC He provided edits and recommendations for the manuscript. RR Treated the patient and reviewed the manuscript. HWT Treated the patient and provided edits and recommendations for manuscript. JLP Treated the patient and provided major edits to manuscript. All authors read and approved the final manuscript.

Competing interests

The authors declare that they have no competing interests.

Author details

[1]Department of Radiation Oncology, Mayo Clinic, 4500 San Pablo Road South, Jacksonville, FL 32224, USA. [2]Department of Neurological Surgery, Mayo Clinic, Jacksonville, Florida, USA. [3]Department of Pathology and Laboratory Medicine, Mayo Clinic, Jacksonville, Florida, USA. [4]Department of Hematology and Medical Oncology, Mayo Clinic, Jacksonville, Florida, USA.

References

1. Almefty RO, Tyree TL, Fusco DJ, Coons SW, Nakaji P. Primary histiocytic sarcoma of the brain mimicking cerebral abscess. J Neurosurg Pediatr. 2013; 12:251–7.
2. Bai J, Li G, Shen M, Sui D, Lin S. Primary central nervous system histiocytic sarcoma mimicking glioma. Neurol India. 2014;62(6):684–5.
3. Bell SL, Hanzely Z, Alakandy LM, Jackson R, Stewart W. Primary meningeal histiocytic sarcoma: a report of two unusual cases. Neuropathol Appl Neurobiol. 2012;38:111–4.
4. Brown AF, Fan H, Floyd JR, Henry JM, Higgins RA. Primary central nervous system histiocytic sarcoma arising after precursor B-cell acute lymphoblastic leukemia. J Neuropathol Exp Neurol. 2015;74(12):1120–6.
5. Campo E, Swerdlow SH, Harris NL, et al. The 2008 WHO classification of lymphoid neoplasms and beyond: evolving concepts and practical applications. Blood. 2011;117:5019–32.
6. Cao M, Eshoa C, Schultz C, Black J, Zu Y, Chang CC. Primary central nervous system histiocytic sarcoma with relapse to mediastinum: a case report and review of the literature. Arch Pathol Lab Med. 2007;131:301–5.
7. Chalasani S, Hennick M, Hocking WG, Shaw GR, Lawler B. Unusual presentation of a rare cancer: histiocytic sarcoma in the brain 16 years after treatment for acute lymphoblastic leukemia. Clin Med Res. 2013;11(1):31–5.
8. Chen CJ, Williams E, McAneney TE, Williams BJ, Mandell JW, Shaffrey ME. Histiocytic sarcoma of the cavernous sinus: case report and literature review. Brain Tumor Pathol. 2015;32(1):66–71.
9. Cheuk W, Walford N, Lou J, Lee AK, Fung CF, Au KH, et al. Primary histiocytic lymphoma of the central nervous system: a neoplasm frequently overshadowed by a prominent inflammatory component. Am J Surg Pathol. 2001;25:1372–9.
10. Devic P, Androdias-Condemine G, Streichenberger N, Berger F, Honnorat J, Broussolle E, et al. Histiocytic sarcoma of the central nervous system: a challenging diagnosis. QJM. 2012;105:77–9.
11. Foster M, Kamaly-Asl I, Stivaros S, Kelsey A, Gattamenini R, Kilday JP. Primary cerebral histiocytic sarcoma in childhood: a case report of protracted survival and review of the literature. Childs Nerv Syst. 2015;31(12):2363–8.
12. Gatalica Z, Bilalovic N, Palazzo JP, et al. Disseminated histiocytoses biomarkers beyond BRAFV600E: frequent expression of PD-L1. Oncotarget. 2015;6(23): 19819–25.
13. Gentzler RD, Kahn D. Histiocytic sarcoma: a case of a 52-year-old female with two synchronous primary malignancies at presentation. Medicine Forum. 2011;11:31–3.
14. Gill-Samra S, Ng T, Dexter M, Wong M, Nahar N, Allsopp K, et al. Histiocytic sarcoma of the brain. J Clin Neurosci. 2012;19:1456–8.
15. Gomi K, Tanaka M, Yoshida M, Ito S, Sonoda M, Iwasaki F, et al. Primary cerebellar histiocytic sarcoma in a 17-month-old girl. J Neurosurg Pediatr. 2012;10:126–9.
16. Hornick JL, Jaffe ES, Fletcher CDM. Extranodal histiocytic sarcoma—clinicopathologic analysis of 14 cases of a rare epithelioid malignancy. Am J Surg Pathol. 2004;28:1133–44. 2004
17. Idbaih A, Mokhtari K, Emile JF, et al. Dramatic response of a BRAF V600E-mutated primary CNS histiocytic sarcoma to vemurafenib. Neurology. 2014; 83(16):1478–80.
18. Kim YH, Yie GH, Kim NR, Jeon I, Cho HY, Seok JY, Kim EY, Lee KC. Pediatric intracerebral histiocytic sarcoma with rhabdoid features: case report and literature review. Neuropathology. 2017;37(6):560–8.
19. Laviv Y, Zagzag D, Fichman-Horn S, Michowitz S. Primary central nervous system histiocytic sarcoma. Brain Tumor Pathol. 2013;30:192–5.
20. Machado ES, de Miranda AC, Escopelli T, Caron R, Escopelli AC. Histiocytic sarcoma. Rev Bras Hematol Hemoter. 2011;33(2):155–7. https://doi.org/10.5581/1516-8484.20110038.
21. Marguet F, Piton N, Adle-Biassette H, Renaud F, Bohers E, Boyer T, Zarea A, Derrey S, Sabourin JC, Laquerriere A. Molecular characteristics of multifocal brain histiocytic sarcoma. Neuropathol Appl Neurobiol. 2018; https://doi.org/10.1111/nan.12490.
22. Moulignier A, Mikol J, Heran F, Galicier L. Isolated III cranial nerve palsies may point to primary histiocytic sarcoma. BMJ Case Rep. 2014; https://doi.org/10.1136/bcr-2014-204663.
23. Pérez-Ruiz E, Delgado M, Sanz A, Gil AM, Domínguez AR. Primary leptomeningeal histiocytic sarcoma in a patient with a good outcome: a case report and review of the literature. J Med Case Rep. 2013;13(7):127.
24. Porkka K, Koskenvesa P, Lundan T, et al. Dasatinib crosses the blood-brain barrier and is an efficient therapy for central nervous system Philadelphia chromosome-positive leukemia. Blood. 2008;112(4):1005–12.
25. So H, Kim S, Yoon DH, et al. Primary histiocytic sarcoma of the central nervous system. Cancer Res Treat. 2015;47(2):322–8.
26. Sun W, Nordberg ML, Fowler MR. Histiocytic sarcoma involving the central nervous system: clinical, immunohistochemical, and molecular genetic studies of a case with review of the literature. Am J Surg Pathol. 2003; 27:258–65.
27. Tagawa M, Maekawa N, Konnai S, Takagi S. Evaluation of costimulatory molecules in peripheral blood lymphocytes of canine patients with

histiocytic sarcoma. PLoS One. 2016;11(2):e0150030. https://doi.org/10.1371/journal.pone.0150030. eCollection 2016

28. Torres CF, Korones DN, Powers JM, Vadasz AG. Primary leptomeningeal histiocytic lymphoma in a young child. Med Pediatr Oncol. 1996;27:547–50.
29. Toshkezi G, Edalat F, O'Hara C, Delalle I, Chin LS. Primary intramedullary histiocytic sarcoma. World Neurosurg. 2010;74:523–7.
30. Ueno T, Nishijima H, Kurotaki H, Kurose A, Tomiyama M. An unusual case of chronic meningitis due to histiocytic sarcoma of the central nervous system with meningeal dissemination. Neurol Sci. 2016;37(11):1875–7.
31. Wang J, Li T, Chen H, Liu Q. A case of primary central nervous system histiocytic sarcoma. Clin Neurol Neurosurg. 2012;114:1074–6.
32. Wu W, Tanrivermis Sayit A, Vinters HV, Pope W, Mirsadraei L, Said J. Primary central nervous system histiocytic sarcoma presenting as a postradiation sarcoma: case report and literature review. Hum Pathol. 2013;44:1177–83.
33. Zanelli M, Ragazzi M, Marchetti G, Bisagni A, Principi M, Fanni D, Froio E, Serra S, Zanetti E, De Marco L, Giangaspero F, Ascani S. Primary histiocytic sarcoma presenting as diffuse leptomeningeal disease: case description and review of the literature. Neuropathology. 2017; https://doi.org/10.1111/neup.12390, 2017.

4

Effect of dose rate on pulmonary toxicity in patients with hematolymphoid malignancies undergoing total body irradiation

Dong-Yun Kim[1], Il Han Kim[1,4], Sung-Soo Yoon[2,4], Hyoung Jin Kang[3,4], Hee Young Shin[3,4] and Hyun-Cheol Kang[1*]

Abstract

Background: This study evaluated the effect of radiation dose rate in patients with hematolymphoid malignancies undergoing myeloablative conditioning with total body irradiation (TBI), for hematopoietic stem cell transplantation.

Methods: The incidence of pulmonary toxicity (PT) and treatment efficacy were compared between the conventional (≥ 6 cGy/min) and reduced dose rate (< 6 cGy/min). Seventy-seven patients receiving once-daily TBI between 2000 and 2016 were reviewed. We compared the cumulative rate of PT, overall survival (OS), relapse, and transplantation-related mortality (TRM) between conventional ($n = 54$) and reduced ($n = 23$) groups. Factors associated with PT were assessed in the presence of competing risks.

Results: The median follow-up time was 40.7 months, and PT occurred in 50 patients (64.9%). On multivariate analyses, the groups classified by the dose rate ($P = 0.010$), total dose ($P = 0.025$), and conditioning regimen ($P = 0.029$) were significant factors for the development of PT. OS was significantly reduced when PT occurred ($P < 0.001$). However, the OS, relapse, and TRM were not different between the two groups.

Conclusions: In summary, about two-thirds of the patients undergoing daily TBI experienced PT, which affected OS. Therefore, reducing the dose rate (less than 6 cGy/min) of TBI can decrease the risk of PT, without compromising the treatment efficacy.

Keywords: Hematolymphoid malignancy, Total body irradiation, Pulmonary toxicity, Dose rate

Background

Total body irradiation (TBI)-based myeloablative conditioning, followed by allogeneic stem cell transplantation, is conducted for patients with high-risk or relapsed hematolymphoid malignancies [1–3]. TBI has been used in 46% to 53% of allogeneic hematopoietic stem cell transplantations (HSCT) as a preconditioning component, with other chemotherapeutic agents [4]. There have been a wide variety of TBI doses and fractionation schedules used by each institution. The American College of Radiology (ACR) and the American Society for Radiation Oncology (ASTRO) recommended some basic principles with competing goals of anti-leukemic effects and toxicity reductions; however, a firm consensus has yet to be established [5].

Several complications limit the success of this treatment. Particularly, pulmonary toxicity (PT) is one of the most harmful sequelae of TBI [6–8]. PT is a life-threatening problem after TBI, followed by bone marrow transplantation (BMT), which together, account for 25–50% non-relapse deaths in prior studies [2, 8–13].

In our institution, we have implemented a TBI regimen with once-daily treatment and have gradually reduced the dose rate, to lower lung toxicities. Since 2014, most patients have been treated with a dose rate of less than 6 cGy/min, based on the availability of the extended source-to-surface distance (SSD). The current study examines the risk factors of PT in the once-daily treatment TBI regimen and confirms whether reducing the

* Correspondence: shule@snu.ac.kr; hermes-shule@hanmail.net
[1]Department of Radiation Oncology, Seoul National University College of Medicine, 101 Daehak-ro, Jongno-gu, Seoul 03080, Republic of Korea
Full list of author information is available at the end of the article

dose rate affects the clinical outcomes, i.e., overall survival rate, relapse rate, and transplantation-related mortality (TRM), after HSCT. Our goal of the study is to suggest an ideal dose rate of TBI at the once-daily treatment setting.

Methods

After the approval of the Institutional Review Board, a retrospective analysis of 92 patients (2–63 years old) with hematolymphoid malignancies, who underwent myeloablative TBI as part of the conditioning regimen between 1998 and 2016 at Seoul National University Hospital, was performed. Seventy-seven patients were eligible for this study, except for single fraction TBI ($n = 9$), the presence of existing lung disease ($n = 3$), or failure to perform the planned fraction of TBI due to poor performance status ($n = 3$).

Patients received 9–12 Gy TBI in 3–4 fractions, once-daily, without a day interval. The TBI technique was based on a two-dimensional radiotherapy plan, with 6- or 15-MV photon beam. Patients were positioned in the lateral decubitus position on a stretcher against the wall of the linear accelerator room, to maximize the SSD and field size so that the entire patient was encompassed. Depending on the patient's height, if the lying position with straightened legs was greater than the field size, the knees posture changed to the bent position. Also, the body thickness of the patient was measured along the entire axis at the prescription point, and thus, the thickness of the compensator at each site was different. In addition to the compensator, a beam spoiler was also used, and both were calibrated as correction factors. The lung shielding technique was not used, but instead, the dose to the anterior lung was attenuated via a lead compensator by 5 to 10% of the prescription dose, and the posterior lung was masked by the arms.

From 1999 to 2013, the dose rate continuously decreased, from a maximum of 17.3 to 6.18 cGy/min, and since 2014, dose rates have been maintained under 6 cGy/min. Our institution has attempted to lower the dose rate of TBI to reduce PT, which has been possible by ensuring an adequate SSD distance (400 cm).

After completing TBI, patients received sequential chemotherapy for conditioning before HSCT. In total, 78.3% of the regimens included chemotherapy, with either cyclophosphamide alone or with one other agent added to cyclophosphamide, such as cytarabine, fludarabine, or etoposide, and the rest used chemotherapy, i.e., cytarabine/fludarabine, busulfan/fludarabine/etoposide, melphalan, melphalan/fludarabine, or thiotepa. There were variations in the pre-HSCT regimen, which was influenced by the type of malignancy, donor source, and prior chemotherapy. Stem cells of the donor source were derived from peripheral blood, bone marrow, or cord blood. Post-transplantation graft-versus-host disease prophylaxis was administered to all patients.

Definition of PT and other clinical outcomes

According to the criteria commonly used in previous studies [3, 7, 8, 12], PT was defined if patients met any one of the following three definitions, after TBI-based HSCT: (1) two of three of the following clinical symptoms: dyspnea/cough or any reference to respiratory symptoms, pyrexia, and hypoxia/ cyanosis; (2) radiographic evidence: chest radiograph with bilateral diffuse shadowing and/or increased density or increased interstitial markings or opacities, or chest computed tomography with diffuse ground glass opacities; or (3) ventilatory defects, as noted on pulmonary function tests with either restrictive patterns or obstructive patterns. The presence of infection was defined by the detection of infectious agents, through media, such as blood culture or bronchoalveolar lavage. TRM was determined as mortality in the absence of any evidence of recurrence until 3 months after HSCT [14]. In previous literatures, TRM was generally defined as death from any cause without leukemia relapse [15, 16]. Many cases of death after HSCT are due to infectious causes [17], and the risk of opportunistic infection is small after 3 months [18]. For this reason, we limited the definition of TRM to 3 months after TBI followed by HSCT.

Statistical analyses

We analyzed factors affecting PT (e.g., group divided by dose rate, total dose (Gy), daily dose (Gy), age at TBI, gender, cancer type, donor type, conditioning regimen, or number of prior chemotherapy regimens) and performed subgroup analyses by the etiology of PT (infection vs. non-infection) in the presence of the competing risks suggested by the Fine–Gray model. After conducting univariate regression of PT, multivariate analysis of PT was done by including covariates in the competing risks regression model with $P < 0.20$. Overall survival, relapse rate, and TRM were examined by the Kaplan-Meier method, with the p-value calculated by the log-rank test. All analyses were performed using Stata/MP 14.2 with a significance level of 0.05.

Results

A total of 77 patients with median age of 19.9 years (range, 1.8–66.4 years) were analyzed for the study. The median follow-up time was 40.7 months. The demographics of the patients are listed in Table 1. We grouped patients by the dose rate of TBI. The dose rate of less than 6 cGy/min was classified as the 'reduced group (n=23)', and the dose rate of ≥6 cGy/min was categorized as the 'conventional group (n=54)'. Median dose rate was 4.8 cGy/min (range, 4.2–5.2 cGy/min) in the reduced group and 8.6 cGy/min (range, 6.2–17.3 cGy/min) in the conventional group.

Table 1 Patient characteristic ($N = 77$)

	Dose rate < 6 cGy/min ($N = 23$)	Dose rate ≥ 6 cGy/min ($N = 54$)	P-value
Age at TBI (year)	29.4 ± 18.6 (1.9–66.4)	15.9 ± 8.9 (1.8–41.7)	0.002[b]
Sex			
Male	14 (60.9%)	32 (59.9%)	0.895[a]
Female	9 (39.1%)	22 (40.1%)	
Type of Cancer			
ALL	15 (65.2%)	32 (59.3%)	0.172[a]
AML	2 (8.7%)	14 (25.9%)	
Others	6 (26.1%)	8 (14.8%)	
Total dose (Gy)	11.7 ± 0.9 (9–12)	10.9 ± 1.1 (9–12)	0.004[b]
Daily dose (Gy)	3.0 ± 0.1 (2.5–3.0)	3.1 ± 0.2 (2.3–3.3)	0.001[b]
Daily dose < 3	1 (4.3%)	2 (3.7%)	
Daily dose ≥3	22 (95.7%)	52 (96.3%)	0.017[a]
Donor type			
Related	16 (69.6%)	22 (40.7%)	0.021[a]
Unrelated	7 (30.4%)	32 (59.3%)	
Conditioning regimen			
Cyclophosphamide	4 (17.4%)	8 (14.8%)	0.271[a]
Cyclophosphamide + other[c]	14 (60.9%)	24 (44.4%)	
Others[d]	5 (21.7%)	22 (40.7%)	
Number of prior chemotherapy regimens			
1	3 (13.0%)	14 (25.9%)	0.193[a]
2	8 (34.8%)	23 (42.6%)	
≥ 3	12 (52.2%)	17 (31.5%)	

[a] P-value by chi-square test. [b] P-value by Mann-Whitney U test

[c] Other: cytarabine, fludarabine, etoposide

[d] Others: cytarabine/fludaraibine, busulfan/fludarabine/etoposide, melphalan, melphalan/fludarabine, thiotepa

There was a statistical difference between the groups, according to the dose rate in age at TBI (year), total dose (Gy), daily dose (Gy), and donor cell type. The median follow-up time was 10.6 months (range, 0.7–30.6 months) in the reduced group, and 12.6 months (range, 0.5–191.9 months) in the conventional group; however, the difference between the two groups was not significant. Overall PT, including both infectious and non-infectious types, developed in 50 patients (64.9%). Ten patients (43.5%) in the reduced group and 40 patients (74.1%) in the conventional group had PT, which was significantly different between the groups ($P = 0.01$) (Table 2).

The median time to onset of PT after TBI was 5.4 months (range, 0.1–30.9 months), and 3.7 and 5.2 months for the reduced and conventional group, respectively, revealing no statistical significance. The

Table 2 Incidence of pulmonary toxicity related to time after total body irradiation according to the groups classified by the dose rate

	Reduced group, dose rate < 6 cGy/min ($N = 23$)	Conventional group, dose rate ≥ 6 cGy/min ($N = 54$)	P-value
Follow-up time (month)	10.6 (0.7–30.6)	12.6 (0.5–191.9)	0.114[b]
Overall Pulmonary toxicity	10 (43.5%)	40 (74.1%)	0.010[a]
Infectious PT	8 (34.8%)	28 (51.9%)	
Non-infectious PT	2 (8.7%)	12 (21.8%)	
3 month - Pulmonary toxicity	5 (21.7%)	20 (37.1%)	0.085[b]
6 month - Pulmonary toxicity	9 (39.7%)	28 (52.3%)	0.085[b]
Time to PT after TBI (month)	3.7 ± 3.4 (0.5–11.8)	5.2 ± 6.5 (0.1–30.9)	0.085[b]

PT Pulmonary toxicity

[a] P by chi-square test

[b] P by log-rank test

incidence of PT during the short-term period of 3 and 6 months after TBI was compared, respectively. The development of PT at 3 and 6 months was 21.7% and 39.7% in the reduced group, and 37.1% and 52.3% in the conventional group, respectively ($P = 0.085$) (Table 2).

Clinical factors associated with PT were analyzed by univariate and multivariate methods, with competing risks regression. On multivariate analysis, overall PT was significantly related to the groups, according to the dose rate (Sub hazard ratio [SHR] 2.61, 95% confidence interval [CI] 1.26–5.40, $P = 0.010$), total dose (Gy) (SHR 1.38, 95% CI 1.04–1.83, $P = 0.025$), and conditioning regimen following TBI (SHR 2.86, 95% CI 1.11–7.38, $P = 0.029$) (Table 3). In subgroup analyses, infectious PT showed a significant association with the groups (SHR 2.38, 95% CI 1.02–5.54, $P = 0.045$), total dose (Gy) (SHR 1.40, 95% CI 1.07–1.85, $P = 0.025$), and daily dose (Gy) (SHR 0.24, 95% CI 0.07–0.83, $P = 0.025$) (Table 4). Also, the groups divided by the dose rate had borderline significance for non-infectious PT (SHR 4.06, 95% CI 0.90–18.28, $P = 0.068$) (Table 4).

Overall survival was significantly reduced when PT occurred ($P < 0.001$). The 2-year overall survival rate was 28.0% with PT, but 81.5% without PT (Fig. 1). However, the dose rate of TBI did not significantly affect overall survival ($P = 0.769$). Furthermore, other factors, such as total dose, daily dose, and conditioning regimen, did not affect the overall survival in the univariate analysis. The 1-year overall survival rate in the reduced group was 39.8% and 40.7% in the conventional group (Fig. 2). There was no statistically significant difference in the relapse rate between the groups, according to the dose rate. Comparing the 1-year relapse rate after TBI with Fine-Gray model, the reduced group had an occurrence of 41.1%, and in the conventional group, this value was 40.2%, respectively ($P = 0.953$) (Fig. 3). In addition, when analyzing the 3-month TRM after HSCT, no significant difference was found between the groups ($P = 0.455$). The 3-month TRM was 13.0% in the reduced group, and 24.1% in the conventional group (Fig. 4).

Table 3 Univariate & multivariate analysis of risk factor for overall pulmonary toxicity

	Univariate analysis			Multivariate analysis		
	SHR	95% CI	*P*-value	SHR	95% CI	*P*-value
Group						
Reduced dose rate group	1 (ref)					
Conventional dose rate group	1.86	0.93–3.71	0.078	2.61	1.26–5.40	0.010
Total dose (Gy)	1.19	0.94–1.51	0.156	1.38	1.04–1.83	0.025
Daily dose (Gy)						
Daily dose < 3	1 (ref)					
Daily dose ≥3	0.67	0.36–1.25	0.205			
Women	1.23	0.70–2.18	0.471	–	–	–
Age at TBI (year)	1.00	0.98–1.02	0.723	–	–	–
Cancer type						
ALL	1 (ref)					
AML	1.47	0.81–2.67	0.210	–	–	–
Others	1.17	0.56–2.44	0.682	–	–	–
Unrelated donor	1.22	0.70–2.10	0.482	–	–	–
Conditioning regimen						
Cyclophosphamide	1 (ref)					
Cy + other[a]	1.92	0.76–4.81	0.165	2.86	1.11–7.38	0.029
Others[b]	1.06	0.40 – 2.81	0.911	1.60	0.54–4.73	0.394
Prior chemotherapy regimens						
1	1 (ref)					
2	0.61	0.29–1.30	0.200	–	–	–
≥ 3	1.32	0.69–2.52	0.409	–	–	–

P-by Fine-Gray

SHR Sub-hazard ratios, *ALL* Acute lymphoblastic leukemia, *AML* Acute myeloid leukemia, *GVHD* Graft-versus-host disease

[a] other: cytarabine, fludarabine, etoposide

[b] others: cytarabine/fludaraibine, busulfan/fludarabine/etoposide, melphalan, melphalan/fludarabine, thiotepa

Table 4 Univariate and multivariate analysis of risk factor for infectious and non-infectious pulmonary toxicity

	Infectious			Non-infectious		
	SHR	95% CI	*P*-value	SHR	95% CI	*P*-value
Univariate analysis						
Group						
Reduced dose rate group	1 (ref)			1 (ref)		
Conventional dose rate group	1.77	0.81–3.85	0.153	4.06	0.90–18.28	0.068
Total dose (Gy)	1.38	1.02–1.87	0.038	0.83	0.55–1.26	0.381
Daily dose (Gy)						
Daily dose < 3	1 (ref)			1 (ref)		
Daily dose ≥3	0.52	0.25–1.10	0.087	0.68	0.37–1.22	0.201
Women	1.22	0.64–2.34	0.545	1.10	0.35–3.44	0.871
Age at TBI (year)	1.00	0.98–1.02	0.854	0.99	0.96–1.02	0.486
Cancer type						
ALL	1 (ref)			1 (ref)		
AML	1.69	0.87–3.31	0.124	1.40	0.30–6.57	0.668
Others	1.22	0.48–3.09	0.671	1.26	0.36–4.44	0.718
Unrelated donor	1.30	0.68–2.48	0.436	0.98	0.34–2.85	0.971
Conditioning regimen						
Cyclophosphamide	1 (ref)			1 (ref)		
Cyclophosphamide + other*	1.65	0.65–4.20	0.290	Cannot be calculated	Cannot be calculated	0.921
Others†	0.80	0.29–2.19	0.659	Cannot be calculated	Cannot be calculated	0.925
Prior chemotherapy regimens						
1	1 (ref)			1 (ref)		
2	0.60	0.27–1.35	0.219	0.45	0.07–2.97	0.405
≥ 3	1.25	0.60–2.60	0.551	2.20	0.42–11.42	0.349
Multivariate analysis						
Group						
Reduced dose rate group	1 (ref)					
Conventional dose rate group	2.38	1.02–5.54	**0.045**			
Total dose (Gy)	1.40	1.07–1.85	**0.016**			
Daily dose (Gy)	0.24	0.07–0.83	**0.025**			
Cancer type						
ALL	1 (ref)					
AML	1.69	0.83–3.42	0.146			
Others	1.41	0.56–3.52	0.463			

*other: cytarabine, fludarabine, etoposide † others: cytarabine/fludaraibine, busulfan/fludarabine/etoposide, melphalan, melphalan/fludarabine, thiotepa

Discussion

PT is a common and severe complication after allogeneic HSCT following TBI, occurring in 25–80% of patients [3, 6, 14, 19–23]. PT after HSCT can develop from either infectious or non-infectious etiologies. PT accounts for approximately 50% of TRM, [3, 6, 19] and many studies have shown that PT leads to a significant reduction in the overall survival rate [3]. Therefore, studies on factors affecting the development of PT have been conducted to reduce lung toxicity, which is detrimental to prognosis after TBI followed by HSCT.

A wide variety of TBI doses and fractionation schedules have been studied in different institutions, to decrease toxicities. Among the factors affecting toxicities during TBI and HSCT, the dose rate of TBI is one of the major components for reducing the development of PT [3, 19, 21]. According to the guidelines published by the ACR and the ASTRO, in 2013, many protocols require a dose rate under 20 cGy/min in the setting of twice-daily treatment

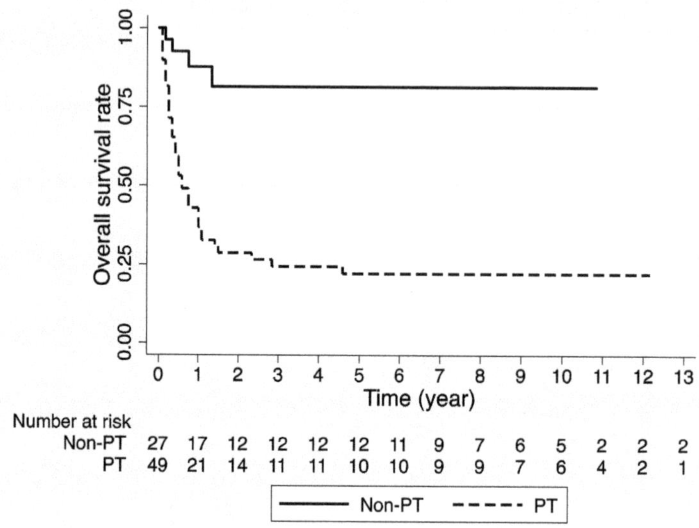

Fig. 1 Actuarial overall survival curves in patients with and without pulmonary toxicity ($P < 0.001$ by log-rank test)

[5]. In previously published data, a large retrospective review of 932 patients undergoing TBI followed by HSCT disclosed that a dose rate less than 6 cGy/min was correlated with a decreased incidence of PT [8]. Also, one retrospective study found that using a TBI dose rate of less than 4 cGy/min was significantly associated with reducing the incidence of interstitial pneumonitis [21]. Furthermore, in a mouse model for BMT, a high TBI dose rate was more toxic than a low dose rate, assessed by a lethal dose for 50% mortality and ventilation rate [24]. However, all these studies were the results of TBI settings that were delivered twice-daily.

Although many studies have been based on TBI for twice-daily, it is practically difficult to treat patients for TBI twice a day in the actual clinical settings. For this reason, many institutions have performed TBI on a single fractional day, such as our hospital [5, 14, 19, 25–27]. According to Soejima et al. [15], there was no significant difference in the 5-year overall survival rate and the relapse-free survival between the once-daily TBI regimen and the twice-daily regimen, and even less lung toxicity in

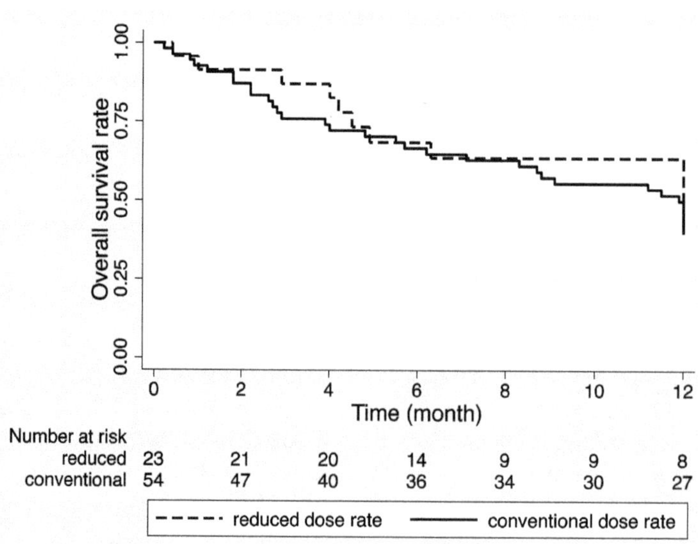

Fig. 2 Actuarial survival curves in patients divided by dose rate of total body irradiation. Reduced dose rate < 6 cGy/min and conventional dose rate ≥ 6 cGy/min ($P = 0.769$ by log-rank test)

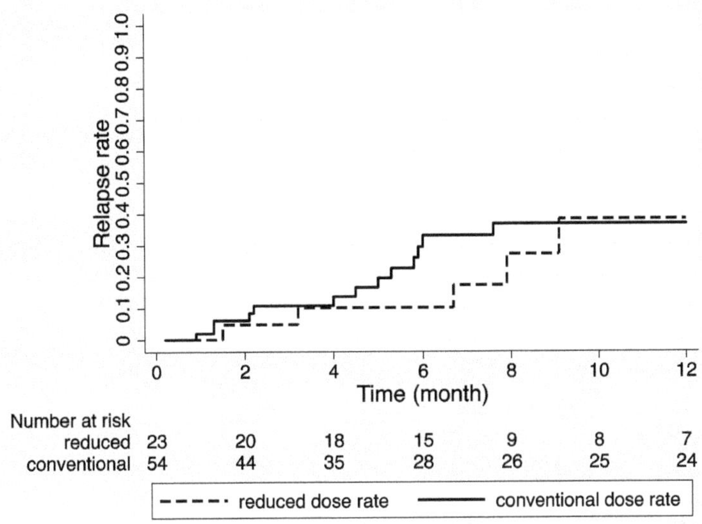

Fig. 3 Probability rates of relapse, according to the groups, divided by the dose rate of total body irradiation ($P = 0.716$ by log-rank test)

the once a day TBI technique. In light of such evidence, our institution has attempted to modify the once-daily TBI protocols to reduce the lung toxicities, by adjusting the total dose, total fraction, dose rate, and SSD, which do not impair the therapeutic effect after HSCT. However, the results of the once-daily based treatment have been scarce, and there are few studies related to clinical outcomes, as well as dose rate and PT, which demands a further investigation. Particularly, since the dose rate is a major factor affecting the development of PT, it is necessary to study the effect of the dose rate on once-a-day treatment and suggest a feasible dose rate that can reduce PT. As mentioned above, guidelines by the ACR and the ASTRO recommended a dose rate under 20 cGy/min in twice-daily regimen, there is no consensus on whether dose rate standard can be applied equally when treating once a day. Furthermore, because twice daily treatment is generally expected to produce less long-term sequelae than once-daily regimen, the criteria for dose rate in once-daily TBI may need to be more stringent than the twice-daily setting.

In the present study, we divided the groups by the TBI dose rate and analyzed the factors affecting lung toxicity

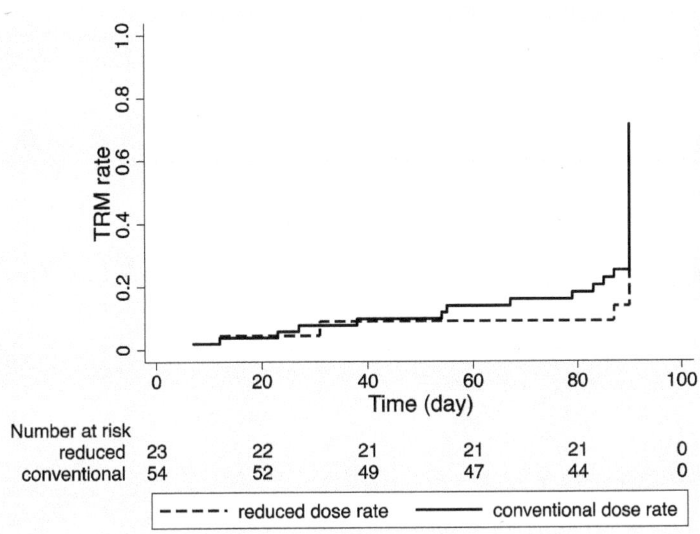

Fig. 4 Probability rates of treatment-related mortality, according to the groups, divided by the dose rate of total body irradiation ($P = 0.131$ by log-rank test)

in each group. The dose rate was divided by 6 cGy/min as the reference value because our institution has treated all the patients at the lowest possible dose rate since 2014, when extended SSD became available, and most of the TBI dose rates have remained below 6 cGy/min. Our study demonstrated that overall PT and infectious PT were associated with the dose rate of TBI, and may also represent a trend in non-infectious PT. These results suggested that the myeloablative regimen, including TBI before HSCT, caused immunodeficiency and neutropenia that made patients fragile to the opportunistic infections [28].

Although it is well known that reducing the dose rate can lower the incidence of lung injuries [3, 20, 21], it has not been clearly discovered whether or not the reduced dose rate affects the clinical outcomes, such as overall survival, relapse, and TRM after HSCT. Our study revealed that a TBI dose rate < 6 cGy/min did not show statistically significant inferiority in the clinical outcomes as conditioning for HSCT after TBI. These findings would be the basis for treating patients using the once a day TBI technique, with the dose rate under 6 cGy/min, and could be demonstrated if the number of enrolled patients increased.

This study has several limitations. Due to the retrospective nature of our research, it has inherent weak points for inhomogeneity of patient's characteristics. The sample size is insufficient to confirm the results from the data. Also, there was a possibility to misjudge the etiology of PT, because infectious and non-infectious causes can overlap in certain situations. Nevertheless, the results obtained from this study are meaningful in the actual clinical setting, where there are not many institutions treating with single fraction per day TBI, and the relevant clinical results are limited. Therefore, suggesting an appropriate TBI dose rate to reduce PT will be helpful in treating patients with single fraction per day TBI. Moreover, given the relatively homogeneous total dose and dose per fraction delivered in this study, the effect of the dose rate has increased reliability.

Conclusions

About two-thirds of the patients undergoing daily TBI for pre-treatment of HSCT experienced PT, which affected overall survival. Reducing the dose rate of TBI decreased the risk of PT, without compromising the treatment efficacy in overall survival, relapse, and TRM. Based on the findings, we suggest reducing the dose rate to less than 6 cGy/min for daily TBI treatment.

Abbreviations

ACR: American College of Radiology; BMT: Bone marrow transplantation; HSCT: Hematopoietic stem cell transplantation; OS: Overall survival; PT: Pulmonary toxicity; SSD: Source-to-surface distance; TBI: Total body irradiation; TRM: Treatment-related mortality

Authors' contributions

DY performed data acquisition, statistical analysis and participated in drafting the manuscript. HC designed the study, participated in treatment of the patients and also revised manuscript critically. IH, SS, HJ, HY participated in treatment and carried out clinical evaluations in follow-up visits. All authors read and approved the final manuscript.

Competing interests

The authors declare that they have no competing interests.

Author details

[1]Department of Radiation Oncology, Seoul National University College of Medicine, 101 Daehak-ro, Jongno-gu, Seoul 03080, Republic of Korea. [2]Department of Internal Medicine, Seoul National University College of Medicine, 101 Daehak-ro, Jongno-gu, Seoul 03080, Republic of Korea. [3]Department of Pediatrics, Seoul National University College of Medicine, 101 Daehak-ro, Jongno-gu, Seoul 03080, Republic of Korea. [4]Seoul National University Cancer Research Institute, 101 Daehak-ro, Jongno-gu, Seoul 110-779, Republic of Korea.

References

1. Wong JYC: Update on the use of radiation therapy for adult leukemia TBI , Total marrow RT and beyond. 2016.
2. Sorror ML, Storer BE, Maloney DG, Sandmaier BM, Martin PJ, Storb R. Outcomes after allogeneic hematopoietic cell transplantation with nonmyeloablative or myeloablative conditioning regimens for treatment of lymphoma and chronic lymphocytic leukemia. Blood. 2008;111(1):446–52.
3. Abugideiri M, Nanda RH, Butker C, Zhang C, Kim S, Chiang KY, Butker E, Khan MK, Haight AE, Chen Z, et al. Factors influencing pulmonary toxicity in children undergoing allogeneic hematopoietic stem cell transplantation in the setting of Total body irradiation-based Myeloablative conditioning. Int J Radiat Oncol Biol Phys. 2016;94:349–59.
4. Niederwieser D, Baldomero H, Szer J, Gratwohl M, Aljurf M, Atsuta Y, Bouzas L, Confer D, Greinix H, Horowitz M. Hematopoietic stem cell transplantation activity worldwide in 2012 and a SWOT analysis of the worldwide network for blood and marrow transplantation group including the global survey. Bone Marrow Transplant. 2016;51(6):778–85.
5. Wolden SL, Rabinovitch RA, Bittner NHJ, Galvin JM, Giap HB, Schomberg PJ, Rosenthal SA. American college of radiology (ACR) and american society for radiation oncology (ASTRO) practice guideline for the performance of total body irradiation (TBI). Am J Clin Oncol: Cancer Clin Trials. 2013;36:97–101.
6. Kelsey CR, Horwitz ME, Chino JP, Craciunescu O, Steffey B, Folz RJ, Chao NJ, Rizzieri DA, Marks LB. Severe pulmonary toxicity after myeloablative conditioning using total body irradiation: an assessment of risk factors. Int J Radiat Oncol Biol Phys. 2011;81:812–8.
7. Depledge MH, Barrett A, Powles RL. Lung function after bone marrow grafting. Int J Radiat Oncol Biol Phys. 1983;9(2):145–51.
8. Weiner RS, Bortin MM, Gale RP, Gluckman E, Kay HE, H-j K, Hartz AJ, Rimm AA. Interstitial pneumonitis after bone marrow transplantation: assessment of risk factors. Ann Intern Med. 1986;104(2):168–75.
9. Fukuda T, Hackman RC, Guthrie KA, Sandmaier BM, Boeckh M, Maris MB, Maloney DG, Deeg HJ, Martin PJ, Storb RF. Risks and outcomes of idiopathic pneumonia syndrome after nonmyeloablative and conventional conditioning regimens for allogeneic hematopoietic stem cell transplantation. Blood. 2003;102(8):2777–85.
10. Sureda A, Robinson S, Canals C, Carella AM, Boogaerts MA, Caballero D, Hunter AE, Kanz L, Slavin S, Cornelissen JJ. Reduced-intensity conditioning compared with conventional allogeneic stem-cell transplantation in relapsed or refractory Hodgkin's lymphoma: an analysis from the lymphoma working Party of the European Group for blood and marrow transplantation. J Clin Oncol. 2008;26(3):455 62.

11. Gogna NK, Morgan G, Downs K, Atkinson K, Biggs J. Lung dose rate and interstitial pneumonitis in total body irradiation for bone marrow transplantation. J Med Imaging Radiat Oncol. 1992;36(4):317–20.
12. Barrett A, Depledge MH, Powles RL. Interstitial pneumonitis following bone marrow transplantation after low dose rate total body irradiation. Int J Rad Oncol Biol Phys. 1983;9(7):1029–33.
13. Crawford SW, Hackman RC. Clinical course of idiopathic pneumonia after bone marrow transplantation. Am Rev Respir Dis. 1993;147:1393.
14. Soejima T, Hirota S, Tsujino K, Yoden E, Fujii O, Ichimiya Y, Mizuno I. Total body irradiation followed by bone marrow transplantation: comparison of once-daily and twice-daily fractionation regimens. Radiat Med. 2007;25:402–6.
15. Törlén J, Remberger M, Le Blanc K, Ljungman P, Mattsson J. Impact of pretransplantation indices in hematopoietic stem cell transplantation: knowledge of center-specific outcome data is pivotal before making index-based decisions. Biol Blood Marrow Transplant. 2017;23(4):677–83.
16. Park J, Choi EK, Kim JH, Lee SW, Song SY, Yoon SM, Kim YS, Kim SS, Park JH, Park J. Effects of total body irradiation-based conditioning on allogeneic stem cell transplantation for pediatric acute leukemia: a single-institution study. Radiat Oncol J. 2014;32(3):198.
17. Sabloff M, Sobecks RM, Ahn KW, Zhu X, de Lima M, Brown JR, Inamoto Y, Holland HK, Aljurf MD, Laughlin MJ. Does Total body irradiation conditioning improve outcomes of Myeloablative human leukocyte antigen–identical sibling transplantations for chronic lymphocytic leukemia? Biol Blood Marrow Transplant. 2014;20(3):421–4.
18. Wingard JR, Hsu J, Hiemenz JW. Hematopoietic stem cell transplantation: an overview of infection risks and epidemiology. Infect Dis Clin. 2010;24(2):257–72.
19. Carruthers SA, Wallington MM. Total body irradiation and pneumonitis risk: a review of outcomes. Br J Cancer. 2004;12:2080–4.
20. Bruno B, Souillet G, Bertrand Y, Werck-Gallois MC, So Satta A, Bellon G. Effects of allogeneic bone marrow transplantation on pulmonary function in 80 children in a single paediatric Centre. Bone Marrow Transplant. 2004; 34:143–7.
21. Beyzadeoglu M, Oysul K, Dirican B, Arpaci F, Balkan A, Surenkok S, Pak Y. Effect of dose-rate and lung dose in total body irradiation on interstitial pneumonitis after bone marrow transplantation. Tohoku J Exp Med. 2004; 202:255–63.
22. Sampath S, Schultheiss TE, Wong J. Dose response and factors related to interstitial pneumonitis after bone marrow transplant. Int J Radiat Oncol Biol Physics. 2005;63:876–84.
23. Chien JW, Maris MB, Sandmaier BM, Maloney DG, Storb RF, Clark JG. Comparison of lung function after myeloablative and 2 Gy of total body irradiation-based regimens for hematopoietic stem cell transplantation. Biol Blood Marrow Trans. 2005;11:288–96.
24. Safwat A, Nielsen OS, El-Badawy S, Overgaard J. Effect of radiation dose rate and cyclophosphamide on pulmonary toxicity after total body irradiation in a mouse model. Int J Radiat Oncol* Biol* Phys. 1996;34(1):85–91.
25. Hill-Kayser CE, Plastaras JP, Tochner Z, Glatstein E. TBI during BM and SCT: review of the past, discussion of the present and consideration of future directions. Bone Marrow Transplant. 2011;46:475–84.
26. Izawa H, Hirowatari H, Yahata Y, Hamano Y, Ito K, Saito AI, Yamamoto H, Miura K, Karasawa K, Sasai K. Effect of dose fractionation on pulmonary complications during total body irradiation. J Radiat Res. 2011;52(4):502–8.
27. Gopal R, Ha CS, Tucker SL, SA G, Khouri IF, Gajewski JL, Andersson BS, Cox JD, Champlin RE. 2223 comparison of two different total body irradiation (TBI) fractionation regimens with respect to acute and late pulmonary toxicity. Int J Radiat Oncol*Biol*Phys. 1999;45:392–3.
28. Toruner M, Loftus EV, Harmsen WS, Zinsmeister AR, Orenstein R, Sandborn WJ, Colombel JF, Egan LJ. Risk factors for opportunistic infections in patients with inflammatory bowel disease. Gastroenterology. 2008;134(4):929–36.

5

Dosimetric analysis and comparison of reduced longitudinal cranial margins of VMAT-IMRT of rectal cancer

Hendrik Dapper[1*†], Markus Oechsner[1*†], Stefan Münch[1,3], Kai Borm[1], Jan Peeken[1], Michael Mayinger[1], Stephanie E. Combs[1,2,3] and Daniel Habermehl[1]

Abstract

Background: The cranial border of the target volume (TV) in rectal cancer patients treated with neoadjuvant chemoradiation (nCRT) is mostly defined at the level of L5/S1. However, current studies have shown that relapse cranially of the target volume after neoadjuvant nCRT and surgery is very rare. A reduction of cranial TV margins could be reasonable to reduce toxicity to the organs at risk (OAR). In this study we compared the dose distribution to the OAR for different cranial longitudinal margins using a dose-volume histogram (DVH) analysis.

Methods: Ten patients with loco regional advanced rectal cancer were analysed retrospectively. All patients were planned for Volumetric Arc Therapy Radiation Therapy (VMAT). Next to the original PTV (PTV0), three new planning target volumes (PTV) were defined for each patient: The PTV0 reduced by 1 cm, 2 cm and 3 cm on cranial extension. For each PTV a treatment plan with a total dose of 50.4 Gy with daily doses of 1.8 Gy was calculated. Dose to the OAR were evaluated and compared.

Results: For the bone marrow, the small bowel and the peritoneal space all clinically relevant relative dose parameters (V10-V50) as well as the Dmedian could be significantly reduced with every cranial target volume reduction of 1 cm. For V10 of the peritoneal space the dose could be nearly halved with a 3 cm shortened TV. After TV reduction of 3 cm also for the urinary bladder a significant dose reduction of the Dmedian could be achieved.

Conclusions: Considering the very low recurrence rates in the TME and IMRT era, the distribution patterns of these relapses as well as the relevant side effects of nCRT, we would agree with existing recommendations of reduction of the cranial target volume in nCRT treated rectal cancer patients.

Keywords: Rectal cancer, Reduced cranial margins, Dosimetric quantification, IMRT

Background

Neoadjuvant short term radiation therapy (RT, 5 × 5 Gy) or conventional chemoradiation (CRT) are the standard treatment protocols for patients with locally advanced rectal cancer (UICC-Stage II or III) for potential curative disease of the lower and middle third [1]. Several studies have demonstrated that with n(C)RT loco regional relapse rates can be significantly reduced and sphincter preservation rates in lower carcinoma can be improved [2–4].

* Correspondence: hendrik-dapper@gmx.de; markus.oechsner@mri.tum.de
†Hendrik Dapper and Markus Oechsner contributed equally to this work.
[1]Department of Radiation Oncology, Klinikum rechts der Isar, TU München, Ismaninger Str. 22, 81675 Munich, Germany
Full list of author information is available at the end of the article

In the last decade there have been significant changes in both, surgery and radiation techniques in the treatment of rectal cancer patients. The total mesorectal excision (TME) alone can provide very good local control rates. In some trials, long term local control, especially for T3 N0 tumors, could reach more than 90% compared with conventional operation techniques [4, 5]. But even though local control rates improved with TME alone, not all institutes can achieve such good results and even with excellent surgical technique, neoadjuvant radiotherapy can usually halve the number of loco regional relapse [4, 6]. Furthermore, intensity modulated radiation therapy (IMRT) of the pelvic is more conformal than conventional radiation therapy and achieves better dose sparing of OAR [7–9]. But though modern n(C)RT techniques can effectively improve loco regional control, it is not without side effects. Especially the hematologic and acute gastrointestinal side effects are still relevant and can lead to treatment breaks [10–12].

Radiation contouring guidelines mainly based on data before the TME era, although studies dealing with patterns of relapse have shown that loco regional relapse is mainly below the level of S1-S2 [13], without primary nodal involvement and a negative circumferential resection margin even below S2-S3 [14]. The RTOG Consensus Panel for elective Clinical Target Volumes (CTV) in Anorectal Cancer recommends an inclusion of the presacral space where common iliac vessels bifurcate into external/internal iliacs (approximate boney landmark: sacral promontory) [15]. In case of positive lymph nodes, the current International Consensus Guidelines on Clinical Target Volume Delineation in Rectal Cancer recommend an inclusion of the prescaral space at the level of the bifurcation of the aorta in common iliac arteries or 5 mm above the last positive lymph node into the CTV [16].

It was shown that lowering the cranial CTV margins reduces the small bowel exposure with 3D and IMRT radiotherapy for long course neo-adjuvant treatment [17]. With this study we want to verify to what extent a reduction of different cranial CTV margins in nCRT treated rectal cancer patients leads to positive effects on dose-volume distribution.

Methods

Patient characteristics

A total of 10 rectal cancer patients with UICC stadium III (T3N+) treated with a conventional nCRT concept (total dose 50.4 Gy, single dose 1.8 Gy) from 2014 to 2017 in our institution were included in this study. We selected patients with tumors 5–12 cm from the anal verge. All patients received at least one pre-therapeutic MRI, a proctorectoscopy and a planning CT scan. Only those patients were included, where the last macroscopic suspected visible tumor (on primary tumour site or suspected lymph nodes) in pre-treatment MRI could be identified 4 cm below the cranial boarder of the pelvic pre-sacral space (bifurcation of the common iliac arteries). All patients received concomitant chemotherapy. Either 5-Fluoruracil (5FU) on day 1–4 and 29–32 with 1000 mg/qm body surface area (BSA) or Capecitabine 825 mg/qm BSA two times a day, 5 days per week. Patients′ characteristics are shown in Table 1.

Contouring

Contouring and treatment planning was performed using Eclipse 13.0 planning system (Varian Medical Systems, Palo Alto, CA, USA). Contouring was performed on planning CTs with 3 mm slice thickness. All patients were immobilized in prone position. For the definition of the target volumes, we also used MRI-scans and the information of the proctorectoscopy as well as PET-CT/MRI information, if available. The clinical target volume (CTV) definition for standard PTV (PTV0) were based on the recommendations of the RTOG Consensus Panel Contouring Atlas [15].

Three new clinical target volumes were defined and extended by 1 cm to create the PTVs. First, the original CTV was reduced by 1, 2 and 3 cm (longitudinal) and if necessary, adjusted to bones and vessels. By using 1 cm safety margin of these CTVs, PTVs were defined for each patient: The standard PTV minus 1 cm cranially (PTV-1), the standard PTV minus 2 cm cranially (PTV-2) and the standard PTV minus 3 cm cranially (PTV-3) (Fig. 1). The goal was to keep the shortest PTV (PTV-3) at least 2 cm above the last macroscopically visible primary tumor or lymph node metastases on MRI scan.

The small bowel, as well as the peritoneal space as a surrogate, the urinary bladder, the bone marrow, the femoral heads and the genitals were contoured as OARs on the planning CT-scans. We defined the pelvic bones as they could be identified on planning CT-scan. Cranial

Table 1 Patient characteristics

Patient	Gender	TNM	Primarius: Localisation from anal verge	Lymph node localisation	Cranial PTV margin
1	f	uT3 cN1b	4–9 cm	fossa obturatoria r.	L5/S1
2	m	uT3 uN1a	5–10 cm	perirectal	L5 sup./post.
3	f	uT3 cN1b	5–10 cm	fasica	L5 sup./post.
4	m	uT3 uN1a	4–7 cm	perirectal	L5 sup./ventral
5	m	uT3 uN2a	5–11 cm	fasica	L5/S1
6	m	uT3 uN1b	6–10 cm	perirectal	L5/S1
7	m	uT2 uN2b	9–12 cm	presacral, perirectal	L4
8	m	cT3 cN2a	6–10 cm	fasica	L4 sup./ventral
9	m	uT3 uN2a	4–9 cm	perirectal	L5 sup./post.
10	f	uT3 cN1a	5–9 cm	perirectal	L5 sup./ventral

r right, *sup* superior, *post* posterior, *m* male, *f* female

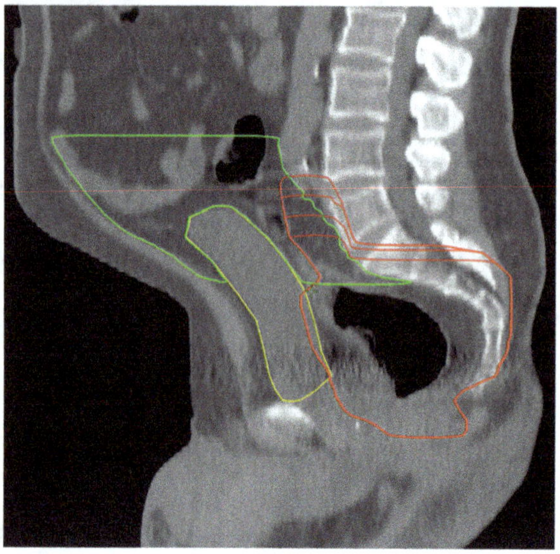

Fig. 1 Rectal cancer - cranial radiation target volume reduced by 1, 2 and 3 cm. Red: Original PTV, PTV -1 cm, PTV-2 cm and PTV-3 cm. Original PTV cranial on level of L4/L5 interspace (posterior), PTV - 3 cm on the level of L5/S1. Green: Peritoneal space, yellow: Urinary bladder

lineation was 2.1 cm above PTV0 and caudal lineation was 2.1 cm below the PTV0. The whole of sacral, iliac, ischial and pubic bone as well as the acetabulum and L5 and L4 were included. The small bowel loops were contoured as they could be identified on planning CT scan. The peritoneal space includes the small bowel, the large bowel, peritonealised large bowel and intraperitoneal vessels. The sexual organs as well as the urinary bladder were excluded. Contouring was done almost analogous to Robyn Banerjee et al. 2012 [18]: Superiorly we used 7 slices above the cranial end of the original PTV. Inferiorly it was 3 mm below the lowest identified small bowel loop or on the level of the peritoneal sigmoid colon. The anterior boarder was the abdominal muscles and posterior the vertebral bodies, vena cava and aorta as well as the psoas muscles. Laterally, the boundary was the pelvic side wall and the muscles.

Treatment planning and evaluation

For all ten patients we optimized four treatment plans for PTV0–3 using Volumetric-modulated arc therapy (VMAT) with two full arcs (358° rotation) and 15 MeV photons. Plans were optimized for treatment with a Varian Clinac DHX linear accelerator (Varian Medical Systems, Palo Alto, CA, USA).

The planning goal was to achieve a homogeneous dose distribution within the PTV and to reduce the dose to OARs, in particular the small bowel, bladder, bone marrow, femoral heads and the genitals.

Dose calculations were performed using the Anisotropic Analytical Algorithm (AAA) and heterogeneity correction. The prescribed dose for the neoadjuvant treatment plans was 50.4 Gy with single doses of 1.8 Gy. All plans were normalized to a median dose of the PTV corresponding to the prescription dose.

To compare dose distribution to the OAR we analysed absolute median dose (Dmedian) and maximum dose (Dmax) on all treatment plans (PTV, PTV-1, PTV-2, PTV-3). For the small bowel loops and the peritoneal space, as a surrogate for the small bowel, we also analysed relative dose parameters (volume receiving 10 Gy, 15 Gy, 20 Gy, 25 Gy, 30 Gy, 35 Gy, 40 Gy, 45 Gy, 50 Gy) for all treatment plans. The volumes receiving 10 Gy, 20 Gy, 30 Gy and 40 Gy (V10 - V40) of the bone marrow and the absolute dose of 65 cc, 100 cc, 180 cc and 830 cc to the peritoneal space were additionally evaluated for all treatment plans.

For all dose parameters of the OAR, a two-sided Wilcoxon test was performed with SPSS 25.0 (SPSS Inc., Chicago, IL, USA) to identify significant differences between the plans for PTV0 and PTV1–3. A p-value < 0.05 was considered to indicate statistical significance.

Results

Dosimetric analysis

The standard PTV (PTV0) (the original planned target volume) differed in the cranial boarder in the 10 patients. The highest extension was at the level of L4 (vertebral middle), the lowest was at the level of L5/S1 (superior/anterior). In mean, it was in the longitudinal middle of L5. The cranial margin of PTV minus 3 cm (PTV-3) varies between the level of L5/S1 (posterior) and the level of S2 (inferior/anterior). Patient characteristics are found in Table 1.

The mean volumes of the PTV0, PTV-1, PTV-2 and PTV-3 were 1524 cc, 1466 cc, 1366 cc and 1255 cc. This is a reduction of just 18% from PTV0 to PTV-3. The dose coverage of all PTVs was performed accurately, which resulted in identical mean Dmean, mean Dmedian and mean Dmax. For the bone marrow, the small bowel loops and the peritoneal space nearly all absolute and relative dose parameters were significantly reduced for the new PTVs (PTV-1, PTV-2, PTV-3) compared to PTV0 (Tables 2 and 3, Fig. 2).

The bone marrow had a mean volume of 1412 cc. Dmedian of the bone volume and all relative dose parameters (V10, V20, V30, V40) for all cranial shortened PTVs (PTV-1, PTV-2 and PTV-3) compared to the PTV0 were significant reduced ($p \le 0.008$). Relatively, the volume in low dose range didn't decrease as much as in high dose range. The V10 of the PTV-3 (70%) was 19% less than of the PTV0 (87%) whereas the V40 was reduced by 29%. As expected, the Dmax did not change within the different plans (all 54.0 Gy).

The peritoneal space had nearly constant caudal extension to the level of S1/S2 in the different patients. The situation

Table 2 Absolute dose parameters of organs at risk for different cranial PTVs of rectal cancer

Structure	Parameter	PTV0	PTV-1	*p*-value	PTV-2	*p*-value	PTV-3	*p*-value
		Dose (Gy)						
Rectum	Median	50.5	50.4	*0.170*	49.9	*0.220*	49.6	*0.185*
	Max	53.4	53.2	*0.110*	53.3	*0.687*	53.3	*0.624*
Sigmoid colon	Median	38.8	37.4	*0.362*	33.1	*0.126*	29.8	*0.093*
	Max	51.9	52.0	*0.575*	51.7	*0.444*	52.0	*0.221*
Femoral head	Median	23.4	23.6	*0.646*	23.9	*0.241*	23.8	*0.646*
	Max	37.9	38.2	*0.441*	38.8	*0.203*	38.6	*0.114*
Bladder	Median	28.0	27.8	*0.153*	27.0	*0.110*	**25.7**	*0.013*
	Max	52.5	52.5	*0.575*	52.7	*0.314*	52.7	*0.221*
Bone	Median	27.6	**26.6**	*0.007*	**24.9**	*0.005*	**21.9**	*0.005*
	Max	53.8	53.8	*0.959*	53.7	*0.594*	53.8	*0.959*
Small bowel loops	Median	2.7	**1.1**	*0.005*	**0.6**	*0.005*	**0.4**	*0.005*
	Max	45.5	45.5	*0.508*	42.8	*0.441*	41.1	*0.445*
Peritoneal space	Median	20.9	**15.5**	*0.005*	**9.9**	*0.005*	**5.0**	*0.005*
	Max	53.6	53.6	*0.721*	53.8	*0.386*	53.4	*0.214*
	65 cc	50.9	50.4	*0.475*	**48.5**	*0.083*	**46.1**	*0.007*
	100 cc	49.3	**48.5**	*0.153*	**46.2**	*0.028*	**44.4**	*0.005*
	180 cc	46.2	**44.2**	*0.038*	**42.8**	*0.009*	**41.6**	*0.005*
	830 cc	18.0	**14.9**	*0.012*	**9.6**	*0.012*	**7.5**	*0.012*

Bold values: statistic significant to PTV0. PTV-1 = PTV minus 1 cm on cranial site. *p*-value = PTV1,2,3 vs. PTV0

was similar for the small bowel. The mean volume of the peritoneal space was 1847 cc. For both, the small bowel loops and for the peritoneal space, a significant reduction of the relative dose parameters (V10, V15, V20, V25, V30, V35, V40, 45, Dmedian, Dmax) and for the peritoneal space also for the evaluated volumes (180 cc, 830 cc) was shown. The Dmedian for the peritoneal space for the PTV0, PTV-1, PTV-2 and PTV-3 was 20.9 Gy, 15.5 Gy, 9.9 Gy and 5.0 Gy (for all $p = 0.005$). The biggest relative differences in dose distribution of the peritoneal space are shown for medium-sized volumes (180 cc). Generally the dose to large volumes changed more than for very small volumes. The dose of 830 cc of the peritoneal space for the PTV-1, PTV-2 and PTV-3 was 14.9 Gy, 9.6 Gy and 7.5 Gy and all decreased significantly compared to 18 Gy of the PTV0 ($p = 0.012$). In contrast, for 65 cc, a significant dose change was just seen for PTV-3. Analogous, the largest differences in the volume of the peritoneal space were seen for low doses. The V10 of the PTV-3 was about halved compared to PTV0 while the V50 could just be reduced by about a quarter.

The mean volume of the small bowel was much higher (2977 cc) and differed much between the patients due to different cranial extensions of the planned CT imaging. This affected the Dmedian but not the relative dose parameters. Compared to the peritoneal space, a similar outcome was found for the relative dose parameters of the small bowel loops. The V10 (18%, 14% and 10%) of PTV-1, PTV-2 and PTV-3 was significant lower (for all $p = 0.008$) compared to PTV0 (21%) while there was not a big change in V50 (all 0%) compared to 1% ($p = 0.028$–0.612). The Dmax still remained high for both, small bowel loops and peritoneal space for all PTVs and did not show statistically significant changes.

A significant reduction of the Dmedian for the urinary bladder was just seen with 3 cm lowered PTV. The PTV-3 was 25.7 Gy compared to PTV0 with 28.0 Gy ($p = 0.013$) while there were no differences in different Dmax. For the sigmoid colon there was a slight decrease in dose distribution with reduced margins of the target volume (not significant) and the Dmax remained almost the same for all PTVs (about 52.0 Gy). Finally, as expected, the Dmedian and Dmax of the femoral head (left) for different PTVs did not differ significantly.

Discussion

Benefit of the reduction of the target volume

We could show that each cranial reduction of 1 cm from the standard PTV in rectal cancer patients of the lower and middle third can significantly reduce the dose to the bone marrow and small bowel (loops & peritoneal space) for almost all relevant dose parameters (Tables 2 and 3, Fig. 2). Also for urinary bladder the Dmedian can be reduced with a 3 cm lowered cranial margin. In similar study approaches, for example in esophageal carcinoma,

Table 3 Relative dose parameters of selected organs at risk for different cranial PTVs of rectal cancer

Structure	Parameter	PTV0	PTV-1	*p*-value	PTV-2	*p*-value	PTV-3	*p*-value
		Volume (%)						
Bone	V10	87	**84**	*0.007*	**78**	*0.005*	**70**	*0.005*
	V20	69	**66**	*0.005*	**62**	*0.005*	**55**	*0.005*
	V30	44	**41**	*0.007*	**39**	*0.005*	**33**	*0.005*
	V40	29	**27**	*0.017*	**24**	*0.007*	**20**	*0.005*
Darm loops	V10	21	**18**	*0.008*	**14**	*0.008*	**10**	*0.008*
	V15	19	**16**	*0.008*	**13**	*0.008*	**8**	*0.008*
	V20	14	**11**	*0.008*	**09**	*0.008*	**06**	*0.008*
	V25	9	**7**	*0.008*	**5**	*0.008*	**4**	*0.008*
	V30	6	**5**	*0.008*	**3**	*0.008*	**3**	*0.008*
	V35	4	**3**	*0.028*	**2**	*0.028*	**2**	*0.018*
	V40	3	**2**	*0.043*	**2**	*0.028*	**1**	*0.028*
	V45	2	**2**	*0.018*	**2**	*0.028*	**1**	*0.028*
	V50	1	**0**	*0.612*	**0**	*0.176*	**0**	*0.028*
Peritoneal space	V10	71	**58**	*0.005*	**47**	*0.005*	**37**	*0.008*
	V15	61	**51**	*0.005*	**42**	*0.005*	**33**	*0.005*
	V20	48	**42**	*0.005*	**34**	*0.005*	**28**	*0.005*
	V25	36	**32**	*0.005*	**27**	*0.005*	**22**	*0.005*
	V30	27	**24**	*0.005*	**21**	*0.005*	**18**	*0.005*
	V35	22	**20**	*0.005*	**17**	*0.005*	**15**	*0.005*
	V40	18	**17**	*0.005*	**15**	*0.005*	**13**	*0.005*
	V45	16	**15**	*0.005*	**13**	*0.005*	**12**	*0.005*
	V50	08	**07**	*0.114*	**06**	*0.005*	**06**	*0.005*

Bold values: statistic significant versus PTV0. PTV-1 = PTV minus 1 cm on cranial site. *p*-value = PTV1,2,3 vs. PTV0

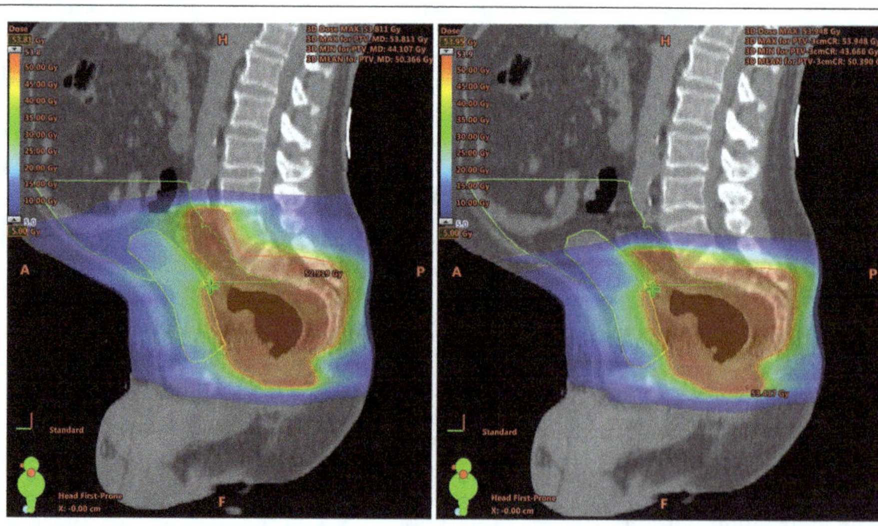

Fig. 2 Change in dose distribution after a target volume reduction of 3 cm. Protection of OARs. Differences in dose distribution (colour-wash) of the original bPTV (left) and the cranial 3 cm reduced PTV (3 cm, right). Especially the low and middle dose range covering less volume of the peritoneal space (green shape) and the bladder (yellow shape)

it has already been shown that a reduction of longitudinal margins would probably lead to an expected lower rate of side effects [19]. So the main question is whether it is to be expected that such margin reductions can also be translated into better therapy tolerance in rectal cancer. In large prospective trials the rate of severe acute enteritis was about 15% [20, 21]. Chronical consequences of small bowel radiation can be obstruction, perforation, fistula, bleeding, persistent diarrhea and malabsorption [22, 23].

The relevance of dose-volume relationships and side effects in different types of pelvic cancer treated with chemoradiation was demonstrated. The importance of dose sparing of bone marrow was required for anal cancer [24]. For anal cancer patients treated with definitive CRT Cheng et al. could proof a highly significant correlation of ≥grade 3 hematologic toxicity with the mean dose and low-dose dose parameters (V5, V10, V15, V20) and recommended dose constraints to the lumbo-sacral-spine with V10 ≤ 80% [25]. In 50 patients treated with IMRT, a higher V20 of the pelvic bone marrow was associated with lower white blood cell nadir ($p = 0.048$) and patients with V40 ≥ 41% of the lumbo-sacral bone marrow had higher risk to develop ≥Grade 3 hematologic toxicity [26]. The most comparable study design was from Wan et al. [27]. Here the V40 of the lumbosacral spine was associated with clinically significant grade ≥ 2 hematologic toxicity in patients receiving conventional concurrent CRT (50 à 2 Gy, IMRT, Capecitabine) (grade ≥ 2hematologic toxicity with V40 ≥ 60% vs. V40 < 60% was 38.3% vs.13%, $p = 0.005$). Interestingly, no case of severe acute toxicity was registered in a radiation dose intensification study in rectal cancer [28].

In our study, V10, V20, V30 and V40 of the whole bone of the pelvis (including lumbosacral spine) would be decreased significantly with each cranial reduction of the PTV of 1 cm compared to the standard PTV (PTV0). The V10 for the bone in the pelvis (mainly lumbosacral spine) was 87% for PTV0, 84% for PTV-1, 78% for PTV-2 and 70% for PTV-3 ($p \leq 0.007$). The effect was less but still significant in high dose range. The V40 was 29% for PTV0, 27% for PTV-1 ($p = 0.017$), 24% for PTV-2 ($p = 0.007$) and 20% for PTV-3 ($p = 0.005$). Even so the definition of the bone marrow and the type of chemotherapy could vary in those studies, with significant reduced relative dose parameters it is to be assumed that acute ≥2 and ≥ 3 hematologic toxicity would be significantly reduced as well.

The survey and evaluation of the dose distribution on the small bowel is complex. A major problem is the definition of small bowel loops on the planning CT scan because of inconsistent position of the small bowel throughout the treatment course. The evidence for relationships between dose distributions and clinical side effects is still limited, therefore clear recommendations concerning small bowel constraints are still difficult [29]. Some authors prefer the definition of the peritoneal space as a more reliable surrogate for the small bowel, whereas other studies have shown that both approaches, small bowel and peritoneal space, can be useful for dose comparison [18]. Therefore, in our study, we defined the small bowel loops and the peritoneal space. Furthermore all of our rectal cancer patients were irradiated in prone position because there is good evidence that prone position is superior to supine position in terms of dose distribution to the small bowel in patients who underwent pelvic irradiation with 3D conformal RT and most likely applies to the VMAT-IMRT as well [30, 31]. Our study design and peritoneal space definition orientated on Banerjee et al.. They have published data of 67 patients who were irradiated with nCRT and compared peritoneal space versus small bowel and evaluated dose parameters to predicting grade ≥ 3 acute toxicity. The mayor findings were, that peritoneal space V15 less than 830 cc and a small bowel V15 less than 275 cc correlated with < 10% risk of grade ≥ 3 acute toxicity [18]. In our study the volume receiving 15 Gy could be roughly halved with a PTV-reduction of 3 cm. The V15 of the peritoneal space decreased significantly with every cm. Furthermore, we had similar findings for V15 of the small bowel (551 cc, 444 cc, 339 cc and 240 cc; $p = 0.008$). Though, only the V15 of the peritoneal space for PTV-2 and -3 cm was below 830 cc and for the small bowel only the V15 of the PTV-3 was below 275 cc.

There are several mathematical models to estimate dose/volume-relationships and probability of acute side effects. Roeske et al. e. a. suggest that the volume of the peritoneal space receiving the prescription dose (45–50 Gy) should be < 195 cc [32]. As mentioned, in our study the relative changes in the dose distribution on high dose range wasn't as high as in low dose range. In our treatment plans the V45 and V50 were 292 cc and 138 cc for the standard PTV whereas it decreased to 213 cc and 103 cc for the PTV-3 (both: $p = 0.005$). Those changes were all statistic significant. In summary of the results and the clinical relationships of the DVH and the toxicity, it should be noted that cranial target volume reduction can significantly reduce all parameters that have been clinically relevant in the literature. That might reduce acute and late intestinal toxicity but has to be proven in prospective trials which use cranially reduced CTV margins.

The opportunity of smaller cranial margins in n(C)RT treated rectal cancer patients

The opportunity of smaller cranial margins in n(C)RT treated rectal cancer patients, especially with IMRT, of the middle and lower third is currently discussed [33]. In a recently published editorial, Te Vuong, Aurelie Garant & Fleure Gallant summarised the situation very well [34]. The TME trial could show a further reduction of local recurrence with short term neoadjuvant RT. After a median follow up of 6.1 years, RT with 5 × 5 Gy local relapse was 5.6% compared to 10.9% with TME alone [4]. Moreover RT is most effective if the quality of TME is high [35]. Next to the fact that loco-regional relapse after RT and TME is very rare, studies dealing with patterns of local relapse have shown that locoregional relapse is mainly below the level of S1-S2. In an update of the TME-trial, patterns of local relapse were published. Local relapse after RT and TME was still very rare (1.1% of all patients) and most likely posterior or laterally of the primary tumor site [36]. A Swedish study analysed the site of recurrence of rectal cancer patients treated with abdominal resection (mostly with n(C)RT). All cases of relapse (155 of 2315) have been in the lower 75% of the pelvis, means below the S1/S2 interspace [13]. Additionally, in a three-dimensional analysis of recurrence patterns in rectal cancer patients with recurrence after TME, Nijkamp et al. could demonstrate that patient without primary node involvement had no recurrences cranially of the S2-S3 interspace [14]. With CTV reduction to the S2-S3 interspace, over 60% (three-field conventional RT) and 80% (IMRT) reduction in absolute small bowel exposure (dose levels from 15 to 35 Gy) could be achieved. A cranial PTV reduction should therefore be possible without an increased risk for locoregional recurrence rates. Ongoing randomized prospective trials on the timing of surgery after IMRT-based neoadjuvant chemoradiation treatment (ClinicalTrials.gov, number NCT03465982; number NCT02551237) could provide a valid contribution to the definition of the patterns of local relapse and acute toxicity, to consolidate the clinical rationale of the reduction of the cranial target volumes for patients with rectal cancer.

Conclusion

Reduction of the cranial target volume in nCRT for patients with rectal cancer of the lower and middle third can lead to a significant reduction of the dose parameters proven to be crucial for toxicity rates, especially acute gastrointestinal and hematologic side effects. Due to the anatomical conditions, meaningful dose restrictions to OAR that other studies have shown can best be achieved by cranial CTV reduction. Considering the very low recurrence rates in the TME and IMRT era, the distribution patterns of these relapses as well as the relevant side effects of the neoadjuvant irradiation, we would agree with existing recommendations of a reduction of the cranial target volumes at least up to the level of S1/S2 interspace.

Abbreviations

2D/3D: 2/3 dimensional; BM: Bone marrow; BSA: Body surface area; CRT: Chemoradiation; CTV: Clinical target volume; E. a.: For example; Gy: Gray; IMRT: Intensity modulated radiotherapy; nCRT: Neoadjuvant chemoradiation; OAR: Organs at risk; PC: Peritoneal Space; PET: Positron Emission Tomography; PTV: Planning target volume; RC: Rectal cancer; RT: Radiation therapy; RT: Radiotherapie; SB: Small bowel; SIB: Simultaneously integrated boost; VMAT: Volumetric modulated arc therapy

Funding

This research did not receive any specific grant from funding agencies in 448 the public, commercial, or not-for-profit sectors.

Authors' contributions

DH and SC treated the patients and provided the data and study infrastructure. DH developed the study design, collected, and interpreted data, performed statistical analysis and drafted the manuscript. DH made substantial contributions to conception and design of the study, interpreted data and revised the manuscript. SM, KB, MM, JP and SC contributed significantly to the discussion and interpretation of the results. MO calculated the therapy plans. HD, MO and DH made the main contributions to conception and design of the study, analysed and interpreted data and drafted the manuscript. All co-authors read and revised the revised the manuscript. The final version of the manuscript was approved by all co-authors.

Competing interests

The authors declare that they have no competing interests.

Author details

[1]Department of Radiation Oncology, Klinikum rechts der Isar, TU München, Ismaninger Str. 22, 81675 Munich, Germany. [2]Institute for innovative Radiotherapie (iRT), Helmholtz Zentrum München, Ingolstädter Landstr. 1, Neuherberg, Germany. [3]Deutsches Konsortium für Translationale Krebsforschung (DKTK), Partner Site Munich, Munich, Germany.

References

1. S3-Leitlinie kolorektales Karzinom. Langversion 2.0 - November 2017 - AWMF-Registernummer: 021/007OL. Stuttgart: Thieme; 2017.
2. Sauer R, Liersch T, Merkel S, et al. Preoperative versus postoperative chemoradiotherapy for locally advanced rectal cancer: results of the German CAO/ARO/AIO-94 randomized phase III trial after a median follow-up of 11 years. J Clin Oncol. 2012;30:1926–33.
3. Cammà C, Giunta M, Fiorica F, Pagliaro L, Craxì A, Cottone M. Preoperative radiotherapy for resectable rectal cancer: a meta-analysis. JAMA. 2000;284: 1008–15.
4. Peeters KCMJ, Marijnen CAM, Nagtegaal ID, et al. The TME trial after a median follow-up of 6 years: increased local control but no survival benefit in irradiated patients with resectable rectal carcinoma. Ann Surg. 2007;246:693–701.
5. Heald RJ, Moran BJ, Ryall RD, Sexton R, MacFarlane JK. Rectal cancer: the Basingstoke experience of total mesorectal excision, 1978-1997. Arch Surg. 1998;133:894–9.
6. Enríquez-Navascués JM, Borda N, Lizerazu A, et al. Patterns of local recurrence in rectal cancer after a multidisciplinary approach. World J Gastroenterol. 2011;17:1674–84.
7. Portelance L, Chao KS, Grigsby PW, Bennet H, Low D. Intensity-modulated radiation therapy (IMRT) reduces small bowel, rectum, and bladder doses in patients with cervical cancer receiving pelvic and Para-aortic irradiation. Int J Radiat Oncol Biol Phys. 2001;51:261–6.

8. Mell LK, Tiryaki H, Ahn K-H, Mundt AJ, Roeske JC, Aydogan B. Dosimetric comparison of bone marrow-sparing intensity-modulated radiotherapy versus conventional techniques for treatment of cervical cancer. Int J Radiat Oncol Biol Phys. 2008;71:1504–10.
9. Wee CW, Kang H-C, Wu H-G, et al. Intensity-modulated radiotherapy versus three-dimensional conformal radiotherapy in rectal cancer treated with neoadjuvant concurrent chemoradiation: a meta-analysis and pooled-analysis of acute toxicity. Jpn J Clin Oncol. 2018;48:458–66.
10. Mitra D, Hong TS, Horick N, et al. Long-term outcomes and toxicities of a large cohort of anal cancer patients treated with dose-painted IMRT per RTOG 0529. Adv Radiat Oncol. 2017;2:110–7.
11. Yang TJ, Oh JH, Apte A, Son CH, Deasy JO, Goodman KA. Clinical and dosimetric predictors of acute hematologic toxicity in rectal cancer patients undergoing chemoradiotherapy. Radiother Oncol. 2014;113:29–34.
12. Fernández-Martos C, Pericay C, Aparicio J, et al. Phase II, randomized study of concomitant chemoradiotherapy followed by surgery and adjuvant capecitabine plus oxaliplatin (CAPOX) compared with induction CAPOX followed by concomitant chemoradiotherapy and surgery in magnetic resonance imaging-defined, locally advanced rectal cancer: Grupo cancer de recto 3 study. J Clin Oncol. 2010;28:859–65.
13. Syk E, Torkzad MR, Blomqvist L, Nilsson PJ, Glimelius B. Local recurrence in rectal cancer: anatomic localization and effect on radiation target. Int J Radiat Oncol Biol Phys. 2008;72:658–64.
14. Nijkamp J, Kusters M, Beets-Tan RGH, et al. Three-dimensional analysis of recurrence patterns in rectal cancer: the cranial border in hypofractionated preoperative radiotherapy can be lowered. Int J Radiat Oncol Biol Phys. 2011;80:103–10.
15. Myerson RJ, Garofalo MC, El Naqa I, et al. Elective clinical target volumes for conformal therapy in anorectal cancer: a radiation therapy oncology group consensus panel contouring atlas. Int J Radiat Oncol Biol Phys. 2009;74:824–30.
16. Valentini V, Gambacorta MA, Barbaro B, et al. International consensus guidelines on clinical target volume delineation in rectal cancer. Radiother Oncol. 2016;120:195–201.
17. Nijkamp J, Marijnen C, van Herk M, van Triest B, Sonke J-J. Adaptive radiotherapy for long course neo-adjuvant treatment of rectal cancer. Radiother Oncol. 2012;103:353–9.
18. Banerjee R, Chakraborty S, Nygren I, Sinha R. Small bowel dose parameters predicting grade ≥ 3 acute toxicity in rectal cancer patients treated with neoadjuvant chemoradiation: an independent validation study comparing peritoneal space versus small bowel loop contouring techniques. Int J Radiat Oncol Biol Phys. 2013;85:1225–31.
19. Münch S, Oechsner M, Combs SE, Habermehl D. DVH- and NTCP-based dosimetric comparison of different longitudinal margins for VMAT-IMRT of esophageal cancer. Radiat Oncol. 2017;12:128.
20. Sauer R, Becker H, Hohenberger W, et al. Preoperative versus postoperative chemoradiotherapy for rectal cancer. N Engl J Med. 2004;351:1731–40.
21. Aschele C, Cionini L, Lonardi S, et al. Primary tumor response to preoperative chemoradiation with or without oxaliplatin in locally advanced rectal cancer: pathologic results of the STAR-01 randomized phase III trial. J Clin Oncol. 2011; 29:2773–80.
22. Vistad I, Kristensen GB, Fosså SD, Dahl AA, Mørkrid L. Intestinal malabsorption in long-term survivors of cervical cancer treated with radiotherapy. Int J Radiat Oncol Biol Phys. 2009;73:1141–7.
23. Ceelen W, Fierens K, van Nieuwenhove Y, Pattyn P. Preoperative chemoradiation versus radiation alone for stage II and III resectable rectal cancer: a systematic review and meta-analysis. Int J Cancer. 2009;124:2966–72.
24. Franco P, Arcadipane F, Ragona R, et al. Hematologic toxicity in anal cancer patients during combined chemo-radiation: a radiation oncologist perspective. Expert Rev Anticancer Ther. 2017;17:335–45.
25. Cheng JC-H, Bazan JG, Wu J-K, Koong AC, Chang DT. Lumbosacral spine and marrow cavity modeling of acute hematologic toxicity in patients treated with intensity modulated radiation therapy for squamous cell carcinoma of the anal canal. Pract Radiat Oncol. 2014;4:198–206.
26. Franco P, Ragona R, Arcadipane F, et al. Dosimetric predictors of acute hematologic toxicity during concurrent intensity-modulated radiotherapy and chemotherapy for anal cancer. Clin Transl Oncol. 2017;19:67–75.
27. Wan J, Liu K, Li K, Li G, Zhang Z. Can dosimetric parameters predict acute hematologic toxicity in rectal cancer patients treated with intensity-modulated pelvic radiotherapy? Radiat Oncol. 2015;10:162.
28. Alongi F, Fersino S, Mazzola R, et al. Radiation dose intensification in pre-operative chemo-radiotherapy for locally advanced rectal cancer. Clin Transl Oncol. 2017;19:189–96.
29. Kavanagh BD, Pan CC, Dawson LA, et al. Radiation dose-volume effects in the stomach and small bowel. Int J Radiat Oncol Biol Phys. 2010;76:S101–7.
30. Martin J, Fitzpatrick K, Horan G, et al. Treatment with a belly-board device significantly reduces the volume of small bowel irradiated and results in low acute toxicity in adjuvant radiotherapy for gynecologic cancer: results of a prospective study. Radiother Oncol. 2005;74:267–74.
31. White R, Foroudi F, Sia J, Marr MA, Lim Joon D. Reduced dose to small bowel with the prone position and a belly board versus the supine position in neoadjuvant 3D conformal radiotherapy for rectal adenocarcinoma. J Med Radiat Sci. 2017;64:120–4.
32. Roeske JC, Bonta D, Mell LK, Lujan AE, Mundt AJ. A dosimetric analysis of acute gastrointestinal toxicity in women receiving intensity-modulated whole-pelvic radiation therapy. Radiother Oncol. 2003;69:201–7.
33. Joye I, Haustermans K. Clinical target volume delineation for rectal cancer radiation therapy: time for updated guidelines? Int J Radiat Oncol Biol Phys. 2015;91:690–1.
34. Vuong, Te; Garant, Aurelie; Gallant, Fleure. Intensity-modulated radiation therapy for patients with rectal cancer: Editorial; 2014. https://www.futuremedicine.com/doi/pdf/10.2217/crc.14.20.
35. Sebag-Montefiore D, Stephens RJ, Steele R, et al. Preoperative radiotherapy versus selective postoperative chemoradiotherapy in patients with rectal cancer (MRC CR07 and NCIC-CTG C016): a multicentre, randomised trial. Lancet. 2009;373:811–20.
36. Kusters M, Marijnen CAM, van de Velde CJH, et al. Patterns of local recurrence in rectal cancer; a study of the Dutch TME trial. Eur J Surg Oncol. 2010;36:470–6.

6

Changes in cardiac volume determined with repeated enhanced 4DCT during chemoradiotherapy for esophageal cancer

Xue Wang[1,2], Jin-Zhi Wang[2*], Jian-Bin Li[2*], Ying-Jie Zhang[2], Feng-Xiang Li[2], Wei Wang[2], Yan-Luan Guo[3], Qian Shao[2], Min Xu[2], Xi-Jun Liu[2] and Yue Wang[4]

Abstract

Background: Concurrent chemoradiotherapy is considered curative intent treatment for patients with non-operative esophageal cancer. Radiation-induced heart damage receives much attention. We performed repeated four-dimensional computed tomography (4DCT) to detect changes in cardiac volume during radiotherapy for esophageal cancer patients, and explored potential factors responsible for those changes.

Methods: Forty-six patients with esophageal cancer underwent enhanced 4DCT and three-dimensional (3D) CT scans before radiotherapy and every 10 fractions during treatment. The heart was contoured on 3DCT images, 4DCT end expiratory (EE) images and 4DCT maximum intensity projection (MIP) images by the same radiation oncologist. Heart volumes and other relative parameters were compared by the SPSS software package, version 19.0.

Results: Compared with its initial value, heart volume was smaller at the 10th fraction (reduction = 3.27%, 4.45% and 4.52% on 3DCT, EE and MIP images, respectively, $p < 0.05$) and the 20th fraction (reduction = 6.05%, 5.64% and 4.51% on 3DCT, EE and MIP images, respectively, $p < 0.05$), but not at the 30th fraction. Systolic and diastolic blood pressures were reduced (by 16.95 ± 16.69 mmHg and 7.14 ± 11.64 mmHg, respectively, both $p < 0.05$) and the heart rate was elevated by 5.27 ± 6.25 beats/min ($p < 0.05$) after radiotherapy. None of the potential explanatory variables correlated with heart volume changes.

Conclusions: Cardiac volume reduced significantly from an early treatment stage and maintained the reduction until the middle stage. The heart volume changes observed on 3DCT and 4DCT were consistent during radiotherapy. The changes in heart volume, blood pressure and heart rate may be valuable indicators of cardiac impairment and target dose changes.

Keywords: Esophageal cancer, Concurrent chemoradiotherapy, Heart volume change, Contrast enhanced four-dimensional computed tomography, Blood pressure

Background

Esophageal cancer ranked ninth for cancer incidence and sixth for cancer death in 2013, with 442,000 new cases and 440,000 deaths [1]. Concurrent chemoradiotherapy (CCRT) is considered to be a curative-intent treatment for patients with medically inoperable esophageal cancer [2]. Radiotherapy is an effective and relatively safe treatment for esophageal cancer [3], but can cause late locoregional complications such as esophageal, pulmonary and cardiac toxicity [4].

Concerns about radiation-related cardiac toxicity have been thoroughly discussed for patients with breast cancer and Hodgkin's disease [5–11]. However, the maximum dose delivered to the heart is usually higher for patients with esophageal cancer than for patients with Hodgkin's disease. Further, the irradiated volume of the heart is larger for esophageal cancer patients than for breast cancer patients [12].

* Correspondence: wjz0603@126.com; lijianbin@msn.com
[2]Department of Thoracic Radiation Oncology, Shandong Cancer Hospital affiliated to Shandong University, Shandong Academy of Medical Sciences, No. 440 Jiyan Road, Jinan 250117, Shandong Province, China
Full list of author information is available at the end of the article

Radiation-induced heart damage in esophageal cancer has received much attention. In a recent prospective analysis, Zhang et al. used single photon emission computed tomography to evaluate cardiac function in patients with esophageal cancer, and determined that cardiac impairment occurred during radiotherapy [3]. Using cone beam computed tomography (CBCT), Haj et al. prospectively investigated the changes in cardiac volume in esophageal cancer patients treated with neoadjuvant chemoradiation. The authors found that the cardiac volume was reduced in the early stage (41.4 Gy/1.8 Gy per fraction) of radiotherapy [13]. However, delineating soft tissue on CBCT is challenging, as the image quality is poorer than that of computed tomography (CT), and not all separate heart components are distinguishable by CBCT [14]. Four-dimensional computed tomography (4DCT) provides better image quality and can reduce artifacts caused by respiratory motion. Moreover, contrast enhancement in 4DCT is helpful for identifying the extent of tissues, which can reduce errors in organ delineation [15]. 4DCT is therefore considered to be a reliable and effective tool for assessing tumor and organ motion, as well as changes in tumor volume [16–21].

A reduction in heart volume suggests that subclinical cardiac damage may have occurred. Furthermore, changes in heart volume may influence the dose distribution of radiation to the tumor target and organs at risk. Consequently, changes in cardiac volume during radiotherapy for esophageal cancer require further exploration. In the present study, we explored the influence of radiotherapy on the heart volume by performing repeated 4DCT scans with intravenous contrast during the course of CCRT in patients with esophageal cancer. In addition, we assessed the correlations of age, gender, body mass index (BMI), disease staging, blood pressure, heart rate at baseline, blood pressure changes and heart rate changes with the cardiac volume reduction during CCRT.

Methods

Patients

Between September 2015 and January 2017, 58 patients with pathologically proven thoracic esophageal squamous cell carcinoma who were scheduled to receive CCRT in our department were consecutively enrolled in this study. None of the patients had a history of cardiovascular disease or chest radiotherapy. All patients had Karnofsky Performance Status values ≥80 and were considered physiologically fit for the therapy. This prospective study was approved by the Local Research and Ethics Committee at Shandong Cancer Hospital & Institute. Written informed consent was obtained from all patients prior to enrollment.

CT simulation and image acquisition

All patients underwent contrast-enhanced three-dimensional CT (CE-3DCT) and CE-4DCT scans sequentially on a 16-slice CT scanner (Philips Brilliance Bores CT, Netherlands) while breathing. During the simulation, vacuum bags were used to immobilize patients in the supine position with their arms extended overhead. Three laser alignment lines were marked on the patients before CT acquisition. During radiotherapy, CE-4DCT and CE-3DCT images were acquired every 10 fractions with the patients in the same position.

During the 4DCT image acquisition, the respiratory signal was recorded with the Varian Real-time Positioning Management (RPM) gating system, which tracks the trajectory of infrared markers placed on the patient's abdomen. The signal was sent to the scanner to label each CT image with a time tag. GE Advantage 4D software (GE Healthcare, Waukesha, WI, USA) sorts the reconstructed 4DCT images into 10 respiratory phases (labeled as 0–90%) on the basis of these tags, with 0% corresponding to end inspiration and 50% corresponding to 4DCT end expiratory (EE). Both the 3DCT and 4DCT images were reconstructed with a thickness of 3 mm, and the images were transferred to the Eclipse Treatment Planning System (Eclipse 8.6) for structure delineation and treatment plan generation. The 4DCT maximum intensity projection (MIP) was created from the 10 phases of 4DCT.

Cardiac delineation and data acquisition

Heart contours were delineated according to the guidelines developed by Feng et al. [22], with the appropriate window settings (window width = 500 Hounsfield units, window level = 50 Hounsfield units). All delineations were performed by the same radiation oncologist to avoid inter-observer variation. For the determination of intra-observer variation, the heart volumes of six patients were delineated five times by the same radiation oncologist at one-week intervals. Together with the heart volume, the maximum heart distance (MHD) in the horizontal direction (reflecting the size of the heart contours) was measured automatically by the planning system.

Blood pressure and heart rate measurement

During treatment, patients' systolic blood pressure, diastolic blood pressure and heart rate were measured every day, according to international guidelines [23].

Radiotherapy

The CE-3DCT and CE-4DCT scans before radiotherapy were registered based on bony landmarks by means of software tools in the Eclipse Treatment Planning System (Varian Medical Systems). The gross tumor volume was contoured on each phase of the 4DCT. The clinical target volume (CTV) was defined as the primary tumor, plus a 3-cm expansion superiorly and inferiorly along the length of the esophagus and a 0.5-cm radial expansion for each phase of 4DCT, then manually excluding the anatomical barriers (lung, trachea, large vessels, bones and heart) when not involved. The internal target volume was then constructed to envelop the CTV (10 CTVs in each phase of the 4DCT). The planning target volume was generated through the expansion of the internal target volume 0.5 cm in all directions.

All radiation treatments were delivered 5 days per week as either three-dimensional conformal radiotherapy or intensity-modulated radiotherapy, with 2.0 Gy per fraction and 6-MV photon beams. The patients were prescribed a total dose of 60 Gy. The main dose constraint was to limit the dose to both lungs to a V20 value (i.e., the percentage of the total lung volume receiving 20 Gy or more) of less than 30%. Other constraints included a V40 value < 50% for the whole heart and a maximum dose to the spinal cord of no more than 45 Gy.

Chemotherapy

Patients in this study received one of two types of chemotherapy concurrently with their radiotherapy. Type A consisted of cisplatin (75 mg/m^2 intravenously on day 1) and 5-fluorouracil (700 mg/m^2 intravenous continuous infusion over 24 h daily on days 1–4) every 21 days. Type B consisted of capecitabine (625 mg/m^2 twice a day by mouth on days 1–14) and oxaliplatin (85 mg/m^2 intravenously on day 1) every 21 days.

Calculation of radiation dose to the heart

The radiation dose to the heart was calculated from the heart volume receiving 20 Gy (V20), 30 Gy (V30), 40 Gy (V40), 45 Gy (V45) or 50 Gy or more (V50), as well as the average heart dose.

Statistical analysis

Since the data were normally distributed, the results are presented as the mean ± standard deviation (mean ± SD). Changes in cardiac volume, MHD, blood pressure and heart rate during radiotherapy were analyzed with paired-sample t-tests. The associations between the change in heart volume and potential explanatory variables were examined by one-way analysis of variance or Pearson's correlation analysis, as appropriate. The heart doses between fragments were analyzed by one-way analysis of variance. The initial heart volumes determined from 3DCT, EE and MIP images were compared through paired-sample t-tests.

Statistical analyses were performed with the SPSS software package, version 19.0, with $p < 0.05$ considered to be statistically significant.

Results

Patients

Patients with thoracic esophageal cancer were scheduled to undergo CE-3DCT and CE-4DCT scanning, with initial scans before radiotherapy and repeated scans at the tenth, twentieth and thirtieth fractions during radiotherapy. Those who failed to complete all the scans were excluded. Thus a total of 46 patients were included in this study. The patients' characteristics are summarized in Table 1.

Changes in heart volume and maximum heart distance during radiotherapy

Between the initial measurement (before radiotherapy) and the tenth fraction, the heart volume and MHD were markedly reduced at the middle location. On 3DCT, EE and MIP images, respectively, the heart volume was reduced by 3.27%, 4.45% and 4.52% ($p = 0.027$, $p < 0.001$ and $p < 0.001$), and the MHD was reduced by 0.98%, 1.40% and 1.29% ($p = 0.035$, $p = 0.001$ and $p < 0.001$). There were no significant changes in heart volume or MHD for the upper and lower locations at the tenth fraction. The results are presented in Table 2.

At the middle location, the heart volume was significantly lower at the twentieth fraction than at the initial measurement, with mean reductions of 6.05%, 5.64% and 4.51% on 3DCT, EE and MIP images, respectively (all $p < 0.001$). The MHD at the twentieth fraction for the middle location was reduced by 1.82%, 1.88% and 1.29% ($p = 0.001$, $p < 0.001$ and $p < 0.001$) on 3DCT, EE and MIP images, respectively. For the upper and lower locations, there were no significant changes in heart volume or MHD on the three types of images at the twentieth fraction.

The heart volume and MHD displayed a tendency to recover to the initial level at the thirtieth fraction. The differences in heart volume and MHD on the three types of images between the initial measurement and the thirtieth fraction were not significant ($p > 0.05$).

Changes in blood pressure and heart rate during radiotherapy

Figure 1 displays the changes in systolic blood pressure, diastolic blood pressure and heart rate during the course of treatment for the patients with mid-thoracic esophageal cancer. Both systolic and diastolic blood pressure exhibited trends of decline during the entire treatment period at the middle location. At the tenth, twentieth and thirtieth fractions, respectively, systolic blood pressure was reduced by 15.64 ± 12.30 mmHg ($p < 0.001$), 17.36 ± 17.96 mmHg ($p < 0.001$) and 16.95 ± 16.69 mmHg ($p < 0.001$), and diastolic blood pressure was reduced by 2.91 ± 6.50 mmHg ($p = 0.048$), 4.32 ± 9.70 mmHg ($p = 0.049$) and 7.14 ± 11.64 mmHg ($p = 0.009$) from

Table 1 Baseline characteristics and potential explanatory variables for cardiac volume reduction

Features	Value	*P*-value
Number of patients	46	
Age (years, Mean ± SD)	66.93 ± 9.76	0.281[a]
Gender (*n*, %)		0.107[b]
Female	14(30.43)	
Male	32(69.57)	
BMI (Mean ± SD)	22.63 ± 3.92	0.606[a]
Smoker (*n*, %)		0.410[b]
Yes	21(45.65)	
No	25(54.35)	
Hypertension (*n*, %)		0.309[b]
Yes	6 (13.04)	
No	40 (86.96)	
Tumor location (*n*)		
Upper	11	
Middle	22	
Lower	13	
Stage		0.137[b]
Stage II	13	
Stage III	33	
BP systolic at baseline (mmHg)	125.05 ± 15.98	0.881[a]
BP diastolic at baseline (mmHg)	75.66 ± 8.17	0.167[a]
HR at baseline (beats/min)	75.32 ± 6.23	0.412[a]
△BP systolic (Mean ± SD)	17.36 ± 17.96	0.160[a]
△BP diastolic (Mean ± SD)	4.32 ± 9.70	0.077[a]
△HR (Mean ± SD)	4.64 ± 4.91	0.448[a]

Abbreviations: *BMI* Body mass index, *BP* Blood pressure, *HR* Heart rate, *P*-value: the correlation between the potential explanatory variables and decline of heart volume. △BP systolic:systolic blood pressure at the twentieth − the initial systolic blood pressure. △BP diastolic: diastolic blood pressure at the twentieth − the initial diastolic blood pressure. △HR: heart rate at the twentieth − the initial heart rate

[a]Pearson's correlation analysis

[b] one-way ANOVA analysis

$P \geq 0.05$ reflects that there was no correlation between the potential explanatory variables and heart volume change. Inversely, $P < 0.05$ reflects that the potential explanatory variables were strongly linked to heart volume change

baseline.On the contrary, the heart rate at the middle location increased significantly from baseline, by 3.91 ± 7.92 ($p = 0.031$), 4.64 ± 4.91 ($p < 0.001$) and 5.27 ± 6.25 ($p = 0.001$) beats per minute at the tenth, twentieth and thirtieth fractions, respectively. However, at the upper and lower locations, no significant changes in blood pressure or heart rate were found during the entire treatment period.

Comparison of cardiac doses among the three locations

As shown in Table 3, the heart dose was significantly greater for patients with mid-thoracic esophageal tumors than for patients with upper tumors ($p < 0.05$). Although the heart dose tended to be higher in the middle location than in the lower location, the difference between these two locations did not reach statistical difference ($p > 0.05$).

Factors potentially relevant to the decrease in heart volume

The age, gender, BMI, disease staging, systolic blood pressure at baseline, diastolic blood pressure at baseline, heart rate at baseline, decrease in blood pressure and increase in heart rate did not correlate significantly with the heart volume changes or the MHD (all $p > 0.05$). The data are summarized in Table 1.

Comparison of heart volumes among the three types of images from the initial scans

Larger heart volumes ($p < 0.05$) were observed on the MIP images (mean value of 716.62 cm^3) than on the 3DCT and EE images (680.96 cm^3 and 685.02 cm^3, respectively). The mean heart volumes on the 3DCT and EE images did not differ significantly from one another ($p > 0.05$). Consistent results were found for the MHD among the three types of images. The data are summarized in Table 4.

Exclusion of intra-observer variation

The heart volumes of six patients were determined five times by the same radiation oncologist. No significant intra-observer variation was found ($p > 0.05$). The intra-observer error (5.40 ± 0.95 cm^3) was significantly lower than the heart volume variation during radiotherapy (23.63 ± 14.11 cm^3, $p = 0.010$).

Discussion

The cardiac volume during radiotherapy was assessed by means of organ delineation through enhanced 4DCT, which can eliminate the effects of respiratory motion on the heart. In the early stages of CCRT, we found that the heart volume had decreased significantly from the initial measurement, with a decline of approximately 6%. Lutkenhaus et al. [14] used CBCT imaging retrospectively to investigate the changes in cardiac volume over the course of chemoradiotherapy for patients with esophageal cancer. Consistent with our study, those authors revealed that the cardiac volume was reduced with a median reduction of 8% between the initial measurement at week 1 and the measurement at week 4. However, they did not analyze the relationship between heart volume and tumor location.

The present study demonstrated that heart volume and MHD were reduced mainly in patients with tumors in the mid-thoracic region, rather than in the upper and lower locations. This was primarily due to the close

Table 2 Change of heart volume and MHD during radiotherapy (rate %, Mean ± SD)

Image	Location	0th–10th		0th–20th		0th–30th	
		HV (%)	MHD (%)	HV (%)	MHD (%)	HV (%)	MHD (%)
3DCT	upper	0.45 ± 4.35	−0.38 ± 2.09	3.06 ± 9.24	1.24 ± 3.29	−6.91 ± 15.34	−2.12 ± 4.81
	middle	3.27 ± 4.32*	0.98 ± 1.41*	6.05 ± 6.99*	1.82 ± 2.13*	2.64 ± 9.99	0.95 ± 3.50
	lower	1.06 ± 5.56	0.27 ± 2.00	−0.19 ± 10.79	−0.19 ± 3.56	2.44 ± 13.65	0.91 ± 4.78
EE	upper	−1.15 ± 4.51	−0.90 ± 1.42	1.10 ± 5.87	0.40 ± 2.28	−3.27 ± 12.11	−0.57 ± 4.38
	middle	4.45 ± 2.07*	1.40 ± 1.03*	5.64 ± 5.30*	1.88 ± 1.79*	2.83 ± 6.85	0.70 ± 2.68
	lower	0.10 ± 6.88	0.06 ± 2.27	1.14 ± 9.96	0.41 ± 3.16	2.72 ± 10.26	1.47 ± 4.03
MIP	upper	−1.54 ± 4.00	−1.24 ± 0.97	1.68 ± 6.17	0.20 ± 2.17	−3.12 ± 15.12	−0.71 ± 4.80
	middle	4.52 ± 2.40*	1.29 ± 0.84*	4.51 ± 5.02*	1.29 ± 1.50*	2.67 ± 7.26	0.62 ± 2.54
	lower	2.65 ± 9.12	0.28 ± 2.05	1.81 ± 9.05	0.52 ± 3.10	3.39 ± 10.96	1.19 ± 3.97

Abbreviation: *0th–10th* Comparison between the initial measure and the tenth fraction, *0th–20th* Comparison between the initial measure and the twentieth fraction, *0th–30th* Comparison between the initial measure and the thirtieth fraction, *HV* Heart volume, *MHD* Maximum heart distance, *EE* End expiratory of 4DCT, *MIP* Maximum intensity projection of 4DCT
*represent the $P < 0.05$

proximity of the mid-esophagus to the heart. These results are also supported by the relative dose data: the V20, V30, V40, V45 and V50 values and the mean heart dose were greater when the esophageal tumor was in the middle region than in an upper or lower location. In a recent report, Zhang et al. observed new myocardial perfusion defects during radiotherapy in eight patients with esophageal cancer, and found that the defects were typically small fraction defects limited to the radiation field. They also discovered that the heart dose of patients with new myocardial perfusion defects were significantly larger than those of patients without new defects [3]. We therefore inferred that a high radiotherapy dose to the heart could be an important contributor to heart volume change. Ogino et al. concluded that the risk of symptomatic cardiac disease increased following high-dose and large-volume irradiation of the heart in long-term esophageal cancer survivors [12]. Based on above studies, precise radiotherapy technology and effective methods should be recommended to reduce the heart dose.

Although the reductions in heart volume and MHD in this study did not necessitate hospitalization or the use of cardiovascular drugs, some studies have suggested that radiotherapy damages the heart at both the cellular and molecular levels. For example, when the prescription dose for esophageal cancer accumulated to 40 Gy/20 fractions, a mild perfusion defect in the left ventricular anterior wall near the apex was found, which confirmed that the

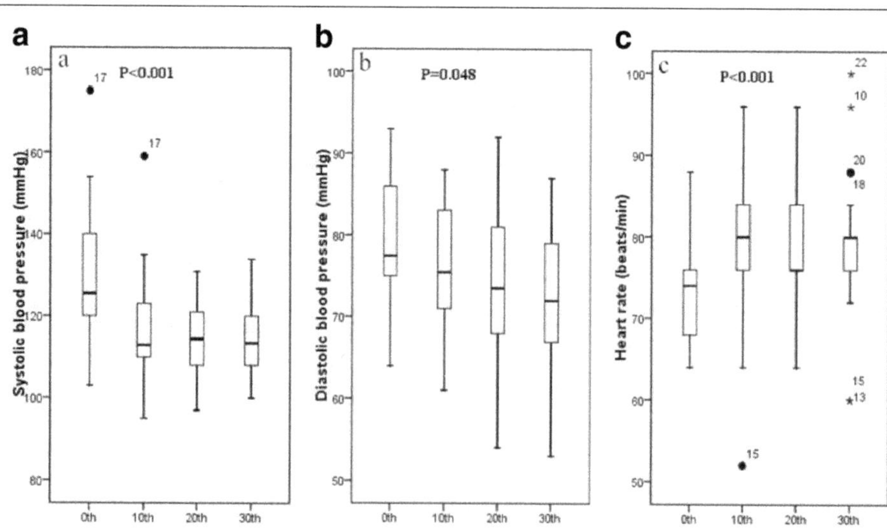

Fig. 1 The changes of blood pressure and heart rate. This figure displays the changes of systolic blood pressure, diastolic blood pressure and heart rate during the course of treatment for the patients with mid-thoracic esophageal cancer. The abscissa represents the course of radiotherapy. The ordinate represents systolic blood pressure (**a**), diastolic blood pressure (**b**) or heart rate (**c**). Abbreviations: 0th = before radiotherapy; 10th = the tenth fraction of radiotherapy; 20th = the twentieth fraction of radiotherapy; 30th = the thirtieth fraction of radiotherapy (after radiotherapy)

Table 3 Comparison of cardiac dose among different locations (rate %, Mean ± SD)

parameter	V20(%)	V30(%)	V40(%)	V45(%)	V50(%)	mean dose (Gy)
upper	17.24 ± 18.85	11.09 ± 12.35	5.15 ± 5.31	2.91 ± 3.15	1.48 ± 1.61	8.09 ± 7.58
middle	52.34 ± 22.13	39.48 ± 19.76	20.39 ± 11.07	12.99 ± 7.09	8.61 ± 5.79	2.49 ± 7.71
lower	41.80 ± 16.31	26.43 ± 9.44	16.73 ± 3.47	11.66 ± 1.17	8.40 ± 0.86	2.08 ± 6.47
P						
upper-middle	0.002	0.003	0.003	0.002	0.005	< 0.001
upper-lower	0.149	0.272	0.127	0.072	0.071	0.053
middle-lower	0.450	0.331	0.606	0.765	0.951	0.510

Abbreviation: *upper-middle* Comparison between the upper location between the middle location, *upper-lower* Comparison between the upper location and the lower location, *middle-lower* Comparison between the middle location and the lower location

myocardium was damaged by radiotherapy [3]. During radiotherapy for esophageal cancer patients, troponin T levels increased significantly (by 0.007 units, $p = 0.001$) from baseline to week 5, providing an early sign of cardiac damage [13]. Additionally, in one study [24], ionizing radiation was reported to cause non-transient alterations in the cardiac mitochondria, which ultimately may have caused heart muscle malfunction. At a microscopic level, not only did collagen levels increase as a whole, but the proportion of type I collagen increased relative to that of type III collagen. This change was thought to alter the compliance of the myocardium, thus contributing to diastolic dysfunction [25].

Diastolic dysfunction is now recognized as a common cause of heart failure and poor outcomes, even when the left ventricular ejection fraction is preserved [26, 27]. Thus, we assumed that reduced cardiac diastolic function could partly explain the reduced heart volume in the present study. Diastolic dysfunction was observed in patients who received mediastinal radiation of > 35 Gy for Hodgkin's disease [28]. Hatakenaka et al. concluded that direct radiation to the left ventricle predominantly impaired diastolic function by restricting wall motion in the radiated areas [2]. Consistently, Zhang et al. found that wall motion and wall thickening decreased significantly during radiotherapy in patients with esophageal cancer [3].

In the present study, we also assessed potential parameters that could predict the observed decline in heart volume. However, we found no correlations between the cardiac volume reduction and the patients' baseline characteristics. On the contrary, Haj et al. found that the decrease in heart volume correlated significantly with the systolic blood pressure at baseline, diastolic blood pressure at baseline and heart rate at baseline in patients with esophageal cancer [13]. The reasons for these differing results are unclear. Larger sample sizes and extensive multivariate analyses will be essential in further research.

The patients in our study had squamous cell carcinomas and received total radiation doses of up to 60 Gy in CCRT, much higher than the neoadjuvant chemoradiation dose for esophageal cancer (approximately 40 Gy) and the CCRT dose for adenocarcinoma (approximately 50.4 Gy). It should be noted that a change in heart volume immediately after CCRT (60 Gy) has not been reported. Our results indicated that the heart volume and MHD tended to recover to the initial level at the thirtieth fraction. Edmunds et al. found that the cardiac volume had increased by 1.7% ($p = 0.747$) 3 months after radical radiotherapy for esophageal cancer [29]. The reasons for this phenomenon are poorly understood, but we have considered several possibilities. Firstly, at the thirtieth fraction, the cardiomyocyte edema became serious and the cardiac repair became more obvious than the injury. Secondly, dehydration was reported to be the main reason for hospital admission during CCRT for esophageal cancer [30]; therefore, the recovery of the depleted intravascular volume in the later stages of CCRT

Table 4 Comparison of heart volume or MHD between the three images (cm^3 or cm, Mean ± SD)

parameter	MIP-3DCT		MIP-EE		EE-3DCT	
	volume	MHD	volume	MHD	volume	MHD
3DCT	680.96 ± 133.75	10.88 ± 0.71	–	–	680.96 ± 133.75	10.88 ± 0.71
EE	–	–	685.02 ± 125.28	10.91 ± 0.66	685.02 ± 125.28	10.91 ± 0.66
MIP	716.62 ± 123.45	11.07 ± 0.64	716.62 ± 123.45	11.07 ± 0.64	–	–
Rate (%)	5.76 ± 4.41	1.71 ± 1.47	4.81 ± 2.45	1.47 ± 0.97	0.91 ± 3.77	0.24 ± 1.33
P	< 0.001	< 0.001	< 0.001	< 0.001	0.294	0.313

Abbreviation: *EE* End expiratory of 4DCT, *MIP* Maximum intensity projection of 4DCT, *MHD* Maximum heart distance, *MIP-3DCT* Comparison between MIP and 3DCT, *MIP-EE* Comparison between MIP and EE, *EE-3DCT* Comparison between EE and 3DCT may have increased the heart volume. Moreover, in our study, the hearts were outlined along the pericardium, so changes in the pericardium may have been responsible for the observed results. Martel et al. [31] studied the effects of the radiation dose and volume on the pericardium in 57 patients with localized esophageal carcinoma. Nonmalignant pericardial effusions occurred in five patients, and the effusions were found at least 3 months post-radiation treatment. However, we did not observe significant pericardial effusion at the end of radiotherapy. Therefore, the mechanisms responsible for the change in heart volume after radiotherapy require further study.

While the heart rate increased during radiotherapy in the present study, both systolic and diastolic blood pressure decreased significantly. Similarly, Haj et al. discovered that systolic and diastolic blood pressure decreased and the heart rate increased in patients treated with neoadjuvant chemoradiation [13]. In Hatakenaka's [2] study, the LV-STVI and heart rate exhibited opposite trends, but the cardiac output index did not change. The authors reasoned that the cardiac output index remained the same because the elevated heart rate had compensated for the reduced LV-STVI. Zhang et al. explained that the acceleration of the heart rate may have been due to radiotherapy-induced damage to the heart conduction system [3]. And many reports concluded that conduction abnormalities such as sick sinus syndrome, ventricular arrhythmias, bundle branch blocks and complete heart blocks can be caused by RT [32–34].

To study the changes in cardiac volume during radiotherapy, we used 4DCT, which explicitly includes temporal changes in anatomy during the imaging process [17], and thus can provide spatial and temporal information on the heart during respiration. Moreover, CE-4DCT is a feasible technology that has been applied in the clinic [35]. The coefficients of variation for the gross tumor volumes delineated on CE-4DCT images are smaller than those delineated on plain scan images, indicating that CE-4DCT can reduce the error of organ delineation [15]. Our results demonstrated that the initial heart volumes determined from MIP images were larger than those determined from 3DCT and EE images, while the heart volumes determined from 3DCT and EE images did not differ significantly from one another. The trends in heart volume changes observed on these three types of images were consistent during radiotherapy. Thus, the volume changes were not due to differences among the various image types, further confirming that the cardiac volume decreased in the early stages of radiotherapy.

Morphological changes resulting from heart volume variation could result in inaccurate dose delivery to the tumor and organs at risk [14]. Since volume changes mainly occurred around the twentieth fraction of radiotherapy, modification of the treatment plan at this time point would probably be beneficial for suppressing the tumor and protecting the heart from radiotherapy.

The patients in the present study received chemotherapy at the same time as radiotherapy. Chemotherapeutic drugs are known to have cardiotoxic effects; for instance, they may cause arrhythmias [36–41]. However, there has been little research on cardiac volume reduction resulting from chemotherapy. Thus, the possible effects of chemotherapy on the cardiac volume should be studied further to determine the generalizability of our findings.

Our study may have been impacted by some limitations. Blood samples were not collected, so we did not use biomarkers to research the function of the heart. In addition, because long-term follow up is not carried out after radiotherapy, the long-term effects of radiotherapy on the cardiac volume could not be determined.

Conclusions

We discovered that the heart volume and MHD decreased significantly in the early stages of CCRT for esophageal cancer, but we found no symptomatic heart disease during treatment. The blood pressure decreased, while the heart rate increased significantly during the course of treatment. The cardiac dose was higher for the middle location than for the upper and lower locations. The observed changes in cardiac volume may have been caused by the relatively high dose of radiation. These changes may be valuable indicators of cardiac impairment necessitating target dose changes.

Abbreviations

3DCT: Three-dimensional computed tomography; 4DCT: Four-dimensional computed tomography; BMI: Body mass index; CBCT: Cone beam computed tomography; CCRT: Concurrent chemoradiotherapy; CE: Contrast-enhanced; CTV: Clinical target volume; EE: End expiratory; MHD: Maximum heart distance; MIP: Maximum intensity projection; RPM: Real-time Positioning Management

Funding

This work was supported by The National Key Research and Development Program of China (2016YFC0904700), the Key Research and Development Program of Shandong province (2016GSF201093), the Science and Technology Plan Projects of Shandong Academy of Medical Sciences (Youth Fund: 2015-51).

Authors' contributions

JB Li, JZ Wang and X Wang participated in the study design, contributed to the data collection, drafted the manuscript and approved the final version to be submitted. YJ Zhang, FX Li, W Wang and YL Guo made important contributions to the design of the study and the revision of the content. Q Shao, M Xu, XJ Liu and Y Wang contributed to the collection and analysis of data. All authors read and approved the final manuscript.

Competing interests

The authors declare that they have no competing interests.

Author details

[1]School of Medicine and Life Sciences, University of Jinan-Shandong Academy of Medical Sciences, Jinan, Shandong Province, China. [2]Department of Thoracic Radiation Oncology, Shandong Cancer Hospital affiliated to Shandong University, Shandong Academy of Medical Sciences, No. 440 Jiyan Road, Jinan 250117, Shandong Province, China. [3]Department of PET-CT Room, Shandong Cancer Hospital affiliated to Shandong University, Shandong Academy of Medical Sciences, Jinan, Shandong Province, China. [4]Medical imaging department, Shandong Cancer Hospital affiliated to Shandong University, Shandong Academy of Medical Sciences, Jinan, Shandong Province, China.

References

1. Fitzmaurice C, Dicker D, Pain A, Hamavid H, Moradi-Lakeh M, MacIntyre MF, Allen C, Hansen G, Woodbrook R, Wolfe C, Hamadeh RR, Moore A, Werdecker A. The global burden of cancer 2013. JAMA Oncol. 2015;1:505–27.
2. Hatakenaka M, Yonezawa M, Nonoshita T, Nakamura K, Yabuuchi H, Shioyama Y, Nagao M, Matsuo Y, Kamitani T, Higo T, Nishikawa K, Setoguchi T, Honda H. Acute cardiac impairment associated with concurrent chemoradiotherapy for esophageal cancer: magnetic resonance evaluation. Int J Radiat Oncol Biol Phys. 2012;83:e67–73.
3. Zhang P, Hu X, Yue J, Meng X, Han D, Sun X, Yang G, Wang S, Wang X, Yu J. Early detection of radiation-induced heart disease using (99m) Tc-MIBI SPECT gated myocardial perfusion imaging in patients with oesophageal cancer during radiotherapy. Radiother Oncol. 2015;115:171–8.
4. Monjazeb AM, Blackstock AW. The impact of multimodality therapy of distal esophageal and gastroesophageal junction adenocarcinomas on treatment-related toxicity and complications. Semin Radiat Oncol. 2013;23:60–73.
5. Brusamolino E, Baio A, Orlandi E, Arcaini L, Passamonti F, Griva V, Casagrande W, Pascutto C, Franchini P, Lazzarino M. Long-term events in adult patients with clinical stage IA-IIA nonbulky Hodgkin's lymphoma treated with four cycles of doxorubicin, bleomycin, vinblastine, and dacarbazine and adjuvant radiotherapy: a single-institution 15-year follow-up. Clin Cancer Res. 2006;12:6487–93.
6. Carmel RJ, Kaplan HS. Mantle irradiation in Hodgkin's disease. An analysis of technique, tumor eradication, and complications. Cancer. 1976;37:2813–25.
7. Hancock SL, Tucker MA, Hoppe RT. Factors affecting late mortality from heart disease after treatment of Hodgkin's disease. JAMA. 1993;270:1949–55.
8. Hull MC, Morris CG, Pepine CJ, Mendenhall NP. Valvular dysfunction and carotid, subclavian, and coronary artery disease in survivors of hodgkin lymphoma treated with radiation therapy. JAMA. 2003;290:2831–7.
9. Konski A, Li T, Christensen M, Cheng JD, Yu JQ, Crawford K, Haluszka O, Tokar J, Scott W, Meropol NJ, Cohen SJ, Maurer A, Freedman GM. Symptomatic cardiac toxicity is predicted by dosimetric and patient factors rather than changes in 18F-FDG PET determination of myocardial activity after chemoradiotherapy for esophageal cancer. Radiother Oncol. 2012;104:72–7.
10. Wei X, Liu HH, Tucker SL, Wang S, Mohan R, Cox JD, Komaki R, Liao Z. Risk factors for pericardial effusion in inoperable esophageal cancer patients treated with definitive chemoradiation therapy. Int J Radiat Oncol Biol Phys. 2008;70:707–14.
11. Cosset JM, Henry-Amar M, Pellae-Cosset B, Carde P, Girinski T, Tubiana M, Hayat M. Pericarditis and myocardial infarctions after Hodgkin's disease therapy. Int J Radiat Oncol Biol Phys. 1991;21:447–9.
12. Ogino I, Watanabe S, Iwahashi N, Kosuge M, Sakamaki K, Kunisaki C, Kimura K. Symptomatic radiation-induced cardiac disease in long-term survivors of esophageal cancer. Strahlenther Onkol. 2016;192:359–67.
13. Haj Mohammad N, Kamphuis M, Hulshof MC, Lutkenhaus LJ, Gisbertz SS, Bergman JJ, de Bruin-Bon HA, Geijsen ED, Bel A, Boekholdt SM, van Laarhoven HW. Reduction of heart volume during neoadjuvant chemoradiation in patients with resectable esophageal cancer. Radiother Oncol. 2015;114:91–5.
14. Lutkenhaus LJ, Kamphuis M, van Wieringen N, Hulshof MC, Bel A. Reduction in cardiac volume during chemoradiotherapy for patients with esophageal cancer. Radiother Oncol. 2013;109:200–3.
15. Wang JZ, Li JB, Qi HP, Li YK, Wang Y, Zhang YJ, Wang W. Effect of contrast enhancement in delineating GTV and constructing IGTV of thoracic oesophageal cancer based on 4D-CT scans. Radiother Oncol. 2016;119:172–8.
16. Rietzel E, Pan T, Chen GT. Four-dimensional computed tomography: image formation and clinical protocol. Med Phys. 2005;32:874–89.
17. Keall P. 4-dimensional computed tomography imaging and treatment planning. Semin Radiat Oncol. 2004;14:81–90.
18. Underberg RW, Lagerwaard FJ, Cuijpers JP, Slotman BJ, van Sörnsen de Koste JR, Senan S. Four-dimensional CT scans for treatment planning in stereotactic radiotherapy for stage I lung cancer. Int J Radiat Oncol Biol Phys. 2004;60:1283–90.
19. Guckenberger M, Wilbert J, Meyer J, Baier K, Richter A, Flentje M. Is a single respiratory correlated 4D-CT study sufficient for evaluation of breathing motion? Int J Radiat Oncol Biol Phys. 2007;67:1352–9.
20. Handels H, Werner R, Schmidt R, Frenzel T, Lu W, Low D, Ehrhardt J. 4D medical image computing and visualization of lung tumor mobility in spatio-temporal CT image data. I nt J Med Inform. 2007;76(Suppl 3):S433–9.
21. Dinkel J, Welzel T, Bolte H, Hoffmann B, Thierfelder C, Mende U, Debus J, Heller M, Kauczor HU, Biederer J. Four-dimensional multislice helical CT of the lung: qualitative comparison of retrospectively gated and static images in an ex-vivo system. Radiother Oncol. 2007;85:215–22.
22. Feng M, Moran JM, Koelling T, Chughtai A, Chan JL, Freedman L, Hayman JA, Jagsi R, Jolly S, Larouere J, Soriano J, Marsh R, Pierce LJ. Development and validation of a heart atlas to study cardiac exposure to radiation following treatment for breast cancer. Int J Radiat Oncol Biol Phys. 2011;79:10–8.
23. Mancia G, Fagard R, Narkiewicz K, Redón J, Zanchetti A, Böhm M, Christiaens T, Cifkova R, De Backer G, Dominiczak A, Galderisi M, Grobbee DE, Jaarsma T. 2013 ESH/ESC guidelines for the management of arterial hypertension: the task force for the management of arterial hypertension of the European Society of Hypertension (ESH) and of the European Society of Cardiology (ESC). J Hypertens. 2013;31:1281–357.
24. Barjaktarovic Z, Schmaltz D, Shyla A, Azimzadeh O, Schulz S, Haagen J, Dörr W, Sarioglu H, Schäfer A, Atkinson MJ, Zischka H, Tapio S. PLoS One. 2011;6: e27811.
25. Chello M, Mastroroberto P, Romano R, Zofrea S, Bevacqua I, Marchese AR. Changes in the proportion of types I and III collagen in the left ventricular wall of patients with post-irradiative pericarditis. Cardiovasc Surg. 1996;4:222–6.
26. Redfield MM, Jacobsen SJ, Burnett JC Jr, Mahoney DW, Bailey KR, Rodeheffer RJ. Burden of systolic and diastolic ventricular dysfunction in the community: appreciating the scope of the heart failure epidemic. JAMA. 2003;289:194–202.
27. Vasan RS, Benjamin EJ, Levy D. Prevalence, clinical features and prognosis of diastolic heart failure: an epidemiologic perspective. J Am Coll Cardiol. 1995; 26:1565–74.
28. Heidenreich PA, Hancock SL, Vagelos RH, Lee BK, Schnittger I. Diastolic dysfunction after mediastinal irradiation. Am Heart J. 2005;150:977–82.
29. Edmunds K, Brooks C, Hansen VN, Harris V, Tait DM. Cardiac volume effects during chemoradiotherapy for esophageal cancer (regarding Lutkenhaus et al. reduction in cardiac volume during chemoradiotherapy for patients with esophageal cancer). Radiother Oncol. 2015;114:128–9.
30. Crosby TD, Brewster AE, Borley A, Perschky L, Kehagioglou P, Court J, Maughan TS. Definitive chemoradiation in patients with inoperable oesophageal carcinoma. Br J Cancer. 2004;90:70–5.
31. Martel MK, Sahijdak WM, Ten Haken RK, Kessler ML, Turrisi AT. Fraction size and dose parameters related to the incidence of pericardial effusions. Int J Radiat Oncol Biol Phys. 1998;40:155–61.
32. Lee PJ, Mallik R. Cardiovascular effects of radiation therapy: practical approach to radiation therapy-induced heart disease. Cardiol Rev. 2005;13:80–6.
33. Camp-Sorrell D. Cardiovascular late effects. Oncology (Williston Park). 2008; 22(2 Suppl Nurse Ed):42–4.
34. Heidenreich PA, Kapoor JR. Radiation induced heart disease: systemic disorders in heart disease. Heart. 2009;95:252–8.
35. Cattaneo GM, Passoni P, Sangalli G, Slim N, Longobardi B, Mancosu P, Bettinardi V, Di Muzio N, Calandrino R. Internal target volume defined by contrast-enhanced 4D-CT scan in unresectable pancreatic tumour: evaluation and reproducibility. Radiother Oncol. 2010;97:525–9.

36. Zhang P, Xi M, Li QQ, Hu YH, Guo X, Zhao L, Liu H, Liu SL, Luo LL, Liu Q, Liu MZ. Concurrent cisplatin and 5-fluorouracil versus concurrent cisplatin and docetaxel with radiotherapy for esophageal squamous cell carcinoma: a propensity score-matched analysis. Oncotarget. 2016;7:44686–94.
37. Kuropkat C, Griem K, Clark J, Rodriguez ER, Hutchinson J, Taylor SG 4th. Severe cardiotoxicity during 5-fluorouracil chemotherapy: a case and literature report. Am J Clin Oncol. 1999;22:466–70.
38. Lieutaud T, Brain E, Golgran-Toledano D, Vincent F, Cvitkovic E, Leclercq B, Escudier B. 5-fluorouracil cardiotoxicity: a unique mechanism for ischaemic cardiopathy and cardiac failure? Eur J Cancer. 1996;32A:368–9.
39. Schöber C, Papageorgiou E, Harstrick A, Bokemeyer C, Mügge A, Stahl M, Wilke H, Poliwoda H, Hiddemann W, Köhne-Wömpner CH. Cardiotoxicity of 5-fluorouracil in combination with folinic acid in patients with gastrointestinal cancer. Cancer. 1993;72:2242–7.
40. Doll DC, List AF, Greco FA, Hainsworth JD, Hande KR, Johnson DH. Acute vascular ischemic events after cisplatin-based combination chemotherapy for germ-cell tumors of the testis. Ann Intern Med. 1986;105:48–51.
41. Içli F, Karaoğuz H, Dinçol D, Demirkazik A, Günel N, Karaoğuz R, Uner A. Severe vascular toxicity associated with cisplatin-based chemotherapy. Cancer. 1993;72:587–93.

7

Reliability of the gamma index analysis as a verification method of volumetric modulated arc therapy plans

Jong Min Park[1,2,3,4†], Jung-in Kim[1,2,3†], So-Yeon Park[5], Do Hoon Oh[6*] and Sang-Tae Kim[7*]

Abstract

Background: We investigate the gamma passing rate (GPR) consistency when applying different types of gamma analyses, linacs, and dosimeters for volumetric modulated arc therapy (VMAT).

Methods: A total of 240 VMAT plans for various treatment sites, which were generated with Trilogy (140 plans) and TrueBeam STx (100 plans), were retrospectively selected. For each VMAT plan, planar dose distributions were measured with both MapCHECK2 and ArcCHECK dosimeters. During the planar dose distribution measurements, the actual multileaf collimator (MLC) positions, gantry angles, and delivered monitor units were recorded and compared to the values in the original VMAT plans to calculate mechanical errors. For each VMAT plan, both the global and local gamma analyses were performed with 3%/3 mm, 2%/2 mm, 2%/1 mm, 1%/2 mm, and 1%/1 mm. The Pearson correlation coefficients (r) were calculated 1) between the global and the local GPRs, 2) between GPRs with the MapCHECK2 and the ArcCHECK dosimeters, 3) and between GPRs and the mechanical errors during the VMAT delivery.

Results: For the MapCHECK2 measurements, strong correlations between the global and local GPRs were observed only with 1%/2 mm and 1%/1 mm ($r > 0.8$ with $p < 0.001$), while weak or no correlations were observed for the ArcCHECK measurement. Between the MapCHECK2 and ArcCHECK measurements, the global GPRs showed no correlations (all with $p > 0.05$), while the local GPRs showed moderate correlations only with 2%/1 mm and 1%/1 mm for TrueBeam STx ($r > 0.5$ with $p < 0.001$). Both the global and local GPRs always showed weak or no correlations with the MLC positional errors except for the GPRs of MapCHECK2 with 1%/2 mm and 1%/1 mm for TrueBeam STx and the GPR of ArcCHECK with 1%/2 mm for Trilogy ($r < -0.5$ with $p < 0.001$).

Conclusions: The GPRs varied according to the types of gamma analyses, dosimeters, and linacs. Therefore, each institution should carefully establish their own gamma analysis protocol by determining the type of gamma index analysis and the gamma criterion with their own linac and their own dosimeter.

Keywords: Gamma passing rate, Volumetric modulated arc therapy, Patient-specific quality assurance, Log file analysis, Modulation degree

* Correspondence: dohoon05@gmail.com; rad21@korea.kr
[†]Jong Min Park and Jung-in Kim contributed equally to this work.
[6]Department of Radiation Oncology, Myongji Hospital, Goyang, South Korea
[7]Nuclear Emergency Division, Radiation Protection and Emergency Preparedness Bureau, Nuclear Safety and Security Commission, Seoul, South Korea
Full list of author information is available at the end of the article

Background

Intensity-modulated radiation therapy (IMRT) enables conformal delivery of prescription doses to target volumes while minimizing radiotherapy-induced complications by reducing the doses to organs at risk (OARs) located nearby the target volumes [1, 2]. This is possible owing to photon beam intensity modulations by mechanical modulations of the multileaf collimator (MLC) positions [3]. Compared to IMRT, volumetric modulated arc therapy (VMAT) is possible to deliver equal to or better dose distributions than those of IMRT more rapidly by simultaneous mechanical modulations of the MLC positions, gantry rotation speeds, and dose rates [4]. The optimal dose distributions of VMAT are also attributed to photon beam modulations. Although the photon beam modulation of VMAT enables to generate an optimal dose distribution, an excessive modulation of a VMAT plan results in discordance between the planned and actually delivered dose distributions to a patient, i.e., patients are not treated as intended with excessively modulated VMAT plans [5–7]. This is because of increases in the dose calculation uncertainty and mechanical uncertainty [5, 6, 8]. For excessively modulated VMAT plans, small or irregularly shaped beam apertures tend to be used more frequently, whose dose calculation accuracy with current dose calculation algorithms is limited; therefore, the calculated dose distribution (intended dose distribution) would not be actually delivered to a patient during treatment due to the increased dose calculation uncertainty [5, 6]. Besides the dose calculation uncertainty of excessively modulated VMAT plans, mechanical movements of MLCs, gantry rotation, and beam delivery system become complicated, which increases the mechanical uncertainty [8–10]. Therefore, the intended mechanical movements of excessively modulated VMAT plans might not be perfectly implemented during the actual plan delivery to a patient. This also causes discordance between the planned and delivered dose distributions. In this respect, pre-treatment verification of the delivered dose distributions of VMAT plans, i.e., pre-treatment patient-specific quality assurance (QA), is highly recommended and routinely performed for each VMAT plan before treatment in the clinical setting [11–13]. The most popular method as patient-specific QA for VMAT is the gamma index analysis [14–16].

Although the gamma index analysis is widely adopted in the clinical setting, some issues on the gamma index analysis have been raised by previous studies [11, 13, 17–19]. The gamma index method evaluates the coincidence between the calculated and measured dose distributions by utilizing the percent dose difference (DD) and distance to agreement [15]. Regarding the calculation of the DD, there are two types of gamma index methods, which are the global and local gamma index analyses [1]. The global gamma index analysis calculates the DDs relative to the maximum dose (or prescription dose), while the local gamma index analysis calculates the DDs relative to the doses at each evaluated point. Because the DD is a percent value, the local gamma index analysis could exaggerate the DDs in the low-dose regions, while the global gamma index method could underestimate the dose discrepancies in the low-dose regions [1]. Since there are no clear guidelines to use the global or local gamma index analysis as pre-treatment patient-specific QA for VMAT, each clinic autonomously decides that which type of gamma index analysis should be used in that clinic; however, it is uncertain that the global gamma index analysis can substitute for the local gamma index analysis or vice versa. For the tolerance levels of the gamma passing rates, Heilemann et al. demonstrated that a global gamma passing rate of 90% with 2%/2 mm could detect clinically unacceptable VMAT plans owing to significant errors by introducing deliberately MLC errors [12]. However, it was also demonstrated that the gamma passing rates of IMRT or VMAT depend on the types of dosimeter [11, 13]. Hussein et al. and Fredh et al. showed dependency of the gamma passing rates on the types of dosimeters for IMRT and VMAT plans [11, 13]. They claimed that the configuration and resolution of the detector have a great impact on the calculation of the gamma passing rates. Therefore, the tolerance levels suggested by previous studies or international guidelines might not be always appropriate for a particular institution's dosimeter. Moreover, it is uncertain that the gamma index analysis could sensitively reflect the VMAT delivery accuracy depending on the modulation degree. Although the gamma index analysis is widely accepted in the clinical setting, its reliability seems to be investigated thoroughly. Therefore, in this study, we investigated the correlation between the global and local gamma passing rates by utilizing 240 VMAT plans with various modulation degrees. In addition, by utilizing two types of dosimeters, we investigated the correlation between the gamma passing rates of those two dosimeters. We also investigated the relationship between the gamma passing rates and the mechanical errors acquired from the log files recorded during the VMAT delivery in the linac control system. Finally, we investigated the relevance between the gamma passing rates and the differences in the dose-volumetric parameters between the original plans and the plans reconstructed with the log files. By doing this, we evaluated the reliability of the gamma index analysis under various conditions.

Methods

Patient selection

For this study, a total of 200 patients with head and neck (H&N) cancer (60 patients), prostate cancer (40 patients), liver cancer (11 patients treated with fractionated radiotherapy and 20 patients treated with stereotactic ablative radiotherapy (SABR)), lung cancer (20 patients treated with SABR), brain tumor (20 patients), and spine tumor (9 patients treated with fractionated radiotherapy and 20 patients with SABR) were retrospectively selected after an institutional review board approval (IRB No. 1802–069-922). Every patient underwent CT scans using Brilliance CT Big Bore™ (Philips, Amsterdam, the Netherlands).

Generation of VMAT plans

A single VMAT plan was generated for each patient except for the patients with prostate cancer. For those patients, two VMAT plans per a patient were generated, which were a primary plan and a boost plan. Plan information is summarized in Table 1. A total of 140 VMAT plans were generated using the C-series linac, Trilogy™ with the Millennium 120™ MLC (Varian Medical Systems, Palo Alto, CA) while a total of 100 VMAT plans were generated with TrueBeam STx™ with the high-definition (HD) 120™ MLC (Varian Medical Systems, Palo Alto, CA, USA). Every VMAT plan in this study was generated with the Eclipse™ system (Varian Medical Systems, Palo Alto, CA). A progressive resolution optimizer (PRO, ver.13.7, Varian Medical Systems, Palo Alto, CA) was used for optimization of the VMAT plans, and the anisotropic analytic algorithm (AAA, ver.13.7, Varian Medical Systems, Palo Alto) was used for dose calculation with a dose calculation resolution of 1 mm.

Gamma index analysis

For the gamma index analysis of each VMAT plan, two types of dosimeters were utilized in this study, which were a MapCHECK2™ dosimeter inserted in a MapPHAN™ (Sun Nuclear Corporation, Melbourne, FL) and an ArcCHECK™ dosimeter (Sun Nuclear Corporation, Melbourne, FL). To generate the reference 2D dose distribution, CT images of both dosimeters were taken and used to generate verification plans in the Eclipse system. The dose distributions were calculated with a dose calculation resolution of 1 mm, which is the finest dose calculation resolution of the Eclipse system. To reduce the volume averaging effect, we calculated the dose distributions with the finest dose calculation resolution [20]. To acquire accurate measured dose distributions, both the MapCHECK2 and ArcCHECK dosimeters were calibrated according to the manufacturer guidelines. Before measuring the 2D dose distributions, the outputs of Trilogy and TrueBeam STx were calibrated according to the American Association of Physicists in Medicine Task Group 51 protocol [21]. For an accurate setup of the dosimeters, cone beam computed tomography images of the dosimeters were acquired to verify the dosimeter setup before the measurements. Both the global and local gamma passing rates with various gamma criteria, which were 3%/3 mm, 2%/2 mm, 2%/1 mm, 1%/2 mm, and 1%/1 mm, were calculated with the absolute doses using the SNC patient™ software (Sun Nuclear Corporation, Melbourne, FL), which linearly interpolates calculated doses less than 1 mm resolution [22]. The SNC

Table 1 - Plan information

	N	Energy	Prescription dose	Fraction number
Trilogy (*N* = 140)				
H&N	40	6 MV	67.5 Gy to $PTV_{67.5Gy}$ 54 Gy to PTV_{54Gy} 48 Gy to PTV_{48Gy}	30
Prostate primary	40	15 MV	50.4	28
Prostate boost	40	15 MV	30.6	17
Liver	11	15 MV	50	25
Spine	9	15 MV	30	10
TrueBeam STx (*N* = 100)				
H&N	20	6 MV	67.5 Gy to $PTV_{67.5Gy}$ 54 Gy to PTV_{54Gy} 48 Gy to PTV_{48Gy}	30
Brain	20	6 MV	30	10
Lung SABR	20	6 MV FFF	60	4
Spine SABR	20	10 MV FFF	19	1
Liver SABR	20	10 MV FFF	42	3

Note: *H&N* Head and neck, *SABR* Stereotactic ablative radiotherapy, *FFF* Flattening filter free patient software was used to calculate gamma passing rates both with the MapCHECK2 measurements and the ArcCHECK measurements. When calculating gamma passing rates, the reference images were measured dose distributions and the evaluated images were calculated dose distributions. To calculate the global gamma passing rates, we calculated the DDs relative to the maximum doses.

Differences in the mechanical parameters between the original VMAT plans and the log files recorded during the VMAT delivery

When measuring the 2D dose distributions of the VMAT plans with the MapCHECK2 and ArcCHECK dosimeters, the log files in the linac control system, which are the records of the actual MLC positions, gantry angles, and delivered monitor units (MUs) at each control point during the VMAT delivery, were acquired. The reliability of the log files was examined by periodic linac QA by international guidelines and previous studies [23–25]. The MU delivery errors at each control point were considered mechanical errors in this study since the MU delivery at each control point is controlled by the linac control system synchronized with the MLC movements and gantry rotation speeds. To compare the values of the mechanical parameters from the log files to the values defined in the original VMAT plans, the log files were reformatted as DICOM-RT files with an in-house program written in MATLAB (Mathworks Inc., Natick, MA). The differences in the MLC positions, gantry angles, and delivered MUs were calculated with the DICOM-RT formatted log files and the original VMAT plans in the DICOM-RT format. Because two log file sets were acquired during the VMAT deliveries for the MapCHECK2 and ArcCHECK measurements, the two sets of the calculated differences were averaged.

Modulation complexity score and the differences in the dose-volumetric parameters between the original VMAT plans and the reconstructed VMAT plans with the log files

We calculated modulation complexity score for VMAT (MCS_v) suggested by Masi et al. to quantify the modulation degrees of each VMAT plan [9]. The MCS_v has values in the range from 0 to 1. As increasing the modulation complexity of a VMAT plan, the value of MCS_v decreases (cf. $MCS_v = 1$ means no modulation of a VMAT plan).

The DICOM-RT formatted files were imported to the Eclipse system and dose distributions were calculated with the patient CT images. After that, we calculated the minimum dose to cover 95% of the planning target volume (PTV) ($D_{95\%}$) as well as the percent volume of the body structure irradiated by at least 50% of the prescription dose ($V_{50\%}$). Since the H&N VMAT plan had a total of three PTVs, only the PTV receiving the highest prescription dose ($PTV_{67.5Gy}$) was analyzed. The values of $D_{95\%}$ of the PTV and $V_{50\%}$ of the body calculated from the reconstructed plans with the log files were compared to those of the original VMAT plans.

Correlation analysis

To evaluate the consistency between the global and the local gamma passing rates, the Pearson correlation coefficient (*r*) with corresponding *p* values was calculated between the global and local gamma passing rates with various gamma criteria. The correlations with *r* values from 0.3 to 0.49 are regarded as weak correlations. Those from 0.5 to 0.69 and 0.7 to 1.0 are regarded as moderate and strong correlations, respectively. The *p* values equal to or less than 0.05 are regarded as statistically significant in this study. To evaluate the dosimeter dependency of the gamma passing rates, the correlations between the gamma passing rates from the MapCHECK2 measurements and those from the ArcCHECK measurements were analyzed. To evaluate the detectability of the gamma passing rates on the mechanical errors during the VMAT deliveries, the correlations between the gamma passing rates and the mechanical errors calculated with the original VMAT plans and the log files were analyzed. The correlations between the gamma passing rates and the MCS_v were calculated to examine changes in the gamma passing rates according to the modulation degree of VMAT plans [9]. To examine relevance of the gamma passing rates to the changes in the dose-volumetric parameters, the correlations between the gamma passing rates and the differences in the PTV $D_{95\%}$ of the original treatment plans from those of the reconstructed plans with the log files were analyzed. In addition, the correlations between the gamma passing rates and the differences in the $V_{50\%}$ of the body structures of the original treatment plans from those of the reconstructed plans with log files were also analyzed.

Results

Global gamma passing rates

The global gamma passing rates with various gamma criteria of the VMAT plans for various treatment sites, measured with the MapCHECK2 and ArcCHECK dosimeters, are shown in Fig. 1.

For the VMAT plans with Trilogy, the prostate primary plans showed the lowest gamma passing rates in general with the MapCHECK2 measurements. For the ArcCHECK measurements, the prostate boost plans showed the lowest gamma passing rates with every gamma criterion tested in this study. The gamma passing rates with MapCHECK2 were not coincident with those with ArcCHECK, sometimes contradictory to each other.

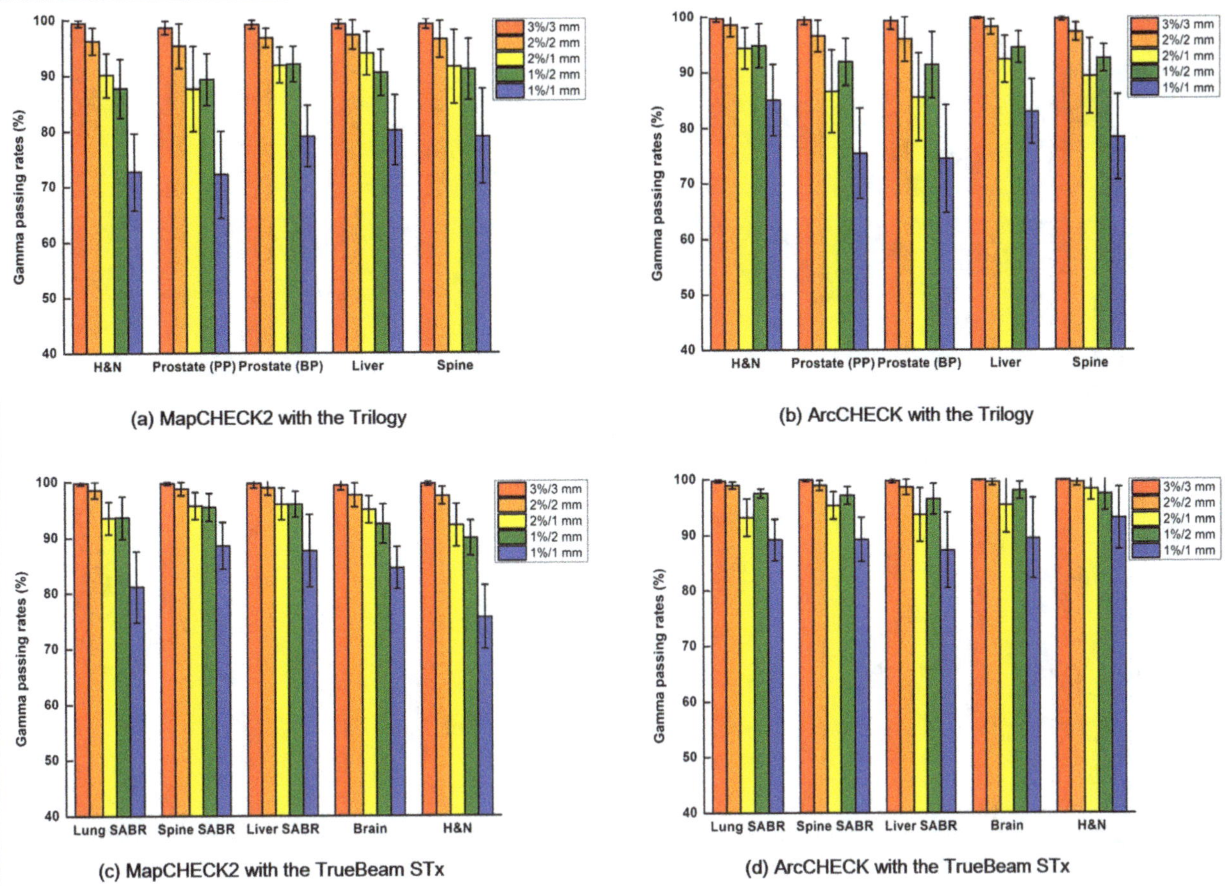

Fig. 1 Global gamma passing rates of the VMAT plans. Global gamma passing rates with various gamma criteria calculated from the measurements with the MapCHECK2 dosimeter are shown for Trilogy (**a**) and TrueBeam STx (**c**). Those with the ArcCHECK dosimeter using Trilogy (**b**) and TrueBeam STx (**d**) are also shown. For the global gamma passing rates with Trilogy, the H&N plans, prostate primary plans (PPs), prostate boost plans (BPs), liver plans, and spine plans were analyzed, while the lung SABR, spine SABR, liver SABR, brain, and H&N plans were analyzed with TrueBeam STx

For the VMAT plans with TrueBeam STx, the H&N plans generally showed the lowest gamma passing rates with the MapCHECK2 measurements, while the liver plans generally showed the highest gamma passing rates. For the ArcCHECK measurements, the lung SABR plans generally showed the lowest gamma passing rates, while the H&N plans generally showed the highest gamma passing rates. The gamma passing rates with MapCHECK2 were not coincident with those with ArcCHECK, sometimes contradictory to each other.

Local gamma passing rates

The local gamma passing rates with various gamma criteria of the VMAT plans for various treatment sites, measured with MapCHECK2 and ArcCHECK, are shown in Fig. 2.

For the VMAT plans with Trilogy, the H&N plans showed the lowest gamma passing rates with 3%/3 mm and 2%/2 mm, while the prostate primary plans showed the lowest gamma passing rates with the rest of the gamma criteria for the MapCHECK2 measurements. However, for the ArcCHECK measurements, the H&N VMAT plans showed the lowest gamma passing rates consistently regardless of the gamma criteria. Both the MapCHECK2 and the ArcCHECK measurements showed the highest gamma passing rates for the liver plans in general. The gamma passing rates with MapCHECK2 were generally coincident with those with those of ArcCHECK, however, not always.

For the VMAT plans with TrueBeam STx, both the MapCHECK2 and ArcCHECK measurements showed the lowest gamma passing rates for the H&N plans. Except for the gamma passing rates with 3%/3 mm, both the MapCHECK2 and ArcCHECK measurements showed the highest gamma passing rates for the spine SABR VMAT plans. Similar to the results with Trilogy, the gamma passing rates of MapCHECK2 were generally coincident with those of ArcCHECK.

Mechanical errors during the VMAT delivery

The differences in the mechanical parameters between the values defined in the original VMAT plans and those

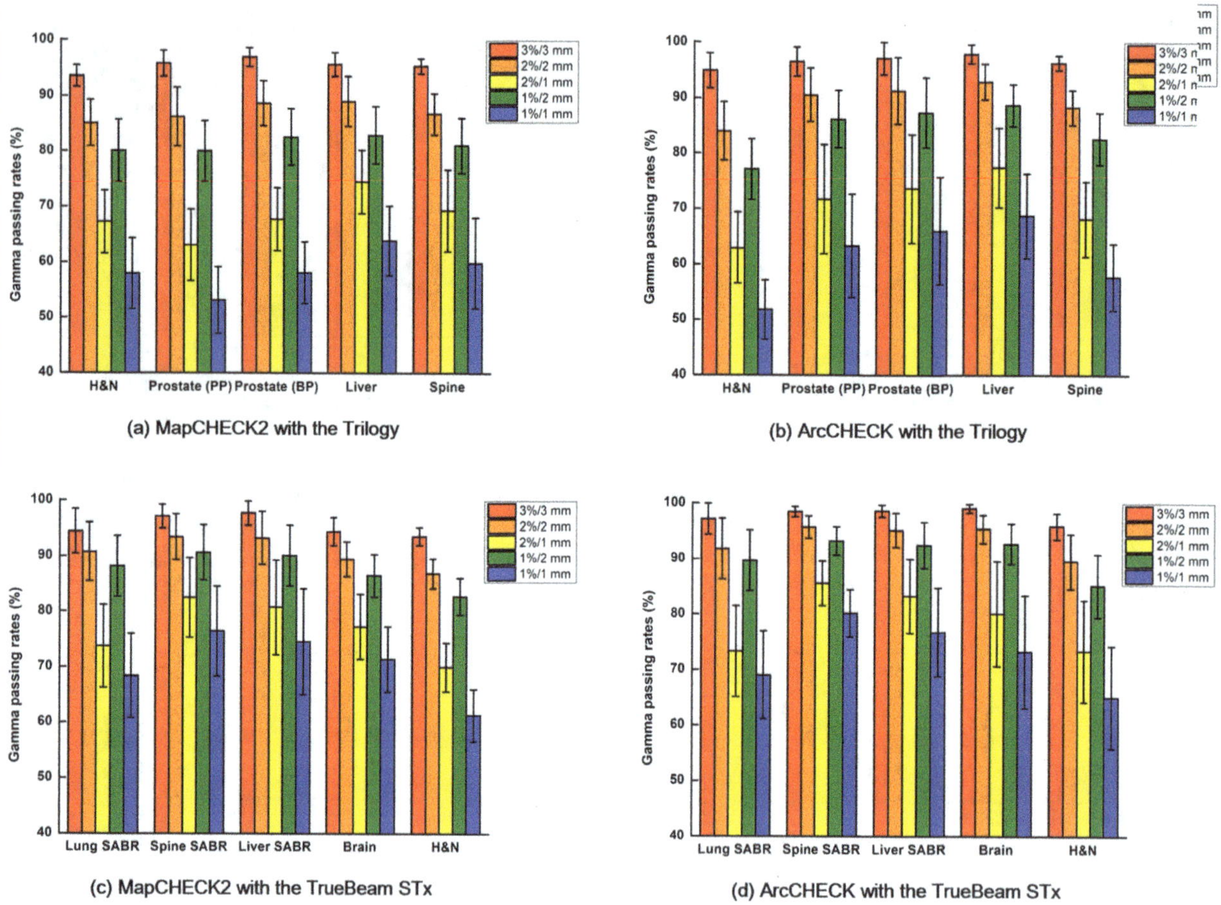

Fig. 2 Local gamma passing rates of the VMAT plans. Local gamma passing rates with various gamma criteria calculated from the measurements with the MapCHECK2 dosimeter are shown for Trilogy (**a**) and TrueBeam STx (**c**). Those with the ArcCHECK dosimeter using Trilogy (**b**) and TrueBeam STx (**d**) are also shown. For the local gamma passing rates with Trilogy, H&N plans, prostate primary plans (PPs), prostate boost plans (BPs), liver plans, and spine plans were analyzed, while the lung SABR, spine SABR, liver SABR, brain, and H&N plans were analyzed with TrueBeam STx

in the log files recorded during the VMAT deliveries are shown in Fig. 3.

For the mechanical errors of Trilogy, the MLC positioning errors were the largest when delivering the H&N VMAT plans (0.19 ± 0.06 mm), while those differences were the lowest when delivering the prostate boost plans (0.03 ± 0.01 mm). The MU delivery errors were the largest for the spine VMAT plans (0.12 ± 0.04 MU), while those were the smallest for the prostate boost plans (0.05 ± 0.01 mm).

For the mechanical errors of TrueBeam STx, the MLC positioning errors were the largest for the H&N VMAT plans (0.09 ± 0.01 mm) same as the results with Trilogy, while those errors were the smallest for the lung SABR VMAT plans (0.01 ± 0.01 mm). However, this was opposite for the MU delivery errors showing the largest errors during the lung SABR VMAT deliveries (0.40 ± 0.03 MU), while showing the smallest errors during the H&N VMAT deliveries (0.02 ± 0.01 MU). The large MU delivery errors were only observed in the SABR VMAT plans. The gantry positional error was the largest for the liver SABR VMAT plans (0.04 ± 0.02°), while that was the smallest for the lung SABR VMAT plans (0.01 ± 0.00°).

In general, the MLC positional errors and the gantry positional errors of TrueBeam STx were much smaller than those of Trilogy. The MU delivery errors of the SABR VMAT plans with TrueBeam STx were generally larger than those with the non-SABR VMAT plans both with TrueBeam STx and Trilogy.

Modulation complexity score for VMAT

The average values of MCS_v calculated from VMAT plans with the Trilogy and TrueBeam STx are shown in Fig. 4. For the Trilogy, the H&N VMAT plans showed the lowest average value of MCS_v ($1.28 \times 10^{-3} \pm 0.26 \times 10^{-3}$) while the prostate boost VMAT plans showed the highest average value of MCS_v ($1.72 \times 10^{-3} \pm 0.39 \times 10^{-3}$). For the TrueBeam STx, the H&N VMAT plans showed the lowest average value of MCS_v ($1.16 \times 10^{-3} \pm 0.27 \times 10^{-3}$) while

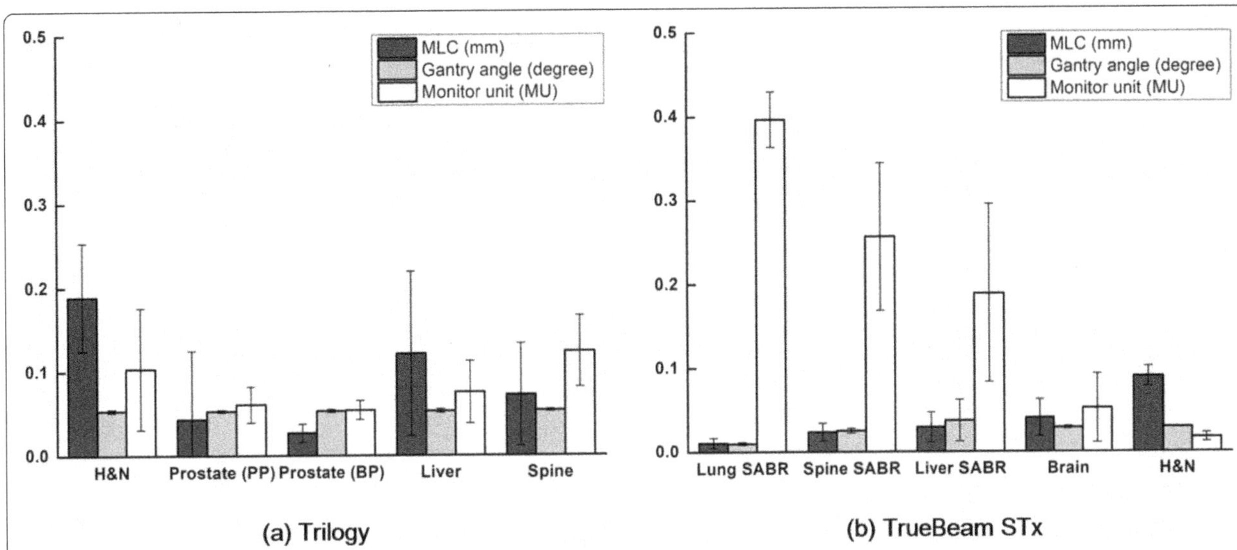

Fig. 3 Differences in the mechanical parameters between those defined in the original VMAT plans and those recorded during the VMAT plan deliveries in the log files. MLC positional errors, gantry angle errors, and MU errors are shown for Trilogy (**a**) and TrueBeam STx (**b**). The units of the MLC errors, gantry angle errors, and MU errors are millimeters, degrees, and MUs, respectively

the lung SABR VMAT plans showed the highest average value of MCS_v ($3.17 \times 10^{-3} \pm 0.36 \times 10^{-3}$).

Correlations between the global and local gamma passing rates

The Pearson correlation coefficients (r) between the global and local gamma passing rates are shown in Table 2 with corresponding p values.

For the MapCHECK2 measurements, the strongest correlations were observed between the global and local gamma passing rates with a gamma criterion of 1%/2 mm for both the Trilogy and TrueBeam STx systems ($r = 0.806$ with $p < 0.001$ for Trilogy and $r = 0.860$ with $p < 0.001$ for TrueBeam STx). The tighter the gamma criteria, the stronger the correlations became in general. With gamma criteria of 2%/1 mm, 1%/2 mm, and 1%/1 mm, moderate or strong correlations were observed between the global and local gamma passing rates with both the Trilogy and TrueBeam STx systems, showing r values larger than 0.5 (all with $p < 0.001$). No correlations were observed between the global and local gamma passing rates with 3%/3 mm. For the TrueBeam STx, no distinctive differences in the correlations were observed between SABR and non-SABR VMAT plans.

For the ArcCHECK measurements, weak or no correlations between the global and local gamma passing rates were observed for every gamma criterion except for 3%/3 mm. With a gamma criterion of 3%/3 mm with the

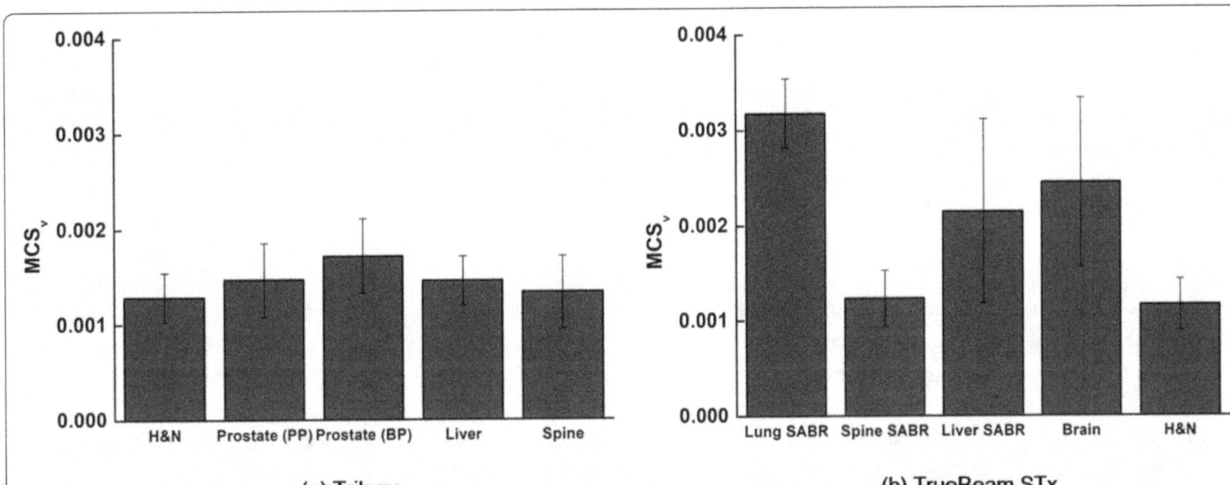

Fig. 4 Modulation complexity score for VMAT plans. Average values of the modulation complexity score for volumetric modulated arc therapy (MCS_v) for each treatment site are shown. The MCS_v of plans with the Trilogy (**a**) and the TrueBeam STx (**b**) are shown

Table 2 - Correlations between the global and local gamma passing rates

Gamma criteria	MapCHECK2 measurements		ArcCHECK measurements	
	r	*p*	*r*	*p*
Trilogy (C-series linac)				
3%/3 mm	0.218	0.010	0.540	< 0.001
2%/2 mm	0.621	< 0.001	0.440	< 0.001
2%/1 mm	0.642	< 0.001	0.339	< 0.001
1%/2 mm	0.806	< 0.001	0.469	< 0.001
1%/1 mm	0.770	< 0.001	0.325	< 0.001
TrueBeam STx (SABR + non-SABR)				
3%/3 mm	–	–	0.271	0.006
2%/2 mm	0.451	< 0.001	0.202	0.043
2%/1 mm	0.510	< 0.001	0.376	< 0.001
1%/2 mm	0.860	< 0.001	0.391	< 0.001
1%/1 mm	0.842	< 0.001	0.383	< 0.001
TrueBeam STx (SABR)				
3%/3 mm	–	–	0.409	0.001
2%/2 mm	0.332	0.010	0.318	0.013
2%/1 mm	0.531	< 0.001	0.519	< 0.001
1%/2 mm	0.845	< 0.001	0.460	< 0.001
1%/1 mm	0.851	< 0.001	0.480	< 0.001
TrueBeam STx (non-SABR)				
3%/3 mm	–	–	–	–
2%/2 mm	0.434	0.005	–	–
2%/1 mm	0.404	0.010	0.454	0.003
1%/2 mm	0.826	< 0.001	0.453	0.003
1%/1 mm	0.758	< 0.001	0.506	0.001

Note: Only *r* values with $p \leq 0.05$ are shown

Trilogy system, a moderate correlation ($r = 0.540$ with $p < 0.001$) was observed between the global and local gamma passing rates. For the SABR plans of the TrueBeam STx, a moderate correlation ($r = 0.519$ with $p < 0.001$) was observed between the global and local gamma passing rates with 2%/1 mm. No clear tendency was observed in the correlations between the global and local gamma passing rates with both the Trilogy and TrueBeam STx systems for the ArcCHECK measurements.

Correlations between the gamma passing rates of the MapCHECK2 and ArcCHECK measurements

The *r* values between the gamma passing rates of the MapCHECK2 and ArcCHECK measurements are shown in Table 3 with corresponding *p* values.

For the global gamma passing rates, no correlations between the gamma passing rates of the MapCHECK2 and ArcCHECK measurements were observed for every gamma criterion (all with $r < 0.3$).

Table 3 - Correlations between the gamma passing rates of MapCHECK2 and ArcCHECK

Gamma criteria	Global gamma passing rates		Local gamma passing rates	
	r	*p*	*r*	*p*
Trilogy (C-series linac)				
3%/3 mm	–	–	0.242	0.004
2%/2 mm	–	–	0.288	0.001
2%/1 mm	–	–	0.260	0.002
1%/2 mm	–	–	0.266	0.001
1%/1 mm	–	–	0.202	0.016
TrueBeam STx (SABR + non-SABR)				
3%/3 mm	–	–	0.365	< 0.001
2%/2 mm	–	–	0.412	< 0.001
2%/1 mm	–	–	0.528	< 0.001
1%/2 mm	–	–	0.468	< 0.001
1%/1 mm	–	–	0.589	< 0.001
TrueBeam STx (SABR)				
3%/3 mm	–	–	0.355	0.005
2%/2 mm	–	–	0.263	0.042
2%/1 mm	0.273	0.035	0.381	0.003
1%/2 mm	–	–	0.275	0.033
1%/1 mm	–	–	0.413	0.001
TrueBeam STx (non-SABR)				
3%/3 mm	–	–	0.369	0.019
2%/2 mm	–	–	0.629	< 0.001
2%/1 mm	–	–	0.729	< 0.001
1%/2 mm	–	–	0.637	< 0.001
1%/1 mm	–	–	0.745	< 0.001

Note: Only *r* values with $p \leq 0.05$ are shown

For the local gamma passing rates with the TrueBeam STx system, moderate correlations were observed between the gamma passing rates of the MapCHECK2 and ArcCHECK measurements with 2%/1 mm and 1%/1 mm ($r = 0.528$ with $p < 0.001$ for 2%/1 mm and $r = 0.589$ with $p < 0.001$ for 1%/1 mm). For the rest of the gamma passing rates with TrueBeam STx, weak correlations were observed (3%/3 mm, 2%/2 mm, and 1%/2 mm). To examine correlations of the non-SABR plans separately, strong correlations were observed except for the gamma passing rates with 3%/3 mm (all with $r > 0.6$ with $p < 0.001$). For the Trilogy system, no correlations were observed between the gamma passing rates of the two dosimeters.

Correlations between the gamma passing rates and the mechanical errors

The *r* values between the gamma passing rates and the MLC positional errors during the VMAT delivery are shown in Table 4 with corresponding *p* values.

Table 4 - Correlations between the gamma passing rates and the MLC positional errors

Gamma criteria	MapCHECK2 measurements				ArcCHECK measurements			
	Global gamma passing rates		Local gamma passing rates		Global gamma passing rates		Local gamma passing rates	
	r	*p*	*r*	*p*	*r*	*p*	*r*	*p*
Trilogy (C-series linac)								
3%/3 mm	0.213	0.011	– 0.447	< 0.001	–	–	–	–
2%/2 mm	–	–	– 0.183	0.031	0.307	< 0.001	–0.355	< 0.001
2%/1 mm	–	–	0.190	0.025	0.536	< 0.001	– 0.211	0.013
1%/2 mm	– 0.334	< 0.001	–	–	0.305	< 0.001	– 0.503	< 0.001
1%/1 mm	–	–	–	–	0.546	< 0.001	–0.374	< 0.001
TrueBeam STx (SABR + non-SABR)								
3%/3 mm	–	–	–0.339	0.001	–	–	–0.382	< 0.001
2%/2 mm	–0.358	< 0.001	–0.478	< 0.001	0.211	0.035	–0.369	< 0.001
2%/1 mm	–0.328	0.001	–0.394	< 0.001	0.458	< 0.001	–0.230	0.021
1%/2 mm	–0.554	< 0.001	–0.542	< 0.001	–	–	–0.478	< 0.001
1%/1 mm	–0.531	< 0.001	–0.502	< 0.001	0.316	0.001	–0.364	< 0.001
TrueBeam STx (non-SABR)								
3%/3 mm	–	–	–	–	–	–	–0.699	< 0.001
2%/2 mm	–0.336	0.034	–0.475	0.002	–	–	–0.593	< 0.001
2%/1 mm	–0.507	0.001	–0.470	0.002	0.463	0.003	–	–
1%/2 mm	–0.577	< 0.001	–0.584	< 0.001	–	–	– 0.619	< 0.001
1%/1 mm	– 0.740	< 0.001	– 0.622	< 0.001	0.348	0.028	–0.365	0.021

Note: Only *r* values with $p \leq 0.05$ are shown

For the MapCHECK2 measurements with Trilogy, both the global and local gamma passing rates always showed weak or no correlations with the MLC positional errors. In the case of TrueBeam STx, both the global and local gamma passing rates also showed weak or no correlations with the MLC positional errors except for the gamma passing rates with 1%/2 mm and 1%/1 mm, which showed moderate correlations ($r < -0.5$ with $p < 0.001$). To examine correlations of the non-SABR plans separately, a strong correlation was observed for the global gamma passing rates with 1%/1 mm ($r = -0.740$ with $p < 0.001$). The correlations of the non-SABR plans were generally higher than those of the SABR plans.

For the ArcCHECK measurements with Trilogy, the global gamma passing rates with 2%/1 mm and 1%/1 mm showed moderate correlations with the MLC errors ($r = 0.536$ with $p < 0.001$ for 2%/1 mm and $r = 0.546$ with $p < 0.001$ for 1%/1 mm). However, this is not reasonable because the *r* values were positive. Since the gamma passing rates should decrease with increasing the MLC errors, there should be negative correlations between the gamma passing rates and the MLC errors. The local gamma passing rate with 1%/2 mm showed a moderate negative correlation with the MLC errors ($r = -0.503$ with $p < 0.001$). In the case of TrueBeam STx, weak or no correlations were observed between the gamma passing rates and the MLC errors. To examine non-SABR plans separately, correlations of the local gamma passing rates with 3%/3 mm, 2%/2 mm, and 1%/2 mm showed moderate correlations to the MLC errors. Similarly to the MapCHECK2 results, the correlations of the non-SABR plans were generally higher than those of the SABR plans.

The *r* values between the gamma passing rates and the gantry angle errors during the VMAT delivery are shown in Table 5 with corresponding *p* values. Weak or no correlations were observed between the gamma passing rates and the gantry angle errors.

The *r* values between the gamma passing rates and the MU delivery errors are shown in Table 6 with corresponding *p* values. For the Trilogy, Weak or no correlations were observed between the gamma passing rates and the MU delivery errors always showing absolute *r* values smaller than 0.34. For the TrueBeam STx, local gamma passing rates of the SABR plans showed weak or moderate correlations to the MU delivery errors ($-0.59 < r < -0.39$ with $p < 0.003$) while both the global and local gamma passing rates of the non-SABR plans showed weak or no correlations to the MU delivery errors.

Correlations between the gamma passing rates and the MCS_v

The *r* values between the gamma passing rates and the MCS_v are shown in Table 7 with corresponding *p* values.

Table 5 - Correlations between the gamma passing rates and the gantry angle errors

Gamma criteria	MapCHECK2 measurements				ArcCHECK measurements			
	Global gamma passing rates		Local gamma passing rates		Global gamma passing rates		Local gamma passing rates	
	r	*p*	*r*	*p*	*r*	*p*	*r*	*p*
TrueBeam STx (SABR + non-SABR)								
2%/2 mm	–	–	–	–	– 0.258	0.010	–	–
1%/2 mm	–	–	–	–	– 0.242	0.015	–	–
TrueBeam STx (SABR)								
2%/2 mm	–	–	–	–	– 0.398	0.002	–	–
1%/2 mm	–	–	–	–	– 0.405	0.001	–	–
1%/1 mm	–	–	–	–	– 0.257	0.048	–	–
TrueBeam STx (non-SABR)								
2%/1 mm	–	–	–	–	0.347	0.028	–	–
1%/1 mm	–	–	–	–	0.333	0.035	–	–

Note: Only r values with $p \leq 0.05$ are shown

For the Trilogy, both the global and local gamma passing rates showed weak or no correlations except for the local gamma passing rates with 2%/1 mm from the ArcCHECK measurements ($r = 0.529$ with $p < 0.001$). For the TrueBeam STx, no correlations were observed.

Correlations of the gamma passing rates to the differences in the dose-volumetric parameters between the original plans and the plans reconstructed with log files

The r values of the gamma passing rates to the differences in the $D_{95\%}$ of the PTVs between the original plans

Table 6 - Correlations between the gamma passing rates and the MU delivery errors

Gamma criteria	MapCHECK2 measurements				ArcCHECK measurements			
	Global gamma passing rates		Local gamma passing rates		Global gamma passing rates		Local gamma passing rates	
	r	*p*	*r*	*p*	*r*	*p*	*r*	*p*
Trilogy (C-series linac)								
3%/3 mm	–	–	– 0.304	< 0.001	–	–	– 0.251	0.003
2%/2 mm	–0.191	0.024	–0.183	0.030	–	–	–0.312	< 0.001
2%/1 mm	–0.238	0.005	–	–	–	–	–0.323	< 0.001
1%/2 mm	–0.211	0.012	–	–	–	–	–0.305	< 0.001
1%/1 mm	–0.216	0.010	–	–	–	–	–0.330	< 0.001
TrueBeam STx (SABR + non-SABR)								
3%/3 mm	–	–	–	–	–0.270	0.007	–	–
2%/2 mm	0.236	0.018	–	–	–0.317	0.001	–	–
2%/1 mm	–	–	–	–	– 0.336	0.001	–	–
1%/2 mm	0.243	0.015	–	–	–	–	–	–
TrueBeam STx (SABR)								
3%/3 mm	–	–	–0.546	< 0.001	–	–	– 0.398	0.002
2%/2 mm	–	–	– 0.456	< 0.001	–	–	– 0.425	0.001
2%/1 mm	–0.452	< 0.001	– 0.581	< 0.001	–	–	– 0.519	< 0.001
1%/2 mm	– 0.491	< 0.001	– 0.441	< 0.001	–	–	– 0.422	0.001
1%/1 mm	– 0.625	< 0.001	– 0.583	< 0.001	–	–	– 0.496	< 0.001
TrueBeam STx (non-SABR)								
1%/2 mm	0.343	0.030	0.323	0.042	–	–	–	–
1%/1 mm	0.369	0.019	–	–	–	–	–	–

Note: Only r values with $p \leq 0.05$ are shown

Table 7 - Correlations between the gamma passing rates and the modulation complexity score

Gamma criteria	MapCHECK2 measurements				ArcCHECK measurements			
	Global gamma passing rates		Local gamma passing rates		Global gamma passing rates		Local gamma passing rates	
	r	*p*	*r*	*p*	*r*	*p*	*r*	*p*
Trilogy (C-series linac)								
3%/3 mm	0.193	0.023	0.448	< 0.001	–	–	0.340	< 0.001
2%/2 mm	0.268	0.001	0.392	< 0.001	–	–	0.378	< 0.001
2%/1 mm	0.433	< 0.001	0.352	< 0.001	–	–	0.529	< 0.001
1%/2 mm	0.311	< 0.001	0.238	0.005	–	–	0.282	0.001
1%/1 mm	0.482	< 0.001	0.268	0.001	–	–	0.453	< 0.001
TrueBeam STx								
3%/3 mm	–	–	–	–	−0.243	0.015	–	–
2%/1 mm	–	–	–	–	− 0.196	0.050	–	–

Note: Only *r* values with $p \leq 0.05$ are shown

and the reconstructed plans with log files are shown in Table 8 with corresponding *p* values. For both the Trilogy and TrueBeam STx, weak or no correlations were observed between the gamma passing rates and the changes in the $D_{95\%}$.

The *r* values of the gamma passing rates to the differences in the $V_{50\%}$ of the body structures between the original plans and the reconstructed plans with log files are shown in Table 9 with corresponding *p* values. Same as the results of the PTV $D_{95\%}$, weak or no correlations were observed for every case.

Discussion

In this study, the global gamma passing rates from the MapCHECK2 measurements contradict with those from ArcCHECK for both measurements with Trilogy and TrueBeam STx as shown in Fig. 1. Therefore, no correlations were observed between the global gamma passing rates of the MapCHECK2 and ArcCHECK measurements as shown in Table 3. In addition, except for the global gamma passing rate with 1%/2 mm, the global gamma passing rates with the Trilogy system indicated that the plan delivery accuracy of the prostate VMAT plans were the lowest showing the lowest gamma passing rates although the mechanical errors during the delivery were the lowest as shown in Fig. 3. The MLC positional errors, which are known to be the most dominant mechanical errors affecting the VMAT delivery accuracy, were always the highest for the H&N VMAT plans for both the Trilogy and TrueBeam STx systems [10, 26]. Furthermore, it is known that the modulation degree of prostate VMAT plans is lower than that of H&N VMAT plans with the SIB technique from various previous studies [5, 6, 12, 27]. In the case of H&N VMAT plans, owing to adjacent multiple target volumes with multiple prescription

Table 8 - Correlations between the gamma passing rates and the differences in the $D_{95\%}$ of PTVs between the original plans and the reconstructed plans with log files

Gamma criteria	MapCHECK2 measurements				ArcCHECK measurements			
	Global gamma passing rates		Local gamma passing rates		Global gamma passing rates		Local gamma passing rates	
	r	*p*	*r*	*p*	*r*	*p*	*r*	*p*
TrueBeam STx (SABR + non-SABR)								
3%/3 mm	–	–	–	–	–	–	− 0.225	0.025
2%/2 mm	–	–	− 0.264	0.008	–	–	− 0.240	0.016
2%/1 mm	–	–	− 0.238	0.017	–	–	− 0.274	0.006
1%/2 mm	−0.283	0.004	−0.294	0.003	–	–	−0.279	0.005
1%/1 mm	−0.333	0.001	−0.313	0.001	–	–	−0.318	0.001
TrueBeam STx (non-SABR)								
2%/2 mm	–	–	−0.326	0.040	–	–	–	–
2%/1 mm	–	–	−0.340	0.032	–	–	–	–
1%/2 mm	–	–	−0.323	0.042	–	–	–	–
1%/1 mm	−0.421	0.007	−0.436	0.005	–	–	–	–

Note: Only *r* values with $p \leq 0.05$ are shown

Table 9 - Correlations between the gamma passing rates and the differences in the $V_{50\%}$ of patient body between the original plans and the reconstructed plans with log files

Gamma criteria	MapCHECK2 measurements				ArcCHECK measurements			
	Global gamma passing rates		Local gamma passing rates		Global gamma passing rates		Local gamma passing rates	
	r	*p*	*r*	*p*	*r*	*p*	*r*	*p*
Trilogy (C-series linac)								
2%/1 mm	–	–	– 0.166	0.050	–	–	–	–
1%/1 mm	–	–	–0.187	0.027	–0.185	0.029	–	–
TrueBeam STx (SABR + non-SABR)								
3%/3 mm	–	–	–	–	–	–	–0.293	0.003
2%/2 mm	–	–	–	–	–	–	–0.327	0.001
2%/1 mm	–0.253	0.011	–	–	–	–	–0.328	0.001
1%/2 mm	–	–	–	–	–	–	–0.332	0.001
1%/1 mm	–0.254	0.011	–	–	–	–	–0.326	0.001
TrueBeam STx (SABR)								
2%/1 mm	–	–	–	–	–	–	–0.293	0.023
1%/2 mm	–	–	0.264	0.042	–	–	–	–
TrueBeam STx (non-SABR)								
3%/3 mm	–	–	–	–	–	–	–0.351	0.027
2%/2 mm	–	–	–	–	–	–	–0.351	0.027
1%/2 mm	–	–	–	–	–	–	–0.335	0.035

Note: Only *r* values with $p \leq 0.05$ are shown

doses, which requires a steep dose gradient between the target volumes, an overlap between the target volumes and OARs, such as parotid glands, and concave-shaped target volumes in the axial view to reduce the doses to the spinal cord and brain stem, the modulation degree of H&N VMAT plans is generally much higher than that of prostate VMAT plans. The values of MCS_v in this study also indicated that the modulation degrees of the H&N VMAT plans were the highest while those of the prostate VMAT plans were the lowest since the values of the MCS_v decrease as increasing the modulation degree of VMAT plans (Fig. 4) [9]. With the TrueBeam STx system, the global gamma passing rates from the ArcCHECK measurements indicated that the modulation degree of the lung SABR VMAT plans were the highest. In the case of lung SABR VMAT plans, because of a small target volume, a generally round-shaped target volume, and OARs generally located far from the target volume, the modulation degree of lung SABR VMAT is known to be low [28]. This can also be clearly identified in Fig. 3, which shows the lowest MLC positional errors and gantry angle errors. In addition, the MCS_v of the lung SABR VMAT plans indicated that the modulation degrees of the lung SABR VMAT plans were the lowest (Fig. 4). Since every VMAT plan analyzed in this study was clinically acceptable according to the previous study showing global gamma passing rates with 2%/2 mm of more than 95% [12], and the power of discrimination of the global gamma evaluation was relatively weak compared to the local gamma evaluation, it seems that the values of the global gamma passing rates could not always show the plan delivery accuracy minutely according to the modulation degree. The contradictory results between MapCHECK2 and ArcCHECK might be attributed to device setup errors or dosimeter response errors. On the contrary, the local gamma passing rates with MapCHECK2 generally showed similar results to those with ArcCHECK, both showing the lowest gamma passing rates of the H&N VMAT plans in general. The local gamma passing rates seem to be more reliable than the global gamma passing rates. The superior reliability of the local gamma passing rates to the global gamma passing rates can also be identified with the higher correlations of the local gamma passing rates between the MapCHECK2 and ArcCHECK dosimeters than those of the global gamma passing rates as shown in Table 3. No correlations were observed between the two dosimeters for the global gamma passing rates (all with $p >$ 0.05); however, weak or moderate correlations were observed for the local gamma passing rates with statistical significance (all with $p < 0.05$). Therefore, when using the gamma index analysis to verify the VMAT delivery accuracy, the local gamma index analysis seems more appropriate than the global gamma analysis in general. However, the local gamma index analysis did not always show consistency between the dosimeters and did not always show superior correlations to the mechanical errors (Tables 4, 5, and 6).

To compare the correlations between the global and local gamma passing rates from the MapCHECK2 measurements to those from the ArcCHECK measurements, the tendencies of those two dosimeters were different from each other. Weak or no correlations were observed for the ArcCHECK measurements, while strong correlations were observed for the MapCHECK2 measurements with tight gamma criteria ($r > 0.7$ with $p < 0.001$ with 1%/2 mm and 1%/1 mm). In addition, the correlations of the gamma passing rates from the MapCHECK2 measurements with the MLC positional errors were different from those from the ArcCHECK measurements. For the MapCHECK2 measurements, both the global and local gamma passing rates with 1%/2 mm and 1%/1 mm of the VMAT plans using TrueBeam STx showed moderate correlations with the MLC errors, while the local gamma passing rates with 1%/2 mm showed moderate correlations with the MLC errors for the ArcCHECK measurements.

Since TrueBeam STx delivers VMAT plans more accurately by the integrated control system, i.e., supervisor, than the C-series linac, the mechanical errors during the VMAT delivery of TrueBeam STx were smaller than those of Trilogy. This can be identified in the MLC and gantry angle errors from the log files shown in Fig. 3. Although the MU delivery errors of the TrueBeam STx system were higher than those of the Trilogy system, this was observed only in the SABR VMAT plans, which used a huge amount of MUs. For the fractionated VMAT plans, the MU delivery errors of TrueBeam STx were smaller than those of Trilogy. In addition, both the global and local gamma passing rates of the H&N VMAT plans with the TrueBeam STx system were always higher than those with Trilogy regardless of the gamma criteria.

To review the correlations of the gamma passing rates to the mechanical errors of SABR and non-SABR VMAT plans, the local gamma passing rates of the SABR VMAT plans showed higher correlations to the MU delivery errors than did the non-SABR VMAT plans (absolute values of $r > 0.39$ with $p < 0.003$) while those of the non-SABR VMAT plans showed higher correlations to the MLC errors than did the SABR VMAT plans (absolute values of $r > 0.36$ with $p < 0.03$ except the MapCHECK2 gamma passing rates with 3%/3 mm and the ArcCHECK gamma passing rates with 2%/1 mm). Since the SABR plans delivered relatively larger MUs at each control point than did the non-SABR plans, the MLC speeds during beam delivery were relatively lower than those of the non-SABR VMAT plans (data are not shown). On the contrary, the non-SABR plans delivered relatively smaller MUs at each control point than did the SABR plans, the MLC speeds during beam delivery were relatively higher than those of the SABR plans (data are not shown). Therefore, uncertainty in the MU delivery increased for the SABR plans while uncertainty in the MLC movements increased for the non-SABR plans (Fig. 3). In this respect, we acquired higher correlations of the gamma passing rates to the MU delivery errors for the SABR plans while higher correlations were observed between the gamma passing rates and the MLC errors for the non-SABR plans (Tables 4 and 6).

To review the correlations of the gamma passing rates to the dose-volumetric parameter differences ($D_{95\%}$ of the PTV and $V_{50\%}$ of the body) between the original treatment plan and the plans reconstructed with the log files, no distinctive correlations were observed same as the results of the previous study [18].

The limitation of the present study is that clinically unacceptable VMAT plans owing to huge discrepancies between the plan and the delivery were not included in the VMAT plans analyzed in this study. Therefore, we could not investigate the tolerance levels for the gamma index analyses in this study. Nevertheless, we found that the gamma passing rates depend on not only the modulation degree or errors in the VMAT plans, but also the types of gamma index analyses, dosimeters, gamma criteria, and types of linacs.

Conclusions

In this study, correlations between the global and local gamma passing rates varied according to the dosimeter type, linac type, and gamma criteria. In addition, the correlations between the gamma passing rates from different dosimeters were not strong and varied according to the type of the gamma index analysis, linac type, and gamma criteria. The correlations of the gamma passing rates with the MLC errors also varied according to the type of gamma analysis, type of dosimeters, and gamma criteria. Therefore, to utilize the gamma index analysis for the verification of the VMAT delivery accuracy, each institution should carefully establish their own gamma analysis protocol by determining the type of the gamma index analysis and gamma criterion with their own linac and dosimeter.

Abbreviations

AAA: Anisotropic analytic algorithm; DD: Dose difference; H&N: Head and neck; HD: High-definition; IMRT: Intensity-modulated radiation therapy; IRB: Institutional review board; MCS_v: Modulation complexity score for volumetric modulated arc therapy; MLC: Multileaf collimator; MU: Monitor unit; OAR: Organ at risk; PRO: Progressive resolution optimizer; QA: Quality assurance; SABR: Stereotactic ablative radiotherapy; VMAT: Volumetric modulated arc therapy

Funding

This study was supported by a grant from the National R&D Program for Cancer Control, Ministry of Health & Welfare, Republic of Korea (No. 1631200).

Authors' contributions

STK and DHO conceived the study concept, designed the study, and oversaw the completion of the study. JMP, JIK, and SYP participated in the experiments and collected the data. JMP and JIK analyzed the data, checked the data, and drafted the manuscript. All the authors read and approved the final manuscript. All the authors had full access to all the data and had final responsibility for the decision to submit for publication. All authors read and approved the final manuscript.

Competing interests

The authors declare that they have no competing interests.

Author details

[1]Department of Radiation Oncology, Seoul National University Hospital, Seoul, South Korea. [2]Institute of Radiation Medicine, Seoul National University Medical Research Center, Seoul, South Korea. [3]Biomedical Research Institute, Seoul National University Hospital, Seoul, South Korea. [4]Institute for Smart System, Robotics Research Laboratory for Extreme Environments, Advanced Institutes of Convergence Technology, Suwon, South Korea. [5]Department of Radiation Oncology, Veterans Health Service Medical Center, Seoul, South Korea. [6]Department of Radiation Oncology, Myongji Hospital, Goyang, South Korea. [7]Nuclear Emergency Division, Radiation Protection and Emergency Preparedness Bureau, Nuclear Safety and Security Commission, Seoul, South Korea.

References

1. Ezzell GA, Galvin JM, Low D, Palta JR, Rosen I, Sharpe MB, Xia P, Xiao Y, Xing L, Yu CX, et al. Guidance document on delivery, treatment planning, and clinical implementation of IMRT: report of the IMRT subcommittee of the AAPM radiation therapy committee. Med Phys. 2003;30:2089–115.
2. Zhang P, Happersett L, Hunt M, Jackson A, Zelefsky M, Mageras G. Volumetric modulated arc therapy: planning and evaluation for prostate cancer cases. Int J Radiat Oncol Biol Phys. 2010;76:1456–62.
3. Brahme A. Optimization of stationary and moving beam radiation therapy techniques. Radiother Oncol. 1988;12:129–40.
4. Otto K. Volumetric modulated arc therapy: IMRT in a single gantry arc. Med Phys. 2008;35:310–7.
5. Du W, Cho SH, Zhang X, Hoffman KE, Kudchadker RJ. Quantification of beam complexity in intensity-modulated radiation therapy treatment plans. Med Phys. 2014;41:021716.
6. Park JM, Park SY, Kim H. Modulation index for VMAT considering both mechanical and dose calculation uncertainties. Phys Med Biol. 2015;60: 7101–25.
7. Park SY, Park JM, Sung W, Kim IH, Ye SJ. Texture analysis on the edge-enhanced fluence of VMAT. Radiat Oncol. 2015;10:74.
8. Li R, Xing L. An adaptive planning strategy for station parameter optimized radiation therapy (SPORT): segmentally boosted VMAT. Med Phys. 2013;40:050701.
9. Masi L, Doro R, Favuzza V, Cipressi S, Livi L. Impact of plan parameters on the dosimetric accuracy of volumetric modulated arc therapy. Med Phys. 2013;40:071718.
10. Nicolini G, Clivio A, Cozzi L, Fogliata A, Vanetti E. On the impact of dose rate variation upon RapidArc implementation of volumetric modulated are therapy. Med Phys. 2011;38:264–71.
11. Fredh A, Scherman JB, Fog LS, Munck af Rosenschold P. Patient QA systems for rotational radiation therapy: a comparative experimental study with intentional errors. Med Phys. 2013;40:031716.
12. Heilemann G, Poppe B, Laub W. On the sensitivity of common gamma-index evaluation methods to MLC misalignments in Rapidarc quality assurance. Med Phys. 2013;40:031702.
13. Hussein M, Rowshanfarzad P, Ebert MA, Nisbet A, Clark CH. A comparison of the gamma index analysis in various commercial IMRT/VMAT QA systems. Radiother Oncol. 2013;109:370–6.
14. Low DA, Dempsey JF. Evaluation of the gamma dose distribution comparison method. Med Phys. 2003;30:2455–64.
15. Low DA, Harms WB, Mutic S, Purdy JA. A technique for the quantitative evaluation of dose distributions. Med Phys. 1998;25:656–61.
16. Van Dyk J, Barnett RB, Cygler JE, Shragge PC. Commissioning and quality assurance of treatment planning computers. Int J Radiat Oncol Biol Phys. 1993;26:261–73.
17. Jin X, Yan H, Han C, Zhou Y, Yi J, Xie C. Correlation between gamma index passing rate and clinical dosimetric difference for pre-treatment 2D and 3D volumetric modulated arc therapy dosimetric verification. Br J Radiol. 2015;88:20140577.
18. Nelms BE, Zhen H, Tome WA. Per-beam, planar IMRT QA passing rates do not predict clinically relevant patient dose errors. Med Phys. 2011;38:1037–44.
19. Rozendaal RA, Mijnheer BJ, van Herk M, Mans A. In vivo portal dosimetry for head-and-neck VMAT and lung IMRT: linking gamma-analysis with differences in dose-volume histograms of the PTV. Radiother Oncol. 2014;112:396–401.
20. Huang JY, Pulliam KB, McKenzie EM, Followill DS, Kry SF. Effects of spatial resolution and noise on gamma analysis for IMRT QA. J Appl Clin Med Phys. 2014;15:4690.
21. Almond PR, Biggs PJ, Coursey BM, Hanson WF, Huq MS, Nath R, Rogers DW. AAPM's TG-51 protocol for clinical reference dosimetry of high-energy photon and electron beams. Med Phys. 1999;26:1847–70.
22. Bailey DW, Spaans JD, Kumaraswamy LK, Podgorsak MB. The MapCHECK measurement uncertainty function and its effect on planar dose pass rates. J Appl Clin Med Phys. 2016;17:165–73.
23. Klein EE, Hanley J, Bayouth J, Yin FF, Simon W, Dresser S, Serago C, Aguirre F, Ma L, Arjomandy B, et al. Task group 142 report: quality assurance of medical accelerators. Med Phys. 2009;36:4197–212.
24. Neal B, Ahmed M, Kathuria K, Watkins T, Wijesooriya K, Siebers J. A clinically observed discrepancy between image-based and log-based MLC positions. Med Phys. 2016;43:2933–5.
25. Kutcher GJ, Coia L, Gillin M, Hanson WF, Leibel S, Morton RJ, Palta JR, Purdy JA, Reinstein LE, Svensson GK, et al. Comprehensive QA for radiation oncology: report of AAPM radiation therapy committee task group 40. Med Phys. 1994;21:581–618.
26. Park JM, Wu HG, Kim JH, Carlson JN, Kim K. The effect of MLC speed and acceleration on the plan delivery accuracy of VMAT. Br J Radiol. 2015;88: 20140698.
27. Kim JI, Choi CH, Wu HG, Kim JH, Kim K, Park JM. Correlation analysis between 2D and quasi-3D gamma evaluations for both intensity-modulated radiation therapy and volumetric modulated arc therapy. Oncotarget. 2016; 8(3):5449–59.
28. Kim JI, Park SY, Kim HJ, Kim JH, Ye SJ, Park JM. The sensitivity of gamma-index method to the positioning errors of high-definition MLC in patient-specific VMAT QA for SBRT. Radiat Oncol. 2014;9:167.

8

A remote EPID-based dosimetric TPS-planned audit of centers for clinical trials: outcomes and analysis of contributing factors

Narges Miri[1], Kimberley Legge[1], Kim Colyvas[1], Joerg Lehmann[1,2], Philip Vial[3,4], Alisha Moore[5], Monica Harris[5] and Peter B. Greer[1,2*]

Abstract

Background: A novel remote method for external dosimetric TPS-planned auditing of intensity modulated radiotherapy (IMRT) and volumetric modulated arc therapy (VMAT) for clinical trials using electronic portal imaging device (EPID) has been developed. The audit has been applied to multiple centers across Australia and New Zealand. This work aims to assess the audit outcomes and explores the variables that contributed to the audit results.

Methods: Thirty audits were performed of 21 radiotherapy facilities, 17 facilities underwent IMRT audits and 13 underwent VMAT audits. The assessment was based on comparisons between the delivered doses derived from images acquired with EPIDs and planned doses from the local treatment planning systems (TPS). Gamma pass-rate (GPR) and gamma mean value (GMV) were calculated for each IMRT field and VMAT arc (total 268 comparisons). A multiple variable linear model was applied to the GMV results (3%/3 mm criteria) to assess the influence and significance of explanatory variables. The explanatory variables were Linac-TPS combination, TPS grid resolution, IMRT/VMAT delivery, age of EPID, treatment site, record and verification system (R&V) type and dose-rate. Finally, the audit results were compared with other recent audits by calculating the incidence ratio (IR) as a ratio of the observed mean/median GPRs for the remote audit to the other audits.

Results: The average (± 1 SD) of the centers' GPRs were: 99.3 ± 1.9%, 98.6 ± 2.7% & 96.2 ± 5.5% at 3%, 3 mm, 3%, 2 mm and 2%, 2 mm criteria respectively. The most determinative variables on the GMVs were Linac-TPS combination, TPS grid resolution and IMRT/VMAT delivery type. The IR values were 1 for seven comparisons, indicating similar GPRs of the remote audit with the reference audits and > 1 for four comparisons, indicating higher GPRs of the remote audit than the reference audits.

Conclusion: The remote dosimetry audit method for clinical trials demonstrated high GPRs and provided results comparable to established more resource-intensive audit methods. Several factors were found to influence the results including some effect of Linac-TPS combination.

Keywords: Auditing, Dosimetry, Electronic portal imaging device

* Correspondence: peter.greer@newcastle.edu.au
[1]University of Newcastle, Newcastle, NSW, Australia
[2]Calvary Mater Newcastle, Newcastle, NSW, Australia
Full list of author information is available at the end of the article

Background

Starting in the mid-1990s, multileaf collimators (MLCs) were introduced to linear accelerators (linacs) to deliver a highly conformal dose to the patients. Inverse planning algorithms were added to treatment planning systems (TPSs) to plan the delivered dose when MLCs were used to modulate the profiles of beams. Intensity modulated beams formed the foundation of intensity modulated radiotherapy (IMRT) and volumetric modulated arc therapy (VMAT) deliveries [1]. Machine and patient specific quality assurance (QA) measurements are taken by local physicists to ensure accuracy and stability of IMRT/VMAT deliveries. The European Society for Radiotherapy and Oncology (ESTRO) recommends an additional external audit for independent verification [2]. Additionally, in the context of clinical trials, a dosimetry audit provides a controlled environment to minimize dependency of the outcome on stochastic and systematic errors that can reduce the trial cost and enhance the outcome reliability [3]. Conventionally, an auditing center performs the assessment by site visit(s) or by mailing phantoms and dosimeters [4, 5].

Remote auditing can significantly reduce the audit costs while enhancing the efficiency. Recently, a novel approach was introduced to remotely audit IMRT and VMAT deliveries [6, 7]. The method is termed the Virtual EPID Standard Phantom Audit (VESPA) and it is based on images from electronic portal imaging devices (EPIDs) and image to dose conversion models [8–11]. In VESPA, the audit center provides instructions and CT data for participants to produce benchmarking plans using their local TPS. These plans are then transferred to two provided virtual water phantoms and the doses exported. The participants deliver the dose in air to their EPID and send the corresponding images together with calibration images and their planning data to the audit center. The image signals are converted to dose in the virtual phantoms using in-house developed software. The method combines the cost and efficiency benefits of remote audits with a standardized measurement and analysis process using EPIDs. Details of the method and feasibility of the approach have been reported in a pilot study for six centers [7].

This work aims to assess the VESPA audit outcomes and explores the contribution of several explanatory variables to the overall outcomes of the audit. Results are presented for 30 audits from 21 treatment centers in terms of gamma analysis for multiple criteria. A multi-variable model was developed to understand whether the audit was sensitive to differences in equipment of the centers or other factors. Finally, the audit outcome was compared with other recent audits to assess whether the VESPA audit is consistent with conventional audit approaches.

Methods

Equipment

Participants were radiotherapy centers from Australia and New Zealand who were already treating patients with IMRT or VMAT and required credentialing for clinical trials by the Trans-Tasman Radiation Oncology Group (TROG). Additional file 1 provides details of the centers and their planning and treatment equipment. Of the 21 centers, 17 participated in the IMRT audit and 13 in the VMAT audit. TROG supplied a head and neck (HN) and a post-prostatectomy (PP) trial benchmarking plan case including CT datasets and planning instructions (TROG trials 12.01 HPV and 08.03 RAVES). Additionally CT datasets of two standard virtual water-equivalent QA phantoms were also provided; a virtual flat phantom (VFP) of 30 cm height, 40 cm width, 40 cm length and a virtual cylindrical phantom (VCP) of 20 cm diameter and 40 cm length. A separate EPID guide was included in the audit instructions to assist with calibration and data acquisition. As centers either submitted one or two plans for their audit, a total of 27 IMRT plans and 19 VMAT plans were submitted resulting in 268 individual IMRT fields or VMAT arcs.

Planning and measurements

Each center planned the HN and PP trial patients on the provided patient datasets for IMRT or VMAT following the benchmarking instructions. A dose of 70 Gy was prescribed in 35 fractions for the HN plan and 64 Gy in 32 fractions for the PP plan. Except for one case at 10 MV these all were planned and delivered at 6 MV energy. The plans were then transferred onto the two supplied virtual phantoms within the local planning system. For 2D planar dose calculations the individual IMRT fields and VMAT arcs were transferred to the VFP at perpendicular incidence (zero gantry angle). This required collapsing all gantry angles to zero for the VMAT plans. For calculation of composite 3D dose the plans were transferred to the VCP at actual gantry angles. The phantoms were positioned at 90 cm source to surface distance (SSD). These verification plan doses were then exported in DICOM format. A DICOM-RT format TPS plan was also provided for calibration purposes.

All EPID measurements were made in-air with no phantom or treatment couch present. For the IMRT audit an integrated image for each field was acquired both at gantry zero and at actual gantry angles. For the VMAT audit EPID cine-images with 5 frames averaged per image were acquired continuously throughout the delivery of each arc and the acquired angle for each cine-image was recorded. These were summed to obtain an integrated image for each arc. A calibration plan was also provided to determine EPID positioning and sag with gantry angle as well as to calibrate EPID signal to dose. The centers exported their images and TPS doses and uploaded them via the cloud to the auditing site for assessment.

Analysis

All analysis was performed by the auditing site using in-house software developed in MATLAB (The Mathworks, Natick, USA). Integrated images of each individual IMRT field and VMAT arc delivery were used to reconstruct 2D dose planes at 10 cm depth in the VFP. Details of the method to calculate dose in phantom from EPID images have been detailed previously [7, 8]. For calculation of composite 3D dose in the VCP, a similar method to Ansbacher [12] was used with the IMRT images at actual gantry angles and the cine images for VMAT delivery. These were converted to dose in the VCP using the same dose conversion model as for the 2D individual field analysis but with additional contour correction and percentage depth dose modelling to derive 3D dose.

An in-house developed gamma (γ) algorithm was used for the dose comparison. All doses above 10% of the maximum dose were assessed with a search region of 0.6 cm radius. The gamma function used a global dose difference criteria defined as a percentage of the maximum dose. For 2D dose planes from individual fields or arcs, 2D gamma analysis was employed with the TPS dose map interpolated to the EPID resolution. Gamma pass-rate (GPR) and gamma mean values (GMV) were calculated for each 2D dose plane comparison for the individual IMRT fields and VMAT arcs (268 comparisons). The GPR is the percentage of assessed points that have a gamma score of less than or equal to 1. The GMV is the mean of the gamma scores of all assessed points in the 2D distribution. Similarly GPR and GMV were calculated for the composite 3D dose distributions using 3D gamma analysis with both dose distributions interpolated to 0.4 times the distance-to-agreement metric.

A multivariable linear model was made for quantitative assessment of the significance/contribution of different (explanatory) variables on the overall outcome of the audit. This is a standard statistical technique to examine the influence of different variables on an overall result. Explanatory variables that were chosen were Linac-TPS combination, TPS calculation grid resolution, IMRT or VMAT delivery, age of EPID, treatment site (HN or PP), record and verification (R&V) system type and nominal dose-rate. The EPID to dose conversion method was developed using measured doses in water and EPID images from Varian Clinac linear accelerator for aS1000 type EPID [8] and Truebeam linear accelerators for aS1200 type EPID [10, 11] at a center with Eclipse planning system. Therefore this will examine whether the Varian and Truebeam combinations with Eclipse produce higher pass-rates than other combinations. The other variables were chosen based on available data from each center for the audit. The linear model was based on analysis of least squares of the GMVs for the 268 *2D dose planes* in the audit. The influence of the explanatory variables was studied through both visual and statistical assessment. The visual assessment was made by scatterplot of the audit GMVs versus each variable. The Tukey-Kramer honest significance test (HSD) and student's t-test were used for assessment of the significance of the differences in results due to the explanatory variables. Statistical studies were performed in JMP software [13].

Finally, to assess the consistency of the VESPA audit with other reported audits, the results were compared with published results. To this purpose, the incidence ratio (IR) was calculated as the ratio of the observed GPR for the VESPA audit to the reference audit. Comparisons should be 'stable' if the range for the 95% confidence interval is 'small', i.e. < 0.5. The 95% confidence interval was calculated using:

$$IR \pm 1.96 \left. \frac{IR}{\sqrt{(\#\text{of observed planes})}} \right)$$

Results

Figure 1(a) and (c) demonstrate the spread of GPRs and GMVs for different criteria for the measured planar IMRT fields and VMAT arcs. Maximum GPRs were 100.0% and minimum GPRs were 84.9%, 76.4% and 62.7% for 3%/3 mm, 3%/2 mm and 2%/2 mm criteria respectively. The mean GPRs and GMVs are shown in Table 1. Normal quantiles are plotted for both GPRs and GMVs in Fig. 1(b) and (d). As these figures suggest, more linearity is visually observed for GMV than GPR, indicating better normal distribution of GMV.

The composite 3D dose distributions were analysed for the HN and PP plans in the VCP. Figure 2(a) illustrates the GPRs and Fig. 2(b) the GMVs for the 3D gamma analysis. The maximum GPRs were 100.0%, 99.9% and 99.1% and the minimum GPRs were 80.6%, 56.6% and 26.4% for 3%/3 mm, 3%/2 mm and 2%/2 mm criteria respectively. Mean GPRs (±1SD) were 97.7 (3.3)%, 92.5 (8.0)% and 80.8 (14.5)% for the same criteria.

A multiple variable linear model was made using the GMVs for the 2D dose plane comparisons. Table 2 summarizes the model outcome for the explanatory variables. The most influential variables in determining the results were Linac-TPS combination, TPS grid resolution and delivery type (IMRT or VMAT). The least

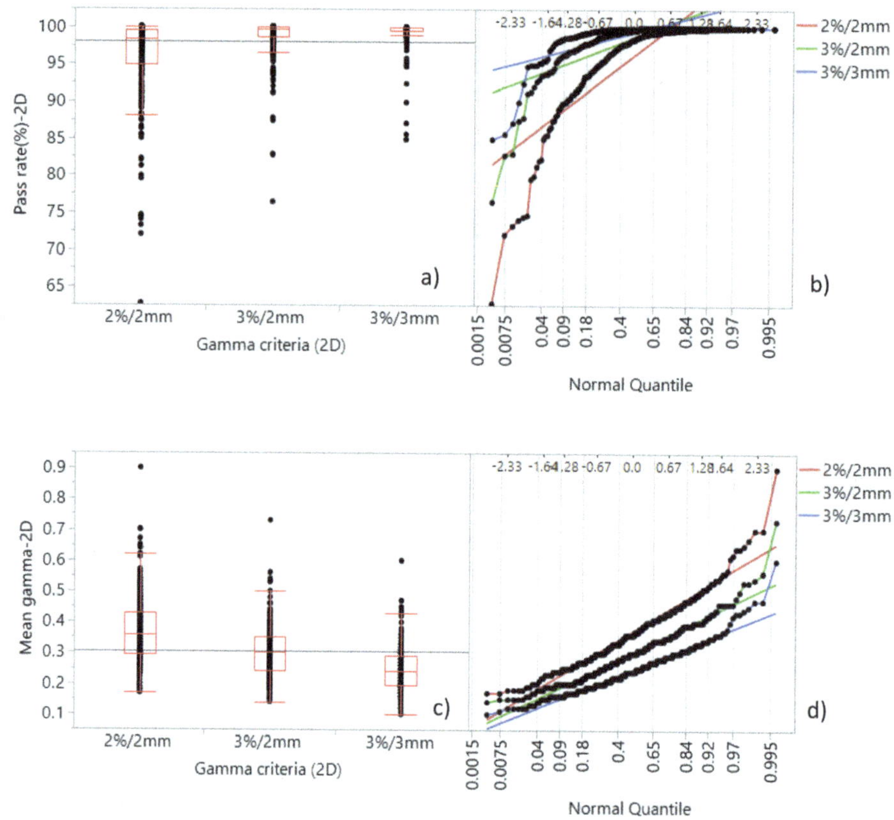

Fig. 1 Gamma analysis results and normal quantile linearity for the 2D dose plane comparisons for 268 IMRT fields and VMAT arcs at 3%/3 mm, 3%/2 mm and 2%/2 mm criteria. The normal quantile linearity indicates normality of distributions. **a** GPRs; **b** GPR normal quantile; **c** GMVs; **d** GMV normal quantile

significant variables were EPID age, treatment site, record and verification system and dose-rate.

Figure 3 shows GPR and GMV scatterplots for the three most significant explanatory variables. The 1st plot for Linac-TPS combination shows some apparent distinctions between results for different combinations of linear accelerator and TPS type. The other two variables were colored according to the Linac-TPS combination.

Figure 4 contains plots of GMVs (3%, 3 mm) estimated marginal means (EMM, named lsmeans in JMP) and 95% CIs for the three variables with significant effects in the model. Follow-up testing of the significant differences (Tukey-Kramer HSD/student's t test) between the means for the significant variables led to the following interpretations. For Linac-TPS, TB-Eclipse had a significantly lower mean than all other combinations (except TB-Pinnacle). The 4 combinations Elekta-Monaco, Elekta-Pinnacle, Varian-Monaco and Varian-Pinnacle were not significantly different to each other and appear to form a group with similarly high levels. There was some support for TB-Pinnacle and Varian-Eclipse having somewhat lower levels than the high group of 4 with 4 instances of significantly lower means (TB-Pinnacle lower than Varian-Monaco, Varian-Pinnacle and Elekta-Pinnacle, Varian-Eclipse lower than Varian-Pinnacle). For TPS grid, resolution 0.25 cm had higher GMV than the other two conditions which were both the same. For delivery, VMAT was higher than IMRT. Additional file 1 lists the test results.

Table 1 Summary of the 2D audit gamma results

Gamma criteria	GPR (1 SD)	GMV (1 SD)
2%,2 mm	96.2 (5.5)%	0.37 (0.11)
3%,2 mm	98.6 (2.7)%	0.30 (0.09)
3%,3 mm	99.3 (1.9)%	0.25 (0.07)

Table 3 summarises the gamma comparisons at 2%/2 mm between VESPA and five conventional audits. Comparisons were made as variable specific as possible based on the published data, resulting in 16 comparisons. For the comparisons, 5 out of 16 were unstable as their interval range was quite 'wide', > = 0.5, and no conclusion was made for them. Among stable comparisons, 7 indicated similar pass rates of the VESPA with other audits (IR = 1) and 4 comparisons demonstrated higher pass rates for VESPA than the other audits (IR > 1).

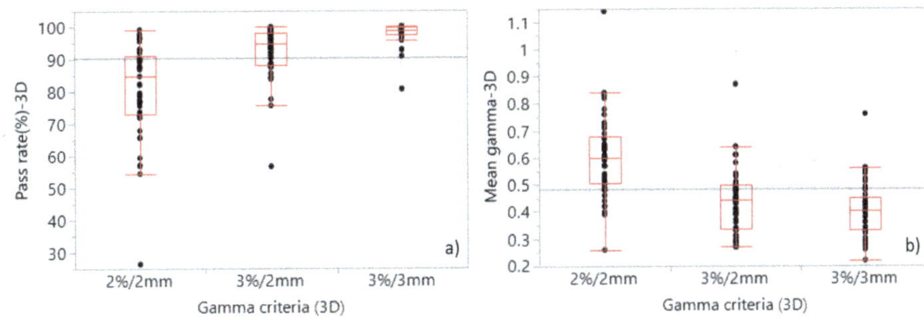

Fig. 2 a GPRs and (**b**) GMVs for composite 3D dose analysis for the plans

Discussion

The 3D composite dose audit results showed lower GPRs and larger GMVs than the 2D individual field/arc dose plane audit results. The 3D analysis could not currently be performed with 3%, 2 mm criteria as recommended by TG218 report for pre-treatment QA methods while the 2D analysis would meet this criteria. However the 3D analysis is sensitive to gantry angle errors as the dose for each image is calculated with the acquired gantry angle and is therefore an important component of the audit. The EPID measurement is inherently 2D and to estimate a 3D dose distribution in the virtual cylindrical phantom requires modelling of percentage depth dose. For the VESPA audit a single field percentage depth dose model was used which was also center independent. Improvement using a field-size specific and/or center-specific depth dose model could be explored. As a result the GMVs from the 2D individual field/arc dose comparisons were used for the statistical analysis in this paper.

Linac-TPS combination was found to influence the audit results. The Linac-TPS combination was used in the analysis rather than as separate variables due to the lack of spread of TPS type across all linac types which could bias results. The TB-Eclipse and TB-Pinnacle combinations were particularly found to result in lower GMV results. There are many potential reasons for this related both to this combination and the audit methodology. The Truebeam systems are a modern linac platform with high specifications for isocentre accuracy and other parameters. They have very accurate EPID positioning with active correction of EPID sag with gantry angle. The newer aS1200 imager does not have significant backscatter artifact which improves their performance for dosimetry. Plan complexity was not captured in the audit but could potentially have an effect. Future audits will include this parameter.

Table 2 Effect of the explanatory variables on overall audit results. The columns have been ordered according the significance of each variable on the results

Variable	LogWorth	*p*
Linac - TPS	12.824	0.00000
TPS grid resolution	4.782	0.00002
IMRT/VMAT Delivery	3.855	0.00014
EPID age-5ys	2.030	0.00933
Treatment site	0.976	0.10561
R&V	0.814	0.15353
Dose rate	0.011	0.97501

Centers were requested to produce the VFP and VCP plans at 0.2 cm or lower resolution although some submitted 0.25 cm resolution plans. The statistical analysis showed that the 0.25 cm resolution gave inferior results. The gamma algorithm used interpolates the TPS data to a high resolution to match the EPID resolution however this is clearly insufficient to counter the effect of the poor TPS resolution. Future audits will mandate the 0.2 cm or lower resolution based on these results. Another interesting finding was that the IMRT results showed lower GMV than the VMAT results. A possible explanation for this could be that the IMRT fields are acquired at fixed gantry angles and the data are corrected for EPID sag at these angles. However the VMAT acquires cine images during rotation and combines these into a single integrated image for 2D analysis. The individual cine images are not corrected for EPID sag and so the effect of this is likely to be greater and result in some blurring of the dose in the integrated image.

The VESPA audit is a TPS-planned audit not and end-to-end audit. These type of audits target a specific technology such as IMRT or VMAT and the CT scan of the phantom is typically provided to the center for planning. Comparing VESPA to other TPS-planned audits, the GPRs were similar to those from Clark et al. [14] for their audit of Varian VMAT deliveries conducted with the Octavius dosimetry system. While the VESPA results were higher for Elekta systems, the variability of these results meant that conclusions could not be drawn. For TPS systems the results were similar except for Pinnacle systems where the VESPA results had higher GPRs. For

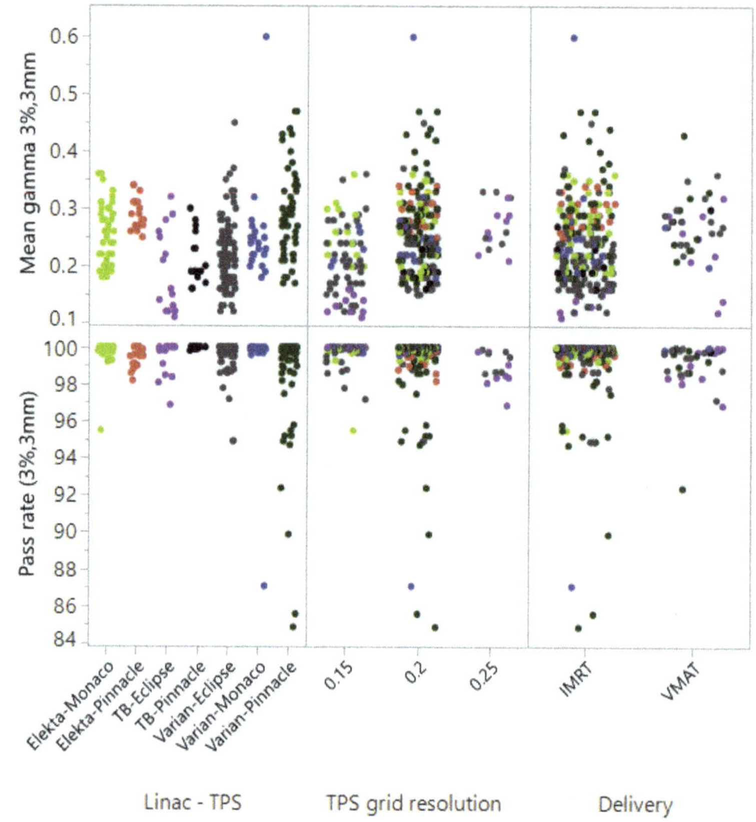

Fig. 3 Scatterplot of the GMVs and the GPRs for the 2D dose plane comparisons of the audit versus the most significant explanatory variables (Linac-TPS combination, dose grid resolution and delivery type)

IMRT audits as well as the Monaco TPS system, significantly higher GPRs were found for VESPA compared to the ArcCheck based audit of Eaton et al. [15].

For the VESPA audit as for most audits and in-house pre-treatment quality assurance the pass/fail criteria were arbitrarily set. It was not possible to know the uncertainties in a particular centers' TPS data or linac measurements. Pass/fail criteria could be set for future audits based on a statistical analysis of the current audit so that outlier centers could be identified. However the future audit would have to use a similar methodology and the same EPID to dose conversion model.

There are some limitations of this study. The measurement equipment are not completely standardized with differences between Varian EPID types (aS1000, aS1200) and Elekta imagers as well as equipment age. Data was collected on EPID response linearity as part of the study to ensure consistent results. 2D dose plane analysis is not ideal particularly for VMAT deliveries where a composite dose analysis would be preferred. By improving

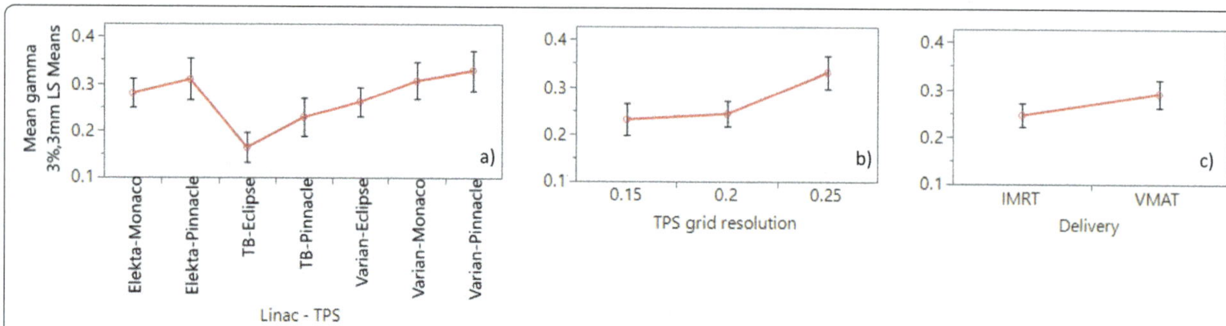

Fig. 4 Plot of GMV for the three explanatory variables that showed most influence on the audit results (Linac-TPS combination, TPS dose grid resolution and IMRT/VMAT delivery)

Table 3 Comparison of the VESPA audit results with other recent audits. The GPRs are compared at 2%/2 mm criteria

Ref	Variable	Compare group γ GPR % (no)	VESPA study γ GPR % (no)	IR (95% CI)	Range	Significance/stability
1- [14]	Linac type	Median				
	Varian	96.7 (25)	96.8 (26)	1.0 (0.8–1.2)	0.4	Insignificant/stable
	TB		96.2 (12)	–		
	TPS type	Median				
	Eclipse	97.3 (22)	96.3 (26)	1.0 (0.8–1.2)	0.4	Insignificant/stable
	Monaco	98.8 (4)	98.5 (2)	1.0 (0.9–1.1)	0.2	Insignificant/stable
	Pinnacle	88.7 (6)	96.1 (10)	1.1 (1.0–1.2)	0.2	Significant/stable
2-[15]	Delivery type	Mean				
	IMRT	90.0 (23)	96.3 (230)	1.1 (0.9–1.3)	0.4	Significant/stable
	VMAT	93.0 (31)	95.5 (38)	1.0 (0.8–1.2)	0.4	Insignificant/stable
	TPS type	Mean				
	Eclipse	95.0 (21)	98.0 (113)	1.0 (0.8–1.2)	0.4	Insignificant/stable
	Monaco	84.0 (5)	96.4 (68)	1.1 (0.9–1.4)	0.5	Significant/unstable
	Pinnacle	91.7 (19)	93.7 (87)	1.0 (0.8–1.2)	0.4	Insignificant/stable
	Treatment site	Mean				
	H&N	90.0 (25)	95.2 (135)	1.1 (0.8–1.3)	0.5	Significant/unstable
	Pelvic	93.0 (10)	97.2 (133)	1.0 (0.8–1.3)	0.5	Insignificant/unstable
5-[21]	Delivery type	Mean				
	IMRT	92.0 (155)	96.3 (230)	1.0 (0.8–1.3)	0.5	Insignificant/unstable
6-[22]	IMRT/VMAT	Mean				
		90.0 (1265)	96.2 (268)	1.1 (0.9–1.3)	0.4	Significant/stable
7-[23]	VMAT	Mean				
		88.0 (118)	95.5 (38)	1.1 (0.9–1.3)	0.4	Significant/stable

the 3D calculation model, it should be possible to audit centers using 3D dose distribution methods with more sensitive criteria (e.g. 3%, 2 mm). Another possibility is to use dose-volume-histogram methods where the ratio of 2D doses is backprojected through the benchmark CT plan and hence percentage depth dose modelling is not required. Elekta linacs are not currently audited for VMAT using VESPA due to difficulties in obtaining cine images and gantry angle information. This is possible with Elekta's newer hardware and software (version 3.41) and a licence to access pixel scaling information, however these were not available at the time of the audit.

The EPID to dose conversion models were developed based on Varian Clinac and Truebeam measured beam data for single linacs and has been applied to multiple linacs of the same type. The model derived on Varian Clinac was applied to the Elekta linacs for this audit. Comparison of the field-size responses for the Elekta and Varian linacs using the TPS calibration plan data (2×2 to 25×25 cm^2 fields) showed that there was a small difference in the average field size factor for the two linac types of maximum 2.1% for the smallest field, and average 0.6%. The field size factors from dose derived from Elekta images of the above fields compared to the TPS data showed greater differences than for Varian/TB centers' data. The average of the absolute difference was 1.2% for Elekta and 0.6% for Varian/TB. Recently a model derived with Elekta measured data was compared to the Varian derived model for Elekta linacs in a separate study that has been submitted for publication. The improvement in results was small and not sufficient to affect the results of the current study.

Though not an end-to-end audit, the VESPA method provides a potentially inexpensive and rapid method to perform dosimetric auditing for specific assessments of new technologies. It takes about 2–4 h to do the planning and delivery. There are several commercial systems available that perform 2D planar EPID dosimetry including but not limited to PortalVision (Varian Medical Systems), Epiqa (Epidose), Epibeam (Dosisoft), and PerFraction (Sun Nuclear) [16, 17]. Some of these systems incorporate simple EPID support-arm backscatter corrections which apply to Varian R and E-Arm systems [18–20]. Currently the analysis is based on in-house software. This software has several advantages over commercial systems in that it has a sophisticated kernel-based backscatter correction; it accounts for EPID sag with gantry angle; and it allows 3D dose determination particularly for VMAT using cine-imaging. This software is not currently commercially available however the authors consider requests from users for the software wherever possible. In principle the VESPA method can be applied in exactly the same way to flattening filter free (FFF) beams however there are currently hardware limitations for imaging these high-dose rate beams on the older EPID systems that are still prevalent. The newer Varian and Elekta EPID systems have FFF imaging capability. The EPID to dose conversion method has also not to date been developed or benchmarked for small field dosimetry auditing.

Conclusion

A new EPID-based remote dosimetric TPS-planned auditing method (VESPA) has been successfully applied to 30 audits of IMRT and VMAT for 21 centers across Australia and New Zealand. 2D dose-plane analysis was found to give more consistent results than 3D analysis. Statistical analysis of the results showed that there was some influence of Linac-TPS combinations on the results. This work shows that the remote EPID method can be used to audit centers with gamma pass-rates comparable or higher than other recent audits.

Abbreviations

2D: Two-dimensional; 3D: Three-dimensional; CI: Confidence interval; CT: Computed tomography; EPID: Electronic portal imaging device; GMV: Gamma mean value; GPR: Gamma pass rate; HN: Head and neck; HSD: Honest significance test; IMRT: Intensity modulated radiation therapy; IR: Incidence ratio; Linac: Linear accelerator; MLC: Multi-leaf collimator; PP: Post-prostatectomy; QA: Quality assurance; R&V: Record and verify; SSD: Source-surface distance; TB: Truebeam; TPS: Treatment planning system; TROG: Trans-Tasman Radiation Oncology Group; VCP: Virtual cylindrical phantom; VESPA: Virtual epid standard phantom audit; VFP: Virtual flat phantom; VMAT: Volumetric modulated arc therapy

Acknowledgements

The authors are grateful for the assistance of the many physicists and therapists at the remote centers who planned the benchmark cases and measured EPID data. The authors are grateful to the University of Newcastle, TROG Cancer research and Calvary Mater Newcastle for funding for NM.

Funding

Narges Miri is a receipient of a University of Newcastle PhD scholarship. PhD stipend funding was also provided by the University of Newcastle, TROG Cancer Research and the Calvary Mater Newcastle Hospital. This study design, collection, analysis and interpretation of data was performed independently of the funding bodies.

Authors' contributions

NM, KL, KC, PBG developed analysis methods, and performed data analysis. NM wrote the manuscript. PV developed audit methodology for Elekta. AM, MH provided data collection and management, audit requirements, liason with centers, interpretation of results. PBG wrote the auditing instructions, developed analysis software, edited the manuscript and liased with centers. All authors read and approved the final manuscript.

Competing interests

The authors declare that they have no competing interests.

Author details

[1]University of Newcastle, Newcastle, NSW, Australia. [2]Calvary Mater Newcastle, Newcastle, NSW, Australia. [3]Liverpool and Macarthur Cancer Therapy Centres and Ingham Institute, Liverpool, NSW, Australia. [4]University of Sydney, Sydney, NSW, Australia. [5]TROG Cancer Research, Newcastle, NSW, Australia.

References

1. Cheung K. Intensity modulated radiotherapy: advantages, limitations and future developments. Biomed Imaging Interv J. 2006;2(1):e19.
2. Alber M, Broggi S, De Wagter C, Eichwurzel I, Engstrom P, Fiorino C, Dietmar G, Hartmann G, Knoos T, Leal A, Marjnissen H, Mijnheer B, Paiusco M, Sanchez-Doblado F, Schmidt R, Tomse M, Welleweerd H. Booklet 9: Guidelines for the verification of IMRT. Brussels: European Society for Radiotherapy and Oncology; 2008.
3. Clark CH, Aird EG, Bolton S, Miles EA, Nisbet A, Snaith JA, Thomas RA, Venables K, Thwaites DI. Radiotherapy dosimetry audit: three decades of improving standards and accuracy in UK clinical practice and trials. Br J Radiol. 2015;88(1055):20150251.
4. Ibbott GS, Molineu A, Followill DS. Independent evaluations of IMRT through the use of an anthropomorphic phantom. Technol Cancer Res Treat. 2006;5(5):481–7.
5. Molineu A, Hernandez N, Nguyen T, Ibbott G, Followill D. Credentialing results from IMRT irradiations of an anthropomorphic head and neck phantom. Med Phys. 2013;40(2):022101.
6. Miri N, Lehmann J, Legge K, Vial P, Greer PB. Virtual EPID standard phantom audit (VESPA) for remote IMRT and VMAT credentialing. Phys Med Biol. 2017;62(11):4293–9.
7. Miri N, Lehmann J, Legge K, Zwan BJ, Vial P, Greer PB. Remote dosimetric auditing for intensity modulated radiotherapy: a pilot study. Phys Imaging Radiat Oncol. 2017;4:26–31.
8. King BW, Morf D, Greer PB. Development and testing of an improved dosimetry system using a backscatter shielded electronic portal imaging device. Med Phys. 2012;39(5):2839–47.
9. King BW, Greer PB. A method for removing arm backscatter from EPID images. Med Phys. 2013;40(7):071703.
10. Miri N, Keller P, Zwan BJ, Greer P. EPID-based dosimetry to verify IMRT planar dose distribution for the aS1200 EPID and FFF beams. J Appl Clin Med Phys. 2016;17(6):292–304.
11. Keller P, Baltes C, Dikaiou K, Zwan B, Greer PB. EPID image to dose conversion on Varian's aS1200. In: 13th annual conference on electronic patient imaging; 2014.
12. Ansbacher W. Three-dimensional portal image-based dose reconstruction in a virtual phantom for rapid evaluation of IMRT plans. Med Phys. 2006; 33(9):3369–82.
13. Schlotzhauer SD. Elementary statistics using JMP. Cary: SAS Institute; 2007.

15. Eaton DJ, Tyler J, Backshall A, Bernstein D, Carver A, Gasnier A, Henderson J, Lee J, Patel R, Tsang Y. An external dosimetry audit programme to credential static and rotational IMRT delivery for clinical trials quality assurance. Phys Med. 2017;35:25–30.
16. Van Esch A, Depuydt T, Huyskens DP. The use of an aSi-based EPID for routine absolute dosimetric pre-treatment verification of dynamic IMRT fields. Radiother Oncol. 2004;71:223–34.
17. Nicolini G, Fogliata A, Vanetti E, Clivio A, Cozzi L. GLAaS: an absolute dose calibration algorithm for an amorphous silicon portal imager. Applications to IMRT verifications. Med Phys. 2006;33(8):2839–51.
18. Nicolini G, Vanetti E, Clivio A, Fogliata A, Boka G, Cozzi L. Testing the portal imager GLAaS algorithm for machine quality assurance. Radiat Oncol. 2008; 3(1):14.
19. Vinall AJ, Williams AJ, Currie VE, Van Esch A, Huyskens D. Practical guidelines for routine intensity-modulated radiotherapy verification: pre-treatment verification with portal dosimetry and treatment verification with in vivo dosimetry. Br J Radiol. 2010;83(995):949–57.
20. Van Esch A, Huyskens DP, Hirschi L, Baltes C. Optimized Varian aSi portal dosimetry: development of datasets for collective use. J Appl Clin Med Phys/Am Coll Med Phys. 2013;14(6):4286.
21. Kim JI, Chung JB, Song JY, Kim SK, Choi Y, Choi CH, Choi WH, Cho B, Kim JS, Kim SJ. Confidence limits for patient-specific IMRT dose QA: a multi-institutional study in Korea. J Appl Clin Med Phys. 2016;17(1):62–9.
22. Crowe SB, Sutherland B, Wilks R, Seshadri V, Sylvander S, Trapp JV, Kairn T. Relationships between gamma criteria and action levels: results of a multicenter audit of gamma agreement index results. Med Phys. 2016;43(3):1501–6.
23. Li G, Wu K, Peng G, Zhang Y, Bai S. A retrospective analysis for patient-specific quality assurance of volumetric-modulated arc therapy plans. Med Dosim. 2015;39(4):309–13.

9

Early toxicity and patient reported quality-of-life in patients receiving proton therapy for localized prostate cancer

Howard J. Lee Jr[1†], Meghan W. Macomber[2†], Matthew B. Spraker[2], Stephen R. Bowen[2], Daniel S. Hippe[3], Angela Fung[4], Kenneth J. Russell[2], George E. Laramore[2], Ramesh Rengan[2], Jay Liao[2], Smith Apisarnthanarax[2] and Jing Zeng[2*]

Abstract

Background: We report prospectively captured clinical toxicity and patient reported outcomes in a single institutional cohort of patients treated for prostate cancer with proton beam therapy (PBT). This is the largest reported series of patients treated mostly with pencil beam scanning PBT.

Methods: We reviewed 231 patients treated on an IRB approved institutional registry from 2013 to 2016; final analysis included 192 patients with > 1-year of follow-up. Toxicity incidence was prospectively captured and scored using CTCAE v4.0. International Prostate Symptoms Score (IPSS), Sexual Health Inventory for Men (SHIM) score, and Expanded Prostate Cancer Index Composite (EPIC) bowel domain questionnaires were collected at each visit. Univariate Cox regression was used to explore associations of grade 2+ toxicity with clinical, treatment, and dosimetric variables.

Results: Median follow-up was 1.7 years. Grade 3 toxicity was seen in 5/192 patients. No grade 4 or 5 toxicity was seen. Patient reported quality-of-life showed no change in urinary function post-radiation by IPSS scores. Median SHIM scores declined by 3.7 points at 1-year post-treatment without further decrease beyond year 1. On univariate analysis, only younger age (HR = 0.61, $p = 0.022$) was associated with decreased sexual toxicity. EPIC bowel domain scores declined from 96 at baseline (median) by an average of 5.4 points at 1-year post-treatment (95% CI: 2.5–8.2 points, $p < 0.001$), with no further decrease over time. Bowel toxicity was mostly in the form of transient rectal bleeding and was associated with anticoagulation use (HR = 3.45, $p = 0.002$).

Conclusions: Grade 3 or higher toxicity was rare at 2-years after treatment with PBT for localized prostate cancer. Longer follow-up is needed to further characterize late toxicity and biochemical control.

Keywords: Prostate cancer, Proton therapy, Quality of life, Patient reported outcomes

* Correspondence: jzeng13@uw.edu

†Howard J. Lee Jr and Meghan W. Macomber contributed equally to this work.

[2]Department of Radiation Oncology, University of Washington School of Medicine, 1959 NE Pacific Street, Campus, Box 356043, Seattle, WA 98195, USA

Full list of author information is available at the end of the article

Background

Numerous treatment options exist for localized prostate cancer. External beam radiation therapy is a non-invasive option that has shown similar disease control rates compared to other approaches such as radical prostatectomy and brachytherapy [1–5], and treatment modality choice is generally a consideration of side effect profile and shared decision making.

Dose escalation has been shown to improve cancer control in prostate cancer [6]. Delivering the high radiotherapy doses to the prostate necessary to improve outcomes can be challenging due to tolerance of surrounding organs at risk, in particular rectum and bladder. Higher radiation doses using conventional external beam techniques have been shown in several retrospective studies to increase the risk of late treatment related toxicity [7, 8]. Proton beam therapy (PBT) has emerged as an external beam radiotherapy treatment option. The unique dosimetric characteristics of PBT allow for dose escalation while reducing dose to surrounding structures, especially in the low-dose bath [7].

While numerous studies have demonstrated this reduction in low dose bath to surrounding normal tissues such as rectum and bladder, the clinical advantage remains unclear [8]. Only a few centers have reported clinical outcomes of patients treated with PBT for prostate cancer [9–18]. Existing proton literature in prostate cancer is mostly based on passive scattering proton technology, while pencil beam scanning (PBS) has some dosimetric advantages [19]. We present our 2-year outcomes regarding toxicity and patient reported quality of life (QOL) for patients receiving PBT at our institution. To our knowledge, this is the largest reported series of patients treated mostly with PBS proton technology.

Methods

Patient details and data collection

We reviewed 231 patients treated consecutively at our institution with PBT for localized prostate cancer on a prospective IRB-approved registry. Patients were excluded for prior radical prostatectomy, prior radiotherapy, treatment with mixed photon and proton radiation, or follow-up < 1-year. Total 192 patients were included in this analysis. Baseline characteristics are outlined in Table 1. All patients underwent institutional pathology review of prostate biopsy to confirm Gleason score. Intermediate risk patients by D'Amico risk groups underwent computed tomography (CT) and/or magnetic resonance imaging (MRI) of the pelvis. Patients with high-risk disease also had technetium bone scans.

Outcome and follow up

All patients were evaluated at pre-treatment, weekly on-treatment, and every 3–4 months for the first year post-treatment, then at 6-month intervals. Acute toxicity

Table 1 Patient characteristics

Variable	No. (%) or Median (Range)
Age, years	68 (50–85)
Race and ethnicity	
African-American	3 (1.6%)
Asian	4 (2.1%)
Hispanic	2 (1.0%)
White	176 (91.7%)
Unknown	7 (3.6%)
T stage	
T1	104 (54.2%)
T2a	49 (25.5%)
T2b	25 (13.0%)
T2c	4 (2.1%)
T3-T4	10 (5.2%)
PSA, ng/ml	7.2 (1.6–69.6)
Gleason score	
6	42 (21.9%)
7 = 3 + 4	80 (41.7%)
7 = 4 + 3	36 (18.8%)
8	14 (7.3%)
9–10	20 (10.4%)
Risk category	
Low	38 (19.8%)
Intermediate	104 (54.2%)
High	50 (26.0%)
Baseline IPSS Bother score[a]	2 (0–7)
Baseline IPSS score[a]	6 (0–28)
Baseline EPIC bowel domain score[a]	96 (61–100)
Baseline SHIM score[ab]	18 (0–25)
Comorbidities	
History of diabetes	19 (9.9%)
History of hypertension	96 (50.0%)
History of inflammatory bowel disease	2 (1.0)
History of hemorrhoids	26 (13.5%)
Smoking status[a]	
Never	103 (57.5%)
Former	65 (36.3%)
Current	11 (6.1%)
Aspirin use	74 (38.5%)
Anticoagulant use	22 (11.5%)
Pre-treatment urologic function	
Alpha blocker use	37 (19.3%)
Alpha reductase inhibitor use	14 (7.3%)
TURP	9 (4.7%)

Table 1 Patient characteristics *(Continued)*

Variable	No. (%) or Median (Range)
Androgen deprivation therapy	71 (37.0%)
Low risk	1/71 (1.4%)
Intermediate risk	27/71 (38.0%)
High risk	43/71 (60.6%)
Pencil beam vs. uniform scanning	144 vs 48 (75.0% vs 25%)
Number of fields/day	
1	92 (48%)
2	100 (52%)
Whole pelvis radiation	19 (9.9%)
US-based prostate volume, cm^3	40 (12–100)

[a]Those with missing values were excluded from the corresponding summary: IPSS bother score ($n = 7$), IPSS score ($n = 4$), EPIC score ($n = 28$), SHIM score ($n = 14$), smoking status ($n = 13$), and US-based prostate volume ($n = 12$);
[b]Based on patients not receiving androgen deprivation therapy ($n = 121$)

was defined as from start of radiation therapy to 90 days after treatment completion, and late toxicity was defined as at any time after 90 days. Patients prospectively completed International Prostate Symptoms Score (IPSS), Sexual Health Inventory for Men (SHIM) score, and Expanded Prostate Cancer Index Composite (EPIC) bowel domain questionnaires. Toxicity was scored using Common Terminology Criteria for Adverse Events, version 4.0 (CTCAE).

Treatment details

Proton therapy treatment included CT simulation at 1.25 mm slice thickness in the supine position using vacuum-locked body mold for immobilization, with instructions for full bladder and empty rectum. All patients had placement of three Visicoil fiducial markers under transrectal ultrasound guidance (IBA Dosimetry GmbH, Schwarzenbruck, Germany). All patients were treated with daily rectal balloons filled with 90 cc of saline. Patients were also instructed to drink 16 oz. of water 30 min to one hour prior to treatment to ensure a full bladder, with adjustments made based on individual urinary function. Treatment planning was categorized according to whether the clinical target volume (CTV) included prostate only, prostate and seminal vesicles, or inclusion of pelvic nodes for high risk disease at the discretion of the treating physician. Planning target volume (PTV) was an expansion of 5 mm in all directions except 4 mm posteriorly. Target coverage goal was 95% of PTV receiving 100% of prescribed dose, and 100% of PTV receiving ≥95% of prescribed dose. All patients received treatment with standard fractionation (1.8–2.0 CGE fractions). Prescribed dose was 79.2–81 CGE in 85% of patients, and 75.6–81 CGE in > 95% of patients. Prescribed doses to pelvic lymph nodes were 45–50.4 CGE. Maximum dose was kept to < 103% of prescribed dose. Organs at risk (OAR) doses are show in Table 2.

Most patients were treated with two lateral beams. Patients were treated with either uniform scanning (UNS) or PBS (our center switched from UNS to PBS in late-2014), with 1- or 2-fields per day. Patients receiving radiation to the pelvic nodes were treated with 2-fields per day. Patients receiving radiation to prostate without pelvic nodes were initially treated two-fields per day and then our center switched to treating one-field per day as the standard in 2015 (alternating between the two lateral beams every other day). This improved efficiency and was not felt to impact treatment quality. For UNS patients, a 0.8–1.2-cm margin was used to account for penumbra. Wax range compensators were designed with an additional range uncertainty of 2.5% + 2 mm added to the distal and proximal ranges, as well as 1–2-cm smearing margins. These were designed using commercially available Xio treatment planning software (Elekta, Stockholm, Sweden).

Dose was verified with an ion chamber measurement performed in water and field shape was verified by comparing the physical shape of the apertures and compensators with the treatment planning system. For PBS delivery, treatment plans were created using the RayStation treatment planning software (RaySearch Laboratories AB, Stockholm, Sweden) with single-field uniform dose optimization. Dose and

Table 2 Patient dosimetry ($N = 192$)

Variable	No. (%) or Median (Range)
Dose	
< 79.2 Gy (RBE)	27 (14.1%)
≥ 79.2 Gy (RBE)	165 (85.9%)
DVH Parameters	
Rectal wall V50, %	30.7 (8.0–56.6)
Rectal wall V75, %	16.2 (0.0–30.6)
Rectum V50, %	18.6 (2.0–39.4)
Rectum V70, %	9.2 (0.0–34.7)
Bladder wall V47, %	19.0 (6.8–56.7)
Bladder wall V75, %	11.5 (0.0–37.0)
Bladder V50, %	11.8 (2.1–58.5)
Bladder V75, %	5.1 (0.0–35.5)
Femoral head mean dose	
Right, Gy	25.8 (15.4–41.1)
Left, Gy	25.1 (11.3–39.9)
Femoral head max dose	
Right, Gy	35.6 (27.5–60.4)
Left, Gy	35.6 (27.8–63.6)
Penile bulb mean dose, Gy	45.1 (1.8–71.3)
Bowel Max Dose, Gy (RBE)[a]	51.4 (46.0–54.0)

[a]Based on patients receiving whole pelvis treatment

fluence were measured pre-treatment using the MatrixxPT ion chamber array device (IBA Dosimetry GmbH, Schwarzenbruck, Germany).

A constant relative biological effectiveness (RBE) factor of 1.1 was used to convert physical dose to RBE adjusted dose. In the present study, CGE and RBE adjusted dose are used interchangeably. The robustness of target and organs at risk (OAR) doses was evaluated by computing the plan with ±3% range uncertainty, as well as simulating setup errors by 3-mm isocenter deviations in the anterior/posterior, superior/inferior, and lateral directions. All patients had daily orthogonal kilovoltage x-rays for image guidance prior to treatment with fiducial localization. A digital imaging positioning system was used to determine optimal table shifts along 3 axes to reproduce fiducial localization within 2 mm of the simulation images. Treatment positioning was re-evaluated if more than 5 min passed before beam availability.

Statistical analysis

Statistical computations were performed with R version 3.1.1 (R Foundation for Statistical Computing, Vienna, Austria). Cumulative incidence of toxicity was estimated using the Kaplan-Meier product limit estimator. Univariate Cox proportional hazards regression was used to assess associations of grade 2 or higher (GR2+) toxicity with potential clinical, treatment-related, and dosimetry variables (listed in Tables 1 and 2). The univariate analysis was considered exploratory and hypothesis-generating, so the P-values were not adjusted to account for the number of comparisons. Changes in QOL scores from before and after treatment were analyzed using generalized estimating equation-based linear regression to account for the repeated measurements per patient. Patients who did not have baseline and at least one follow up QOL responses were excluded from that analysis. Throughout the data analysis, two-sided P values < 0.05 were considered statistically significant.

Results

Patient-reported quality of life

Patient reported quality-of-life (QOL) results are detailed in Fig. 1 and Table 3. Urinary function did not change significantly after treatment, as measured by IPSS. Bowel function as measured by EPIC bowel domain scores showed a small decline from 96 at baseline (median) by an average of 5.4 points at 1-year post-treatment (95% CI: 2.5–8.2 points, $p < 0.001$), and then remained stable beyond 1-year ($p = 0.57$). Erectile function as measured by SHIM scores also showed a small decline from 18/25 at baseline (mild ED) by 3.7 points at 1-year post-treatment (95% CI: 1.4–5.9 points, $p = 0.001$). Again, there was no further statistically significant decline beyond 1-year ($p = 0.25$). Treatment with PBS versus UNS did not show a statistically significant difference in toxicity rates, nor did treatment with one-field per day versus two-fields per day.

Genitourinary (GU) toxicity

One grade 3 (GR3) event was seen within the acute window, an episode of gross hematuria that was found on cystoscopy to be likely related to irritation of a scar from previous TURP. In the acute period (< 90 days from treatment completion), 86 patients (44.8%) required medication for management of urinary irritation (i.e. anti-inflammatory drugs or anti-α1 adrenoceptor blockers), defined as GR2 toxicity, with two patients requiring intermittent self-catheterization. Majority (61/86 patients) reported resolution of symptoms by 6-months post-treatment, and 73/86 had resolution of symptoms by 18 months. Most common symptoms included frequency (50 patients), urgency (44 patients), and dysuria (24).

Two patients experienced late GR3 GU toxicity, both radiation cystitis presenting with gross hematuria: one patient required hospitalization for cystoscopy although no intervention was ultimately performed and symptoms resolved; the other patient underwent multiple hyperbaric oxygen treatments with eventual resolution of his symptoms. No patients experienced GR 4 or 5 GU toxicity. Actuarial rate of GR2+ GU toxicity at 2-years was 26.4% (95% CI: 19.4–32.9%), mostly consisting of patients remaining on anti-α1-adrenoceptor blockers for urinary symptoms (Fig. 2). Worsening incontinence was seen in 4 patients, three of whom had some leakage pre-treatment. Of the 51 patients with GR2+ late GU toxicity, 21/51 had resolution of their symptoms within 3–6 months, 24/51 had resolution within 18 months, while the rest remained on anti-α1-adrenoceptor blockers at last follow-up.

Univariate analysis (without adjustment for repeated testing) showed a significant correlation between late GR2+ GU toxicity and increased age (HR = 1.50, $P = 0.004$), higher baseline IPSS score (HR = 1.45, $P = 0.0046$) and higher baseline IPSS bother score (HR = 1.35, $p = 0.016$). No statistically significant associations were found with any other clinical features—including alpha blocker use ($p = 0.19$), ADT ($p = 0.84$), or pre-treatment TURP ($p = 0.14$)—or dosimetric variables. When p-values were adjusted for repeated testing, no statistically significant associations were found between toxicity and any variables.

Gastrointestinal (GI) toxicity

One patient experienced late GR3 toxicity, which was managed with admission for transfusion and resolved after argon plasma coagulation. There were no GR 4 or 5 events. In the acute window, 5 patients reported transient GR2 bowel toxicity, mostly in the form of diarrhea and urgency. Late GR2+ bowel toxicity was seen in 34 patients with an actuarial two-year rate of 21.3% (95% CI: 13.9–28.0%) (Fig. 2). Most observed bowel toxicity

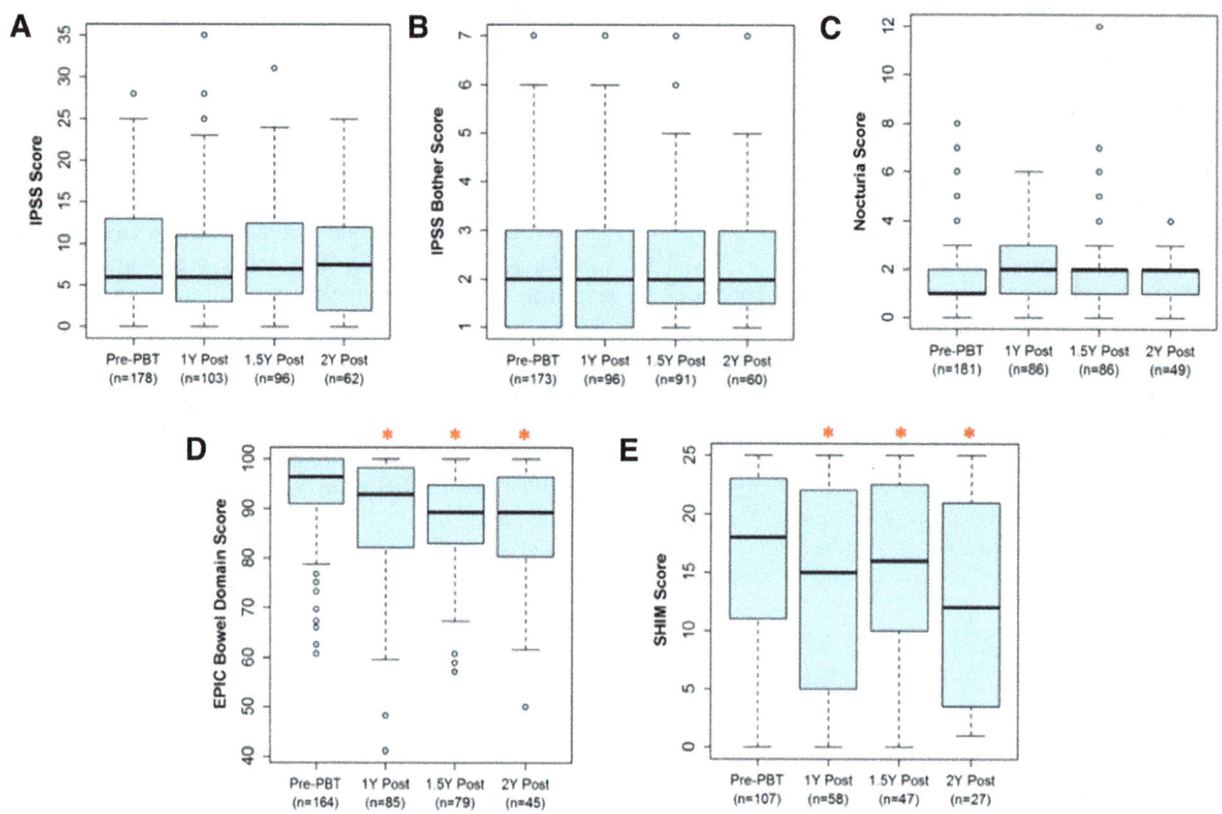

Fig. 1 Patient-reported quality-of-life measures. Box-whisker representation of QOL scores at pre-treatment, 1-year, 1.5-year, and 2-years post-treatment (**a**)=IPSS score, (**b**)=IPSS bother score, (**c**)=Nocturia score, (**d**)=EPIC bowel domain score, and (**e**)=SHIM score

was in the form of transient rectal bleeding (32/39 patients) treated with enemas/suppositories or laser coagulation, with the remaining 7 events were due to isolated rectal discomfort or diarrhea. Of the 32 patients who experienced GR2+ rectal bleeding, all events occurred in the late window. Seventeen received medical management with enemas or suppositories, while 15 underwent argon photocoagulation or electrocautery. Bowel toxicity was associated with anticoagulation use (HR = 3.45, $p = 0.002$ without adjustment for repeated testing).

Erectile dysfunction (ED)

Actuarial two-year rate of late GR2+ ED was 23.0% (95% CI: 13.8–31.3%) (Fig. 2), defined as worsening ED requiring new medical therapies (e.g. sildenafil, tadalafil, vardenafil), with erections firm enough for penetration after medical therapy. Only two patients reported GR3 ED, defined as poor erectile function not responding to oral or injectable medication; both had baseline ED requiring oral medications. On univariate analysis of ED among men not on androgen deprivation therapy, only younger

Table 3 Patient-reported QOL results

	Baseline			Follow Up		Mean Change at 1 Year after Treatment			Mean Annualized Change after 1 Year		
QOL Measure	No. of Patients	Median (Range)	Mean ± SD	No. of Patients	No. of Visits	Value	(95% CI)	P-value[a]	Value	(95% CI)	P-value[a]
EPIC Bowel	164	96 (61–100)	93.4 ± 8.5	100	183	−5.4	(−8.2, −2.5)	< 0.001	−1.2	(−5.2, 2.9)	0.57
IPSS	178	6 (0–28)	8.7 ± 6.6	130	241	0.5	(−0.7, 1.8)	0.40	−0.5	(−1.9, 1.0)	0.54
IPSS Bother	173	2 (1–7)	2.5 ± 1.4	125	221	0.3	(−0.1, 0.7)	0.12	−0.2	(−0.6, 0.2)	0.32
Nocturia	181	1 (0–8)	1.8 ± 1.5	123	217	0.3	(−0.0, 0.5)	0.077	−0.2	(−0.5, 0.2)	0.33
SHIM[a]	107	18 (0–25)	16.5 ± 7.1	66	123	−3.7	(−5.9, −1.4)	0.001	1.8	(−1.3, 5.0)	0.25

[a]Only assessed in patients not on androgen deprivation therapy

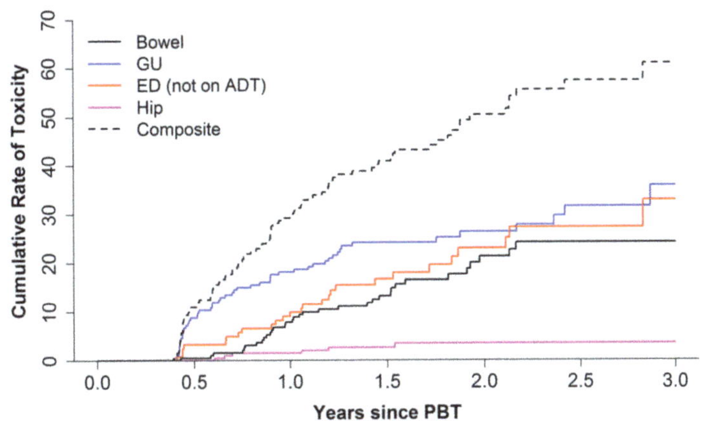

No. at Risk							
Bowel:	192	191	176	107	61	36	11
GU:	192	175	156	96	59	34	8
ED:	121	117	108	64	39	22	7
Hip:	192	192	188	119	75	46	14
Composite:	192	171	134	77	43	22	4

Fig. 2 Cumulative actuarial rates for late grade 2+ toxicity (> 90 days post-treatment). Grade 3 toxicity was seen in 5/192 patients, there were no grade 4/5 toxicity. Grade 2 bowel toxicity was mostly transient rectal bleeding managed by enemas/suppositories or laser coagulation. Grade 2 GU toxicity mostly consisted of urinary symptoms managed by α1 adrenoceptor blockers. Grade 2 erectile dysfunction was defined as requiring medications for erectile function. Grade 2 hip pain was pain requiring anti-inflammatory medications

age (HR = 0.6, $p = 0.022$ without adjustment for repeated testing) was associated with decreased late GR2+ toxicity. Mean dose to the penile bulb was not significantly associated with erectile dysfunction.

Hip toxicity

In the acute window, there were 2 cases of GR2 hip pain requiring anti-inflammatory medication. In the late window, 3 patients reported GR2 hip pain. Three patients reporting maximum GR3 hip pain experienced resolution of symptoms with either cortisone shots to the hip joint, opioid therapy, or eventual hip replacement in one case. The one patient who underwent hip replacement had significant preexisting degenerative changes on pre-treatment imaging. Median time to incidence in those who reported hip pain was 9 months (range 2–29 months). There were no hip fractures. Hip toxicity was not significantly associated with any clinical or dosimetric parameters.

Discussion

This is one of few contemporary studies that evaluates outcomes and toxicity of PBT for localized prostate cancer with prospectively collected data, including patient reported outcomes. This is the largest series to our knowledge that includes patients treated mostly with PBS, which has dosimetric advantages over older passive scattering proton technology in some scenarios [19]. Although PBT offers known dosimetric advantages over photon radiation, especially in the low to intermediate-dose region (such as volume receiving up to 50 Gy), the clinical impact of this is unclear [7, 20].

In our study population, with median follow up of 1.7 years, we found that rates of GR2+ toxicity outcomes were comparable to other reported data. The low rate of GR3 GU toxicity in this study (5/192 patients) is comparable to other evaluations of PBT, with rates generally < 3% [9]. In the largest prospectively captured data of PBT outcomes for prostate cancer to date, Bryant et al. at the University of Florida found a late GR3 GU actuarial 5-year toxicity rate at of 2.9% [9]. Prior retrospective studies from this group found 1.0% GR3 GU toxicity [13], while other groups have reported a range of 0–2% [15, 17].

As shown in Table 4, reports including the present study consistently show that the risk of grade 3+ GU and GI toxicity is generally low after both PBT and IMRT [9, 13, 15, 17, 21–24]. However, wide variations can be seen in GR2+ toxicity rates with both IMRT and PBT. For example, in two IMRT studies, GU and GI GR2+ toxicity rates reported by Vora et al. were 24.4% and 10.9% respectively, while Spratt et al. reported rates of 8.5% and 2.0% [22, 23]. Multiple factors illustrated in Table 4 may explain this variability and also make true comparison across standalone studies difficult. First, using RTOG versus CTCAE scoring criteria can significantly impact physician-reported toxicity rates, since RTOG criteria depend on subjective assessments of what qualifies as mild (grade 1) versus moderate (grade 2) toxicity, whereas CTCAE criteria require medical or procedural intervention to qualify as grade 2. Second, many studies report observed toxicity rates (numbers of patients experiencing toxicity) with varying lengths of median follow-up [22–24]. This can be addressed by

Table 4 Literature review of toxicity data

Study	No. of Patients	Therapy	Median RT Dose Gy or CGE	Median Follow-Up Years	Toxicity Grading Scale	G3+ GU Toxicity	G2+ GU Toxicity	G3+ GI Toxicity	G2+ GI Toxicity
Liauw et al., 2009 [21]	130	IMRT	76	4.4	RTOG	6%[b]	37.0%[b]	5%[b]	14.0%[b]
Spratt et al., 2013 [22]	1002	IMRT	86.4	5.5	CTCAE	2.2%	8.5%	0.7%	2.0%
Vora et al., 2013 [23]	302	IMRT	75.6	7.6	CTCAE	2.6%	24.4%	1%	10.9%
Fang et al., 2015 [24]	94	IMRT	79.2	3.9	CTCAE	0%	18.3%	2.1%	10.8%
Fang et al., 2015 [24]	94	PS PBT	79.2	2.4	CTCAE	2.1%	12.8%	0%	12.8%
Slater et al., 2004 [17]	1255	PS PBT	74	5.3	RTOG	1.0%[a]	–	1.0%[a]	–
Pugh et al., 2013 [15]	291	PS > PBS PBT	76	2.0	RTOG	0%[c]	13.4%[c]	0.3%[c]	9.6%[c]
Mendenhall et al., 2014 [13]	211	PS PBT	78–82	5.2	CTCAE	1.0%[a]	–	0.5%[a]	–
Bryant et al., 2016 [9]	1215	PS PBT	78	5.5	CTCAE	2.9%[a]	–	0.6%[a]	–
Present study, 2017	192	PBS > PS PBT	79.2	1.7	CTCAE	1.0%	26.4%[c]	0.5%	21.3%[c]

Abbreviations: PS passive scatter, *PBS* pencil beam scanning, *PBT* proton beam therapy, *IMRT* intensity-modulated radiation therapy, *RTOG* radiation therapy oncology group, *CTCAE* common terminology criteria for adverse events, version 4.0

[a] = 5-year actuarial rate, [b] = 4-year actuarial rate, [c] = 2-year actuarial rate. No symbol next to a toxicity rate % indicates a rate reported as the number of toxicity events observed over the total number of patients, with varying median follow-up across studies

comparing actuarial toxicity rates at specific time intervals, such as 5-years, but these are only inconsistently reported, and at varying time-points themselves [9, 13, 15, 17, 21]. Third, the dose to which patients are treated often varies from study to study. Fourth and finally, treatment planning and patient setup vary from institution to institution.

There is a clear need for studies that can compare PBT and IMRT in a standardized fashion. Although level one evidence comparing IMRT and PBT in patients with prostate cancer is currently being collected in the PARTIQoL and COMPPARE trials (NCT01617161, NCT03561220), results will not be available for years. Thus far, there is conflicting evidence regarding comparative toxicities. In a case-matched comparison of intensity-modulated radiotherapy (IMRT) or PBT based treatment matched for age, GI and GU co-morbidity, and risk group, Fang et al. report that at 2 years there were no differences in GR2 or higher GU or GI toxicities [24]. A Medicare-based comparative study found lower GU toxicity for PBT at 6 months, but no difference at 12 months [18]. Gray et al. compared three dimensional conformal radiotherapy (3D CRT), IMRT, and PBT and found worse acute patient-reported QOL for urinary symptoms for patients treated with 3D CRT but there were no differences by 2 years [12]. A comparison of patient-reported QOL after PBT with patient-reported QOL from the Prostate Cancer Outcomes and Satisfaction (PROSTQA) treatment assessment study of men treated with high-dose photon radiation, showed no differences in any toxicity domain at 2 years [25]. However, a more recent study using private commercial insurance claims reported that PBT was associated with significant reductions in urinary toxicity but increased bowel toxicity three years after treatment [26].

The dosimetric improvement with PBT over IMRT lies in reductions to low and moderate-dose range exposures of normal tissue and not high dose range (70–80 Gy), therefore it is important to qualify the differences that one might expect from PBT in comparison to IMRT [20]. Some of these benefits may be recognized as a decrease in long term toxicity and changes, including the risk of secondary malignancy, and will require much longer follow up with large patient numbers to fully realize [25]. We found no association of toxicity incidence with PBS versus UNS technique in our patient cohort. This is consistent with a previous study that also showed no associations in a cohort treated with mostly passive scatter, and some pencil beam technique [15]. Thus, PBS treatment technique may not clinically affect toxicity rates in prostate cancer treatment, despite potential dosimetric advantages.

Previous retrospective studies have reported excellent biochemical outcomes with PBT [9, 17]. At this time, we did not have enough patient events or follow up time to comment on control rates in this group. We plan to report updated outcomes in the future as patients accrue to the registry and follow up data matures.

Limitations of this study include the patient selection bias for those treated at a single institution. There could also be a selection bias for those patients who sought access to PBT. The follow up period is short, and radiation toxicity is known to develop years after radiotherapy [27]. However, we believe the present study is an important addition to the literature, to assess early outcomes with modern treatment techniques including daily image guidance with intraprostatic fiducials and PBS approach. Strengths include the rigor of prospectively collected toxicity and outcome data, and data that is both patient and physician reported. Future analysis will include continued patient accrual with longer median follow up. The larger patient numbers will allow us to better assess late treatment toxicities and PSA trends amongst patients treated with PBT for prostate cancer at our institution.

Conclusions

We report toxicity rates in patients treated with contemporary PBT techniques (mostly PBS) at our institution with median 1.7 years of follow up. Grade 3+ toxicities were rare. Patient reported quality-of-life are excellent, with no change in urinary function post-radiation, and small declines in erectile function and bowel QOL by 1-year post-treatment. Larger patient numbers and longer follow up are anticipated to add robustness to our data.

Abbreviations

CGE: Cobalt gray equivalent; CI: Confidence interval; CT: Computed tomography; CTCAE: Common Terminology Criteria for Adverse Events; CTV: Clinical target volume; ED: Erectile dysfunction; EPIC: Expanded Prostate Cancer Index Composite; GI: Gastrointestinal; GR2: Grade 2; GR2+: Grade 2 or higher; GR3: Grade 3; GR4: Grade 4; GU: Genitourinary; Gy: Gray; HR: Hazard ratio; IMRT: Intensity-modulated radiotherapy; IPSS: International Prostate Symptoms Score; IRB: Institutional review board; MRI: Magnetic resonance imaging; OAR: Organs at risk; PBS: Pencil beam scanning; PBT: Proton beam therapy; PS: Passive scatter; PSA: Prostate specific antigen; PTV: Planning target volume; QOL: Quality of life; RBE: Relative biological effectiveness; SHIM: Sexual Health Inventory for Men; UNS: Uniform scanning; US: Ultrasound

Acknowledgments

The authors would like to acknowledge Jordan Dickson BA and Prachie Banthia BA, who assisted in the formatting of blinded datasets containing results from our patient database.

Funding

Study data were collected and managed using REDCap electronic data capture tools hosted at the University of Washington, supported by Institute of Translational Health Science (ITHS) grant support (UL1 TR002319 from NCATS/NIH).

Authors' contributions

HJL and MWM contributed equally to this work and share first authorship. HJL, MWM, MBS, and AF performed the data collection. SRB and DSH contributed to the data analysis. JZ was responsible for the design of this study. All authors contributed to the writing, approved the final manuscript, and have given approval for the manuscript to be published.

Competing interests

Mr. Hippe reports grants from the NIH/NCI, and Dr. Russell reports a scientific advisory position with Varian Medical Corporation during the conduct of this study. All remaining authors of this publication declare no competing interest.

Author details

[1]Duke University School of Medicine, 10 Duke Medicine Circle, Durham, NC 27710, USA. [2]Department of Radiation Oncology, University of Washington School of Medicine, 1959 NE Pacific Street, Campus, Box 356043, Seattle, WA 98195, USA. [3]Department of Radiology, University of Washington School of Medicine, 1959 NE Pacific Street, Campus, Box 357115, Seattle, WA 98195, USA. [4]Seattle Cancer Care Alliance Proton Therapy Center, 1570 N 115th St, Seattle, WA 98115, USA.

References

1. Hamdy FC, et al. 10-Year Outcomes after Monitoring, Surgery, or Radiotherapy for Localized Prostate Cancer. N Engl J Med. 2016;375(15):1415–24.
2. Chen L, et al. Comparison on efficacy of radical prostatectomy versus external beam radiotherapy for the treatment of localized prostate cancer. Oncotarget. 2017;8(45):79854–63.
3. Chen RC, et al. Association between choice of radical prostatectomy, external beam radiotherapy, brachytherapy, or active surveillance and patient-reported quality of life among men with localized prostate Cancer. JAMA. 2017;317(11):1141–50.
4. Potosky AL, et al. Five-year outcomes after prostatectomy or radiotherapy for prostate cancer: the prostate cancer outcomes study. J Natl Cancer Inst. 2004;96(18):1358–67.
5. Wolff RF, et al. A systematic review of randomised controlled trials of radiotherapy for localised prostate cancer. Eur J Cancer. 2015;51(16):2345–67.
6. Zietman AL, et al. Randomized trial comparing conventional-dose with high-dose conformal radiation therapy in early-stage adenocarcinoma of the prostate: long-term results from proton radiation oncology group/ american college of radiology 95-09. J Clin Oncol. 2010;28(7):1106–11.
7. Trofimov A, et al. Radiotherapy treatment of early-stage prostate cancer with IMRT and protons: a treatment planning comparison. Int J Radiat Oncol Biol Phys. 2007;69(2):444–53.
8. Tepper JE. Protons and parachutes. J Clin Oncol. 2008;26(15):2436–7.
9. Bryant C, et al. Five-year biochemical results, toxicity, and patient-reported quality of life after delivery of dose-escalated image guided proton therapy for prostate Cancer. Int J Radiat Oncol Biol Phys. 2016;95(1):422–34.
10. Coen JJ, et al. Acute and late toxicity after dose escalation to 82 GyE using conformal proton radiation for localized prostate cancer: initial report of American College of Radiology Phase II study 03-12. Int J Radiat Oncol Biol Phys. 2011;81(4):1005–9.
11. Colaco RJ, et al. Rectal toxicity after proton therapy for prostate cancer: an analysis of outcomes of prospective studies conducted at the university of Florida proton therapy institute. Int J Radiat Oncol Biol Phys. 2015;91(1):172–81.
12. Gray PJ, et al. Patient-reported outcomes after 3-dimensional conformal, intensity-modulated, or proton beam radiotherapy for localized prostate cancer. Cancer. 2013;119(9):1729–35.
13. Mendenhall NP, et al. Five-year outcomes from 3 prospective trials of image-guided proton therapy for prostate cancer. Int J Radiat Oncol Biol Phys. 2014;88(3):596–602.
14. Nihei K, et al. Multi-institutional phase II study of proton beam therapy for organ-confined prostate cancer focusing on the incidence of late rectal toxicities. Int J Radiat Oncol Biol Phys. 2011;81(2):390–6.
15. Pugh TJ, et al. Quality of life and toxicity from passively scattered and spot-scanning proton beam therapy for localized prostate cancer. Int J Radiat Oncol Biol Phys. 2013;87(5):946–53.
16. Sheets NC, et al. Intensity-modulated radiation therapy, proton therapy, or conformal radiation therapy and morbidity and disease control in localized prostate cancer. JAMA. 2012;307(15):1611–20.
17. Slater JD, et al. Proton therapy for prostate cancer: the initial Loma Linda University experience. Int J Radiat Oncol Biol Phys. 2004;59(2):348–52.
18. Yu JB, et al. Proton versus intensity-modulated radiotherapy for prostate cancer: patterns of care and early toxicity. J Natl Cancer Inst. 2013; 105(1):25–32.

19. Yeung D, McKenzie C, Indelicato DJ. A dosimetric comparison of intensity-modulated proton therapy optimization techniques for pediatric craniopharyngiomas: a clinical case study. Pediatr Blood Cancer. 2014;61(1):89–94.
20. Vargas C, et al. Dose-volume comparison of proton therapy and intensity-modulated radiotherapy for prostate cancer. Int J Radiat Oncol Biol Phys. 2008;70(3):744–51.
21. Liauw SL, et al. Biochemical control and toxicity after intensity-modulated radiation therapy for prostate Cancer. Technol Cancer Res Treat. 2009;8(3): 201–6.
22. Spratt DE, et al. Long-term survival and toxicity in patients treated with high-dose intensity modulated radiation therapy for localized prostate cancer. Int J Radiat Oncol Biol Phys. 2013;85(3):686–92.
23. Vora SA, et al. Outcome and toxicity for patients treated with intensity modulated radiation therapy for localized prostate cancer. J Urol. 2013; 190(2):521–6.
24. Fang P, et al. A case-matched study of toxicity outcomes after proton therapy and intensity-modulated radiation therapy for prostate cancer. Cancer. 2015;121(7):1118–27.
25. Hoppe BS, Bryant C, Sandler HM. Radiation for prostate cancer: intensity modulated radiation therapy versus proton beam. J Urol. 2015;193(4):1089–91.
26. Pan HY, et al. Comparative toxicities and cost of intensity-modulated radiotherapy, proton radiation, and stereotactic body radiotherapy among younger men with prostate Cancer. J Clin Oncol. 2018;36(18):1823–30.
27. Gardner BG, et al. Late normal tissue sequelae in the second decade after high dose radiation therapy with combined photons and conformal protons for locally advanced prostate cancer. J Urol. 2002;167(1):123–6.

10

Imaging dose and secondary cancer risk in image-guided radiotherapy of pediatric patients

Yvonne Dzierma*, Katharina Mikulla, Patrick Richter, Katharina Bell, Patrick Melchior, Frank Nuesken and Christian Rübe

Abstract

Background: Daily image-guided radiotherapy (IGRT) can contribute to cover extended body volumes with low radiation dose. The effect of additional imaging dose on secondary cancer development is modelled for a collective of children with Morbus Hodgkin.

Methods: Eleven radiotherapy treatment plans from pediatric patients with Hodgkin's lymphoma were retrospectively analyzed, including imaging dose from scenarios using different energies (kV/MV) and planar/cone-beam computed tomography (CBCT) techniques. In addition to assessing the effect of imaging dose on organs at risk, the excess average risk (EAR) for developing a secondary carcinoma of the lung or breast was modelled.

Results: Although the variability between the patients is relatively large due to the different target volumes, the additional EAR due to imaging can be consistently determined. For daily 6MV CBCT, the EAR for developing a secondary cancer at age 50 is over 3 cases per 10^4 PY (patient-years) for the female breast and 0.7–0.8 per 10^4 PY for the lungs. This can be decreased by using only planar images (< 1 per 10^4 PY for the breast and 0.1 for the lungs). Similar values are achieved by daily 360° kV CBCT (0.44–0.57 per 10^4 PY for the breast and 0.08 per 10^4 PY for the lungs), which is again reduced for daily 200° kV CBCT (0.02 per 10^4 PY for the lungs and 0.07–0.08 per 10^4 PY for the breast). These values increase if an older attained age is considered (e.g., for 70 years, by a factor of four for the lungs).

Conclusions: Daily imaging can be performed with an additional secondary cancer risk of less than 1 per 10^4 PY if kV CBCT is applied. If MV modalities must be chosen, a similar EAR can be achieved with planar images. A further reduction in risk is possible if the imaging geometry allows for sparing of the breast by a partial rotation underneath the patient.

Keywords: Secondary cancer risk, Radiotherapy for Hodgkin lymphoma, Image-guided radiotherapy, Imaging dose in pediatric patients

Background

Modern radiotherapy offers ever improved techniques for optimal target coverage associated with utmost sparing of neighbouring tissues and organs at risk (OAR's). As dose conformity and dose gradients are increasing, image-guided radiotherapy (IGRT) is a prerequisite, and frequent to daily image-guided positioning verification is common. Since most IGRT systems rely on ionizing radiation for EPID-based (electron portal imaging device) projection or cone-beam computed tomography (CBCT) imaging, an evaluation of the contribution of imaging dose to the treatment plan should be performed, and has been presented for a number of indications in the recent literature. This need is particularly pronounced since there exists a variety of different imaging systems using different photon energy (kV or MV), with 2D or 3D imaging, the dose of which is generally not included in the treatment planning system (TPS). While it is undisputed that the general benefit of image-guided positioning surmounts the possibly deteriorating effects of additional imaging dose on plan quality, particularly sensitive patient collectives such as pediatric patients with good prognosis should not receive excessive imaging dose to

* Correspondence: Yvonne.dzierma@uks.eu
Department of Radiotherapy and Radiation Oncology, Saarland University Medical Centre, Kirrberger Str. Geb. 6.5, 66421 Homburg, Saar, Germany

avoid OAR complications or – in the even lower dose regime – risk of developing secondary malignancies.

The aim of this study is therefore to analyse and compare several common linac-based imaging scenarios (6MV and 121 kV energies for planar and CBCT imaging with daily or non-daily frequency) with regard to their influence on OAR dose and secondary cancer risk in children with Morbus Hodgkin irradiated at the Saarland University Medical Centre. This collective was chosen because of good long-term survival of children with Hodgkin's lymphoma, so that there is a high probability that they will live long enough so that a secondary cancer might develop. Furthermore, secondary cancer induction by irradiation of Morbus Hodgkin patients has been extensively studied for the same reason, so that mathematical model parameters for secondary cancer risk are better known for this type of irradiation.

To assess imaging dose contribution, the summation dose from the complete treatment including different imaging scenarios is calculated and secondary cancer risk is estimated. Although other studies have previously estimated secondary cancer risk for the irradiation of children, they have mainly concentrated on the imaging dose or treatment dose separately. This approach is problematic since the secondary cancer risk from these two contributions cannot be expected to be additive – in fact, the secondary cancer risk estimated for imaging dose would normally use a linear model, which only applies in the low-dose regime. Conversely, the secondary cancer risk model for higher doses of the order of a radiotherapy treatment protocol is generally expected to fall out of the linear range, where either bell-shaped or plateau-like models are assumed to account for cell sterilization. In these cases, adding a linearly estimated secondary cancer risk from imaging dose to the risk calculated for the treatment plan separately might yield quite a different result than directly estimating the total risk from the combined dose distribution. A priori, it cannot be known how the two effects interact, which will also be discussed in this study.

Methods

Patient collective

We included in the analysis all children treated for Hodgkin's lymphoma at the Department of Radiotherapy and Radiation Oncology, Saarland University Medical Centre, in the years 2011 through 2015, which are seven children aged 5–17 years (mean age 14 years) with 11 different target sites (analysed separately, see Table 1 for details). After obtaining written informed consent of the patients and the patients' parents, the patients received involved-field irradiation with 19.8–29.8 Gy in fractions of 1.0–1.8 Gy using an intensity modulated radiotherapy technique (IMRT) with 6 MV photons. In total 134 treatment fractions were delivered, with image-guidance in 63 fractions.

For image-guidance, the following systems are available at our department:

1. 6 MV treatment beam (TBL) at two Siemens Artiste and one Siemens Oncor (Siemens Healthcare, Erlangen, Germany) linear accelerators,
2. 1 MV image beam line (IBL) at two Siemens Artiste linear accelerators [1–3], and
3. 121 kV system kVision at one Siemens Artiste linear accelerator [4–7].

All systems can be used to acquire planar or CBCT images. Planar MV axial images are taken using 1 monitor unit (MU) each from two orthogonal views. For MV CBCT images, either a full 360° or a shortened arc (200°) can be used with different MU settings depending on the patient anatomy and geometry (7–11 MU), with a square field of 27.4 cm width at source-to-surface distance (SSD) 100 cm [1]. The kVision system applies a "pre-shot" to automatically optimize the exposure (the mAs value is displayed and protocolled, generally less than 10 mAs for planar images and between 200 and 700 mAs for CBCT in our collective). While the MV CBCT gantry rotates above the head of the patient, the kV CBCT geometry with a reduced arc is inverted, rotating below the back of the patient because the X-ray tube is installed opposite the treatment head. The field size at SSD 100 cm is 28×28 cm^2 for the kV system [4].

The realistic imaging scenarios applied for the patients depended to some degree on the availability of the techniques for imaging – in 2011, only the 6 MV energy was available, the kVision system was installed last (end 2012). When available, the lower-energy systems were preferentially used for imaging; the percentage use of each imaging system is shown in Fig. 1a. A no-action-level protocol of online positioning correction was followed, so that all deviations observed in pre-treatment imaging (unless smaller than 1 mm) were always corrected for. An analysis of the performed couch shifts after imaging (Fig. 1b) agrees with a normal distribution, although the patient collective is too small to allow for statistical significance. It was checked in a phantom study that the different imaging modalities are in agreement regarding the detected positioning errors [8].

Dose calculation and secondary cancer risk model

The three imaging systems are all commissioned in the Philips Pinnacle treatment planning system (Philips Healthcare, Koninklijke, Netherlands) [1, 4, 9], so that the imaging dose can be calculated together with the patient treatment plan. For each patient, the dose distribution of the original treatment plan (as it was accepted for treatment = Scenario 1) without inclusion of imaging dose is compared with the following imaging scenarios:

Table 1 Patients and target volumes analysed. PTV: planning target volume

Case	Patient	Age at treatment	PTV	Prescription	Imaging
1	1	16	1st series: right lung; 2nd series: right lung and infraclavicular/ pectoral/ mediastinal lymphatics	1st series: 3x100cGy; 2nd series: 11 × 100 cGy; 11x166cGy	1 x 6MV axes 11 x IBL axes
2	2	15	bilateral neck cervical, supra- and infraclavicular lymphatics and mediastinum	11x180cGy	1 x 6MV axes 3 x IBL axes
3	3	17	Right cervical/mediastinal lymphatics	11x180cGy	4 x 6MV axes 1 x 6MV CBCT (7.2 MU)
4	4	16	1st series: Mediastinum 2nd series: Boost Mediastinum	1st series: 11x180cGy; 2nd series: 5x200cGy	1 x 6MV axes 4 x IBL axes
5	4	16	Spleen	11x180cGy	1 x 6MV axes 4 x IBL axes
6	5	16	1st series: Mediastinum; 2nd series: Boost macroscopic residual disease (Mediastinum)	1st series: 11x180cGy; 2nd series: 5x200cGy	6 x kV axes 1 x kV CBCT (414 mAs)
7	5	16	Spleen	11x180cGy	1 x 6MV/IBL axes 1 x kV axes 1 x kV CBCT (621 mAs)
8	6	5	bilateral neck, supra-infraclavicular, mediastinal and paraaortic lymphatics, spleen	11x180cGy	3 x 6MV axes 5 x 6MV CBCT (54 MU in total)
9	6	5	Os ileum	11x180cGy	5 x 6MV portal images
10	7	13	Left cervical lymphatics	11x180cGy	1 x kV axes 2 x kV CBCT (458 mAs in total)
11	7	13	Spleen	11x180cGy	2 x kV axes 3 x kV CBCT (1103 mAs in total) 1 x IBL CBCT (11 MU)

- Scenario 2: treatment plan with real imaging performed for the patient, with imaging device and frequency differing between the individual patients (details listed in Table 1)
- Scenario 3: treatment plan with daily 121 kV 200° CBCT
- Scenario 4: treatment plan with daily 121 kV 360° CBCT
- Scenario 5: treatment plan with daily 6 MV planar imaging
- Scenario 6: treatment plan with daily 360° 6 MV CBCT.

The hypothetical scenarios 3–6 are chosen to analyse the effect of daily imaging, which is more and more becoming the norm [10]. For the kV and 6 MV CBCT scenarios, the average mAs or MU per rotation was calculated for all patients and applied for the hypothetical scenarios: 360° kV CBCT with 377 mAs, 200° kV CBCT with 99 mAs, 6 MV CBCT (360°) with 11 MU. Evidently, kV imaging is the most desirable scenario; however, this is not available at every clinic. This is why we include 6 MV imaging to see how daily imaging can be achieved if only this modality is available. While it is clear that daily 6 MV CBCT would entail too high imaging dose, we include this scenario as the maximum possible imaging dose; contrarily, daily planar images with 6 MV are included as example of the lowest achievable imaging dose for daily MV images. Reality will range in between these two scenarios as occasional CBCT may be used to acquire 3D views. As kV planar images involve very little dose in comparison with all other modalities (lower than kV CBCT or planar MV images by at least an order of magnitude), this modality is not included in our analysis.

Dose calculation of the summation plans was carried out in the Philips Pinnacle TPS Version 9.0–9.6 on a 2 mm dose grid using the collapsed cone algorithm (for a detailed explanation of the procedure, compare [11]). Dose-volume histogram (DVH) values are considered to assess dose to the organs at risk (OARs). For secondary cancer risk calculation, the dose distribution was exported together with the regions of interests (ROIs) of the OARs and imported into Matlab R2015a (MathWorks, Natick, Massachusetts, USA). An in-house software was created to calculate the organ-specific risk for developing secondary carcinoma using Schneider's mechanistic model [12]. This gives the organ excess absolute risk as

$$EAR_{org}(age_x, age_a) = \beta_{org} \cdot OED \cdot \mu(age_x, age_a),$$

where age_x and age_a are the age at exposure and age attained (when developing the secondary malignancy), respectively,

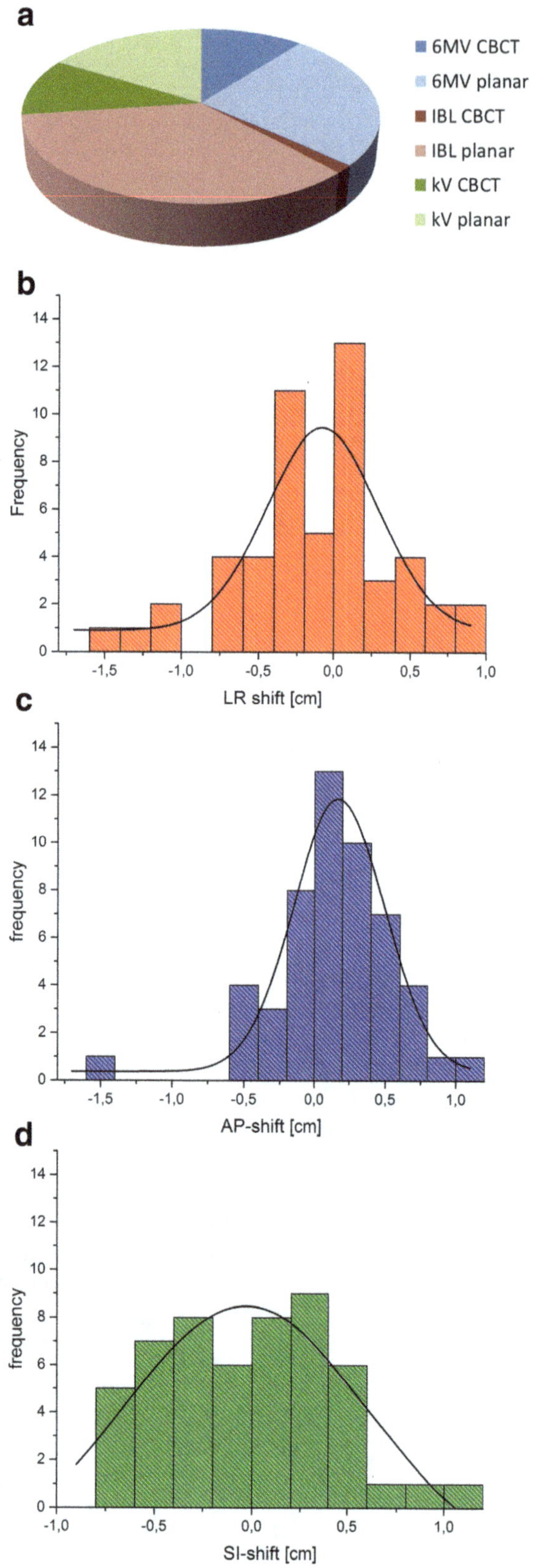

Fig. 1 a Percentage use of each imaging modality in the patient collective. **b** Frequency distribution of couch shifts in left-right (LR), (**c**) anterior-posterior (AP) and (**d**) superior-inferior (SI) direction

$$\mu(age_x, age_a) = \exp\left(\gamma_e(age_x\text{-}30) + \gamma_a \ln\frac{age_a}{70}\right)$$

is a modifying function for adjusting the risk to the ages age_x and age_a and β is a model scaling parameter between the organ effective dose (OED) and the EAR. The organ effective dose is calculated according to [12] as the risk-equivalent-dose (RED)-weighted average of the total volume V_T

$$OED = \frac{1}{V_T}\cdot\sum_i V(D_i)RED(D_i),$$

with the organ-specific dose-response relationship given by the mechanistic model for carcinoma induction including cell killing and fractionation effects:

$$RED(D) = \frac{\exp(-\alpha' D)}{\alpha' R}\left(1\text{-}2R + R^2\exp(\alpha' D)\text{-}(1\text{-}R^2)\exp\left(-\frac{\alpha' R}{1\text{-}R}\right)D\right).$$

Fractionation is taken into account using the linear quadratic model with parameters α and β and a fractionation with target volume prescribed dose D_T in fraction doses of d_T:

$$\alpha' = \alpha + \beta d = \alpha + \beta\frac{D}{D_T}d_T.$$

The main two organs at risk for secondary cancer development in our patient collective are the lungs and the breast, for which the model parameters are given in Table 2.

The software uses the DICOM (Digital Imaging and Communications in Medicine) structure sets, RT dose and CT data set as input together with the organ specific model parameters to calculate the excess absolute cancer risk. In each case, the age of the patient at exposure was included; the secondary cancer risk was modelled for an attained age of 50 years.

A statistical analysis was carried out in Origin Pro 2015G (OriginLab, Northampton, Massachusetts, USA) for descriptive statistics. To assess differences between the planning scenarios, the plans were pair-wise compared against the original plan ("gold standard" without imaging dose) using the Wilcoxon signed-rank test. Please note that "gold standard" is taken to mean the optimal dose distribution (no deterioration from imaging

Table 2 Parameters for modelling the excess absolute risk (from [12])

Model parameter	Female breast	Lung
α in Gy^{-1}	0.044	0.042
R	0.15	0.83
β_{org} in excess cases per 10,000 PY Gy	8.2	8.0
γ_e	−0.037	0.002
γ_a	1.7	4.23

dose), as it was accepted for treatment – this is *not* suggested as the optimal verification scenario, just as a baseline for dose comparisons (see Discussion).

Results

Visualization of dose distributions – Example

Figure 2 shows an example of the imaging dose distribution and the planned dose, where differences between the imaging scenarios become apparent. We selected this patient example because several issues can be observed here: Firstly, the dose distribution from imaging only differs strongly from the original treatment plan. Secondly, the dose distributions of the different imaging scenarios are quite different from each other, both in absolute dose (all imaging dose distributions are scaled to their respective maximum dose, ranging from 11.1 cGy for daily kV CBCT to 240.9 cGy in total for daily 6 MV CBCT) and in dose distribution. For this patient (patient 6), two target volumes were irradiated (lymphatics and os ileum), so that two series of imaging scenarios were simulated. The overlapping region between both imaging sets creates a higher-dose "belt" in the simulated scenarios. In the actual verification, most sessions only imaged the larger cranial planning target volume (PTV), so that most imaging dose is accumulated here. Furthermore, the actual verification used a combination of axial and CBCT imaging, which explains the square shape of the isodoses in this scenario.

If the combined dose from the radiotherapy treatment and imaging is considered, the differences between the scenarios are less obvious. Some small increases in the lower-dose isolines and an increased maximum dose are observed, particularly for those imaging scenarios with higher additional dose (e.g., 6 MV). For this patient, the actual imaging performed contributed rather high dose because this patient was treated among the first in the collective, when kV imaging was not yet installed at our department.

Dose to organs at risk – DVH analysis

An example DVH for the patient shown above is given in Fig. 3. It is obvious that the dose is markedly increased by daily 360° 6MV CBCT, as well as (to a smaller degree) by the actual mixed CBCT-planar 6 MV imaging performed. The other imaging scenarios do not result in a visible increase in the DVH dose. The fact that neither dose to the parotids nor the pharynx appear to change with the imaging scenarios is due to the imaging geometry visible in Fig. 2, in which the imaging beam does not reach up as far cranially to involve these organs.

All DVH parameters are listed in Table 3; an example for the left lung is displayed in Fig. 4. The statistical tests for significance using Wilcoxon's signed-rank test for paired data gave positive results for all organs for which more than 5 patient cases with DVH values existed, because the comparison of any plan with imaging vs. the original plan without imaging always gave positive ranks. Only for those DVH measures such as the D20Gy for the parotid could significance not be reached because of the variability of the plans, which meant that more than half of the patients had D20Gy = 0% for this organ.

As the target volumes and hence treatment plans vary considerably between the patients, the DVH parameters are also very different. Figure 4 shows the variation in DVH parameters for the left lung for the whole patient collective only for the original treatment plan without imaging. The additional dose from imaging creates less absolute difference than the variation between the individual patients, as can be seen for the example of the left lung values in Figs. 5 and 6. For the parotid mean and D2% values, even the extreme imaging scenario with daily 6 MV CBCT only increases dose by less than 1 Gy. For the spinal cord, the D2% dose increases from 19.7 Gy without imaging to at most 21.2 Gy (daily 6 MV), and by only 0.1 Gy for scenarios with kV imaging. Similar results are obtained for the pharynx and maximum (D2%) and mean lung doses. For the lower-dose DVH values, the differences increase somewhat, e.g. by more than 5% for the lung V20Gy and V5Gy. If the individual patient values (range) are considered rather than the average over the patient collective, strong variations appear, with V20% for the lung ranging from 0% to over 46% and V5Gy from 56 to 100% within the collective.

Imaging effect on secondary cancer risk

Secondary cancer risk reflects the behavior of DVH values in varying more between individual patients than between imaging scenarios (Fig. 6, Table 4). Considering the original plan only (no imaging), the absolute excess cancer risk from treatment for the lungs is of the order of 5–6 cases per 10^4 PY (range 1.3–10 per 10^4 PY) and for the breast ranges between 2.4 and 26 per 10^4 PY.

To concentrate on the effect of imaging rather than the inter-individual differences in target volume, we consider the differences between the original plan and the plans including imaging. The absolute excess risk from imaging only (disregarding the "baseline risk" from radiotherapy treatment) is given in Table 5 and shown in Fig. 7 for the left lung. Comparing this with Fig. 6 shows that the variability between the patients is drastically decreased, so that the systematic effect from imaging becomes visible. We can therefore now calculate the average additional risk over the patient collective (Fig. 8), which is considered in the following.

As was expected, daily 6 MV CBCT causes most additional cancer risk (more than 3 cases per 10^4 PY for the female breast and 0.7–0.8 cases per 10^4 PY for the lungs). If only 6 MV imaging is available, the secondary cancer risk can be drastically decreased by preferentially performing planar images; in the case of daily planar 6

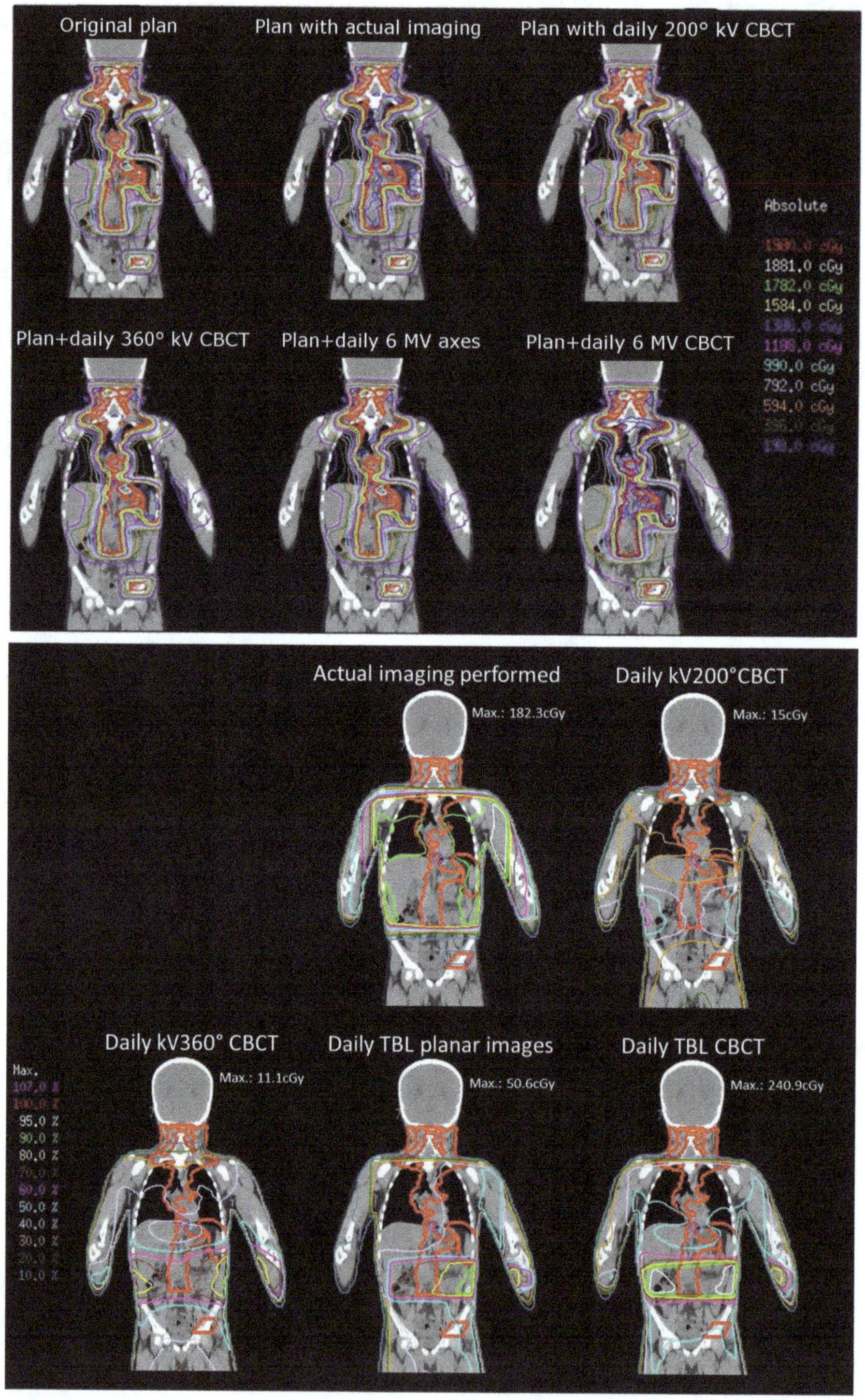

Fig. 2 Upper panel: dose distribution for the original treatment plan and summation plan including different imaging scenarios. Lower panel: dose distribution for different imaging scenarios only

MV imaging the additional excess absolute cancer risk for the breast is decreased to 0.4–0.8 cases per 10^4 PY (a factor of 3.9–5.8) and to 0.1 cases for the lungs (more than a factor of 5). Slightly lower values are achieved by daily 360° kV CBCT (0.44–0.57 per 10^4 PY for the breast and 0.08 per 10^4 PY for the lungs), which is again reduced for daily 200° kV CBCT. For this scenario, the additional excess absolute cancer risk for the lungs is 0.02 per 10^4 PY

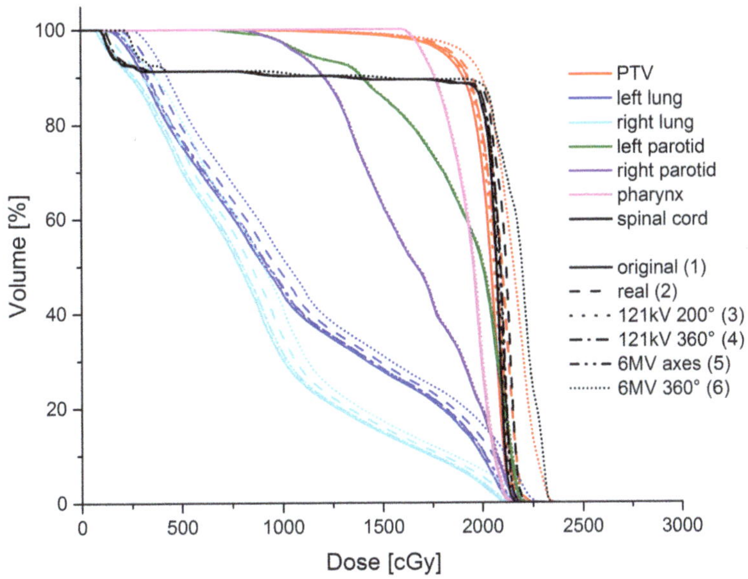

Fig. 3 Example DVH for original plan and different imaging scenarios (same patient as in Fig. 2)

(lower than 360° by a factor of 4) and 0.07–0.08 per 10^4 PY for the breast (decreased by a factor of 6–7 with respect to the 360° kV CBCT scenario). The reason for this more pronounced improvement in the secondary cancer risk for the breast as compared with the lung is the geometry of the imaging system: The 200° kV CBCT is taken rotating the X-ray source under the back of the patient, so that the breast only receives the much attenuated exit dose. As the lungs are located more centrally, the difference between a full CBCT rotation and a partial one does not produce such a pronounced effect. On average, the real imaging performed contributed about as much to secondary cancer risk as daily kV CBCT with mixed 200° and 360° kV CBCT would have.

Discussion

We have mathematically estimated the risk for developing secondary cancers of the lung and female breast for a collective of eight pediatric patients (11 radiotherapy treatment plans) with Morbus Hodgkin based on the dose distribution from the treatment plan and several clinically relevant IGRT scenarios. Although there is relatively large variability between the patients, the additional risk from imaging could be determined. Depending on the imaging scenario used, the excess average risk at age 50 for developing a secondary cancer of the lungs ranged between 1.3 and 10 cases per 10^4 PY (0–2.3 per 10^4 PY only from imaging) and 2.4–27.5 cases per 10^4 PY (0.1–4.8 per 10^4 PY from imaging) for a secondary cancer of the female breast.

Influence of assumed age at secondary cancer incidence

Our estimates for the EAR of secondary cancer development depend on the age attained included in the model. We have opted for a relatively young age of 50 years, since this is already more than 30 years after treatment (age of exposure was set to the real age of the patients at treatment) and since this would be an age at which all possible therapeutic measures would most probably still be taken to cure the secondary malignancy.

The value assumed for the age attained only influences the risk estimate via the modifying function μ, which directly scales with the EAR. For our patient collective and an assumed age attained of 50 years, μ for the lungs is of the order of 0.23, but strongly increases with age attained to 0.95–0.97 for 70 years and about 2.8 for 90 years. This explains to some degree the relatively small EAR values obtained in our study. By considering an attained age of 70 rather than 50 years, all presented risk values would be increased about fourfold, and up to a factor 12 if a long life expectancy as 90 years is assumed. For breast cancer, μ varies more between the patients, as the dependence on the age at exposure is stronger. For an attained age of 50 years, μ is between 0.95 and 1.32, increasing to 1.7–2.3 for an attained age of 70 years and to 2.5–3.6 for 90 years. Here, the age attained only increases the estimated EAR by a factor of less than 3.

Influence of modelling approach

All models for secondary cancer induction are simplified estimates based on the available evidence, which is complicated by the long latency periods and the existence of a large number of confounding factors influencing the risk of secondary cancer induction (e.g., additional chemotherapy, life-style and other exposures such as smoking, etc.). While a numbers of models are available

Table 3 Dose metrics for the organs at risk in the imaging scenarios (mean ± standard deviation, range)

Organ	Criteria	Scenario1	Scenario 2	Scenario 3	Scenario 4	Scenario 5	Scenario 6
Lung le	D mean [Gy]	9.13 ± 4.88 (2.62–17.43)	9.27 ± 4.90 (2.74–17.54)	9.17 ± 4.90 (2.65–17.53)	9.28 ± 4.96 (2.74–17.80)	9.39 ± 5.01 (2.81–17.98)	10.46 ± 5.62 (3.59–20.25)
	V20Gy [%]	9.72 ± 12.07 (0.00–32.26)	11.04 ± 12.55 (0.00–32.55)	9.91 ± 12.20 (0.00–32.54)	10.33 ± 12.52 (0.00–33.34)	10.73 ± 12.74 (0.00–33.84)	14.63 ± 15.05 (0.00–40.55)
	V10Gy [%]	39.27 ± 27.78 (2.33–88.37)	40.03 ± 27.99 (2.44–88.88)	39.46 ± 27.92 (2.35–88.85)	39.89 ± 28.27 (2.43–90.16)	40.36 ± 28.54 (2.49–91.08)	44.55 ± 30.80 (3.20–98.92)
	V5Gy [%]	59.29 ± 29.06 (11.03–100)	60.2 ± 29.24 (11.92–100)	59.46 ± 29.06 (11.23–100)	59.9 ± 28.97 (11.92–100)	60.38 ± 29.01 (12.38–100)	67.28 ± 30.31 (20.45–100)
	D 2% [Gy]	20.81 ± 6.98 (3.33–31.78)	20.96 ± 6.96 (3.43–31.84)	20.85 ± 6.99 (3.37–31.84)	20.98 ± 7.03 (3.45–32.05)	21.14 ± 7.07 (3.47–32.11)	22.12 ± 7.39 (4.33–34.14)
Lung ri	D mean [Gy]	9.2 ± 6.10 (1.58–18.66)	9.33 ± 6.12 (1.65–18.72)	9.24 ± 6.12 (1.61–18.74)	9.29 ± 6.08 (1.68–18.60)	9.38 ± 6.18 (1.65–18.99)	10.43 ± 6.62 (2.26–20.98)
	V20Gy [%]	10.1 ± 13.08 (0.00–38.70)	10.6 ± 13.14 (0.00–38.89)	10.2 ± 13.68 (0.00–38.92)	10.62 ± 13.44 (0.00–39.56)	10.9 ± 13.52 (0.00–39.67)	15.32 ± 16.26 (0.00–46.67)
	V10Gy [%]	41.13 ± 35.44 (0.00–98.93)	41.86 ± 35.30 (0.00–98.94)	41.26 ± 35.47 (0.00–98.93)	41.52 ± 35.55 (0.00–98.95)	41.70 ± 35.51 (0.00–98.96)	45.4 ± 36.36 (0.00–99.12)
	V5Gy [%]	56.29 ± 35.96 (0.00–100)	57.13 ± 36.30 (0.00–100)	56.45 ± 35.96 (0.00–100)	56.8 ± 35.90 (0.00–100)	57.03 ± 35.95 (0.00–100)	62.4 ± 36.23 (0.00–100)
	D 2% [Gy]	20.5 ± 8.66 (3.33–31.78)	20.64 ± 8.65 (3.43–31.84)	20.54 ± 8.67 (3.37–31.48)	20.65 ± 8.70 (3.45–32.05)	20.72 ± 8.73 (3.47–32.11)	21.72 ± 9.24 (4.33–34.14)
Breast le	D mean [Gy]	3.10 ± 2.84 (0.74–7.06)	3.19 ± 2.81 (0.87–7.10)	3.13 ± 2.86 (0.76–7.11)	3.29 ± 2.95 (0.89–7.44)	3.38 ± 3.01 (0.94–7.62)	4.27 ± 3.53 (1.60–9.34)
	D 2% [Gy]	12.60 ± 5.65 (8.85–20.89)	12.67 ± 5.53 (9.01–20.75)	12.56 ± 5.59 (8.86–20.75)	12.76 ± 5.66 (9.02–21.05)	12.86 ± 5.70 (9.08–21.21)	13.93 ± 6.12 (9.90–22.89)
Breast ri	D mean [Gy]	5.81 ± 4.80 (1.37–11.53)	5.89 ± 4.82 (1.41–11.67)	5.83 ± 4.81 (1.38–11.56)	6.0 ± 4.85 (1.49–11.73)	6.01 ± 4.86 (1.50–11.75)	6.97 ± 5.13 (2.16–12.82)
	D 2% [Gy]	16.08 ± 6.12 (9.84–21.41)	16.18 ± 6.12 (9.90–21.43)	16.09 ± 6.12 (9.85–21.43)	16.28 ± 6.17 (9.99–21.43)	16.34 ± 6.19 (10.03–21.70)	17.41 ± 6.46 (10.83–23.31)
Parotid le	D mean [Gy]	5.25 ± 7.94 (0.17–18.71)	5.29 ± 7.92 (0.20–18.75)	5.28 ± 7.93 (0.20–18.71)	5.36 ± 7.91 (0.27–18.72)	5.38 ± 7.92 (0.21–18.72)	5.98 ± 7.82 (0.55–18.78)
	D 2% [Gy]	6.68 ± 9.76 (0.24–21.78)	6.74 ± 9.53 (0.36–21.82)	6.71 ± 9.75 (0.28–21.78)	6.66 ± 9.70 (0.40–21.78)	6.86 ± 9.71 (0.41–21.79)	7.62 ± 9.52 (1.20–21.86)
Parotid ri	D mean [Gy]	3.77 ± 5.96 (0.39–16.50)	3.81 ± 5.95 (0.43–16.53)	3.80 ± 5.95 (0.42–16.50)	3.89 ± 5.92 (0.50–16.51)	3.90 ± 5.92 (0.45–16.51)	4.51 ± 5.74 (0.77–16.57)
	D 2% [Gy]	5.50 ± 7.92 (0.62–21.41)	5.48 ± 7.92 (0.73–21.46)	5.48 ± 7.91 (0.66–21.42)	5.58 ± 7.88 (0.78–21.43)	5.59 ± 7.87 (0.79–21.43)	6.37 ± 7.60 (1.59–21.49)
	OED	0.79 ± 0.82 (0.14–2.20)	0.81 ± 0.81 (0.20–2.20)	0.81 ± 0.82 (0.16–2.20)	0.84 ± 0.80 (0.22–2.20)	0.84 ± 0.80 (0.22–2.20)	1.05 ± 0.70 (0.36–2.20)
	EAR	0.43 ± 0.47 (0.08–1.31)	0.43 ± 0.47 (0.09–1.31)	0.43 ± 0.47 (0.09–1.28)	0.45 ± 0.46 (0.11–1.31)	0.45 ± 0.46 (0.10–1.31)	0.55 ± 0.42 (0.16–1.31)
Pharynx	D mean [Gy]	6.51 ± 7.52 (0.72–19.34)	6.56 ± 7.50 (0.84–19.38)	6.53 ± 7.49 (0.75–19.34)	6.62 ± 7.49 (0.87–19.35)	6.66 ± 7.48 (0.93–19.36)	7.38 ± 7.28 (2.05–19.43)
	D 2% [Gy]	12.28 ± 7.29 (1.06–21.05)	12.37 ± 7.24 (1.18–21.11)	12.31 ± 7.28 (1.09–21.06)	12.48 ± 7.25 (1.22–21.06)	12.39 ± 7.19 (1.27–21.07)	13.33 ± 6.95 (2.41–21.15)
Spinal cord	D 2% [Gy]	19.66 ± 7.97 (6.36–29.53)	19.8 ± 7.97 (6.46–29.60)	19.71 ± 7.99 (6.40–29.61)	19.81 ± 8.02 (6.48–29.80)	19.89 ± 8.05 (6.50–29.90)	21.17 ± 8.43 (7.41–31.67)

with parametrizations for different OAR's, it is as yet unclear which class of model (linear-non-threshold, plateau or bell-shaped) should be considered the most realistic. The full model by Schneider et al. [12] has the intuitive plausibility that high doses leading to cell kill would not be expected to be as cancerogenetic as lower doses resulting only in DNA damage without cell death. However, this hypothesis is not unanimously adopted, as some studies have also supported a linear relationship (compare Filippi et al. for a recent review [13]).

If the assumption of a bell-shaped model should hold true, however, it is highly relevant that all dose contributions

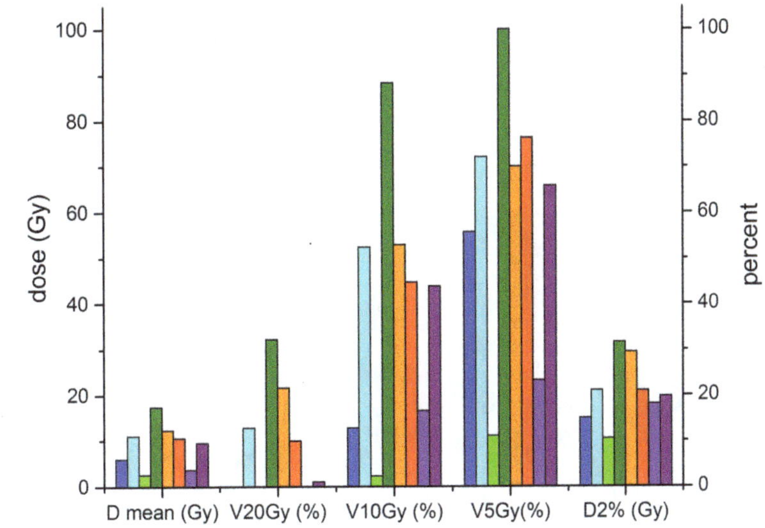

Fig. 4 Dose metrics for the left lung (all patients). Shown are 8 separate data sets because one patient received two separate planning CTs for the two target sites

should be summed together for secondary cancer estimation, rather than considering the effects individually. If the secondary cancer risk from imaging and from treatment were assessed separately from one another, the linear model would be applied to the small doses implicated from imaging. In principle, this approach would be invalid if the treatment dose is far from the linear dose-risk regime, so that the contributions from imaging and treatment are not additive in the simple sense. However, in some cases there is no way of performing a combined imaging plus treatment dose assessment for secondary cancer risk, e.g. if no information on the treatment dose exists and just general conclusions about different imaging systems and their comparison with each other are drawn [14].

While emphasizing that this approach should be avoided because of the presumed non-linear shape of the dose-risk

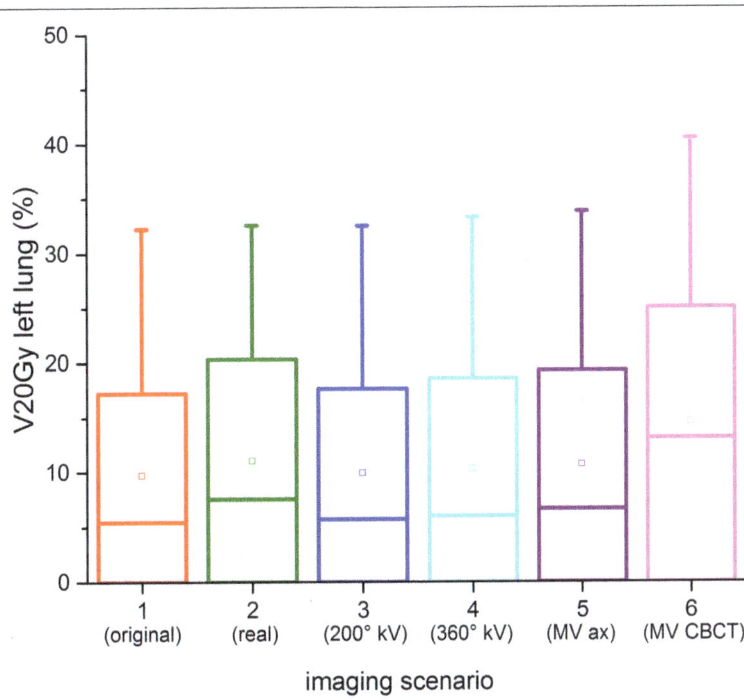

Fig. 5 Spread of the V20Gy dose metric for the left lung across the patient collective. The box gives the 25% and 75% quartile, the horizontal line the median, the square the average. Whiskers reach to the maximum

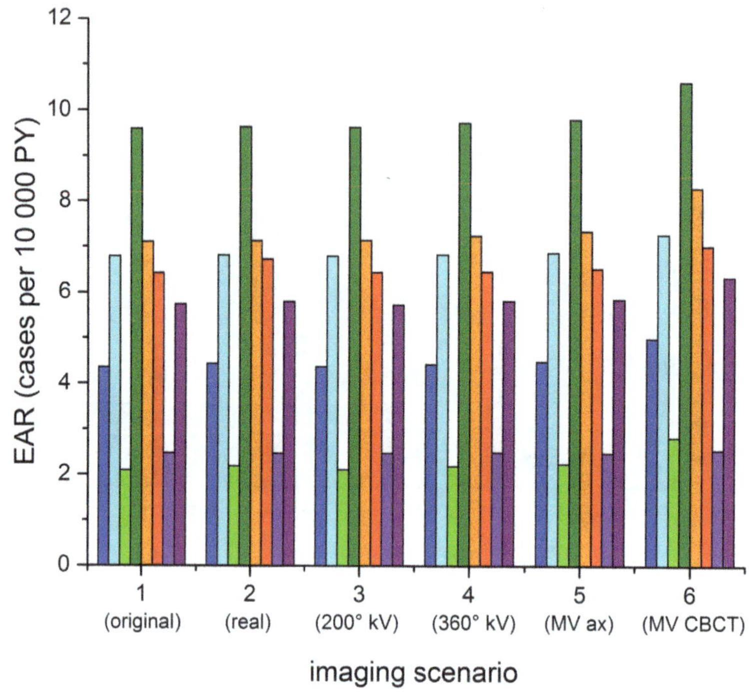

Fig. 6 Excess absolute cancer risk for the left lung for the patient collective modelled for different imaging scenarios (each colour bar corresponds to an individual patient CT data set)

curve, we perform this estimation to demonstrate in how far the results would be influenced by following this approach, as it is sometimes adopted in the literature. Table 6 gives the average dose to the lung and breast from imaging only for the different scenarios, and the resulting secondary cancer risk from the linear model (RED(D) = D). The estimated risk from this method is considerably higher (by a factor 3–4) than the risk resulting from the clinically realistic scenario in

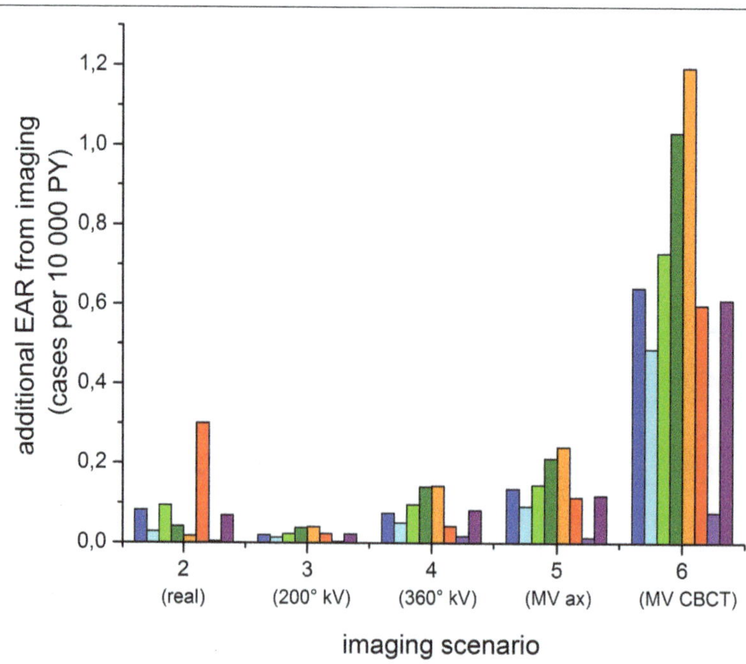

Fig. 7 Additional EAR from imaging only (difference between total EAR as shown in Fig. 6 and EAR from the original plan, each colour bar corresponds to an individual patient CT data set)

Table 4 Excess absolute risk (in cases per 10^4 PY): average ± standard deviation (min-max)

	Scenario 1 (original)	Scenario 2 (real)	Scenario 3 (200° kV-CBCT)	Scenario 4 (360° kV-CBCT)	Scenario 5 (6MV axes)	Scenario 6 (6MV CBCT)
Left lung	5.58 ± 2.5 (2.1–9.6)	5.66 ± 2,5 (2.2–9.6)	6.25 ± 2.7 (2.6–10.6)	5.72 ± 2.6 (2.2–9.9)	5.65 ± 2.5 (2.2–9.7)	5.60 ± 2.5 (2.1–9.6)
Right lung	5.54 ± 3.2 (1.3–10.0)	5.62 ± 3,2 (1.4–10.0)	6.17 ± 3.3 (1.9–10.8)	5.64 ± 3.2 (1.4–10.1)	5.62 ± 3.2 (1.4–10.1)	5.56 ± 3.2 (1.3–10.0)
Left breast	8.73 ± 6.9 (2.4–17.9)	9.03 ± 6,8 (2.8–18.0)	11.87 ± 7.7 (5.3–22.7)	9.53 ± 7.1 (3.0–19.2)	9.30 ± 7.0 (2.9–18.8)	8.81 ± 6.9 (2.4–18.0)
Right breast	14.12 ± 10.3 (4.8–26.0)	14.29 ± 10.2 (5.0–26.2)	16.63 ± 10.0 (7.7–27.5)	14.56 ± 10.2 (5.3–26.3)	14.57 ± 10.2 (5.3–26.3)	14.19 ± 10.2 (4.9–26.1)

which imaging dose and treatment dose act together simultaneously. The possible non-linearity in the risk curve thus plays a significant role and different coinciding contributions to dose should be analysed together, if this is possible.

Comparison with previous studies

A number of studies have estimated imaging dose for MV and kV modalities in either planar or CBCT geometries, although relatively few have considered pediatric patients. For the Varian On-Board Imager (OBI) system (Varian Medical Systems, Palo Alto, California, USA), Ding et al. [15] obtained doses to soft tissue of the order of 4–10 cGy (half-fan) and 3–9 cGy (full-fan mode) for pediatric patients with imaging in the head-and-neck region using the Vanderbilt-Monte-Carlo-Beam-Calibration algorithm. Similar dose values (1.9–10.5 cGy depending on the organ) were reported by Deng et al. [16] for 125 kVp voltage based on Monte Carlo methods. Measurements in an anthropomorphic phantom (adult and pediatric) [17] confirm this order of magnitude. Our calculated average organ doses for the kV imaging scenarios are larger than the original treatment plan dose by up to 20 cGy for daily imaging (up to 16 fractions, which means a few cGy per image). This is in good agreement with previous studies, which can be expected since dose calculations for our system also agreed well with those from Varian and Elekta (Elekta, Stockholm, Sweden) for other tumor indications.

Regarding secondary cancer risk estimates, the results from previous studies are rather varied depending on the assumed target localization, dose distribution and secondary cancer model (for reviews, see [18, 19] and references therein). Comparing our predictions with clinical data, Dörffel et al. [20] observed an absolute excess risk of developing secondary malignancies at the breast of 14.9 per 10,000 PY in a cohort study of 2548 patients treated for Hodgkin's Lymphoma within 30 years' follow-up, which agrees well with the range of values obtained in our study (2–26 cases per 10,000 PY). In their review, Kamran et al. [21] list an absolute risk for breast cancer after Hodgkin lymphoma of 37 per 10,000 PY; Schaapveld et al. [22] estimate an EAR of 20.5–29.3 per 10,000 PY for the lung and 44.7–65.0 per 10,000 PY for the breast. Since our prediction is for an attained age of 50 years and increases with higher age, the agreement is still plausible.

Only few studies have focused on secondary cancer risk from imaging in radiotherapy. Zhang et al. [23] presented imaging dose from Varian kV CBCT as a function of patient chest circumference, where organ mean dose per scan was of the order of 0.8–3 cGy (in agreement with our results), but used the BEIR VII model to transfer these values into relative risks for secondary cancer. As we have pointed out, the non-linear behaviour of the cancer risk curve should be accounted for by considering the combination of treatment and imaging dose where this is possible. For this high-dose regime, it is more common to use Schneider's full mechanistic model; however, this is usually applied to treatment plans rather than IGRT scenarios [24]. To our knowledge, our study is the first one to include imaging scenarios in the radiotherapy treatment plan for an accurate assessment of additional cancer risk in the dose regime used for treatment.

Limitations and implications of this study

In addition to the relatively small patient collective available for our study, it must be born in mind that the treatment plans were not particularly optimized to minimize secondary cancer risk, neither for optimal

Table 5 Additional EAR from imaging only (in cases per 10^4 PY, average ± standard deviation, range in braces)

Organ	Scenario 2 (real)	Scenario 3 (200° kV-CBCT)	Scenario 4 (360° kV-CBCT)	Scenario 5 (6MV axes)	Scenario 6 (6MV CBCT)
Left lung	0.08 ± 0.09 (0.00–0.30)	0.02 ± 0.01 (0.00–0.04)	0.08 ± 0.04 (0.02–0.14)	0.13 ± 0.07 (0.01–0.24)	0.67 ± 0.34 (0.08–1.19)
Right lung	0.07 ± 0.11 (0.00–0.07)	0.02 ± 0.01 (0.00–0.04)	0.08 ± 0.05 (0.02–0.16)	0.1 ± 0.06 (0.01–0.21)	0.75 ± 0.66 (0.08–2.31)
Left breast	0.29 ± 0.16 (0.11–0.46)	0.08 ± 0.03 (0.06–0.12)	0.57 ± 0.22 (0.38–0.88)	0.8 ± 0.33 (0.55–1.29)	3.14 ± 1.19 (1.99–4.81)
Right breast	0.18 ± 0.09 (0.09–0.31)	0.07 ± 0.02 (0.04–0.09)	0.44 ± 0.16 (0.25–0.64)	0.43 ± 0.13 (0.27–0.58)	2.51 ± 0.77 (1.50–3.33)

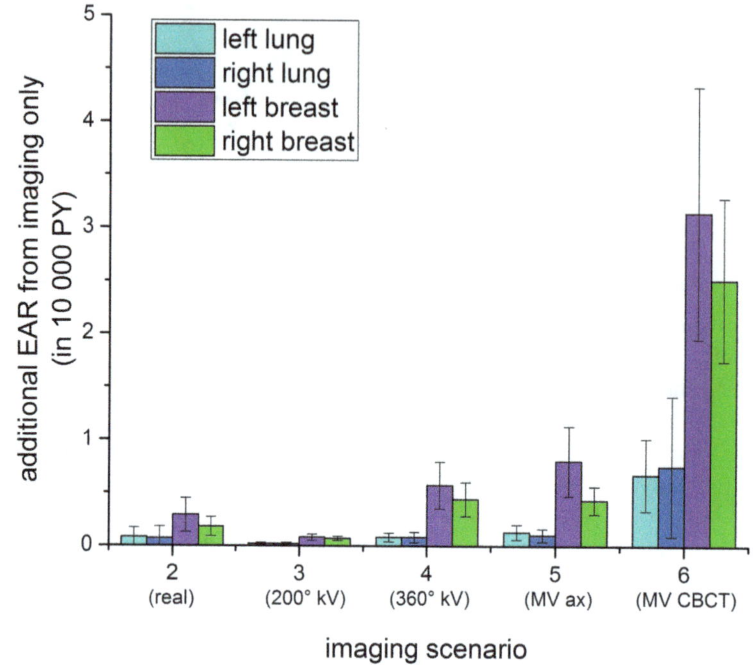

Fig. 8 Additional EAR from imaging only, average (with standard deviation) over all patients

sparing of the female breast. Although these organs are taken into account as an organs at risk in our planning process, a compromise was made for best sparing of all healthy organs, so that the two sites at most risk for secondary cancer incidence were not prioritized over the other OAR's. While all patients were treated with the involved field technique, the target volumes showed strong variation (PTV volumes 54–2419 cm^3, average 1145 cm^3). Most patients were treated using step-and-shoot IMRT (4–14 beams with between 30 and 70 segments), only very small target volumes (e.g., case 9, os ileum) were treated using 3D conformal radiotherapy (3D CRT with 2 beams). Volumetric modulated arc therapy (VMAT) plans were never used. The number of beams and segments used in the IMRT plans varied individually. In addition to setting objectives for the organs at risk, ring and normal tissue structures were created to form a dose gradient around the target volume.

Despite the large variability between the patients, the DVH metrics correspond to those reported by other authors. For example, Maraldo et al. [25] assessed normal tissue doses for different radiotherapy targets for patients with Hodgkin's lymphoma. For the lungs, they found mean doses in the range of 30–52% of the prescribed dose (30 Gy in their study, i.e. 11.7–15.6 Gy) for mantle field and mediastinal irradiation and 2.2–4.0 Gy for neck and axilla irradiation, which agrees with the range of doses from our collective (1.6–18.7 Gy mean lung dose). Similarly, their values for the female breast were between 1.4 and 17 Gy depending on the treatment fields, corresponding to our dose range between 0.7 and 11.5 Gy.

Regarding margins for the PTV, in a previous unpublished study (similar to [8]) we analyzed positioning errors for a collective of children, resulting in a systematic population setup error of 0.7/1.0/− 0.2 mm in the anterior-posterior (AP)/left-right (LR) and superior-/inferior (SI) directions, a variation of population setup error of 1.7/2.6/2.5 mm (AP/LR/SI) and a population random error or 3.9/4.9/3.9 mm (AP/LR/SI), which yields a CTV-PTV margin of 8.2/11.4/10.2 mm according to the margin recipe by van Herk et al.

Table 6 Additional EAR from imaging only if imaging was considered separately from the treatment plan

	Scenario 2 (real)	Scenario 3 (200° kV-CBCT)	Scenario 4 (360° kV-CBCT)	Scenario 5 (6 MV axes)	Scenario 6 (6MV CBCT)
Left lung	0.26 ± 0.34 (0–5.25)	0.08 ± 0.59 (0–5.25)	0.29 ± 0.21 (0.06–5.25)	0.48 ± 0.31 (0.04–5.25)	2.48 ± 1.62 (0.26–5.25)
Right lung	0.25 ± 0.34 (0–1.07)	0.07 ± 0.48 (0–0.15)	0.18 ± 0.17 (0–0.48)	0.34 ± 0.21 (0.04–0.63)	2.28 ± 1.38 (0.24–4.32)
Left breast	0.89 ± 0.57 (0.31–1.41)	0.24 ± 0.10 (0.16–0.39)	1.74 ± 0.83 (1.05–2.96)	2.51 ± 1.27 (1.45–4.35)	10.27 ± 5.08 (6.37–17.7)
Right breast	0.78 ± 0.61 (0.23–1.52)	0.23 ± 0.11 (0.08–0.33)	1.71 ± 0.65 (0.97–2.33)	1.80 ± 0.70 (1.05–2.41)	10.60 ± 3.68 (6.37–13.98)

This table assumes that imaging was considered separately from the treatment dose. In this case, a linear risk model would be applied as imaging dose is in the low dose regime. Data are given as cases per 10^4 PY, average ± standard deviation, range in braces

[26]. In the clinical practice, between 10 and 15 mm margin are used at our department. In fact, the use of daily imaging would be expected to reduce the required margins, as the daily statistical error could be corrected before treatment and position close to the planned "ideal" position could be attained. In this case, a margin reduction would allow for better sparing of organs at risk and a possible decrease in secondary cancer risk. Therefore, the increase in dose from daily imaging might be counterbalanced by an sparing in dose due to improved positioning accuracy. Such a trade-off would be interesting to perform, but remains outside the scope of this study as a number of combinations (margin vs. imaging scenario) would need to be compared. Similar approaches have been presented for other treatment sites [11, 27]. As a rule-of-thumb, dose from kV imaging is relatively small and it might be expected that the positive influence of dose sparing from margin reduction would be dominant in this scenario. Regarding daily MV imaging, however, this might no longer be the case, and it is generally believed that a daily 6 MV CBCT scenario should be avoided unless in very limited indications (e.g., direct vicinity of critical OAR and high-risk target volume).

Finally, the present study focusses on a highly vulnerable collective (children with good long-term prognosis treated with relatively large fields and wide margins), so that the resulting estimated risk can be expected to be larger than for the most frequent radiotherapy treatments (adult patients with small fields), where improved positioning accuracy and small margins achieved by daily (kV) imaging might considerably reduce normal tissue complications without detrimentous effects on secondary cancer risk.

Conclusions

If daily imaging is required, this can be performed with less than 1 case per 10^4 PY additional cancer risk using kV CBCT or – if no other option exists – 6 MV as long as planar images are taken. Depending on the geometry of the X-ray tube (e.g., opposite to the treatment head), a further reduction on dose can be achieved for superficial organs such as the breasts by applying only a reduced-arc rotation (in our case, behind the patient's back). When analyzing secondary cancer risk from imaging modalities, this should in the best case be combined with the treatment plan, as a separate analysis of only imaging dose in the linear range leads to an overestimation of the secondary cancer risk.

Abbreviations

AP: Anterior-posterior; CBCT: Cone-beam CT; CRT: Conformal radiotherapy; CT: Computed tomography; DICOM: Digital Imaging and Communications in Medicine; DVH: Dose-volume histogram; EAR: Excess absolute risk; EPID: Electron portal imaging device; IBL: Imaging beam line; IGRT: Image-guided radiotherapy; LR: Left-right; MU: Monitor units; OAR: Organ at risk; OBI: On-Board Imager; PTV: Planning target volume; PY: Patient-years; RED: Risk equivalent dose; ROI: Region of interest; SI: Superior-inferior; SSD: Source-to-surface distance; TBL: Treatment beam line; TPS: Treatment planning system; VMAT: Volumetric modulated arc therapy

Acknowledgements

We thank three anonymous reviewers for their very constructive and helpful suggestions, which we believe have greatly improved this manuscript.

Funding

The authors did not receive any funding for this study or work related to this study.

Authors' contributions

YD, PM and FN designed the study. KB and KM performed all data handling, with support by PM regarding the medical records. PR wrote and validated the Matlab code. KM, KB and YD performed the data analysis; the interpretation of the results was performed by YD, PM, FN and CR. YD wrote and revised the manuscript. All authors read and approved the final manuscript.

Competing interests

The authors declare that they have no competing interests.

References

1. Dzierma Y, Nuesken FG, Licht NP, Ruebe C. Dosimetric properties and commissioning of cone-beam CT image beam line with a carbon target. Strahlenther Onkol. 2013;189:566–72.
2. Faddegon BA, Wu V, Pouliot J, et al. Low dose megavoltage cone beam computed tomography with an unflattened 4 MV beam from a carbon target. Med Phys. 2008;35(12):5777–86.
3. Faddegon BA, Aubin M, Bani-Hashemi A, et al. Comparison of patient megavoltage cone beam CT images acquired with an unflattened beam from a carbon target and a flattened treatment beam. Med Phys. 2010;37(4):1737–41.
4. Dzierma Y, Nuesken F, Otto W, Alaei P, Licht N, Rübe C. Dosimetry of an in-line Kilovoltage imaging system and implementation in treatment planning. Int J Radiation Oncol Biol Phys. 2014;88(4):913–9.
5. Fast MF, Krauss A, Oelfke U, et al. Position detection accuracy of a novel linac-mounted intrafractional x-ray imaging system. Med Phys. 2012;39:109–18.
6. Stützel J, Oelfke U, Nill S. A quantitative image quality comparison of four different image guided radiotherapy devices. Radiother Oncol. 2008;86:20–4.
7. Fast MF, Koenig T, Oelfke U, et al. Performance characteristics of a novel megavoltage cone-beam-computed tomography device. Phys Med Biol. 2012;57:N15–24.
8. Dzierma Y, Beyhs M, Palm J, et al. Set-up errors and planning margins in planar and CBCT image-guided radiotherapy using three different imaging systems: a clinical study for prostate and head-and-neck cancer. Phys Med (EJMP). 2015;31(8):1055–9.
9. Dzierma Y, Ames E, Nuesken F, Palm J, Licht N, Rübe C. Image quality and dose distributions of three linac-based imaging modalities. Strahlenther Onkol. 2015;191:365–74.
10. Alcorn SR, Chen MJ, Claude L, Dieckmann K, Ermoian RP, Ford EC, et al. Practice patterns of photon and proton pediatric image guided radiation treatment: results from an international pediatric research consortium. Pract Radiat Oncol. 2014;4:336–41.

11. Bell K, Heitfeld M, Licht N, Rübe C, Dzierma Y. Influence of daily imaging on plan quality and normal tissue toxicity for prostate cancer radiotherapy. Radiat Oncol. 2017;12:7.
12. Schneider U, Sumila M, Robotka J. Site-specific dose-response relationships for cancer induction from the combined Japanese A-bomb and Hodgkin cohorts for doses relevant to radiotherapy. Theoretical Biol Medical Modell. 2011;8:27.
13. Filippi AR, Vanoni V, Meduri B, Cozzi L, Scorsetti M, Ricardi U, Lohr F. Intensity modulated radiation therapy and second Cancer risk in adults. Int J Radiat Oncol Biol Phys. 2018;100(1):17–20.
14. Dzierma Y, Minko P, Ziegenhain R, Bell K, Buecker A, Rübe C, Jagoda P. Abdominal imaging dose in radiology and radiotherapy – phantom point dose measurements, effective dose and secondary cancer risk. Phys Med (EJMP). 2017;43:49–56.
15. Ding GX, ChW C. Radiation dose from kilovoltage cone beam computed tomography in an image-guided radiotherapy procedure. Int J Radiation Oncology Biol Phys. 2009;73(2):610–7.
16. Deng J, Chen Z, Roberts KB, Nath R. Kilovoltage imaging doses in the radiotherapy of pediatric cancer patients. Int J Radiation Oncol Biol Phys. 2012;82(5):1680–8.
17. Son K, Kim JS, Lee H, Cho S. Imaging dose of human organs from kV-CBCT in image-guided radiation therapy. Radiat Protect Dosim. 2017;175(2):194–200.
18. Hess CB, Thompson HM, Benedict SH, Seibert JA, Wong K, Vaughan AT, Chen AM. Exposure risks among children undergoing radiation therapy: considerations in the era of image guided radiation therapy. Int J Radiation Oncol Biol Phys. 2016;94(5):978–92.
19. Chargari C, Goodman KA, Diallo I, Guy J-B, Rancoule C, Cosset J-M, Deutsch E, Magne N. Risk of second cancers in the era of modern radiotherapy: does the risk/benefit analysis overcome theoretical models? Cancer Metastasis Rev. 2016;35:227–88.
20. Dörffel W, Riepenhausen M, Lüders H, Brämswig J, Schellong G. Secondary malignancies following treatment for Hodgkin's lymphoma in childhood and adolescence – a cohort study with more than 30 years' follow-up. Dtsch Arztebl Int. 2015;112:320–7.
21. Kamran SC, Berrington de Gonzalez A, Ng A, Haas-Kogan D, Viswanathan AN. Therapeutic radiation and the potential risk of second malignancies. Cancer. 2016;122:1809–21.
22. Schaapveld M, Aleman BMP, van Eggermond AM, Janus CPM, Kron ADG, et al. Second Cancer risk up to 40 years after treatment for Hodgkin's lymphoma. N Engl J Med. 2015;373(26):2499–511.
23. Zhang Y, Wu H, Chen Z, Knisely JP, Nath R, Feng Z, Bao S, Deng J. Concomitant imaging dose and Cancer risk in image guided thoracic radiation therapy. Int J Radiat Oncol Biol Phys. 2015;93(3):523–31.
24. Tamura M, Sakurai H, Mizumoto M, Kamizawa S, Murayama S, et al. Lifetime attributable risk of radiation-induced secondary cancer from proton beam therapy compared with that of intensity-modulated X-ray therapy in randomly sampled pediatric cancer patients. J Radiat Res. 2017;58(3):363–71.
25. Maraldo MV, Lundemann M, Vogelius IR, Specht L. A new method to estimate dosest o the normal tissues after past extended and involved field radiotherapy for Hodgkin lymphoma. Radiother Oncol. 2015;114:206–11.
26. Van Herk M. Errors and margins in radiotherapy. Semin Radiat Oncol. 2004; 14:52–64.
27. Bell K, Licht N, Rübe C, Dzierma Y. Image guidance and positioning accuracy in clinical practice: Influence of positioning errors and imaging dose on the real dose distribution for head and neck cancer treatment. Radiat Oncol, under review.

11

Clinical outcomes of image-guided proton therapy for histologically confirmed stage I non-small cell lung cancer

Koichiro Nakajima[1,2*], Hiromitsu Iwata[1,2], Hiroyuki Ogino[1,2], Yukiko Hattori[1], Shingo Hashimoto[1], Toshiyuki Toshito[3], Kensuke Hayashi[4], Kenji Akita[5], Fumiya Baba[6], Katsumi Nakamae[7], Jun-etsu Mizoe[1,8] and Yuta Shibamoto[2]

Abstract

Background: Two prospective phase II trials were designed to assess the efficacy and safety of image-guided proton therapy (IGPT) for either medically inoperable or operable stage I non-small cell lung cancer (NSCLC). The present study reports the interim results of these trials.

Methods: Fifty-five patients with histologically confirmed stage I NSCLC (IA in 33 patients and IB in 22 patients; inoperable in 21 patients and operable in 34 patients) who received IGPT between July 2013 and February 2017 were analyzed. The median patient age was 71 years (range: 48–88 years). IGPT with fiducial metallic marker matching was performed for suitable patients, and a respiratory gating method for motion management was used for all treatments. Peripherally located tumors were treated with 66 Gy relative biological effectiveness equivalents (Gy(RBE)) in 10 fractions ($n = 49$) and centrally located tumors were treated with 72.6 Gy(RBE) in 22 fractions ($n = 6$). Treatment associated toxicities were evaluated using Common Toxicity Criteria for Adverse Events (v.4.0).

Results: Median follow-up was 35 months (range: 12–54 months) for survivors. For all patients, the 3-year overall survival, progression-free survival, and local control rates were 87% (95% confidence interval: 73–94%), 74% (58–85%), and 96% (83–99%), respectively. Fiducial marker matching was used in 39 patients (71%). Grade 2 toxicities observed were radiation pneumonitis in 5 patients (9%), rib fracture in 2 (4%), and chest wall pain in 5 (9%). There were no grade 3 or higher acute or late toxicities.

Conclusions: IGPT appears to be effective and well tolerated for all patients with stage I NSCLC.

Keywords: Stage I non-small cell lung cancer, Proton therapy, Image-guided proton therapy, Fiducial metallic marker, Respiratory gating system

Background

For stage I non-small cell lung cancer (NSCLC), surgical resection is the current standard treatment. Stereotactic body radiotherapy (SBRT) has been adopted as an alternative treatment modality for medically inoperable patients with stage I NSCLC, and has increasingly been used for operable patients as well [1–4]. In recent years, proton therapy (PT) has been attracting attention as a new and effective treatment option. The greatest advantage of PT over photon-based SBRT is the improved dose distribution that results from the physical properties of proton beams, and in particular the Bragg peak phenomenon. Theoretically, PT enables a reduction in the unnecessary dose delivered to multiple sensitive critical organs at risk (OAR) while facilitating homogenous delivery of higher doses for the tumor [5–7].

In clinical practice, excellent outcomes of PT have been reported for stage I NSCLC [8–11]. There are, however, several outstanding technical improvements that might be made, including the use of image guidance

* Correspondence: k.nakajima.ncu@gmail.com
[1]Department of Radiation Oncology, Nagoya Proton Therapy Center, Nagoya City West Medical Center, 1-1-1 Hirate-cho, Kita-ku, Nagoya 462-8508, Japan
[2]Department of Radiology, Nagoya City University Graduate School of Medical Sciences, 1 Kawasumi, Mizuho-cho, Mizuho-ku, Nagoya 467-8601, Japan
Full list of author information is available at the end of the article

techniques and respiratory motion management. In contrast to SBRT, the optimal irradiation method for a moving target in the body has not been well established because proton beams have more sensitive physical characteristics. Although fiducial marker implantation for image guidance and respiratory gating are widely used for SBRT, neither have been commonly used for PT. In 2013, therefore, we started phase II clinical trials of image-guided PT (IGPT) for stage I NSCLC using fiducial markers with a respiratory gating method.

In the recent several years, dozens of PT facilities have been built and their prevalence will rapidly increase over the next few years [12]. Although its efficacy has been gradually revealed by many investigators, more data is necessary to justify the recent increasing demand for PT. In Japan, medical insurance coverage of PT for stage I NSCLC is now being actively discussed and further evidence is being requested by the government. In this context, we consider that reporting the interim results of our trials is of value, especially given the promising results to date. The purpose of this study was to evaluate 3-year results from our prospective trials of IGPT for stage I NSCLC.

Methods

Study design

An interim analysis of ongoing prospective phase II clinical trials, named "Lung-001" and "Lung-002" and approved by the Institutional Review Board (IRB) of Nagoya City Hospital, was carried out. The IRB numbers are 13–02-09 (9) and 13–02-10 (10), respectively. The former was for medically inoperable patients, and the latter was for operable patients who refused surgery.

The sample size for these trials was calculated based on Simon's two-stage minimax clinical phase II design [13] with a significance level of 0.05 ($\alpha = 0.05$) and a power of 80% ($\beta = 0.20$). For Lung-001, the primary endpoint is incidence of grade 3 or higher radiation pneumonitis (RP) occurring within 180 days from the first date of PT. The acceptable incidence is considered to be less than 5%, and the unacceptable incidence is considered to be more than 15%. It was planned that 39 patients were to be included in Stage 1. If 3 patients or fewer experienced grade 3 or higher RP, the trial was scheduled to move on to Stage 2, with recruitment of an additional 18 patients (a total of 57 patients is required for completion of the trial). For Lung-002, the primary endpoint is 3-year overall survival (OS) rate. The acceptable and unacceptable rates are 65% and 45%, respectively. It was planned that 30 patients were to be included in Stage 1. If 17 or more survived 3 years, the trial was scheduled to move on to Stage 2, with recruitment of an additional 9 patients (a total of 39 patients is required for the trial).

Although the timing of interim analyses had not been defined at the outset, we carried out the interim analysis in response to the request from the Japanese government for up-to-date data, since the Lung-002 study has moved on to Stage 2. In the present study, only patients followed for a minimum of 12 months or until death were enrolled.

Patient eligibility and disease staging

The inclusion criteria were as follows: 1) histologically confirmed NSCLC; 2) clinical stage IA or IB (7th edition of TNM staging of Union for International Cancer Control); 3) Eastern Cooperative Oncology Group performance status of 0–2; 4) no OARs exceeding dose constraints; 5) no previous irradiation of the treatment region; 6) no history of chemotherapy; 7) age ≥ 20 years (Lung-001), or ≥ 20 and ≤ 80 years (Lung-002), 8) forced expiratory volume 1.0 ≥ 700 mL and PaO_2 in room air ≥ 60 Torr (Lung-001), or ≥ 800 mL and ≥ 65 Torr (Lung-002); and 9) written informed consent.

The exclusion criteria were: 1) pregnancy; 2) synchronous or metachronous cancer within 5 years; 3) active infectious disease; 4) other severe comorbidities, e.g., hypertension or diabetes mellitus; 5) severe psychological disorder; and 6) apparent interstitial pneumonitis or pulmonary fibrosis detectable by chest X-ray radiography. Medical inoperability was determined by multidisciplinary thoracic specialists, including a thoracic surgeon.

In all cases, staging was performed with magnetic resonance imaging (MRI) of the brain, computed tomography (CT) of the chest and upper abdomen, and ^{18}F-deoxyglucose-positron emission tomography-CT (PET-CT) within 1 month before the start of PT.

PT and treatment planning

The prescribed dose to the isocenter was 66 Gy relative biological effectiveness equivalents (Gy(RBE)) in 10 fractions for peripherally located tumors and 72.6 Gy(RBE) in 22 fractions for centrally located tumors. The biologically effective dose calculated with an α/β ratio of 10 Gy (BED_{10}) was 110 and 97 Gy(RBE), respectively. All irradiation was given once a day, 5 days a week. The RBE value for our proton beams was determined to be 1.1 [14].

The treatment machines and planning system at our institution were described in detail previously [15]. Briefly, proton treatments were delivered by PROBEAT III (Hitachi, Ltd., Tokyo, Japan) and planned with VQA (Hitachi, Ltd., Tokyo, Japan). A passive scattering technique with mainly 120- to 200-MeV proton beams was used for all treatments. Two to four beam portals were used for each treatment.

Prior to treatment, all patients were evaluated for their respiratory stabilities and tumor motions. In patients with a highly movable tumor, 3 or 4 fiducial markers were implanted near the tumor. The majority of markers were 1.5-mm-diameter gold markers (Olympus, Tokyo, Japan), implanted through bronchoscopy. 0.5-mm-diameter VISICOIL (RadioMed, Barlett, TN, USA) and 0.28-mm-diameter Gold Anchor (Naslund Medical Inc., Chicago, IL, USA) were percutaneously implanted in 2 and 1 patients, respectively. Patients were immobilized in the supine position using an ESFORM immobilization system (Engineering System, Nagano, Japan), and 2-mm-thick CT images were taken using a 16-row multi-detector CT (Aquilion LB; Toshiba Medical Systems, Tochigi, Japan) during the expiration phase for treatment planning. All patients underwent CT simulation with 4-dimensional (4D) CT to account for tumor motion with deformation. Patient respiratory waveforms were monitored throughout the procedures and recorded with an AZ-733 V respiratory gating system (Anzai Medical, Tokyo, Japan). After CT simulation, the 4D-CT images were reconstructed into ten respiratory phases, with end of expiration defined as phase 50% and end of inspiration as phase 0% (=100%). The tumor detected under the lung window was defined as the gross tumor volume (GTV). In addition to the GTV, GTVs from 4D-CT were contoured on CT images of each respiratory phase (GTV_0, GTV_{10} to GTV_{90}). The internal gross tumor volume (IGTV) was defined as the envelope of the GTVs. The IGTV was divided into two; IGTV-all consisted of the GTV and GTVs across all respiratory phases, and IGTV-gate consisted of the GTV and all GTVs within the gating window around phase 50%, e. g., GTV_{20} to GTV_{70} (Fig. 1a). The gating window was chosen with reference to the amplitude of marker and tumor movement. IGTV-gate was only used for patients whose tumor moved more than 10 mm in any direction. For each beam, the IGTV was expanded laterally from the perspective of the beam to encompass the setup error margin (SM) and internal motion margin (IM). The lateral margin was 6 mm for fiducial marker matching plans which included SM and only intrafractional IM. In contrast, the lateral margin for vertebral bone matching plans was 9 mm including SM and intrafractional plus interfractional IM. In addition, beam-specific distal and proximal margins to the IGTV were assigned

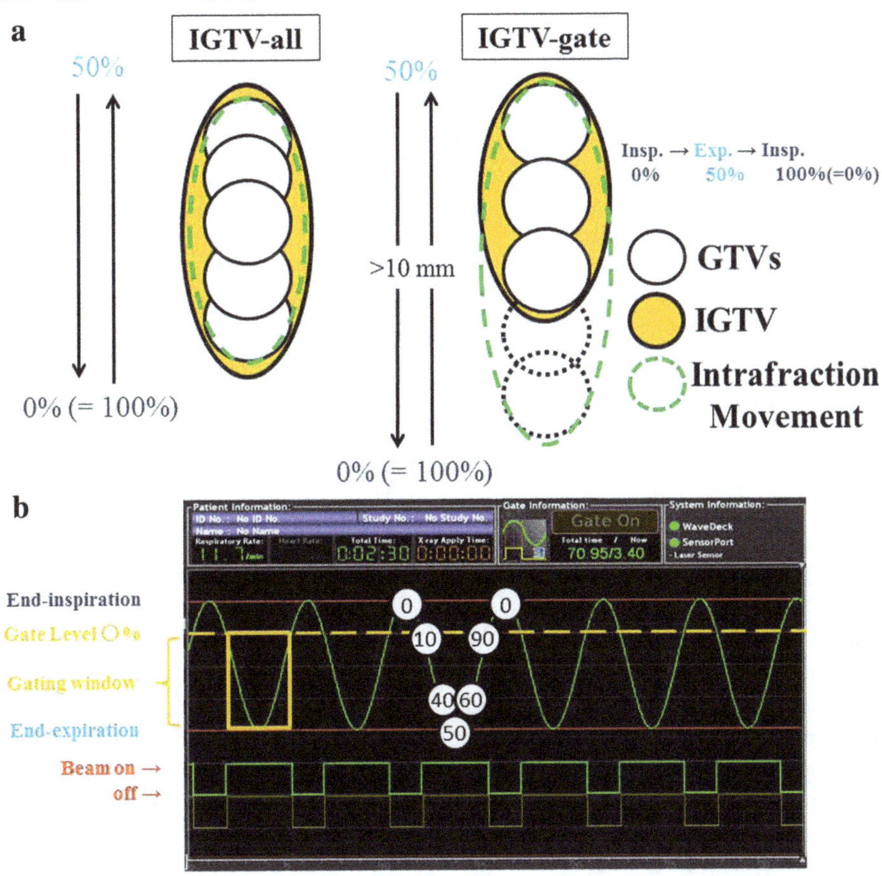

Fig. 1 **a** IGTV volume definition. IGTV-all consisted of GTV and GTVs across all respiratory phases. IGTV-gate consisted of GTV and all GTVs within the gating window around phase 50%. The latter was only used for patients whose tumor moved more than 10 mm in any direction. **b** Schema of the respiratory gating system. Beams turned on only when the monitored respiratory phase was within the predefined gating window. The gate level was defined for each patient by reference to the amplitude of tumor movement

along the beam path axis to account for uncertainties in the range of proton beams. The margins were typically 4–8 mm based on the definition of Moyers et al. [16]. To adjust the proton beam range, compensation boluses were used, and the bolus smearing margins were typically 10–18 mm [16]. The lateral and beam-specific margins were slightly adjusted to meet the dose constraints.

Image-guidance with fiducial markers and respiratory gating irradiation

IGPT was provided for all patients. Daily patient alignments were achieved by matching fiducial markers or vertebral bones. All procedures were performed with 2D/2D matching methods using the PIAS system (Hitachi, Ltd., Tokyo, Japan) [17]. The reference digitally reconstructed radiographs (DRR) and contours for the fiducial markers were developed from the planning CT images. The procedure for fiducial marker matching was as follows: 1) patients were aligned to the isocenter using skin markers and a laser; 2) vertebral bony structure matching was performed with radiographs; 3) radiographs were taken at end-expiration and the couch was manually shifted to align the fiducial marker with the contour of the marker on the DRR, which was developed from 50% phase CT images; 4) radiographs were taken at the inspiration phase to check the correlation between the respiratory waveform and the gating window. All radiographs comprised two sets of orthogonal kilo-voltage digital radiographs.

Respiratory gating irradiation was performed by monitoring patient the waveform under free-breathing. Abdominal surface motion was used as a surrogate for tumor motion, and the beam was turned on only when the monitored respiratory phase fell within the predefined gating window (Fig. 1b).

Treatment evaluation, follow-up, and statistical analysis

The patients were observed at 6-week intervals until 6 months after PT, and at least once every 3 months until 2 years. Thereafter, our protocol policy was to follow-up at 6-month intervals, though most patients were followed up at 3-month intervals. Regular follow-up studies included chest and upper abdominal CT scans and tumor marker examinations. MRI and PET-CT were usually performed once a year or whenever necessary. Acute and late treatment-related toxicities were assessed using the National Cancer Institute Common Toxicity Criteria for Adverse Events (v.4.0). Local recurrence was indicated by expansion of a consolidated fibrotic mass within the irradiated area on CT images, and PET-CT and biopsy were performed when recurrence was strongly suspected.

OS, local control (LC), and progression-free survival (PFS) rates were calculated using the Kaplan-Meier method from the first date of PT. Univariate associations of patient and treatment characteristics with OS, LC and PFS were examined with the log-rank test. Evaluated factors included sex, age, stage, histology, tumor site, radiation dose, position matching method and IGTV definition. A *P*-value of <.05 was considered to be significant. All statistical analyses were performed with EZR version 1.35 [18].

Results

Patient, tumor and treatment characteristics

Characteristics of the patients and tumors are summarized in Table 1 and treatment characteristics are summarized in Table 2. Between July 2013 and February

Table 1 Patient and Tumor Characteristics

Characteristic	All	Inoperable	Operable
No. of patients	55	21	34
Age (y), median (range)	71 (48–88)	81 (65–88)	70 (48–79)
Sex			
Male	32 (58%)	15 (71%)	17 (50%)
Female	23 (42%)	6 (29%)	17 (50%)
Histology			
Adenocarcinoma	44 (80%)	13 (62%)	31 (91%)
Squamous cell carcinoma	10 (18%)	8 (38%)	2 (6%)
NSCLC	1 (2%)	0 (0%)	1 (3%)
ECOG performance status			
0	46 (84%)	12 (57%)	34 (100%)
1	7 (13%)	7 (33%)	0 (0%)
2	2 (4%)	2 (10%)	0 (0%)
Clinical stage (UICC 7th)			
Stage IA	33 (60%)	13 (62%)	20 (59%)
Stage IB	22 (40%)	8 (38%)	14 (41%)
Longest tumor diameter (mm), median (range)	27 (10–50)	27 (14–46)	27 (10–50)
Tumor location			
Center (72.6 Gy(RBE)/22 Fr)	6 (11%)	5 (24%)	1 (3%)
Periphery (66 Gy(RBE)/10 Fr)	49 (89%)	16 (76%)	33 (97%)
Tumor site			
Upper and middle lobe	41 (75%)	16 (76%)	25 (74%)
Lower lobe	14 (25%)	5 (24%)	9 (26%)
Smoking			
Yes	23 (42%)	12 (57%)	11 (32%)
No	32 (58%)	9 (43%)	23 (68%)

Abbreviations, *NSCLC* unclassified non-small cell lung cancer, *ECOG* Eastern Cooperative Oncology Group; UICC 7th, Union for International Cancer Control 7th edition, *Gy(RBE)* grays relative effectiveness, Fr fraction

Table 2 Treatment Characteristics

Characteristic	All	Inoperable	Operable
No. of patients	55	21	34
No. of portals, 2/3/4	3/41/11	0/18/3	3/23/8
Position matching method			
Fiducial marker	39 (71%)	14 (67%)	25 (74%)
Vertebral bone	16 (29%)	7 (33%)	9 (26%)
IGTV definition			
IGTV-all	48 (87%)	18 (86%)	30 (88%)
IGTV-gate	7 (13%)	3 (14%)	4 (13%)
GTV (cc), median (range)	11 (1.1–53)	12 (1.7–38)	10 (1.1–53)
IGTV (cc), median (range)	17 (1.8–80)	22 (2.8–53)	15 (1.8–80)
DVH parameters			
IGTV V95% (%), median (range)	100 (97–100)	100 (99–100)	100 (97–100)
IGTV D95% (%), median (range)	100 (97–100)	99 (98–100)	100 (97–100)
Lung-GTV V5 (%), median (range)	14 (4.3–28)	14 (4.3–28)	13 (5.2–25)
Lung-GTV V20 (%), median (range)	9.3 (3.0–21)	9.6 (3.0–21)	8.7 (3.7–18)

Abbreviations, IGTV internal gross tumor volume, *GTV* gross tumor volume, DVH dose-volume histogram. V95% = volume receiving > 95% of the prescribed dose, D95% = minimum doses covering 95% of the volume, V5, 20 = volume receiving dose > 5/20 Gy(RBE)

2017, 85 patients clinically diagnosed with stage I NSCLC received PT; 21 inoperable patients were included in the Lung-001 study, and 34 operable patients in Lung-002. The participant study flow is depicted in Fig. 2.

Survival and local control

At the time of analysis, 48 patients were alive and 7 patients were dead. Six of the dead patients were in the inoperable group, including 3 deaths from lung cancer and 3 deaths from other causes, while 1 patient in the operable group died of another cause. The median follow-up was 31 months (range: 9–54 months) for all patients and 35 months (range: 12–54 months) for the patients who remained alive. Local recurrence occurred in 2 patients: one with T1a tumor in the inoperable group at 20 months after PT, diagnosed without biopsy; and another with T2a tumor in the operable group at 16 months after PT, diagnosed with biopsy. Regional lymph node recurrence was observed in 2 patients and distant metastasis was observed in 5. The patterns of failure are shown in Table 3.

For all patients, the 3-year OS, PFS, and LC rates were 87% (95% confidence interval [CI]: 73–94%), 74% (58–85%), and 96% (83–99%), respectively (Fig. 3). For inoperable patients ($n = 21$), the 3-year OS, PFS and LC were 75% (95% CI: 50–89%), 66% (42–82%), and 94% (63–99%), respectively. For operable patients ($n = 34$), the 3-year OS, PFS and LC were 95% (70–99%), 80%

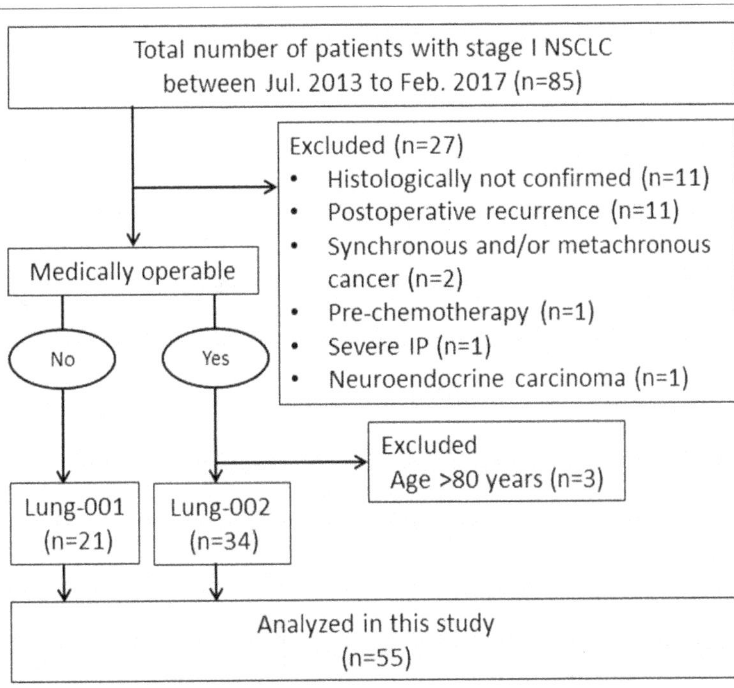

Fig. 2 Study flow diagram. Lung-001 was for medically inoperable patients and Lung-002 was for operable patients who refused surgery

Table 3 Patterns of Failure

Pattern	All(n = 55)	Inoperable(n = 21)	Operable(n = 34)
Local	2 (4%)	1 (5%)	1 (3%)
LN	2 (4%)	2 (10%)	0 (0%)
Distant	5 (9%)	2 (10%)	3 (9%)

Abbreviations, *LN* regional lymph nodes. Distant metastases included ipsilateral (*n* = 1), contralateral (n = 1), bilateral (n = 2), and pleural dissemination (n = 1)

(95% CI: 57–91%), and 97% (79–100%), respectively. In univariate analysis, tumor site (3-year OS: 95% for upper/middle lobe tumors and 75% for lower lobe tumors; $P = .021$), age (3-year OS: 100% for ≤71 years and 77% for >71 years; $P = .018$) and operability ($P = .0066$) were associated with OS. Tumor site (3-year PFS: 86% for upper/middle lobe tumors and 39% for lower lobe tumors; $P = .0020$), histology (3-year PFS: 82% for adenocarcinomas and 43% for squamous cell carcinomas; $P = .040$), and age (3-year PFS: 90% for ≤71 years and 63% for >71 years; $P = .037$) were associated with PFS. No factors were correlated with LC.

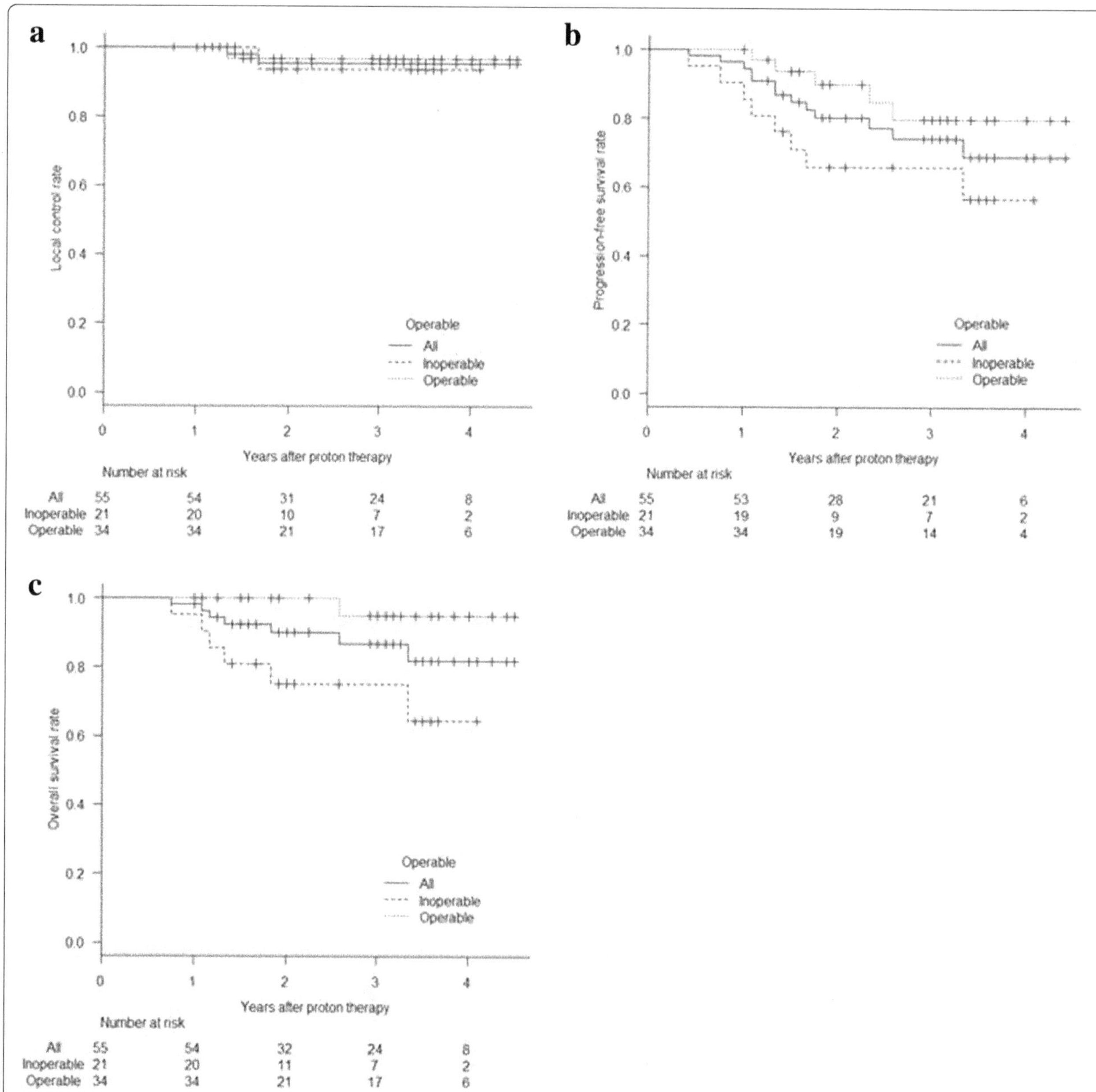

Fig. 3 Kaplan-Meier curves for local control **a**, progression-free survival (**b**) and overall survival (**c**) for all patients, medically inoperable and operable groups

Toxicities

Table 4 summarizes toxicities associated with treatments. No grade 3 or higher toxicities were observed. Five patients (9%) developed grade 2 symptomatic RP at 2 to 7 months from the beginning of PT. All patients received steroids and their symptoms improved. Grade 2 rib fracture and chest wall pain caused by soft tissue inflammation were observed in 2 (4%) and 5 patients (9%), respectively. No symptomatic dermatitis was observed. In addition, there were no other grade 2 toxicities noted during either acute or late observation periods.

Discussion

This study reported clinical outcomes of IGPT using fiducial markers and respiratory gating for operable and inoperable histologically-confirmed stage I NSCLC. IGPT provided 3-year OS and LC rates of 87% and 96%, respectively, with low incidence of toxicities. A systematic review of 9 studies on particle beam therapy (including 6 PT and 5 carbon-ion radiotherapy (CIRT) studies) and 72 SBRT studies has previously been carried out. The 3-year OS, PFS, and LC rates for particle beam therapy were 70, 64, and 88%, respectively, compared to 59, 51, and 86%, respectively for SBRT [19]. No statistically significant survival benefit from particle beam therapy over SBRT was observed after adjusting for potential confounding variables. Our results obtained using IGPT compare favorably with the results of the aforementioned analysis. In addition, we observed no grade 3 toxicities. Although the incidence of severe toxicity was low in both PT or SBRT groups, grade 3 or higher RP was less frequent (PT vs. SBRT, 0.9% vs. 3.4%; $P < .001$) whereas chest wall toxicity was more frequent (1.9% vs. 0.9%; $P = .03$) in the PT group [19]. Furthermore, any-grade rib fractures were observed more frequently in PT (13% vs. 3.2%; $P < .001$). Chest wall toxicity and rib fracture in PT could be problems of critical importance because they compromise patient quality-of-life (QOL). To clarify the advantages of PT, randomized trials should be conducted, but this is practically difficult. Chest wall toxicities and rib fractures after PT may be reduced by employing more portals, and the physical characteristics of PT should be advantageous in reducing toxicities so that it may be possible to further escalate doses to the tumors [5–7, 20].

Table 4 Toxicities

Toxicity	All ($n = 55$)	Inoperable ($n = 21$)	Operable ($n = 34$)
Grade 2			
Radiation pneumonitis	5 (9%)	2 (10%)	3 (9%)
Rib fracture	2 (4%)	0 (0%)	2 (6%)
Chest wall pain	5 (9%)	1 (5%)	4 (12%)
Dermatitis	0 (0%)	0 (0%)	0 (0%)

The toxicities were evaluated according to the Common Terminology Criteria for Adverse Events version 4.0. There were no grade 3 or greater toxicities

The best strategy to employ when using PT for stage I NSCLC remains open to discussion, particularly with respect to the IGPT method and optimal fractionation schedule. We employed fiducial marker matching for suitable patients. Fiducial marker or tumor matching are widely used in SBRT for lung or liver tumors [21, 22], but they have not been commonly used in PT, probably because changes in surrounding anatomical structures (especially the bone) affect the PT dose distribution. Reports from a CIRT group suggested, however, that fiducial marker or tumor matching was better than bony structure matching [23, 24]. We adopted a respiratory gating method, which has been performed in SBRT and other PT facilities, though most PT facilities have uniformly defined IGTV as enveloped GTVs from all respiratory phases with or without 4D-CT. As is well documented in a report about SBRT [25], the IGTV might be unnecessarily large in some cases. In our strategy, choosing IGTV-all or IGTV-gate depending on the amplitude of tumor movement can help to reduce unnecessary doses to critical OAR for specific patients. We selected suitable patients who could possibly benefit from these irradiation methods because PT has several uncertainties and should be operated as personalized treatment [26]. This might have resulted in the absence of severe toxicities and the low rate of local recurrence in the present study. Moreover, this policy might have yielded the results that no factors were associated with LC or grade 2 toxicities (data not shown).

Current PT involves various emerging technologies, including pencil-beam or spot scanning, real-time imaging and gating system, and in-room or cone beam CT among others [27–29]. The current study suggests, however, that in terms of both efficacy and safety, PT is suitable for adoption as a standard treatment option for stage I NSCLC even without such technologies. To confirm the therapeutic benefit of PT, more cases and longer follow-up will be needed. Furthermore, the optimal fractionation regimens with possible dose escalation should be investigated further. Using fewer fraction numbers, especially for central tumors, would increase patient throughput, and this approach may be adopted in the next study. To determine an optimal fractionation regimen, both physical high-precision technology and reasonable biological knowledge are necessary [30]. Over time, the unique biological effects of proton beams, compared to photon beams, have been gradually clarified [14, 31–33]. We will evaluate more effective fractionation regimens focused on PT from both physical and biological aspects.

This study has several limitations. This is an interim analysis of ongoing prospective phase II clinical trials. As such, the sample size was relatively small and the follow-up period relatively short. In addition, to perform IGPT with our method, we have carried out physical analysis of dose distribution, margin definition and respiratory motion effects; the results could not be reported in this article and will be reported in future. Another limitation of the present study is the lack of patient QOL and cost-effectiveness assessment. We have collected the QOL data, but as the data on patients with short follow-up are not yet obtained, we will include the data in the final reports.

Conclusions

Our results indicate that PT is an effective and safe treatment option for stage I NSCLC. Patient-specific optimal irradiation methods may contribute to better clinical outcomes. It is important to select suitable treatment strategies for each patient because patients and tumors are heterogeneous and PT has uncertain sensitive characteristics. Further studies are needed to demonstrate the true value of PT.

Abbreviations

CIRT: Carbon-ion radiotherapy; DRR: Digitally reconstructed radiographs; GTV: Gross tumor volume; Gy(RBE): Gray relative biological effectiveness equivalents; IGPT: Image-guided proton therapy; IGTV: Internal gross tumor volume; IM: Internal motion margin; OAR: Organs at risk; PT: Proton therapy; RP: Radiation pneumonitis; SBRT: Stereotactic body radiotherapy; SM: Setup error margin

Acknowledgements

The authors thank all patients and their family. We are also thankful to Dr. Chihiro Omachi as a member of proton therapy physics, and Rie Muramatsu, Atsushi Yoshida, Kumiko Asai, Kenichiro Tanaka and Akira Shimomura as a member of proton therapy technology, for their valuable help in this research.

Authors' contributions

Each author contributed sufficiently to the work. KN designed the study and wrote the manuscript. HI and HO designed the study and implemented the treatments. YH, SH, TT, KH, KA, FB and KN implemented the treatments and helped collect the data. JM supervised the study. YS helped to write the manuscript. All authors have read and approved the final manuscript.

Competing interests

The authors declare that they have no competing interests.

Author details

[1]Department of Radiation Oncology, Nagoya Proton Therapy Center, Nagoya City West Medical Center, 1-1-1 Hirate-cho, Kita-ku, Nagoya 462-8508, Japan. [2]Department of Radiology, Nagoya City University Graduate School of Medical Sciences, 1 Kawasumi, Mizuho-cho, Mizuho-ku, Nagoya 467-8601, Japan. [3]Department of Proton Therapy Physics, Nagoya Proton Therapy Center, 1-1-1 Hirate-cho, Kita-ku, Nagoya 462-8508, Japan. [4]Department of Proton Therapy Technology, Nagoya Proton Therapy Center, 1-1-1 Hirate-cho, Kita-ku, Nagoya 462-8508, Japan. [5]Department of Respiratory Medicine, Thoracic Oncology Center, Nagoya City West Medical Center, 1-1-1 Hirate-cho, Kita-ku, Nagoya 462-8508, Japan. [6]Department of Radiation Therapy, Nagoya City West Medical Center, 1-1-1 Hirate-cho, Kita-ku, Nagoya 462-8508, Japan. [7]Department of Thoracic Surgery, Thoracic Oncology Center, Nagoya City West Medical Center, 1-1-1 Hirate-cho, Kita-ku, Nagoya 462-8508, Japan. [8]Osaka Heavy Ion Therapy Center, 3-1-10 Otemae, Chuo-ku, Osaka 540-0008, Japan.

References

1. Solda F, Lodge M, Ashley S, et al. Stereotactic radiotherapy (SABR) for the treatment of primary non-small cell lung cancer; systematic review and comparison with a surgical cohort. Radiother Oncol. 2013;109:1–7.
2. Eriguchi T, Takeda A, Sanuki N, et al. Stereotactic body radiotherapy for operable early-stage non-small cell lung cancer. Lung Cancer. 2017;109:62–7.
3. Chang JY, Senan S, Marinus AP, et al. Stereotactic ablative radiotherapy versus lobectomy for operable stage I non-small-cell lung cancer: a pooled analysis of two randomised trials. Lancet Oncol. 2015;16:630–7.
4. Shibamoto Y, Hashizume C, Baba F, et al. Stereotactic body radiotherapy using a radiobiology-based regimen for stage I non-small-cell lung cancer: five-year mature results. J Thorac Oncol. 2015;10:960–4.
5. Macdonald OK, Kruse JJ, Miller JM, et al. Proton beam radiotherapy versus three-dimensional conformal stereotactic body radiotherapy in primary peripheral, early-stage non-small-cell lung carcinoma: a comparative dosimetric analysis. Int J Radiat Oncol Biol Phys. 2009;75:950–8.
6. Kadoya N, Obata Y, Kato T, et al. Dose-volume comparison of proton radiotherapy and stereotactic body radiotherapy for non-small cell lung cancer. Int J Radiat Oncol Biol Phys. 2011;79:1225–31.
7. Roelofs E, Engelsman M, Rasch C, et al. ROCOCO consortium. Results of a multicentric in silico clinical trial (ROCOCO): comparing radiotherapy with photons and protons for non-small cell lung cancer. J Thorac Oncol. 2012;7:165–76.
8. Iwata H, Demizu Y, Fujii O, et al. Long-term outcome of proton therapy and carbon-ion therapy for large (T2a-T2bN0M0) non-small-cell lung cancer. J Thorac Oncol. 2013;8:726–35.
9. Chang JY, Zhang W, Komaki R, et al. Long-term outcome of phase I/II prospective study of dose-escalated proton therapy for early-stage non-small cell lung cancer. Radiother Oncol. 2017;122:274–80.
10. Hatayama Y, Nakamura T, Suzuki M, et al. Clinical outcomes and prognostic factors of high-dose proton beam therapy for peripheral stage I non-small-cell lung cancer. Clin Lung Cancer. 2015;17:427–32.
11. Kanemoto A, Okumura T, Ishikawa H, et al. Outcomes and prognostic factors for recurrence after high-dose proton beam therapy for centrally and peripherally located stage I non-small-cell lung cancer. Clin Lung Cancer. 2014;15:e7–12.
12. Particle Therapy Co-Operative Group. https://www.ptcog.ch. Accessed 18 Aug 2018.
13. Simon R. Optimal two-stage designs for phase II clinical trials. Control Clin Trials. 1989;10(1):10.
14. Iwata H, Ogino H, Hashimoto S, et al. Spot scanning and passive scattering proton therapy: relative biological effectiveness and oxygen enhancement ratio in cultured cells. Int J Radiat Oncol Biol Phys. 2016;95:95–102.
15. Toshito T, Omachi C, Kibe Y, et al. A proton therapy system in Nagoya proton therapy center. Australas Phys Eng Sci Med. 2016;39:645–54.
16. Moyers MF, Miller DW, Bush DA, et al. Methodologies and tools for proton beam design for lung tumors. Int J Radiat Oncol Biol Phys. 2001;49:1429–38.
17. Arjomandy B, Sahoo N, Zhu XR, et al. An overview of the comprehensive proton therapy machine quality assurance procedures implemented at the University of Texas M. D. Anderson Cancer center proton therapy center-Houston. Med Phys. 2009;36:2269–82.

18. Kanda Y. Investigation of the freely available easy-to-use software "EZR" for medical statistics. Bone Marrow Transplant. 2013;48:452–8.
19. Chi A, Chen H, Wen S, et al. Comparison of particle beam therapy and stereotactic body radiotherapy for early stage non-small cell lung cancer: a systematic review and hypothesis-generating meta-analysis. Radiother Oncol. 2017;123:346–54.
20. Wink KC, Roelofs E, Solberg T, et al. Particle therapy for non-small cell lung tumors: where do we stand? A systematic review of the literature. Front Oncol. 2014;4:292.
21. Imura M, Yamazaki K, Shirato H, et al. Insertion and fixation of fiducial markers for setup and tracking of lung tumors in radiotherapy. Int J Radiat Oncol Biol Phys. 2005;63:1442–7.
22. Wunderink W, Romero AM, Seppenwoolde Y, et al. Potentials and limitations of guiding liver stereotactic body radiation therapy set-up on liver-implanted fiducial markers. Int J Radiat Oncol Biol Phys. 2010;77:1573–83.
23. Abe S, Kubota Y, Shibuya K, et al. Fiducial marker matching versus vertebral body matching: Dosimetric impact of patient positioning in carbon ion radiotherapy for primary hepatic cancer. Phys Med. 2017;33:114–20.
24. Sakai M, Kubota Y, Saitoh J, et al. Robustness of patient positioning for interfractional error in carbon ion radiotherapy for stage I lung cancer: bone matching versus tumor matching. Radiother Oncol. 2017; [Epub ahead of print].
25. Zhao B, Yang Y, Li T, et al. Image-guided respiratory-gated lung stereotactic body radiotherapy: which target definition is optimal? Med Phys. 2009;36: 2248–57.
26. Chang JY, Jabbour SK, Ruysscher DD, et al. Consensus statement on proton therapy in early-stage and locally advanced non-small cell lung cancer. Int J Radiat Oncol Biol Phys. 2016;95:505–16.
27. Chang JY, Zhang X, Knopf A, et al. Consensus guidelines for implementing pencil-beam scanning proton therapy for thoracic malignancies on behalf of the PTCOG thoracic and lymphoma subcommittee. Int J Radiat Oncol Biol Phys. 2017;99:41–50.
28. Shimizu S, Miyamoto N, Matsuura T, et al. A proton beam therapy system dedicated to spot-scanning increases accuracy with moving tumors by real-time imaging and gating and reduces equipment size. PLoS One. 2014;9: e94971.
29. Liu W, Zhang X, Li Y, et al. Robust optimization of intensity modulated proton therapy. Med Phys. 2012;39:1079–91.
30. Shibamoto Y, Miyakawa A, Otsuka S, et al. Radiobiology of hypofractionated stereotactic radiotherapy: what are the optimal fractionation schedules? J Radiat Res. 2016;57:i76–82.
31. Mohan R, Peeler CR, Guan F, et al. Radiobiological issues in proton therapy. Acta Oncol. 2017;56:1367–73.
32. Paganetti H. Relative biological effectiveness (RBE) values for proton beam therapy. Variations as a function of biological endpoint, dose, and linear energy transfer. Phys Med Biol. 2014;59:R419–72.
33. Hashimoto S, Sugie C, Iwata H, et al. Recovery from sublethal damage and potentially lethal damage: proton-beam irradiation vs. X-ray irradiation. Strahlenther Onkol. 2018;194:343–51.

12

Nodal failure patterns and utility of elective nodal irradiation in submandibular gland carcinoma treated with postoperative radiotherapy

Cheng-En Hsieh[1,7,11,12], Li-Yu Lee[2,7], Yung-Chih Chou[1], Kang-Hsing Fan[1,7], Ngan-Ming Tsang[1,7,9], Joseph Tung-Chieh Chang[1,7,10], Hung-Ming Wang[3,7], Shu-Hang Ng[4,7], Chun-Ta Liao[5,7], Tzu-Chen Yen[6,7], Ku-Hao Fang[5,7,8] and Chien-Yu Lin[1,7,13*]

Abstract

Background: The patterns of nodal relapse in submandibular gland carcinoma (SMGC) patients treated with postoperative radiotherapy (PORT) remain unclear. This study aims to investigate the nodal failure patterns and the utility of elective nodal irradiation (ENI) in SMGC patients undergoing PORT.

Methods: We retrospectively enrolled 65 SMGC patients who underwent PORT between 2000 and 2014. The nodal failure sites in relation to irradiation fields and pathological parameters were analyzed. ENI regions were categorized into three bilateral echelons (first, levels I–II; second, level III; and third, levels IV–V). Extended ENI was defined as coverage of at least the immediately adjacent uninvolved echelons bilaterally; otherwise, limited ENI was administered.

Results: Thirty patients (46%) were stage III–IV, and 18 (28%) were pN+. Neck irradiation included limited (72%) and extended ENI (28%). With a median follow-up of 79 months, 11 patients (17%) developed nodal failures (ipsilateral, $N = 6$; contralateral, $N = 7$), 7 (64%) of whom relapsed in the adjacent uninvolved echelons. We identified pN+ ($P = 0.030$), extranodal extension (ENE, $P = 0.002$), pT3–4 ($P = 0.021$), and lymphovascular invasion (LVI, $P = 0.004$) as significant predictors of contralateral neck recurrence. Extended ENI significantly improved regional control (RC) in patients with pN+ ($P = 0.003$), ENE ($P = 0.022$), pT3–4 ($P = 0.044$), and LVI ($P = 0.014$), and improved disease-free survival (DFS) in patients with pN+ ($P = 0.034$). For patients with ≥2 coincident adverse factors, extended ENI significantly increased RC ($P < 0.001$), distant metastasis-free survival ($P = 0.019$), and DFS ($P = 0.007$); conversely, no nodal recurrence was observed in patients without these adverse factors, even when only the involved echelon was irradiated.

Conclusions: Nodal failure is not uncommon in SMGC patients treated with PORT if pN+, ENE, pT3–4, and LVI are present. Extended ENI should be considered, particularly in patients with multiple pathological adverse factors.

Keywords: Submandibular gland cancer, Postoperative radiotherapy, Elective nodal irradiation, Nodal failure pattern

* Correspondence: qqvirus1022@gmail.com
[1]Radiation Oncology, Chang Gung Memorial Hospital at Linkou and Chang Gung University, No. 5, Fuxing St., Guishan Dist, Taoyuan City 33305, Taiwan, Republic of China
[7]Head and Neck Oncology Group, Chang Gung Memorial Hospital at Linkou and Chang Gung University, Taoyuan City, Taiwan, Republic of China
Full list of author information is available at the end of the article

Background

Submandibular gland carcinomas (SMGCs) are rare malignancies, accounting for less than 10% of salivary gland neoplasms and 1% of head and neck cancers [1–3]. *En bloc* radical resection is the mainstay of treatment [4], and postoperative radiotherapy (PORT) has been utilized in patients with adverse pathological factors including advanced stage, high-grade tumors, positive surgical margins, bone invasion, and perineural invasion (PNI) [5–9]. The behavior of SMGC and the optimal PORT treatment remain unclear. Data on combined-modality treatments usually encompass parotid gland cancer patients, and the nodal failure patterns and clinical utility of elective nodal irradiation (ENI) for SMGC remain vague [6, 10–13]. The currently recommended nodal irradiation fields are based on the treatment experience of different salivary gland malignancies (most of them arising from the parotid gland).

The incidence of neck metastases in parotid gland carcinoma is reportedly 12–25% [6, 8, 11, 14, 15], with no risk to the contralateral neck [11, 16]. However, the submandibular gland has more extensive lymphatic drainage; hence, SMGC is more amenable to nodal metastasis [6, 10, 17]. According to a detailed study by the Dutch Head and Neck Oncology Group, pathologically positive nodes were detected in 42% of SMGC patients, and the nodal metastasis rate approached 60% for high-grade and advanced T-stage tumors [6]. Even when a unique histology entity (adenoid cystic carcinoma, ACC) is considered, the rates of nodal metastases from submandibular gland malignancies are higher than those observed for parotid gland tumors (22.5% vs 14.5%, respectively) [18]. Furthermore, increased risks of contralateral neck metastasis (12.4-fold) and occult nodal metastasis have been reported in oral cavity squamous cell carcinoma that directly invades into the floor of the mouth [19–21]. As the submandibular glands are proximal to the floor of the mouth and midline of the neck, it is unclear whether contralateral neck treatment should be omitted as it is for parotid gland cancer patients. Therefore, we conducted this retrospective multicenter study to review the long-term outcomes of SMGC patients treated with radical resection and PORT. Additionally, we investigated the use and treatment outcomes of ENI, and identified patients who would most benefit from extended ENI.

Methods

Patients and clinical workup

A total number of 74 patients with SMGC treated with radical surgery and PORT at Linkou, Kaohsiung, Keelung, and Chiayi Chang Gung Memorial Hospitals between January 2000 and December 2014 were identified. Patients with distant metastasis at diagnosis ($N = 5$), history of prior irradiation ($N = 3$), and lymphoma histology ($N = 1$) were excluded; 65 patients were ultimately enrolled. The staging workups and follow-up schedules were described previously [22]. The cancer staging was revised according to the seventh edition (2010) of the American Joint Committee on Cancer staging criteria, and the tumor histology was defined according to 2005 World Health Organization classification.

Treatment

All subjects were treated with radical submandibulectomy, and neck dissection was performed for those with clinical nodal involvement or locally advanced tumors. PORT was administered using megavoltage photon irradiation, 1.8–2 Gy per fraction, five times per week using either three-dimensional conformal radiotherapy, intensity-modulated radiation therapy, or volumetric modulated arc therapy delivery systems. The prophylactic dose of ENI was 46–50 Gy with a 60–66 Gy boost to high-risk regions. ENI was generally administered to patients presenting with adverse pathological features. The neck irradiation regions were categorized into 3 consecutive bilateral echelons according to the lymphatic drainage anatomy of the submandibular gland: the first echelon was for levels I–II, the second for level III, and the third for levels IV–V (Fig. 1a, b). Extended ENI encompassed the adjacent uninvolved echelons bilaterally according to the pathological tumor extension (Fig. 1c). Otherwise, limited ENI, defined as the irradiation of the involved echelon alone or ipsilateral ENI for adjacent uninvolved echelons without prophylactic contralateral neck treatment, was administered. Concurrent chemotherapy was generally applied for patients with adverse pathological features [23]; intravenous cisplatin was the most commonly used agent (typically at 100 mg/m^2 once every 3 weeks or 40 mg/m^2 once per week) [24, 25].

Statistical analysis

Intergroup differences in continuous variables were tested using independent Student's *t*-tests. Categorical data were compared using the Pearson's chi-squared or the Fisher's exact test, as appropriate. Local control (LC), regional control (RC), distant metastasis-free survival (DMFS), disease-free survival (DFS), and overall survival (OS) were calculated from the date of surgery to the date of detection of the relevant events, respectively. Survival curves were plotted using the Kaplan-Meier method and compared using the log-rank test. Multivariate analysis was performed using Cox proportional hazards regression models with a stepwise forward conditional manner. Variables were retained in the model if their significance levels were < 0.05. Results are expressed as hazard ratios with their 95% confidence intervals. All data analyses were performed using the SPSS 20.0 statistical software (IBM Corporation, Armonk, New York, USA).

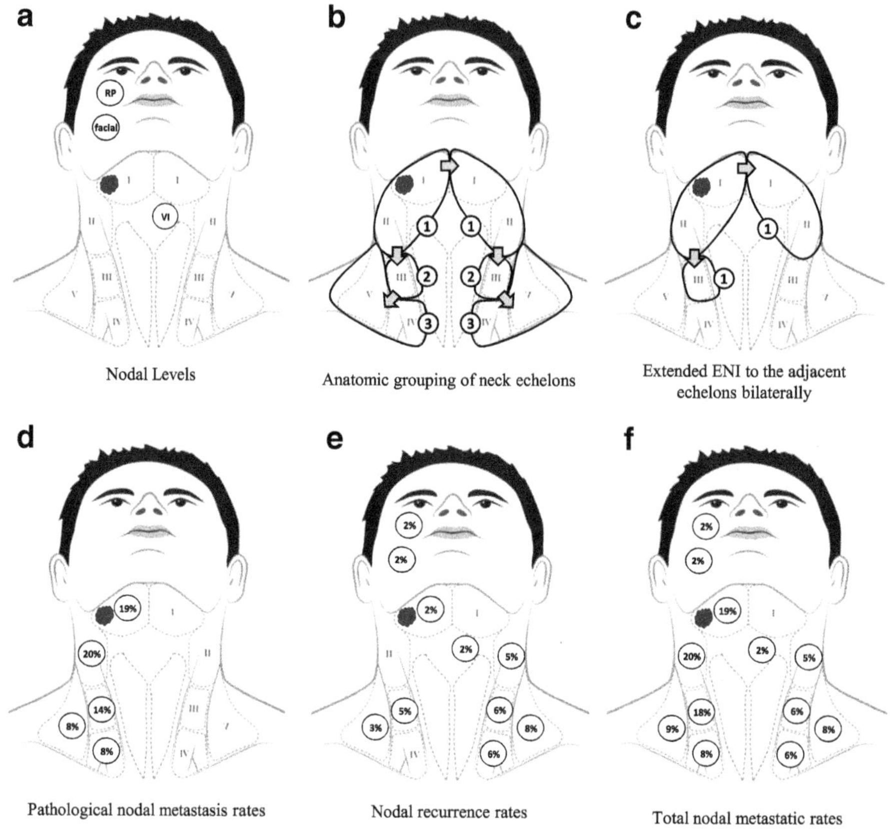

Fig. 1 **a** Depiction of each of Level I–V, retropharyngeal (RP) and facial nodes. **b** The neck irradiation regions were categorized into 3 consecutive bilateral echelons according to lymphatic drainage: the first echelon for levels I–II, the second for level III, and the third for levels IV–V. **c** Taking a submandibular gland carcinoma (SMGC) patient with multiple risk factors as an example, if the tumor invades level I, extended elective nodal irradiation (ENI) of the adjacent bilateral echelons involves the ipsilateral levels I–III and contralateral levels I–II. **d** Pathological nodal metastatic rates in 24 patients who received ipsilateral neck dissection. **e** Nodal recurrent rates and **(F)** total nodal metastatic rates in 65 SMGC patients treated with surgery and postoperative radiotherapy

Results

Patient characteristics

Patient characteristics are demonstrated in Table 1. The median age was 53 years, and the most common histological subtypes were ACC, carcinoma ex pleomorphic adenoma, and mucoepidermoid carcinoma.

Clinically positive nodes were observed in 15 patients (23%); 24 patients (37%) received ipsilateral neck dissection while none received contralateral neck surgery. Consequently, pathological nodal metastasis was detected in 18 patients (28%). The distribution of pathological positive nodes is illustrated in Fig. 1d.

Adjuvant treatments

The median cumulative radiation dose was 66 Gy, and only one patient received a dose less than 50 Gy due to poor health. The median time from surgery to PORT initiation was 34 (range, 11–71) days; the median time was 35 (range, 11–71) days and 29 (range, 14–49) days among those with limited ENI and extended ENI, respectively. Concurrent chemoradiotherapy was administered to 24 patients (limited ENI, $N = 16$; extended ENI, $N = 8$), the most commonly used regimen was intravenous cisplatin-based ($N = 23$). Single-agent cisplatin was administered to 18 patients, whereas concurrent oral uracil-tegafur and cisplatin were administered to the remaining 5 patients. The median cumulative cisplatin dose was 200 mg/m^2. Sixteen of the 23 patients (70%) completed their planned chemotherapy course; one patient received concurrent cetuximab treatment. Neither neoadjuvant nor adjuvant chemotherapy was administered.

Neck irradiation fields

Extended ENI was performed in 18 patients (28%), covering the next adjacent uninvolved echelons bilaterally ($N = 8$) or ≥ 2 additional echelons ($N = 10$). Otherwise, limited ENI was performed in the remaining 47 patients; the irradiated neck regions consisted of involved echelons alone in 30 patients (46%) and of ipsilateral adjacent uninvolved echelons in 17 (26%). Notably, 12 of these patients received unintentional irradiation doses to the

Table 1 Patient characteristics

Characteristic	*N*	%
Sex		
Female/Male	35/30	54/46
Age (years)		
Median (range)	53 (24–79)	
Performance score		
ECOG 0–1	65	100
T stage		
pT1	15	23
pT2	24	37
pT3	20	31
pT4a	6	9
Tumor size (cm)		
Median (range)	2.9 (0.5–8.0)	
N stage		
pN0	6	9
pN1	3	5
pN2b	15	23
cN0/pNx[a]	41	63
Disease stage		
I	13	20
II	22	34
III	11	17
IVa	19	29
Staging modality		
CT	49	75
MRI	6	9
^{18}F-FDG-PET	23	35
Surgical margin		
< 1 mm/≥1 mm	46/19	71/29
Histology		
Adenoid cystic carcinoma	29	45
Carcinoma ex pleomorphic adenoma	11	17
Mucoepidermoid carcinoma	8	12
Lymphoepithelial carcinoma	6	9
Squamous cell carcinoma	4	6
Salivary duct carcinoma	4	6
Adenocarcinoma	2	3
Myoepithelial carcinoma	1	2
Histology grading		
Low to intermediate/High	6/59	9/91
Pathological features		
Perineural invasion	35	54
Extranodal extension	12	19
Bone invasion	2	3

Table 1 Patient characteristics *(Continued)*

Characteristic	*N*	%
Skin invasion	1	2
Lymphovascular invasion	18	28
Neck dissection		
None	41	63
Ipsilateral elective	9	14
Ipsilateral therapeutic	15	23
Contralateral	0	0
< 18 nodes	22	34
≥18 nodes	17	26
Nodal irradiation		
Extended ENI	18	28
Limited ENI	47	72
Concurrent chemotherapy	24	37
Radiotherapy technique		
3D-CRT	19	29
IMRT	31	48
VMAT	15	23
Radiotherapy dose (Gy)		
Median (range)	66 (32–72)	

Abbreviations: *3D-CRT* three-dimensional conformal radiotherapy, *CT* computed tomography, *ECOG* Eastern Cooperative Oncology Group, *ENI* elective nodal irradiation, *^{18}F-FDG-PET* 18F-fluorodeoxyglucose positron emission tomography, *IMRT* intensity-modulated radiation therapy, *MRI* magnetic resonance imaging, *VMAT* volumetric modulated arc therapy
[a],no elective neck dissection in cN0 patients

contralateral levels I ($N = 7$) or I/II ($N = 5$) that encountered the radiation beam paths.

Treatment outcomes and nodal failure patterns

The median follow-up time for the survivors was 79 (range, 19–183) months. By the end of the study, 21 patients (32%) had died owing to cancer recurrence in 16 and intercurrent diseases in five (coronary artery disease, $N = 2$; pneumonia, $N = 2$; and cerebral hemorrhage, $N = 1$). Three patients developed secondary malignancies (gum squamous cell carcinoma, ovarian adenocarcinoma, and cholangiocarcinoma, respectively); the patient with secondary cholangiocarcinoma died of uncontrolled tumor bleeding resulting from SMGC locoregional recurrence (patient #11), and the two other patients were alive with controlled secondary malignancies. The five- and 10-year OS rates were 72 and 63% for the entire cohort, respectively.

Cancer recurrence was recorded in 21 patients (32%). The five- and 10-year DFS rates were 64 and 64%, respectively. The predominant form of treatment failure was distant metastasis (20 patients), and the five- and 10-year DMFS rates were both 66%. Three patients had local recurrence; among them, perineural tumor recurrence was recorded in two ACC patients who were treated with surgical bed irradiation alone (hypoglossal nerve, $N = 1$, #11; facial and lingual nerves, $N = 1$, #12; Table 2, Additional file 1: Figure S1). When we investigated the highest margin of the irradiation fields, we identified that coverage up to the transverse process of the first cervical vertebrae (for level II neck coverage only), mastoid tip, and skull base were performed in 10 (35%), 1 (3%), and 18 (62%) patients while 2 (20%), 0 (0%), and 0 (0%) had outfield recurrence ($P = 0.180$). The five- and 10-year LC rates 96 and 92%, respectively.

Eleven patients (17%) experienced neck recurrence, with five- and 10-year RC rates of 80% and 80%, respectively. The median time to nodal recurrence was 25 (range, 6–57) months in 10 patients with limited ENI and 52 months in 1 patients with extended ENI. Ipsilateral and contralateral neck failures were documented in six and seven patients, respectively; the distributions of recurrent nodes and total nodal metastatic rates are shown in Fig. 1e-f. Seven patients (64%) developed nodal recurrence in the adjacent uninvolved echelons. The detailed neck nodal failure sites and corresponding radiation fields are shown in Table 2. Ten of the 11 patients who experienced nodal relapse also developed uncontrolled distant metastases.

Univariate and multivariate analyses of adverse pathological factors

On univariate analysis (Table 3), the presence of pN+, ENE, pT3–4, LVI, and PNI was significantly correlated with inferior RC, LC, DMFS, and DFS. A significantly worse five-year LC rate was observed in patients with pN+. The presence of pN+, ENE, pT3–4, and LVI was each a significant predictor of poorer OS.

Multivariate analyses revealed that pT3–4 and LVI significantly correlated with poorer RC. No statistically significant prognosticator for LC was identified (Table 3). Notably, pT3–4, LVI, and PNI were identified as significant independent predictors of DMFS, whereas pN+, PNI, and pT3–4 were significantly correlated with worse DFS; pN+ and pT3–4 were significant predictors of inferior OS.

Predictors of nodal recurrence

Neither univariate nor multivariate analyses revealed significant predictors of ipsilateral nodal recurrence; only a trend toward worse ipsilateral nodal failure was observed in patients with pN+ or pT3–4 (Table 4). However, pN+, ENE, pT3–4, and LVI were significant predictors of contralateral neck recurrence on univariate analysis; whereas ENE and LVI were significant independent prognosticators of the same on multivariate analysis.

Table 2 Neck irradiation fields and failure patterns in 12 submandibular gland carcinoma patients who developed locoregional recurrence after postoperative radiotherapy

									Local	Ipsilateral neck							Contralateral neck						
Case	Histology	pT	N stage	Stage	ENE	PNI	LVI	M		I	II	III	IV	VA	VB	Others	I	II	III	IV	VA	VB	Others
1	CXPA	3	pN2b	IVa	+	+	+	+		N	N	N	N	N				F	F	F	F	F	
2	CXPA	3	pN0	III	-	-	+	-												F		F	
3	SDC	3	pN2b	IVa	+	+	+	-		N	N			NF	F	RP					F	F	VI
4	CXPA	2	cN0/pNx†	II	-	+	+	+							F				F	F		F	
5	SCC	4a	pN2b	IVa	+	+	+	-	F		N							F	F				
6	CXPA	3	pN2b	IVa	+	+	+	+			N	N						F					
7	ACC	3	pN0	III	-	+	-	+											F	F		F	
8	ACC	3	pN1	III	-	+	+	+			N					facial							
9	ACC	4a	pN0	IVa	-	+	-	+				F											
10	ACC	4a	pN0	IVa	-	+	-	+				F											
11	ACC	1	pN2b	IVa	-	+	-	+	F*	NF		F											
12	ACC	3	pN0	III	-	+	-	+	F#														

Gray screentones: areas of neck irradiation. Frames: areas of nodal dissection

Abbreviations: *ACC* adenoid cystic carcinoma, *ENE* extranodal extension, *CXPA* carcinoma ex pleomorphic adenoma, *F* site of failure, *LVI* lymphovascular invasion, *M* surgical margins, *N* pathologically involved nodal region, *PNI* perineurial invasion, *pT* pathological T stage, *RP* retropharyngeal nodal failure, *SCC* squamous cell carcinoma, *SDC* salivary duct carcinoma

†, no elective neck dissection in cN0 patients; Perineural tumor recurrence at *hypoglossal nerve (Additional file 1: Figure S1B) and #facial and lingual nerves (Additional file 1: Figure S1A).

Table 3 Univariate and multivariate analyses of adverse pathological factors

Univariate analysis		RC (%)		LC (%)		DMFS (%)		DFS (%)		OS (%)	
Variable	*N*	5-year	*P*	5-year	*P*	5-year	*P*	5-year	*P*	5-year	*P*
N stage											
pN+	18	49.6	0.002	75.0	0.015	31.1	< 0.001	24.5	< 0.001	37.5	< 0.001
pN0 & cN0/pNx[a]	47	87.7		100		77.5		77.8		85.2	
Extranodal extension											
Yes	12	55.4	0.004	83.3	0.149	21.2	< 0.001	21.8	< 0.001	30.0	< 0.001
No	53	84.2		97.3		74.2		72.0		81.0	
T stage											
pT3–4	26	57.9	< 0.001	93.8	0.104	33.2	< 0.001	35.1	< 0.001	45.9	< 0.001
pT1–2	39	93.1		96.7		85.5		82.2		88.9	
Lymphovascular invasion											
Yes	15	51.0	< 0.001	90.0	0.569	29.6	< 0.001	30.5	< 0.001	44.4	< 0.001
No	50	89.4		96.9		78.6		75.0		82.7	
Perineural invasion											
Yes	35	66.2	0.007	92.0	0.084	48.9	0.002	45.7	0.001	66.3	0.092
No	30	95.7		100		87.9		87.9		78.0	
Margin < 1 mm											
Yes	47	79.1	0.910	96.6	0.794	68.7	0.418	66.0	0.449	75.7	0.475
No	18	80.9		91.7		57.0		57.5		61.1	
High-grade histology											
Yes	59	77.1	0.204	94.9	0.466	63.0	0.324	61.3	0.287	68.4	0.079
No	6	100		100		85.7		85.7		100	

Multivariate analysis							
Variable	HR	95% CI	*P*	Variable	HR	95% CI	*P*
Regional control				Disease-free survival			
T stage (pT3–4 vs pT1–2)	8.129	1.661–39.779	0.010	N stage (pN+ vs pN0 & cN0/pNx[a])	4.026	1.464–11.075	0.007
Lymphovascular invasion (Yes vs No)	4.130	1.165–14.643	0.028	Perineural invasion (Yes vs No)	5.377	1.512–19.121	0.009
Local control	–	–	NS	T stage (pT3–4 vs pT1–2)	3.762	1.262–11.213	0.017
Distant metastasis-free survival				Overall survival			
T stage (pT3–4 vs pT1–2)	5.171	1.715–15.591	0.004	N stage (pN+ vs pN0 & cN0/pNx[a])	4.363	1.710–11.127	0.002
Perineural invasion (Yes vs No)	4.337	1.234–15.236	0.022	T stage (pT3–4 vs pT1–2)	4.841	1.671–14.020	0.004
Lymphovascular invasion (Yes vs No)	2.719	1.065–6.942	0.037				

Abbreviations: *CI* confidence interval, *DFS* disease free survival, *DMFS* distant metastasis free survival, *HR* Hazard ratio, *LC* local control, *NS* not statistically significant, *OS* overall survival, *RC* regional control

[a],no elective neck dissection in cN0 patients

Extended elective nodal irradiation

To identify specific populations of SMGC patients who might benefit from extended ENI, we performed subgroup analyses to examine each pathological parameter. As demonstrated in Table 5 and Fig. 2a-d, extended ENI significantly improved RC rates for patients with pN+ ($P = 0.003$), ENE ($P = 0.022$), pT3–4 ($P = 0.044$), and LVI ($P = 0.014$). For patients with pN+, we observed a significant improvement in five-year DFS in those treated with extended ENI (52% vs 0%, $P = 0.034$, Fig. 2e). Although higher five-year DMFS rates were observed for pN+ patients treated with extended ENI (52% vs 13%, $P = 0.166$), as well as higher five- and 10-year OS rates (44 and 44% vs 28 and 0%, $P = 0.333$), the differences were not significant.

To identify the subgroups of patients who might benefit the most from extended ENI, we stratified patients according to pN+, ENE, LVI, and pT3–4 (the patient characteristics between the treatment groups are listed in Additional file 2: Table S1). In patients with ≥1 adverse pathological factor(s), extended ENI to ≥1 adjacent echelons significantly increased five- and 10-year RC rates (86 and 86% vs 45 and 45%, respectively, $P = 0.039$;

Table 4 Univariate and multivariate analyses of clinicopathological risk factors for neck failure

Variables	Ipsilateral neck failure						Contralateral neck failure					
	Univariate analysis			Multivariate analysis			Univariate analysis			Multivariate analysis		
	HR	95% CI	*P*	HR	95% CI	*P*	HR	95% CI	*P*	HR	95% CI	*P*
N stage (pN+ vs pN0 & cN0/pNx[a])	4.491	0.888–22.717	0.069	–	–	NS	5.305	1.176–23.925	0.030	–	–	NS
Extranodal extension (Yes vs No)	1.607	0.185–13.984	0.667	–	–	NS	11.479	2.519–52.305	0.002	6.018	1.203–30.104	0.029
T stage (pT3–4 vs pT1–2)	5.102	0.903–28.819	0.065	–	–	NS	12.293	1.472–102.668	0.021	–	–	NS
Lymphovascular invasion (Yes vs No)	3.738	0.751–18.597	0.107	–	–	NS	22.007	2.643–183.267	0.004	14.920	1.694–131.385	0.015
Perineural invasion (Yes vs No)	63.645	0.089–45,483	0.215	–	–	NS	5.274	0.635–43.827	0.124	–	–	NS
Margin (< 1 mm vs ≥ 1 mm)	1.860	0.217–15.951	0.571	–	–	NS	0.441	0.099–1.974	0.285	–	–	NS
High-grade histology (Yes vs No)	24.834	0.001–872,589	0.548	–	–	NS	24.431	0.001–526,351.9	0.530	–	–	NS
Ipsi. elective neck dissection (Yes vs No)	0.039	0.000–876.767	0.526	–	–	NS	–	–	–	–	–	–
Ipsi. elective nodal irradiation (Yes vs No)	0.402	0.073–2.203	0.294	–	–	NS	–	–	–	–	–	–
Cont. elective nodal irradiation (Yes vs No)	–	–	–	–	–	–	0.778	0.151–4.013	0.764	–	–	NS

Abbreviations: *CI* confidence interval, *Cont.* contralateral, *HR* hazard ratio, *Ipsi.* ipsilateral, *NS* not statistically significant

[a], no elective neck dissection in cN0 patients

Table 5 Survival outcomes of submandibular gland carcinoma patients bearing adverse pathological risk factors, treatment with or without postoperative bilateral elective nodal irradiation

Variable		RC (%)			DMFS (%)			DFS (%)			OS (%)		
	N	5-y	10-y	*P*	5-y	10-y	*P*	5-y	10-y	*P*	5-y	10-y	*P*
Entire cohort													
Extended ENI	18	90.0	90.0	0.207	59.3	59.3	0.700	59.3	59.3	0.871	70.3	61.6	0.636
Limited ENI	47	76.6	76.6		67.6	67.6		65.4	65.4		72.3	63.6	
pN+													
Extended ENI	9	100	100	0.003	51.9	51.9	0.166	51.9	51.9	0.034	44.4	44.4	0.333
Limited ENI	9	0	–		12.5	–		0	–		27.8	0	
Extranodal extension													
Extended ENI	6	100	100	0.022	44.4	44.4	0.328	44.4	44.4	0.161	50.0	50.0	0.319
Limited ENI	6	20.0	–		0	–		0	–		0	–	
pT3–4													
Extended ENI	8	100	100	0.044	40.0	40.0	0.694	40.0	40.0	0.579	37.5	18.8	0.288
Limited ENI	18	41.0	41.0		32.7	32.7		34.3	34.3		49.1	32.8	
Lymphovascular invasion													
Extended ENI	9	80.0	80.0	0.014	32.4	32.4	0.472	32.4	32.4	0.351	55.6	44.4	0.392
Limited ENI	9	25.0	25.0		25.0	25.0		25.0	25.0		33.3	22.2	
Perineural invasion													
Extended ENI	9	80.0	–	0.353	25.9	–	0.195	25.9	–	0.300	55.6	41.7	0.270
Limited ENI	26	66.3	66.3		57.0	57.0		52.6	52.6		69.4	52.9	
Margin < 1 mm													
Extended ENI	12	83.3	83.3	0.512	61.1	61.1	0.905	61.1	61.1	0.763	71.4	53.6	0.374
Limited ENI	35	78.0	78.0		70.3	70.3		66.8	66.8		77.1	65.4	
High grade histology													
Extended ENI	41	88.9	88.9	0.179	63.3	63.3	0.899	63.3	63.3	0.650	68.4	58.6	0.721
Limited ENI	17	73.1	73.1		63.0	63.0		60.4	60.4		68.6	58.8	
0 risk factor[a]													
Extended ENI	6	100	100	–	100	100	0.533	100	100	0.533	100	100	0.449
Limited ENI	26	100	100		91.1	91.1		91.1	91.1		87.9	87.9	
≥1 risk factor[a]													
Extended ENI	12	85.7	85.7	0.039	43.2	43.2	0.558	43.2	43.2	0.349	58.3	48.6	0.752
Limited ENI	21	45.1	45.1		38.2	38.2		31.5	31.5		52.4	32.7	
≥2 risk factors[a]													
Extended ENI	11	83.3	83.3	< 0.001	36.8	36.8	0.019	36.8	36.8	0.007	54.5	43.6	0.117
Limited ENI	8	14.3	–		0	0		0	0		16.7	0	

Abbreviations: *DFS* disease free survival, *DMFS* distant metastasis free survival, *ENI* elective nodal irradiation, *OS* overall survival, *RC* regional control
[a]***Risk factors:*** pN+, extranodal extension, pT3–4, and lymphovascular invasion

Table 5 and Fig. 2f). However, the DMFS, DFS, and OS rates did not significantly differ between each group. For patients with ≥2 coincident adverse pathological factors, extended ENI to the adjacent echelons bilaterally increased five-year RC (83% vs 14%, $P < 0.001$, Fig. 2g), DMFS (37% vs 0%, $P = 0.019$, Fig. 2h), and DFS (37% vs 0%, $P = 0.007$, Fig. 2i) rates significantly. However, the five- and 10-year OS rates were not significantly higher in patients treated with extended ENI (55 and 44% vs 16.7 and 0%, respectively; $P = 0.117$, Fig. 2j). On the other hand, the five- and 10-year RC rates were 100% and 100% in patients who did not receive extended ENI ($N = 26$) but had none of the aforementioned adverse pathological factors; neither elective nodal dissection nor irradiation of the adjacent echelons was performed in 14 of these patients. Furthermore, no significant differences were observed in terms of RC, DMFS, DFS, and OS rates in these low-risk patients whether treated with extended ENI or not.

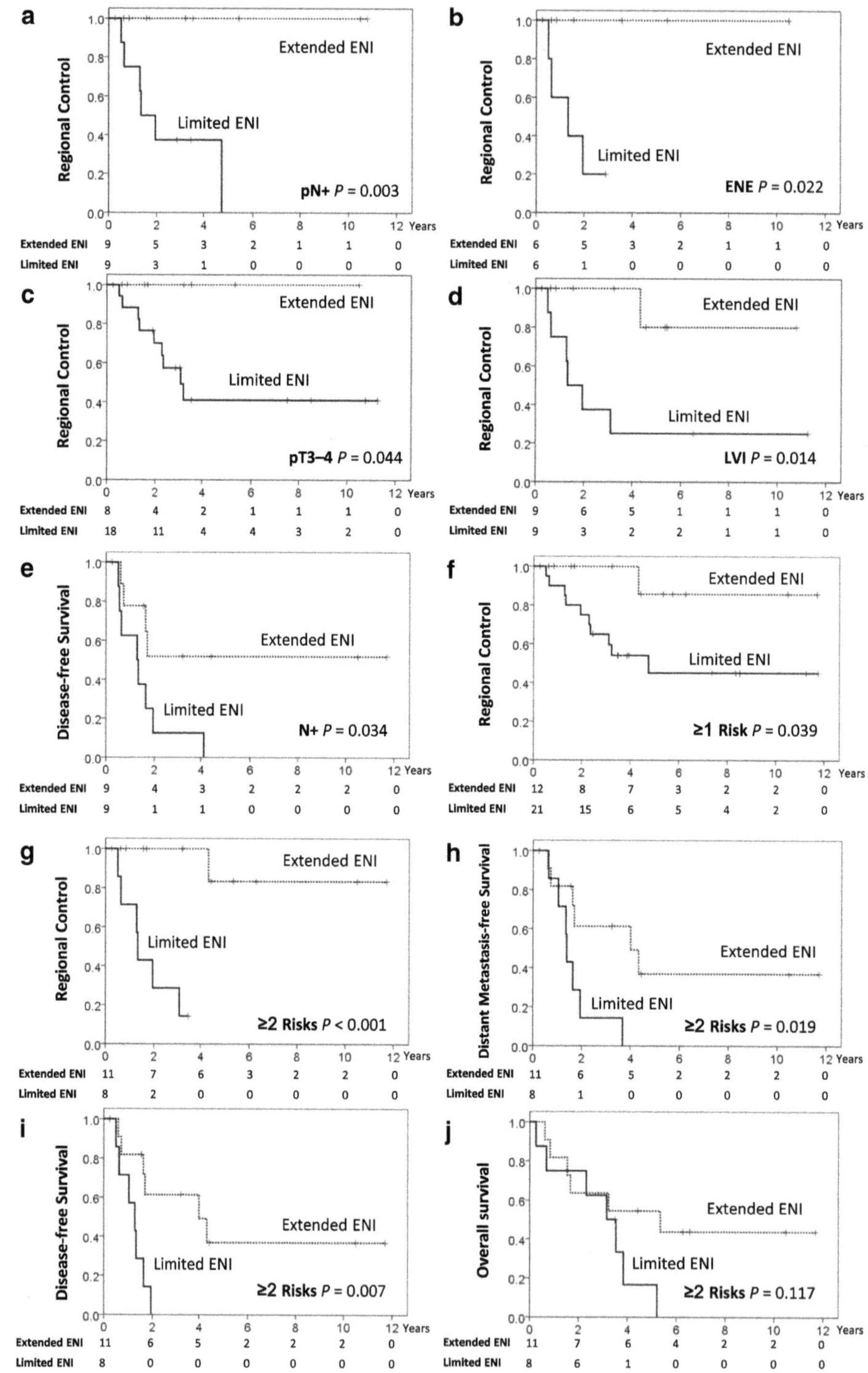

Fig. 2 a–d Regional control curves in patients with pN+, extranodal extension (ENE), pT3–4, and lymphovascular invasion (LVI); and (**e**) disease-free survival curves in pN(+) patients; treated with extended vs limited elective nodal irradiation (ENI). **f** Regional control curves in patients with ≥1 adverse factors, and (**g**–**j**) regional control, distant metastasis-free survival, disease-free survival, and overall survival curves in patients with ≥2 adverse factors treated with extended or limited ENI. (Adverse factors: pN+, ENE, pT3–4, and LVI)

Discussion

Despite their generally indolent clinical course, nodal and distant recurrences remain a major clinical concern in SMGC patients who carry adverse pathological factors, even following combined-modality treatment [1, 2, 6, 8, 26]. The recommended ENI fields of PORT for SMGC derive from the indications outlined for parotid cancer, where ipsilateral level I–V irradiation is adopted for patients with advance T-stage, pN(+), high-grade histology, PNI, and recurrent disease. Ipsilateral upper neck ENI is recommended for cases with early high-risk tumors [6, 10–13].

However, the submandibular gland has a rich lymphocapillary network. A large surgical series revealed that submandibular malignancies had a significantly higher risk of occult nodal metastasis (21%) than parotid gland cancers (9%) [10]. In our previous study of salivary gland cancer patients treated with PORT, those with SMGC exhibited a significantly lower five-year RC rate (73.9%) compared to patients with tumors originating from other salivary glands (parotid, 91.2%; sublingual, 100%; and minor salivary, 100%) [23]. These data suggest that the nodal spreading behavior of SMGCs differs from that of parotid gland tumors, and more aggressive treatment may be warranted for select high-risk SMGC patients.

In the present study, the overall incidence of neck metastasis was as high as 35% (pN+, $N = 18$ [27%]; neck recurrence in patients with pN0 or cN0/pNx [i.e., no elective neck dissection performed for clinically negative necks], $N = 5$, [8%]; Fig. 1d–f) which is consistent with other series [1, 17, 27–29]. Occult metastasis was documented in 9% of our patients (pN+ in cN0 patients, $N = 1$; neck recurrence in pN0 or cN0/pNx, $N = 5$). Our data indicated that contralateral nodal metastasis was not uncommon in SMGC patients (Fig. 1d), particularly in the presence of pN+, ENE, pT3–4, and LVI (Table 4), suggesting that ipsilateral ENI of the neck may be inadequate for these high-risk subgroups. However, our data did not identify predictors for ipsilateral neck relapse, possibly owing to the small number of events and the fact that ipsilateral neck prophylactic treatment was frequently performed for patients with adverse pathological factors. Importantly, we found that 64% of nodal recurrences were located in the adjacent uninvolved echelons, suggesting that ENI of the adjoining echelons might be warranted in selected patients. Notably, 10 of the 11 patients who experienced nodal relapse (91%) also developed distant metastases; this strong correlation implies that reducing nodal recurrence might in turn decrease the risk of distant failure.

Positive surgical margins are a poor prognostic factor and have been reported in 36–46% of SMGC patients [17, 28]. Compared to other surgical series, we observed a higher incidence of surgical margins < 1 mm (71%). This might be attributed to more conservative resections as well as the clinical aggressiveness of SMGC. Intriguingly, our data demonstrated that resection margins < 1 mm were not significantly associated with poor outcomes in the setting of adjuvant radiotherapy; this was comparable to our previous findings with parotid cancer [30]. This may indicate the high efficacy of adjuvant radiotherapy in eradicating microscopic tumors, especially as only two patients experienced nodal relapses within the initial irradiation fields.

We hypothesized that the anatomic proximity of SMGCs to the floor of the mouth and midline of the neck increases the risk of contralateral neck and occult metastasis, and that ipsilateral or limited ENI is inadequate in such cases. Therefore, we categorized the ENI fields into three consecutive bilateral echelons accordingly to anatomical lymphatic drainage. We found no statistically significant differences in disease control and survival rates between patients treated with or without extended ENI. However, in subgroup analyses, extended ENI significantly improved RC rates in patients exhibiting adverse pathological factors. In pN+ patients in particular, a significantly higher DFS rate was observed in those treated with extended ENI, suggesting that a reduced nodal failure rate might translate into a DFS benefit.

To identify SMGC patients who may benefit most from extended ENI, we stratified our patients according to the aforementioned adverse factors. For patients with ≥1 risk factor(s), bilateral ENI extension to the adjacent echelons significantly improved the five-year RC rate; however, there were no significant differences in DMFS, DFS, and OS rates between the groups. Importantly, for patients with ≥2 coincident risk factors, extended ENI significantly increased the five-year RC, DMFS, and DFS rates. The five- and 10-year OS rates were also (non-significantly) higher in patients treated with extended ENI, suggesting that patients bearing multiple coincident adverse factors may derive the most benefit from extended ENI. Conversely, for patients without any of the aforementioned risk factors, irradiation of the involved echelon alone appears to be sufficient for decreasing treatment-related morbidities.

Concordant with the published literature [17, 31], our multivariate analysis identified PNI as an independent predictor for worse DMFS and DFS, but not for inferior RC. Additionally, no significant RC improvement was observed in patients with perineural invasion treated with extended ENI, suggesting that the presence of PNI alone may not warrant the use of extended ENI. Nonetheless, the current study documented that 19 (66%) out of 29 ACC patients presented with PNI, and two (11%) of the 19 developed outfield perineural tumor recurrence. Since a higher propensity of perineural invasion/spread in ACC has been documented [32, 33], prophylactic irradiation to the nerve tract should be strongly recommended particularly in the presence of PNI and locally-advanced disease. However, the distance from the tumor at which radiation treatment should be administered cannot be determined by this limited data. Coverage of the nerve tract of the lingual nerve, hypoglossal nerve, and facial nerve (marginal mandibular branch) to the skull base might be adequate in preventing morbidity as a result of brain irradiation. Additionally, it is warranted to extend outwards to cover the angle of the jaw and the plane between the plasma for the marginal mandibular branch.

We observed a high nodal recurrent rate (17%) in SMGC patients treated with PORT. Additionally, failures at contralateral neck nodes and uninvolved adjacent echelons were frequently observed, particularly in patients with pN+, ENE, pT3–4, and LVI. To our knowledge, we are the first to demonstrate the indications and clinical utility of extended ENI for the bilateral treatment of adjacent echelons of SMGC. However, there are some limitations inherent to this retrospective study. While ours was the largest long-term series of SMGC patients treated with PORT, the relatively small number of subjects may have biased our results. The median follow-up of 79 months was relatively short for accurately evaluating the survival outcomes for SMGC. Additionally, we cannot fully account for all potential biases due to the non-randomized retrospective nature of the study. The subjective treatment decisions and the diverse irradiation fields used may also be regarded as limitations. However, because of the low prevalence and indolent nature of salivary gland malignancies, conducting a decade-long prospective randomized trial would be difficult. The only ongoing randomized trial, RTOG 1008, is designed to investigate the efficacy of postoperative cisplatin-based chemoradiation in patients with salivary gland carcinomas; the target enrollment size is 120 patients. Importantly, this trial does not specifically assess SMGC patients; the neck irradiation field for SMGC is based on empirical experience. Hence, we believe that our multicenter experience is valuable and provides a rationale for the design of future prospective trials.

Conclusion

Our long-term study showed that nodal recurrence on the contralateral side of the neck and adjacent uninvolved echelons was not uncommon in SMGC patients treated with PORT, and that this should be considered during radiotherapy planning. Extended ENI appears to improve RC and DFS rates in patients with certain (or multiple) adverse pathological factors. Conversely, limited ENI to the involved echelons alone appears to be adequate for low-risk patients without risk factors.

Acknowledgements

We are grateful to the members of the Head and Neck Oncology Group at Linkou Chang Gung Memorial Hospital for their invaluable help.

Funding

This study was financially supported by Research Grants CMRPG3F0061, CMRPG3F0061-2, CMRPG3F0861 and CORPG3G0961 from the Chang Gung Medical Foundation.

Honors

Portions of these data were presented at the ASTRO's 56th Annual Meeting (2014; San Francisco, CA, USA). This study was awarded the Outstanding Research Prize by the Chinese Oncology Society in 2014.

Authors' contributions

CEH and CYL conceived of the study. CEH and CYL carried out the manuscript writing and revision for important intellectual content. LYL and CEH performed histology specimen collection and review. CEH and CYL carried out the statistical analyses. KHF, CTL, JTCC, NMT, HMW, KHF, SHN and TCY participated in data collection and patient clinical care. All authors have read and approved the final manuscript.

Competing interests

The authors declare that they have no competing interests.

Author details

[1]Radiation Oncology, Chang Gung Memorial Hospital at Linkou and Chang Gung University, No. 5, Fuxing St., Guishan Dist, Taoyuan City 33305, Taiwan, Republic of China. [2]Pathology, Chang Gung Memorial Hospital at Linkou and Chang Gung University, Taoyuan City, Taiwan, Republic of China. [3]Medical Oncology, Chang Gung Memorial Hospital at Linkou and Chang Gung University, Taoyuan City, Taiwan, Republic of China. [4]Diagnostic Radiology, Chang Gung Memorial Hospital at Linkou and Chang Gung University, Taoyuan City, Taiwan, Republic of China. [5]Otorhinolaryngology, Head and Neck Surgery, Chang Gung Memorial Hospital at Linkou and Chang Gung University, Taoyuan City, Taiwan, Republic of China. [6]Nuclear Medicine and Molecular Imaging Center, Chang Gung Memorial Hospital at Linkou and Chang Gung University, Taoyuan City, Taiwan, Republic of China. [7]Head and Neck Oncology Group, Chang Gung Memorial Hospital at Linkou and Chang Gung University, Taoyuan City, Taiwan, Republic of China. [8]Graduate Institute of Clinical Medical Science, Chang Gung University, Taoyuan City, Taiwan, Republic of China. [9]School of Traditional Chinese Medicine, Chang Gung University, Taoyuan City, Taiwan, Republic of China. [10]Radiation Oncology, Xiamen Chang Gung Hospital, Xiamen City, Fujian Province, China. [11]Departments of Experimental Radiation Oncology, Division of Radiation Oncology, The University of Texas MD Anderson Cancer Center, Houston, Texas, USA. [12]The University of Texas MD Anderson Cancer Center-UT Health Graduate School of Biomedical Sciences, Houston, Texas, USA. [13]Particle Physics and Beam Delivery Core Laboratory, Institute for Radiological Research, Chang Gung Memorial Hospital at Linkou and Chang Gung University, Taoyuan City, Taiwan, Republic of China.

References

1. Bhattacharyya N. Survival and prognosis for cancer of the submandibular gland. J Oral and Maxillofac Surg. 2004;62:427–30.
2. Wahlberg P, Anderson H, Biörklund A, et al. Carcinoma of the parotid and submandibular glands—a study of survival in 2465 patients. Oral Oncol. 2002;38:706–13.
3. Spiro RH. Salivary neoplasms: overview of a 35-year experience with 2,807 patients. Head Neck Surg. 1986;8:177–84.
4. Adelstein DJ, Koyfman SA, El-Naggar AK, Hanna EY. Biology and Management of Salivary Gland Cancers. Semin Radiat Oncol. 2012;22:245–53.
5. Mendenhall WM, Morris CG, Amdur RJ, et al. Radiotherapy alone or combined with surgery for salivary gland carcinoma. Cancer. 2005;103:2544–50.
6. Terhaard CH, Lubsen H, Rasch CR, et al. The role of radiotherapy in the treatment of malignant salivary gland tumors. Int J Radiat Oncol Biol Phys. 2005;61:103–11.

7. Zeidan YH, Pekelis L, An Y, et al. Survival benefit for adjuvant radiation therapy in minor salivary gland cancers. Oral Oncol. 2015;51:438–45.
8. Terhaard CH, Lubsen H, Van der Tweel I, et al. Salivary gland carcinoma: independent prognostic factors for locoregional control, distant metastases, and overall survival: results of the Dutch head and neck oncology cooperative group. Head Neck. 2004;26:681–93.
9. Armstrong JG, Harrison LB, Spiro RH, et al. Malignant tumors of major salivary gland origin. A matched-pair analysis of the role of combined surgery and postoperative radiotherapy. Arch Otolaryngol Head Neck Surg. 1990;116:290–3.
10. Armstrong JG, Harrison LB, Thaler HT, et al. The indications for elective treatment of the neck in cancer of the major salivary glands. Cancer. 1992;69:615–9.
11. Ferlito A, Pellitteri PK, Robbins KT, et al. Management of the neck in cancer of the major salivary glands, thyroid and parathyroid glands. Acta Otolaryngol. 2002;122:673–8.
12. Chen AM, Garcia J, Lee NY, et al. Patterns of nodal relapse after surgery and postoperative radiation therapy for carcinomas of the major and minor salivary glands: what is the role of elective neck irradiation? Int J Radiat Oncol Biol Phys. 2007;67:988–94.
13. Chen AM, Granchi PJ, Garcia J, et al. Local-regional recurrence after surgery without postoperative irradiation for carcinomas of the major salivary glands: implications for adjuvant therapy. Int J Radiat Oncol Biol Phys. 2007;67:982–7.
14. Zbären P, Schüpbach J, Nuyens M, Stauffer E. Elective neck dissection versus observation in primary parotid carcinoma. Otolaryngol Head Neck Surg. 2005;132:387–91.
15. Vander Poorten VL, Balm AJ, Hilgers FJ, et al. The development of a prognostic score for patients with parotid carcinoma. Cancer. 1999;85:2057–67.
16. Régis De Brito Santos I, Kowalski LP, Cavalcante De Araujo V, et al. Multivariate analysis of risk factors for neck metastases in surgically treated parotid carcinomas. Arch Otolaryngol Head Neck Surg. 2001;127:56–60.
17. Han MW, Cho K-J, Roh J-L, et al. Patterns of lymph node metastasis and their influence on outcomes in patients with submandibular gland carcinoma. J Surg Oncol. 2012;106:475–80.
18. Group IHaNS. Cervical lymph node metastasis in adenoid cystic carcinoma of the major salivary glands. J Laryngol Otol. 2017;131:96–105.
19. Lin T-C, Tsou Y-A, Bau D-T, Tsai M-H. Factors influencing contralateral neck metastasis in oral squamous cell carcinoma. Formos J Surg. 2012;45:83–7.
20. Dias FL, Lima RA, Kligerman J, et al. Relevance of skip metastases for squamous cell carcinoma of the oral tongue and the floor of the mouth. Otolaryngol Head Neck Surg. 2006;134:460–5.
21. Pimenta Amaral TM, da Silva Freire AR, Carvalho AL, et al. Predictive factors of occult metastasis and prognosis of clinical stages I and II squamous cell carcinoma of the tongue and floor of the mouth. Oral Oncol. 2004;40:780–6.
22. Liao C-T, Chang J-C, Wang H-M, et al. Analysis of risk factors of predictive local tumor control in oral cavity cancer. Ann Surg Oncol. 2008;15:915–22.
23. Hsieh C-E, Lin C-Y, Lee L-Y, et al. Postoperative radiotherapy with or without concurrent chemotherapy for salivary gland carcinomas. Therapeut Radiol Oncol. 2015;22:89–91.
24. Tsan D-L, Lin C-Y, Kang C-J, et al. The comparison between weekly and three-weekly cisplatin delivered concurrently with radiotherapy for patients with postoperative high-risk squamous cell carcinoma of the oral cavity. Radiat Oncol. 2012;7:215.
25. Hsieh C-E, Lin C-Y, Lee L-Y, et al. Adding concurrent chemotherapy to postoperative radiotherapy improves locoregional control but not overall survival in patients with salivary gland adenoid cystic carcinoma—a propensity score matched study. Radiat Oncol. 2016;11:1–10.
26. Johnston ML, Huang SH, Waldron JN, et al. Salivary duct carcinoma: treatment, outcomes, and patterns of failure. Head Neck. 2016;38:E820–6.
27. Stennert E, Kisner D, Jungehuelsing M, et al. High incidence of lymph node metastasis in major salivary gland cancer. Arch Otolaryngol Head Neck Surg. 2003;129:720–3.
28. Mallik S, Agarwal J, Gupta T, et al. Prognostic factors and outcome analysis of submandibular gland cancer: a clinical audit. J Oral Maxillofac Surg. 2010; 68:2104–10.
29. Storey MR, Garden AS, Morrison WH, et al. Postoperative radiotherapy for malignant tumors of the submandibular gland. Int J Radiat Oncol Biol Phys. 2001;51:952–8.
30. Huang B-S, Chen W-Y, Hsieh C-E, et al. Outcomes and prognostic factors for surgery followed by modern radiation therapy in parotid gland carcinomas. Jpn J Clin Oncol. 2016;46:832–8.
31. Bjorndal K, Krogdahl A, Therkildsen MH, et al. Salivary gland carcinoma in Denmark 1990-2005: a national study of incidence, site and histology. Results of the Danish head and neck Cancer group (DAHANCA). Oral Oncol. 2011;47:677–82.
32. Barrett AW, Speight PM. Perineural invasion in adenoid cystic carcinoma of the salivary glands: a valid prognostic indicator? Oral Oncol. 2009;45:936–40.
33. Chen AM, Bucci MK, Weinberg V, et al. Adenoid cystic carcinoma of the head and neck treated by surgery with or without postoperative radiation therapy: prognostic features of recurrence. Int J Radiat Oncol Biol Phys. 2006;66:152–9.

13

Accelerated vs. conventionally fractionated adjuvant radiotherapy in high-risk head and neck cancer

Christiane Matuschek[1†], Jan Haussmann[1†], Edwin Bölke[1*], Stephan Gripp [1], Patrick J. Schuler[2], Bálint Tamaskovics[1], Peter Arne Gerber[3], Freddy-Joel Djiepmo-Njanang[1], Kai Kammers[4], Christian Plettenberg[5], Bahar Anooshahr[6], Klaus Orth[1] and Wilfried Budach[1]

Abstract

Background: Adjuvant radiotherapy in advanced head and neck squamous cell cancer (HNSCC) reduces the risk of local-regional failure and most likely increases the survival rate. Patients at high risk for tumor recurrence may benefit from more aggressive altered fractionation schedules in order to reduce the overall time from surgery to completion of radiotherapy. Here, we reviewed the results of six randomized trials addressing the above hypothesis.

Methods: In the six trials of interest, a total of 988 patients with locally advanced HNSCC were randomly assigned to receive either accelerated or conventionally fractionated adjuvant radiotherapy. Hazard ratios (HR) were extracted from available publications for local-regional control, distant metastasis as well as overall-, cancer specific- and disease-free survival. Meta-analysis of the effect sizes was performed using fixed and random effect models. Acute and late side effects were categorized and summarized for comparison.

Results: Accelerated radiotherapy did not improve the loco-regional control (n = 988, HR = 0.740, CI = 0.48–1.13, p = 0.162), progression-free survival (HR = 0.89, CI = 0.76–1.04, p = 0.132) or overall survival (HR = 0.88, CI = 0.75–1.04, p = 0.148) significantly. Acute confluent mucositis occurred with significant higher frequency with accelerated radiotherapy. Late side effects did not differ significantly in either group.

Conclusion: Accelerated radiotherapy does not result in a significant improvement of loco-regional control or overall survival in high-risk patients. Acute but not late radiation toxicity were more frequent with the accelerated RT technique. In clinical practice accelerated postoperative radiation therapy might be a suitable option only for a subset of patients.

Keywords: Radiation therapy, Head and neck cancer, High risk, Adjuvant therapy, Conventional fractionation, Accelerated fractionation

Background

Head and neck squamous cell carcinoma (HNSCC) is a common tumor and accounts for approximately 3% of all cancers in the United States. About 40% of patients have locally advanced disease at the time of diagnosis. Surgery, radiation therapy (RT), or both have been used for decades to improve loco-regional control (LRC) and overall survival (OS). The most common schedule for normofractionated RT alone is given as 1.6–2.0 Gy per fraction per day, 5 days a week, for 6–7 weeks. Despite all efforts, the prognosis of patients with locally advanced HPV-negative HNSCC is still disappointing, with 5-year OS rates of 30–35% [1–11].

The role of unconventionally fractionated RT in HNSCC has been studied in numerous trials within different schedules which are usually separated into hyperfractionated (HF) where the treatment is administered in two smaller fractions twice per day and accelerated fractionation (AF) where the overall

* Correspondence: boelke@med.uni-duesseldorf.de
†Christiane Matuschek and Jan Haussmann contributed equally to this work.
[1]Department of Radiotherapy and Radiooncology, Medical Faculty, Heinrich Heine University, Moorenstr. 5, 40225 Dusseldorf, Germany
Full list of author information is available at the end of the article

treatment time is reduced by applying more than 5 fractions per week [12–14].

The rational for this approach is that a shortening of overall treatment time might result in improved local tumor control rates as it counteracts tumor repopulation. Secondly smaller fractions are also believed to result in a reduction in late toxicities as normal tissue, in contrast to tumors, are able to repair RT-induced damages within 6 h [1–4, 15–17]. Thirdly there are also economic and patient convenience arguments to shorten the overall treatment time on a linear accelerator time slot. As surgical interventions have significant impact on morbidity and quality of life it is important to study the influence of different fractionation regimes on adverse events in the postoperative setting [5].

The MARCH meta-analysis published by Bourhis et al. demonstrated that altered fraction schedules are a valuable alternative to chemoradiation as they provide similar gains in reduction of overall mortality compared to standard radiation alone in the definitive therapeutic setting. However between the subgroups of altered fractionation only the hyperfractionated, and not the accelerated, schedules appear to provide a substantial mortality benefit beyond a reduction in local recurrence [14].

However it is currently not established whether this is also true for the postoperative / adjuvant situation. This setting is accompanied by a smaller tumor volume and density, different tumor microenvironment, local inflammation and a potentially different radiobiology i.e. lesser extent of hypoxic cells. These observations allow an investigation of accelerated schedules in the postoperative setting and to the best of our knowledge no meta-analysis has focused on this aspect yet. The results of six randomized trials addressing this question in adjuvant RT were retrieved and analyzed [6–11, 18].

Methods

We thoroughly investigated the electronic databases MEDLINE and EMBASE from inception through July 23, 2017, with no restriction for language or publication status. We also searched the Evidence Based Medicine Reviews database combining searches of Cochrane Database of Systematic Reviews, Database of Abstracts of Reviews of Effects, Cochrane CENTRAL, Cochrane Methodology Register, Health Technology Assessment, NHS Economic Evaluation Database, and ACP Journal Club. Patients with locally advanced HNSCC were randomly assigned to receive either accelerated or conventionally fractionated postoperative RT. Studies that included concurrent or sequential chemotherapy were not allowed. Published hazard ratios and hazard ratios extracted from available survival curves were the basis of the meta-analysis. Additionally, we extracted and categorized the published acute and late side effects from the published papers [6–11, 18, 19]. The idea for this meta-analysis was originally generated in 2016. By the time the literature search was completed and the manuscript was prepared the individual patient meta-analysis by Lacas et al. was published and generated superior estimates of the investigated effect size on overall survival for the include trials [18]. Moreover the extraction of these published data allowed the inclusion of multiple other endpoints beyond locoregional control and overall survival. Additionally the CHARTWEL study, as an unpublished trial, could be included which was otherwise unavailable.

Heterogeneity between trials was assessed using Chi-square test and I statistics. Estimations of the pooled effect sizes were performed using a fixed effect model. When I-statistics showed significant heterogeneity ($p = < 0.1$) a random effect model was applied. Meta-analyses of the effect sizes on locoregional-, local- and regional recurrence, distant failure, progression-free survival, overall survival, cancer- and non-cancer mortality were performed using fixed or random effects models based on hazard ratios and their standard errors using the Microsoft Excel add-in Meta-XL (Version 5.3).

As hazard ratios of clinical endpoints were extracted from the analysis of Lacas et al. all considerations in their paper apply equally to our results [18]. The most important ones are: overall survival was defined as time from randomization to death from any cause. Living patients were censored at the time of the last follow-up. Cancer mortality is defined as death with previous diagnosis of progression and of the treated head and neck cancer as well as death from unknown cause within 5 years after randomization. Time from randomization to first local or distant recurrence or death from any cause was defined as progression-free survival. All events were recorded as first events.

The Cairo 1990 trial reported only combined locoregional recurrence and was not included in the separate analysis of local and regional recurrence [11]. The analysis of locoregional failure consisted of pooled effect sizes of both endpoints from the other trials by a fixed effect model as no heterogeneity was observed. Statistical difference level was set at p-values lower than 0.05 for all evaluations.

Results

We found five publications testing the effect of accelerated vs conventional fractionated postoperative RT in high-risk HNSCC patients [6–11]. Extraction of the single trial data from Lacas et al. allowed the inclusion of six trials [18]. All staging was defined by pathology.

Table 1 (Reported) Study Inclusion criteria and radiation schedules in the included trials. All Staging is defined by pathology

	Ang et al. 2001 [9]	Awwad et al. 2002 [11]	Langendijk et al. 2015 [7]	Sanguineti et al. 2005 [8]	Suwinski et al. 2008 [10]	CHARTWEL unpublished[a]
N patients	151	70	148	226	279	114
Median Follow-up (years; IQR)	13.8 (8.0–16.9)	3.8 (1.6–4.7)	6.3 (5.3–8.0)	4.5 (3.4–6.2)	7.2 (6.3–8-0)	4.8 (3.9–5.4)
Histology	squamous cell carcinoma					n.a.
Localisation	oral cavity / oropharynx / hypopharynx / larynx	oral cavity / hypopharynx / larynx	n.a.	oral cavity / oropharynx / hypopharynx / larynx	oral cavity / oropharynx / larynx	oral cavity / oropharynx / hypopharynx / larynx /other
ECOG PS	≤ 2	≤ 2	n.a.	≤ 2	≤ 1	≤ 2
Age (years)	n.a.	≤ 65	n.a.	18–80	n.a.	n.a.
Resection	planned	surgical resection without macroscopic residual (R0/R1)				n.a.
Definition of "High Risk" situation	ECE or any two of following: - > 1 nodal group - ≥2 positive nodes - > 3-cm node - Oral cavity - Microscopic pos. Margin - Perineural invasion (Pn1)	- T2/N1–2 or - T3–4/any N	- positive surgical margins and/or - extranodal spread (ECE)	one or more of following risk factors: - pT4 - close margin (< 3 mm) - V1 - L1 - pN2–3 - ECE - time from surgery: ≤ 8 w	all non-laryngeal tumors (except T1 N0) or R1 or ECE+ or pN2/3 or two of following minor risk factors: - close margin - V1 - G3 - Pn1	n.a.
Metastases	no distant metastases (M0)					n.a.
Other criteria	n.a.	liver, kidney and other function normal	n.a.	n.a.	n.a.	n.a.
Dose in CF Arm	1.8Gyx35Fx =63Gy 5×/week in 7 weeks	2Gyx30Fx = 60Gy 5×/week in 6 weeks	2Gyx33Fx = 66Gy 5×/week in 7 weeks	2Gyx30Fx = 60Gy 5×/week in 6 weeks	1.8Gyx35Fx = 63Gy 5×/week in 7 weeks	2Gyx30-32Fx = 60-64Gy 5×/week in 7 weeks
Dose in AF Arm	1.8Gyx15Fx = 27Gy; 5×/week+ 2 × 1.8Gy/d × 10; 5×/week = 63Gy in 35Fx in 5 weeks	3 × 1,4Gy/d = 46,2Gy; 6×/week in 12 days	2Gy×10Fx = 20Gy;5×/week + (1,8Gy + 1,3Gy/d)×15 = 66,5Gy in 40 Fx; in 5 weeks	(1.8Gy + 1.4Gy/d)x5Fx +2Gyx 15Fx + (2Gy + 1.6Gy/d)x5Fx = 64Gy in 35 Fx 5×/week in 5 weeks	1.8Gyx35Fx = 63Gy; 7×/week in 5 weeks	(1.5Gyx3/d)x30Fx = 51-54Gy; 5×/week in 2.4 weeks

ECE Extracapsular extension, *CF* Conventional fractionation, *AF* Accelerated fractionation, *n.a.* Not available, *Fx* Fractions
[a]Data from the CHARTWEL trial were retrieved from [18]

Table 2 Patient characteristics of the included trials

	Ang et al. 2001 [9]		Awwad et al. 2002 [11]		Langendijk et al. 2015 [7]		Sanguineti et al. 2005 [8]		Suwinski et al. 2008 [10]		CHARTWEL unpublished[a]
	$n = 151$		$n = 70$		$n = 148$		$n = 226$		$n = 279$		$n = 114$
	CF $n = 75$	AF $n = 76$	CF	AF	CF $n = 74$	AF $n = 74$	CF	AF	CF	AF	
Age (years)											
median (range)	57 (20–83)		50 (25–65)	50 (29–65)	n.a.		61.5 (30–82)		57 (36–77)		n.a.
Gender											
male	163		32	24	111		209		127	122	88
female	50		7	7	37		17		13	17	26
Performance status	(ECOG)										
0	23		0	0	n.a.	n.a.	28	32	279		74
1	114		23	13	n.a.	n.a.	80	73			37
2	14		16	18	n.a.	n.a.	5	8	0		3
3	0		0	0	n.a.	n.a.	0	0	0		
Tumor site											
oral cavity	80	14	14	14	n.a.	n.a.	25	19	59	62	n.a.
oropharynx	66	0	0	0	23		13	27			30
hypopharynx	29	5	5	7	n.a.	n.a.	20	31	0	0	n.a.
larynx	38	20	20	10	10		55	36	81	77	16.
TNM: tumor stage											
T1/T2	84		5	3	21		3	4	36	35	20
T3	129		22	18	n.a.	n.a.	43	56	104	104	n.a
T4			12	10	n.a.	n.a.	67	53			n.a.
TNM: nodal stage											
N0	90		25	16	n.a.	n.a.	41	39	54	39	n.a.
N1			14	15	n.a.	n.a.			86	100	
N2/N3	123						72	74			
Histological grade											
G1	n.a.	15	15	13	n.a.	n.a.	n.a.	n.a.	30	16	n.a.
G2	n.a.	20	20	16	n.a.	n.a.	n.a.	n.a.	66	79	n.a.
G3	n.a.	4	4	2	n.a.	n.a.	n.a.	n.a.	31	37	n.a.
uncertain	213	0	0	0	n.a.	n.a.	113	113	13	7	n.a.
Stage (UICC 7th ed.)											
I	0		2		21		1	1	n.a.	n.a.	20
II	9						2	3	n.a.	n.a.	
III	81		42		23		8	13	n.a.	n.a.	13
IV	103		26		104		102	96	n.a.	n.a.	62
unknown	20	39	39	31	n.a.	n.a.	0	0	140	139	n.a.
Positive (or close)	resection margins										
yes	n.a.	17	17	15	n.a.	n.a.	48	48	78	77	n.a.
no	n.a.	20	20	16	n.a.	n.a.	65	65	50	54	n.a.
uncertain	213	2	2	0	n.a.	n.a.	0	0	12	8	n.a.

Table 2 Patient characteristics of the included trials *(Continued)*

	Ang et al. 2001 [9]		Awwad et al. 2002 [11]		Langendijk et al. 2015 [7]		Sanguineti et al. 2005 [8]		Suwinski et al. 2008 [10]		CHARTWEL unpublished[a]
	n = 151		n = 70		n = 148		n = 226		n = 279		n = 114
	CF n = 75	AF n = 76	CF	AF	CF n = 74	AF n = 74	CF	AF	CF	AF	
Extracapsular extension											
yes	104	n.a.	n.a.	n.a.	n.a.	n.a.	38	37	17	27	n.a.
no	109	n.a.	n.a.	n.a.	n.a.	n.a.	75	76	83	67	n.a.
uncertain	0	39	39	31	n.a.	n.a.	0	0	40	45	n.a.

CF Conventional fractionation group, *AF* Accelerated fractionation group
[a]Data from the CHARTWEL trial were retrieved from [18]

The first paper, published in 2005, was a multicenter Phase III study by Sanguineti et al. [8]. Between 1994 and 2000, 226 patients were enrolled. They found a 2-year LRC of 80% +/− 4% for conventional RT and 78% +/− 5% for accelerated RT ($p = 0.52$). The 2-year OS were 67% +/− 5% for conventional and 64% +/− 5% for accelerated RT ($p = 0.84$). No difference in the clinical outcome among the two treatment arms was detected in a multivariate analysis. Nevertheless, interaction analysis with median values as cut-offs showed a tendency for improved LRC in patients treated with accelerated fractionation (HR = 0.5, CI = 0.2–1.1). Fifty percent of patients treated with accelerated RT had confluent mucositis, compared with only 27% of those treated with conventional fractionation ($p = 0.006$). However, the duration of mucositis did not differ in the two groups. Actuarial Grade 3+ late toxicity rates at 2 years were 18% +/− 4% and 27% +/− 6% for conventional and accelerated RT ($p = 0.10$) [8].

The second paper was published in 2001 by K. Ang et al. from MD Anderson [9]. The group performed a multi-institutional, prospective, randomized trial. In this trial they investigated multiple variables including pathologic risk features, the RT-dose required in the adjuvant setting and the the impact of accelerating RT using a concomitant boost schedule as well as the importance of the overall combined treatment duration on the treatment outcome. Two hundred thirteen patients with advanced disease were divided into three groups based on a set of pathologic risk features. The high-risk group received 63 Gy, by random assignment, for 5 weeks ($n = 76$) or 7 weeks ($n = 75$). Patients were irradiated with standard protocols applicable to the disease site and expected areas of tumor spread. The endpoints were LRC, OS and morbidity. Patients with high-risk patients tended to have a better LRC and OS when postoperative RT was administered in 5 rather than 7 weeks. A longer interval between surgery and postoperative RT in the 7-week timetable led to considerably lower LRC ($p = 0.03$) and OS ($p = 0.01$) rates. As a result, the cumulative length of combined therapy significantly impacted the LRC ($p = 0.005$) and OS ($p = 0.03$) rates. The shorter radiation time, achieved by administering the boost simultaneously did not increase toxicities [9].

Awwad et al. published the third paper in the *British Journal of Cancer* [11]. The trial included 70 patients who had had radical surgery for (T2/N1-N2) or (T3–4/any N) squamous cell carcinoma of the oral cavity, larynx, and hypopharynx. Patients were assigned at random to receive either (a) accelerated hyperfractionation: 46.2 Gy per 12 days, 1.4 Gy per fraction, three fractions per day with 6 h interfraction interval, treating 6 days per week or (b) conventional fractionation: 60 Gy per 6 weeks, 2 Gy per fraction, treating 5 days per week. The researchers found a significant improvement in 3-year LRC in the accelerated hyperfractionation as opposed to conventional fractionation (88 +/− 4% vs 57+/− 9%) ($p = 0.01$). There was, however, no significant difference in the OS (60 +/− 10% vs 46 +/− 9%) ($p = 0.29$). Further, the accelerated hyperfractionated radiotherapy was most beneficial when it started within 6 weeks after surgery and the total treatment time was completed within 10 weeks. Mucositis emerged earlier and was more severe in the accelerated hyperfractionation group. Accelerated hyperfractionation caused more xerostomia, fibrosis and edema. In comparison to conventional fractionation, accelerated hyperfractionation did not seem to offer a survival advantage in patients with rapidly growing tumors. A better local control, however, was achieved in these patients. For slow growing tumors, there was no significant difference in tumor control and survival rate between the two radiation schedules [11].

Suwinski performed a randomized clinical trial on 7-days-a-week postoperative RT for high-risk HNSCC [10]. Between 2001 and 2004, 279 patients with high-risk squamous cell cancer of the larynx ($n = 158$) or cancer of the oral cavity/oropharynx ($n = 121$) were registered. Patients received 63 Gy in 35 fractions given 5-days-a-week ($n = 140$: conventional fraction group) or 7-days-a-week ($n = 139$: accelerated group). Acute and late toxicity were considered acceptable,

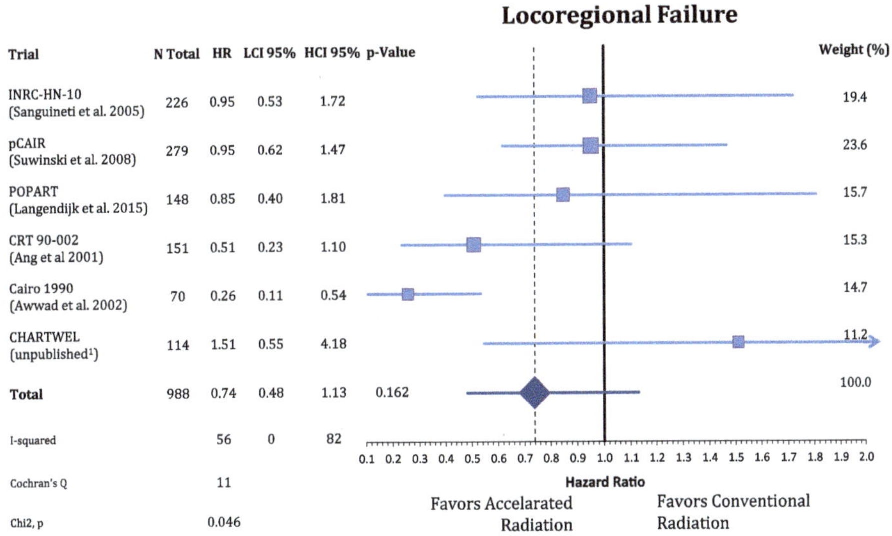

Fig. 1 Forest plot of comparison of locoregional failure between accelerated and conventional radiation using random effect model. Horizontal bars indicate the amount of variation (95% confidence intervals of the parameter estimates). Sizes of squares indicate weight in the pooled effect size

although the proportion of patients with confluent mucositis was higher in the accelerated group compared to conventional fractionation (60% vs. 33.3%). The actuarial 3-year LRC were not significantly different with 64% for conventional vs. 70% for accelerated fractionation ($p = 0.32$) for the whole population. However accelerated treatment yielded a statistically significant improvement in the 3-year LRC for patients with cancer of the oropharynx/oral cavity (74% vs. 53% conventional fractionated, $p = 0.02$). No improvement was found for the local-regional control for patients with cancer of the larynx ($p = 0.46$) [10].

At the European Society for Radiotherapy and Oncology annual meeting in 2015, Langendijk et al. presented their final trial results [6, 7]. Patients with high-risk advanced HNSCC (i.e., positive surgical margins and/or extranodal spread) treated with curative surgery were randomly assigned to receive either standard postoperative RT (2 Gy/fraction/day, 5 days/week to 66 Gy/33 fractions/7 weeks) or postoperative accelerated RT (2 Gy/fraction/day, 5 days per week, to 20 Gy followed by 1.8 Gy/fraction/day and 1.3 Gy/fraction per day to a boost field as a second daily treatment to 66.5 Gy/40 fractions/5 weeks). Endpoints were LRC, OS, acute and late toxicity, and quality of life. A total of 148 patients were registered in this trial (74 pts. for conventional radiotherapy and 74 pts. for the accelerated group). No significant changes were found for acute and late

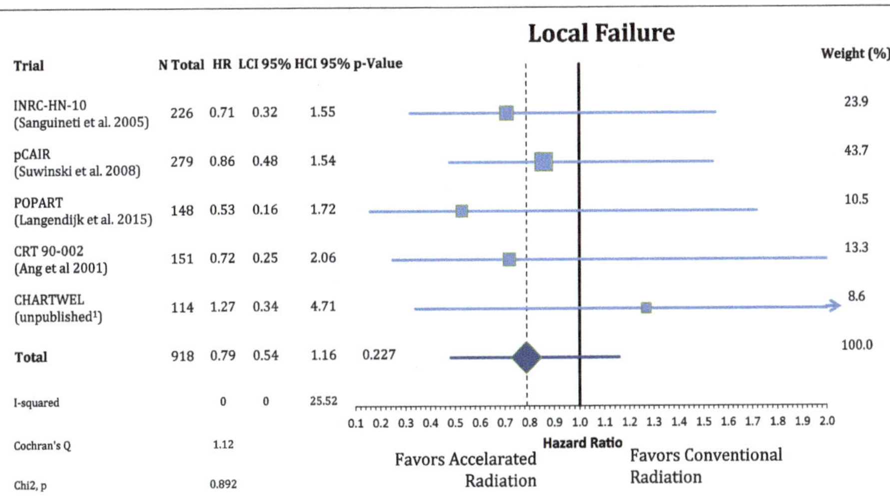

Fig. 2 Forest plot of comparison of local failure between accelerated and conventional radiation using fixed effect model

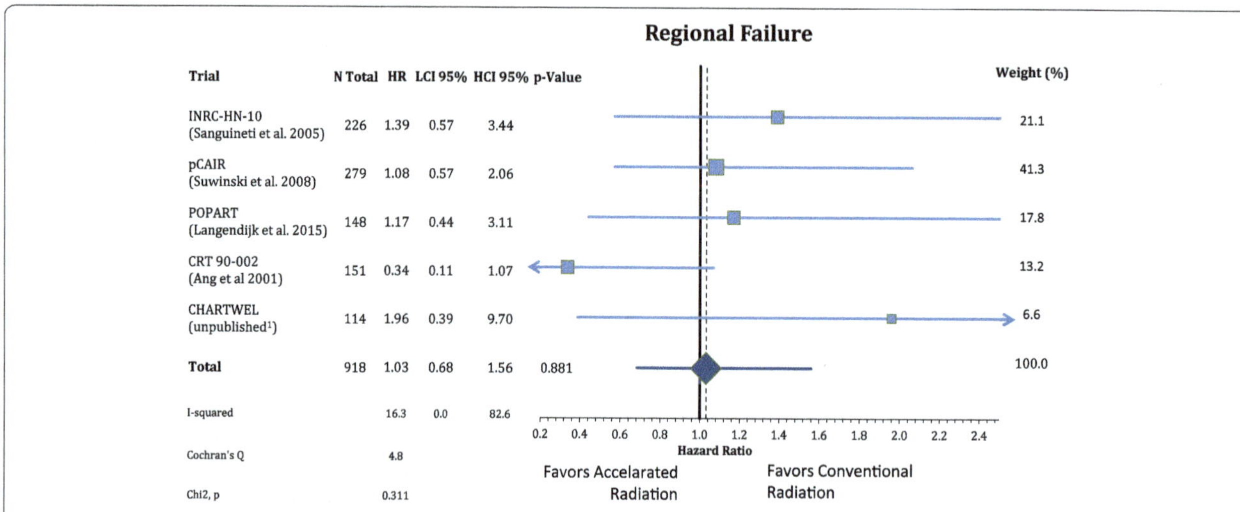

Fig. 3 Forest plot of comparison of regional failure between accelerated and conventional radiation using fixed effect model

toxicity, although there was a trend towards increased need for pain medication among patients in the accelerated group. After 3 years, the LRC rate was 77% in the accelerated group compared to 76% for patients with conventional fractionation (HR = 0.86, CI = 0.42–1.76; p = 0.68). The 3-year OS was not significantly different for the accelerated group vs. the conventionally treated group (71% vs. 63% HR = 0.93, CI = 0.54–1.61; p = 0.81) [7].

The data from the unpublished CHARTWEL trial was available from the updated MARCH meta-analysis [18]. Between 2001 and 2005 114 eligible patients with stage I-IV HNSCC of the oral cavity, oropharynx, hypopharynx, larynx or other sites were randomized to CF RT of 60–64 Gy in 6–6.5 weeks or 51–54 Gy with 1.5 Gy three times daily for 2.4 weeks. Trials results are reported after a median follow-up of 4.8 years.

The patients' characteristics and inclusion criteria are summarized in Tables 1 and 2. All trials included patients with high risk squamous cell carcinoma of the head and neck region randomized to AF or CF without concomitant chemotherapy in both arms. Median follow-up ranges from 3.8–13.8 years. Overall 988 patients were analyzed in eight different oncological endpoints. Figure 1 shows that postoperative accelerated RT did not result in a significant improvement of LRC (n = 988, HR: 0.740, CI = 0.48–1.13, p = 0.162). Differential analysis of local and regional control separately (Figs. 2 and 3) demonstrates a

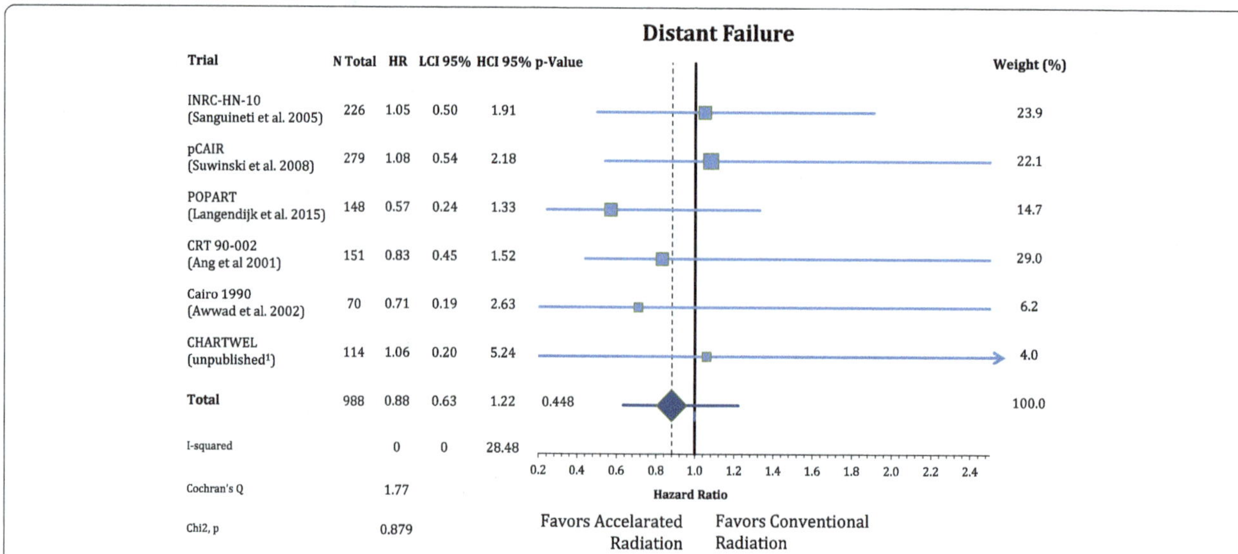

Fig. 4 Forest plot of comparison of distant failure between accelerated and conventional radiation using fixed effect model

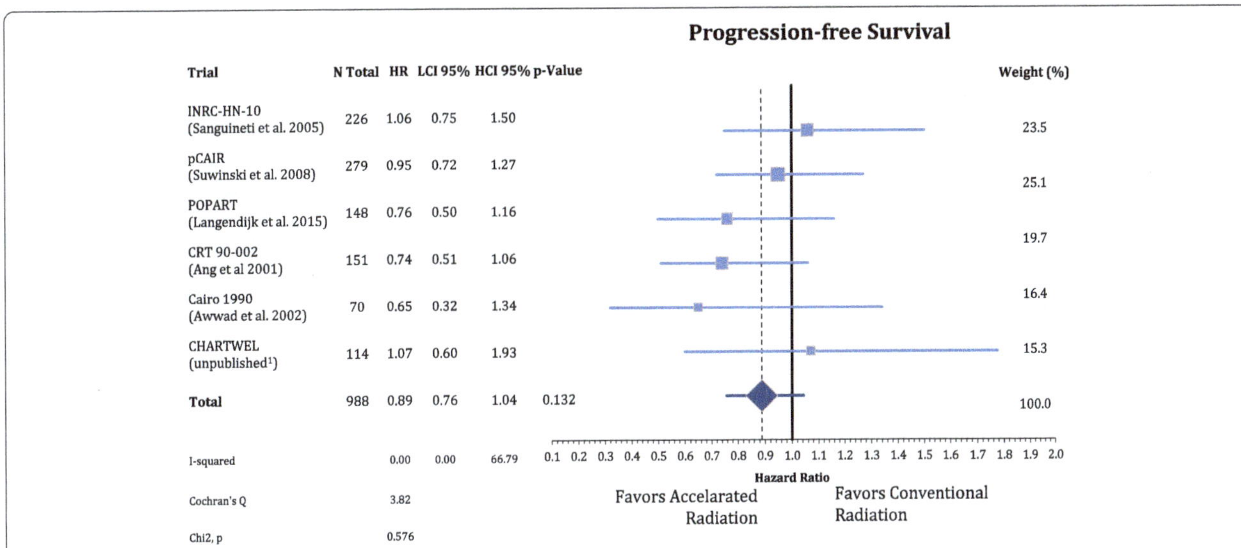

Fig. 5 Forest plot of comparison of progression-free survival between accelerated and conventional radiation using fixed effect model

non-significant reduction in local recurrence (n = 918, HR = 0.79, CI = 0.54–1.16, p = 0.227) and no effect on regional control (n = 918, HR = 1.03, CI = 0.68–1.56, p = 0.881). Likewise there is also no difference in distant metastasis (n = 988, HR = 0.88, CI = 0.63–1.22, p = 0.448) in Fig. 4 and progression free survival (n = 988, HR = 0.89, CI = 0.76–1.04, p = 0.132) (Fig. 5).

Postoperative accelerated RT did not result in a significant improvement of OS (n = 988, HR = 0.88, CI = 0.75–1.04, p = 0.148). The results are depicted in Fig. 6. Further analysis of the causes of death of the trial participants shows that accelerated radiation had not a significant effect in reducing cancer mortality (n = 988, HR = 0.83, CI = 0.68–1.02, p = 0.077) and nor on non-cancer related deaths (n = 988, HR = 0.98, CI = 0.74–1.30, P = 0.891) (Figs. 7 and 8).

In terms of side effects we summarized and categorized acute and late effects from the published trial results in Table 3. We found significantly more acute adverse events like mucositis and need for tube feeding in the patients treated with AF RT. The rate of late side effects did not significantly correlate with accelerated radiotherapy.

We also performed a subgroup analysis comparing moderate accelerated radiation and very accelerated

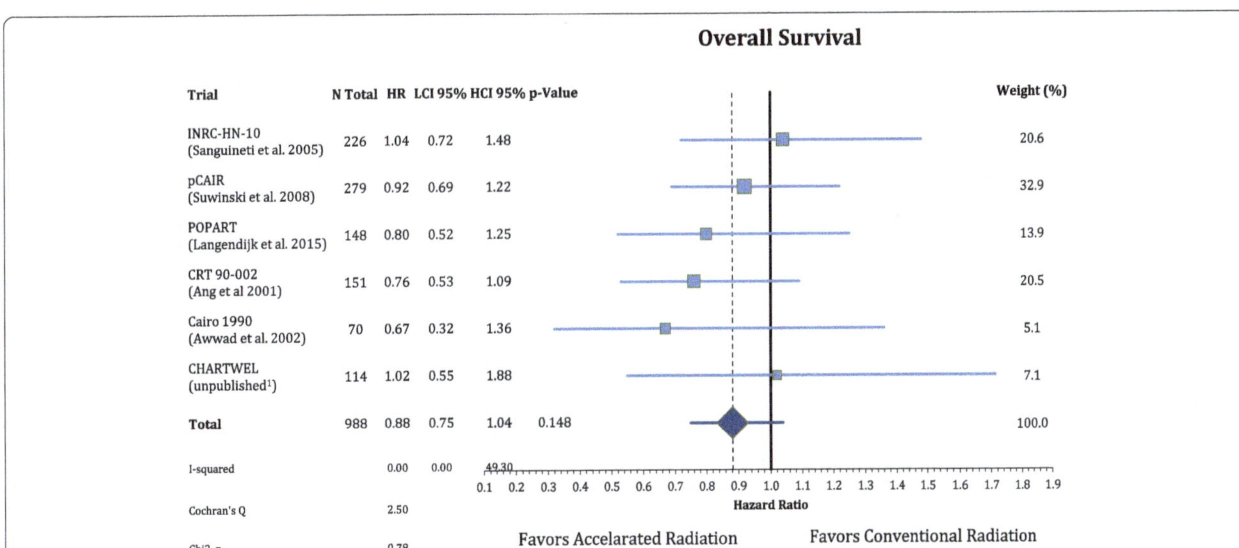

Fig. 6 Forest plot of comparison of overall survival between accelerated and conventional radiation using fixed effect model

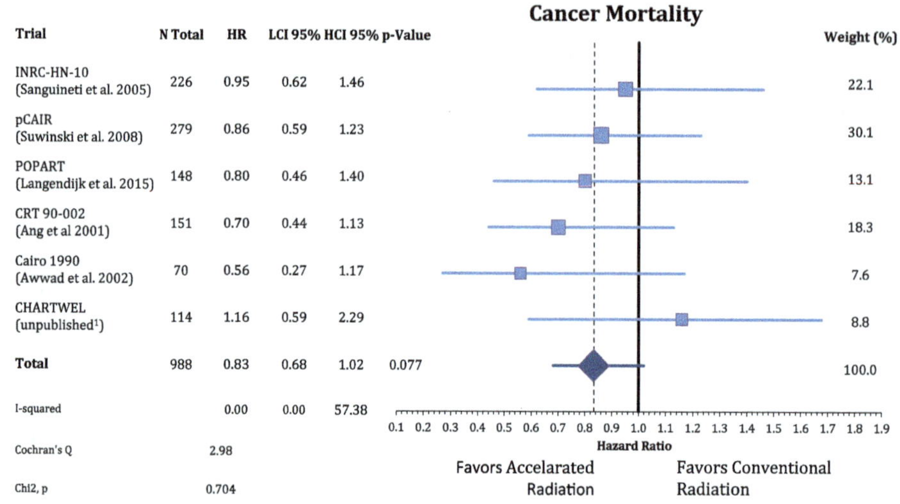

Fig. 7 Forest plot of comparison of cancer mortality between accelerated and conventional radiation using fixed effect model

radiotherapy as defined by the MARCH Meta-analyses [14, 18]. We did not find a significant influence of these subgroups on any of the investigated endpoints (not reported in detail).

Discussion

Despite advances in staging, surgical procedures, radiation techniques and systemic treatment options the clinical outcomes of patients with advanced HNSCC are still disappointing [20–26]. Radiobiological considerations as well as retrospective observational data rendered acceleration in head and neck radiation schedules as an attractive option to improve results [27, 28].

This meta-analysis addressed this question in the adjuvant setting using published effect sizes based on individual patient data with an average median follow-up of about 6 years. We found no significant effect of accelerated fractionated radiation compared to conventional fractionated radiation in the postoperative setting in any of the investigated endpoints.

The current standard of care for high risk HNSCC is concurrent adjuvant chemoradiation (CRT). This is based on the results of two large randomized trials using cisplatin concurrently with radiation [27, 28]. A pooled analysis of the two studies demonstrated a significant benefit in local control and overall survival especially in patients with close surgical margins or extracapsular lymphonodal extension [29].

Altered fractionation schedules as an alternative to systemic therapies to improve the therapeutic ratio in comparison to conventional RT have been intensively investigated.

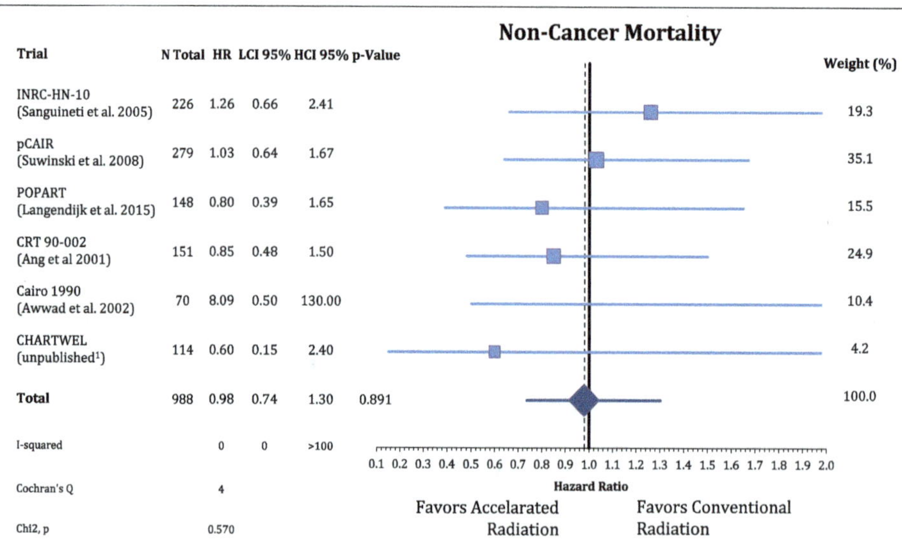

Fig. 8 Forest plot of comparison of non-cancer mortality between accelerated and conventional radiation using fixed effect model

Table 3 Acute and late side effects

Trial	Ang et al. 2001 [9] $n = 151$			Awaad et al. 2002 [11] $n = 70$			Langendijk et al. 2015 [7] $n = 148$			Sanguineti et al. 2005 [8] $n = 226$			Suwinski et al. 2008 [10, 19] $n = 275$			CHARTWEL unpublished[a] $n = 114$		
Acute Toxicity	CF	AF	p	CF	AF	p	CF	AF	p	CF	AF	p	CF	AF	p	CF	AF	p
Mucositis during RT ≥ grade II	n.r.	n.r.		67%	90%	0.04	n.r.	n.r.		74,7%	84,6%	0.007	n.r.	n.r.		n.r.	n.r.	
Mucositis during RT ≥ grade III	36%	62%	0.001	8%	16%		n.r.	n.r.		27%	53%		33.3%	60%	0.02	n.r.	n.r.	
Acute dysphagia ≥ grade III	n.r.	n.r.		10%	23%	0.007	n.r.	n.r.		6,3%	9,1%	n.c.	2%.	5%	n.c.	n.r.	n.r.	
Tube feeding	47%	51%	n.s.	n.r.	n.r.		n.r.	n.r.		8%	14%	0.13	$n = 3$	$n = 5$	n.c.	n.r.	n.r.	
Mean weight loss	n.r.	n.r.		n.r.	n.r.		n.r.	n.r.		0.9%	1.6%	0.3	3.3%	3.1%	n.c.	n.r.	n.r.	
Acute skin reaction, ≥ grade III	n.r.	n.r.		"Low in both groups "		n.s.	n.r.	n.r.		35.1%	38.2%	n.c.	n.r.	n.r.		n.r.	n.r.	
Mucositis 6 weeks after RT	n.r.	n.r.		n.r.	n.r.		n.r.	n.r.		12%	9%	0.84	n.r.	n.r.		n.r.	n.r.	
Late toxicity:																		
Xerostomia grade II/III	n.r.	n.r.		39/ 13%	33/ 42%	0.17	n.r.	n.r.		$n = 14$	$n = 16$	n.c.	$n = 14$	$n = 18$	n.c.	n.r.	n.r.	
Lymphedema grade II/III	n.r.	n.r.		10%	16%	0.7	n.r.	n.r.		n.r.	n.r.		n.r.	n.r.		n.r.	n.r.	
Subcutaneous fibrosis or connective tissue grade II/III	n.r.	n.r.		13%	26%		n.r.	n.r.		$n = 35$	$n = 36$	n.c.	$n = 13$	$n = 16$	n.c.	n.r.	n.r.	
Dysphagia ≥ grade III	$n = 13$	$n = 16$	n.c.	n.r.	n.r.		n.r.	n.r.		$n = 1$	$n = 3$	n.c.	n.r.	n.r.		n.r.	n.r.	
Myelopathy, any grade	n.r.	n.r.		$n = 0$	$n = 1$	n.c.	n.r.	n.r.		$n = 0$	$n = 1$	n.c.	$n = 0$	$n = 1$	n.c.	n.r.	n.r.	
Any late side effects	No difference		n.s.	n.r.	n.r.		n.r.	n.r.		$n = 49$	$n = 56$	0.15	$n = 51$	$n = 64$	n.c.	n.r.	n.r.	
Any late side effects ≥ grade III	$n = 25$	$n = 26$	n.c.	n.r.	n.r.		n.r.	n.r.		$n = 17$	$n = 24$	n.c.	$n = 8$	$n = 18$	n.c.	n.r.	n.r.	
Any side effects							No difference		n.s.							n.r.	n.r.	

CF Conventional fractionation, *AF* Accelerated fractionation; values are reported as number of events or percent (%). *n.c.* Not calculated, *n.r.* Not reported, *n.s.* Not significant

[a]Data from the CHARTWEL trial were retrieved from [18]

In the combined primary and postoperative setting Lacas et al. report that altered fractionation compared to conventional RT results in an improvement in almost all clinically important endpoints, including overall mortality (absolute difference at 5 years of 3.1%, CI 1.3–4.9) [18]. However alternate fractionation was associated with a significant increase in acute toxicity. In a subgroup analysis AF decreased local recurrence significantly. The mortality benefit though derived mainly from the trials using hyperfractionated instead of accelerated RT schedules.

In the sole primary setting of definitive radiotherapy Budach et al. previously published a meta-analysis assessing the effects of accelerated RT [30]. Over 10,000 patients were included in this analysis. They found a significant improvement in LRC with accelerated RT, but no significant benefit in OS. These results are in accordance to the MARCH meta-analysis by Bourhis and colleagues [14].

In the present meta-analysis we investigated whether the improvement in the primary setting for alternative fractionation translates into the postoperative setting. A subgroup analysis of timing of radiotherapy revealed no significant effect on OS or PFS in the updated MARCH meta-analysis [18]. However a complete analysis on postoperative accelerated RT had not been attempted. Our results showed that accelerated radiation fractionation does not significantly improve the studied endpoints. If any, the analyses of local control and cancer specific survival showed a minor trend for an effect of AF. These results are matching the established effects in the definitive radiation setting. Like in the updated MARCH meta-analysis AF has no effect on regional control despite a minor influence on local control. This is again in contrast to HF radiation schedules where its effects extend to both local and regional failures demonstrating a possible way to explain the superiority of HF to AF in survival endpoint.

Worsening of the acute toxicities is a well-established finding throughout the literature investigating alternative fractionation regimes [13, 18]. The analysis of the reported side-effects in Table 3 confirms a worsening of acute toxicities by AF. The acute mucositis rate was significantly higher and appeared earlier during treatment in the accelerated fractionated RT group. Similarly to other trials and meta-analyses we also did not find an increase in late side effects. Therefore prior surgery does not appear to have a noticeable influence on the pattern of adverse events.

This meta-analysis has some strengths as well as limitations to address. The average median trial follow-up of about 6 years provides robust long-term oncological results. The use of pooled trial results of individual patient data allows for a more sophisticated estimation method compared to extracting hazard ratios from published survival curves. Yet the clinical applicability is limited by the relatively small number of analyzable patients (n = 988). Certain analyses might be underpowered to show a benefit of AF in postoperative radiation. Furthermore we were unable to perform any subgroup analysis. Especially as p16-status, a surrogate marker for human papilloma virus (HPV) infection, is an important prognostic marker in HNSCC, studying the effect on fractionation with respect to HPV status would be interesting. Moreover all included trials used conventional radiation techniques which are currently non-standard with the introduction of volumetric arc therapy and image-guided radiation therapy. Another limitation is that the median follow-up time is unequal between the included trials which might lead to heterogeneity in the outcome of the clinical endpoints.

Concurrent chemoradiation or hyperfractionated radiation therapy is both an accepted standard in the definitive treatment of HNSCC and was indirectly shown to be equally effective [31]. Adding chemotherapy to HF RT schedules could provide additional benefits [32, 33]. However this has not been demonstrated for AF [12]. At least in the primary setting, HF, and not AF, should therefore be used as the preferred alternate fractionation schedule. However the Radiation Therapy Oncology Group (RTOG) has implemented a moderately accelerated RT schedule in their comparison of cisplatin vs. cetuximab (RTOG 1016).

In the adjuvant situation the comparison of AF and HF to CRT has not been successfully reported. There is equally a lack of data for adjuvant HF RT compared to standard RT schedules which leaves CRT, CF RT and AF RT as studied options. The clinical scenario where one might consider an accelerated postoperative radiation schedule is difficult to identify. As chemotherapy is very likely superior to adjuvant accelerated radiation only patients who are unable to tolerate concurrent CRT are possible candidates. Further they would need to be at very high risk of local failure and additionally be able to comply with the accompanied aggravated acute toxicities. Our study was not able to identify any potential subgroup that could derive a profound profit from AF.

Future studies using modern RT techniques and simultaneous integrated boost (SIB) might improve the risk benefit ratio in this setting. Intensity modulated radiotherapy was already shown to improve acute and late toxicities compared to conventional RT [34, 35]. Likewise SIB might add a reduction in the incidence of late adverse events compared to sequential boost techniques [36].

Conclusion

Concurrent chemoradiotherapy (conventionally-fractionated) is the standard-of-care as adjuvant intervention for resected and high-risk HNSCC. Postoperative accelerated radiotherapy does not result in a significant improvement of overall survival in high-risk patients. Clinical decision of adjuvant accelerated radiotherapy must be made on case to case basis weighing overall risks and benefits. Future studies with the use of modern radiation techniques might change the risk-benefit ratio in the treatment of squamous cell carcinoma of the head and neck.

Abbreviations

AF: Accelerated fractionation; CF: Conventional fractionation; CI: 95% confidence interval; CL: Confindence limits; CRT: Chemoradiation; ECE: Extracapsular extension; HF: Hyperfractionated; HNSCC: Squamous cell carcinomas of the head and neck; HR: Hazard ratio; IGRT: Image-guided radiation therapy; IMRT: Intensity-modulated radiation therapy; LRC: Locoregional control; n.c.: Not calculated; n.r.: Not reported; n.s.: Not significant; OS: Overall survival rate; QoL: Quality of life; RT: Radiotherapy

Authors' contributions

CM, EB and WB had the idea, coordinated the work, and wrote parts of the manuscript. EB did the literature research, prepared the data for analysis and wrote parts of the manuscript. KK, WB and JH did the statistical analysis. JH and PAG wrote parts of the manuscript. JH, BT contributed significantly to the discussion on the interpretation of the results. CM, JH, ST, and PJS prepared the figures and tables and wrote parts of the manuscript. All authors read and approved the final manuscript.

Competing interests

The authors declare that they have no competing interests.

Author details

[1]Department of Radiotherapy and Radiooncology, Medical Faculty, Heinrich Heine University, Moorenstr. 5, 40225 Dusseldorf, Germany . [2]Department of Oto-Rhino-Laryngology, Head and Neck Surgery, Ulm University Medical

Center, Ulm, Germany. [3]Department of Dermatology, Medical Faculty Heinrich Heine University Dusseldorf, Dusseldorf, Germany. [4]Division of Biostatistics and Bioinformatics, Department of Oncology, The Sidney Kimmel Comprehensive Cancer Center at Johns Hopkins, The Johns Hopkins University School of Medicine, Baltimore, MD, USA. [5]Department of Oto-Rhino-Laryngology, Head and Neck Surgery, Heinrich Heine University Dusseldorf, Dusseldorf, Germany. [6]Vincere Cancer Center, Scottsdale, AZ, USA.

References

1. Tarnawski R, Fowler J, Skladowski K, et al. How fast is repopulation of tumor cells during the treatment gap? Int J Radiat Oncol Biol Phys. 2002;54:229–36.
2. Trott KR. Cell repopulation and overall treatment time. Int J Radiat Oncol Biol Phys. 1990;19:1071–5.
3. Maciejewski B, Withers HR, Taylor JM, Hliniak A. Dose fractionation and regeneration in radiotherapy for cancer of the oral cavity and oropharynx: tumor dose-response and repopulation. Int J Radiat Oncol Biol Phys. 1989; 16:831–43.
4. Withers HR, Maciejewski B, Taylor JM, Hliniak A. Accelerated repopulation in head and neck cancer. Front Radiat Ther Oncol. 1988;22:105–10.
5. Mehanna H, Wong WL, McConkey CC, et al. PET-CT surveillance versus neck dissection in advanced head and neck Cancer. N Engl J Med. 2016;374:1444–54.
6. Langendijk JA, Kaanders JH, Doornaert P, et al. Postoperative accelerated radiotherapy (POPART) versus conventional postoperative radiotherapy (CPORT) in squamous cell head and neck cancer: a multicenter prospective randomized study of the Dutch head and neck cooperative study group. J Clin Oncol. 2010;28:5508.
7. Langendijk H, Kaanders JH, Doornaert P, et al. OC-008: POPART vs CPORT in squamous cell head and neck cancer: results of a multicenter randomised study of the Dutch head and neck study group. Radiother Oncol. 2015;114:9–10.
8. Sanguineti G, Richetti A, Bignardi M, et al. Accelerated versus conventional fractionated postoperative radiotherapy for advanced head and neck cancer: results of a multicenter phase III study. Int J Radiat Oncol Biol Phys. 2005;61:762–71.
9. Ang KK, Trotti A, Brown BW, et al. Randomized trial addressing risk features and time factors of surgery plus radiotherapy in advanced head-and-neck cancer. Int J Radiat Oncol Biol Phys. 2001;51:571–8.
10. Suwinski R, Bankowska-Wozniak M, Majewski W, et al. Randomized clinical trial on 7-days-a-week postoperative radiotherapy for high-risk squamous cell head and neck cancer. Radiother Oncol. 2008;87:155–63.
11. Awwad HK, Lotayef M, Shouman T, et al. Accelerated hyperfractionation (AHF) compared to conventional fractionation (CF) in the postoperative radiotherapy of locally advanced head and neck cancer: influence of proliferation. Br J Cancer. 2002;86:517–23.
12. Bourhis J, Sire C, Graff P, et al. Concomitant chemoradiotherapy versus acceleration of radiotherapy with or without concomitant chemotherapy in locally advanced head and neck carcinoma (GORTEC 99-02): an open-label phase 3 randomised trial. Lancet Oncol. 2012;13:145–53.
13. Overgaard J, Mohanti BK, Begum N, et al. Five versus six fractions of radiotherapy per week for squamous-cell carcinoma of the head and neck (IAEA-ACC study): a randomised, multicentre trial. Lancet Oncol. 2010;11:553–60.
14. Bourhis J, Overgaard J, Audry H, et al. Hyperfractionated or accelerated radiotherapy in head and neck cancer: a meta-analysis. Lancet. 2006;368: 843–54.
15. Harriss-Phillips WM, Bezak E, Yeoh EK. Monte Carlo radiotherapy simulations of accelerated repopulation and reoxygenation for hypoxic head and neck cancer. Br J Radiol. 2011;84:903–18.
16. Marcu L, van Doorn T, Olver I. Modelling of post-irradiation accelerated repopulation in squamous cell carcinomas. Phys Med Biol. 2004;49:3767–79.
17. Bentzen SM. Repopulation in radiation oncology: perspectives of clinical research. Int J Radiat Biol. 2003;79:581–5.
18. Lacas B, Bourhis J, Overgaard J, et al. Role of radiotherapy fractionation in head and neck cancers (MARCH): an updated meta-analysis. Lancet Oncol. 2017;18:1221–37.
19. Suwinski R, Bankowska-Wozniak M, Majewski W, et al. Randomized clinical trial on continuous 7-days-a-week postoperative radiotherapy for high-risk squamous cell head-and-neck cancer: a report on acute normal tissue reactions. Radiother Oncol. 2005;77:58–64.
20. Lu G, Little JV, Wang X, et al. Detection of head and neck Cancer in surgical specimens using quantitative hyperspectral imaging. Clin Cancer Res. 2017; 23(18):5426–36.
21. Ringash J, Waldron JN, Siu LL, et al. Quality of life and swallowing with standard chemoradiotherapy versus accelerated radiotherapy and panitumumab in locoregionally advanced carcinoma of the head and neck: a phase III randomised trial from the Canadian Cancer trials group (HN.6). Eur J Cancer. 2017;72:192–9.
22. Schmitt NC, Page BR. Chemoradiation-induced hearing loss remains a major concern for head and neck cancer patients. Int J Audiol. 2017:1–6. https://doi.org/10.1080/14992027.2017.1353710.
23. Svider PF, Blasco MA, Raza SN, et al. Head and neck Cancer. Otolaryngol Head Neck Surg. 2017;156:10–3.
24. Tao Y, Auperin A, Graff P, et al. Very accelerated radiotherapy or concurrent chemoradiotherapy for N3 head and neck squamous cell carcinoma: pooled analysis of two GORTEC randomized trials. Oral Oncol. 2017;71:61–6.
25. Wang HM, Lin CY, Hsieh CH, et al. Induction chemotherapy with dose-modified docetaxel, cisplatin, and 5-fluorouracil in Asian patients with borderline resectable or unresectable head and neck cancer. J Formos Med Assoc. 2017;116:185–92.
26. Wong BY, Fischer S, Cruickshank HE. Clinical outcome of head and neck cancer patients: a comparison between ENT patients referred via the 2 weeks wait pathway and alternative routes in the UK health system. Eur Arch Otorhinolaryngol. 2017;274:415–20.
27. Bernier J, Domenge C, Ozsahin M, et al. Postoperative irradiation with or without concomitant chemotherapy for locally advanced head and neck cancer. N Engl J Med. 2004;350:1945–52.
28. Cooper JS, Pajak TF, Forastiere AA, et al. Postoperative concurrent radiotherapy and chemotherapy for high-risk squamous-cell carcinoma of the head and neck. N Engl J Med. 2004;350:1937–44.
29. Bernier J, Cooper JS, Pajak TF, et al. Defining risk levels in locally advanced head and neck cancers: a comparative analysis of concurrent postoperative radiation plus chemotherapy trials of the EORTC (#22931) and RTOG (# 9501). Head Neck. 2005;27:843–50.
30. Budach W, Hehr T, Budach V, Belka C, Dietz K. A meta-analysis of hyperfractionated and accelerated radiotherapy and combined chemotherapy and radiotherapy regimens in unresected locally advanced squamous cell carcinoma of the head and neck. BMC Cancer. 2006;6:28.
31. Gupta T, Kannan S, Ghosh-Laskar S, Agarwal JP. Concomitant chemoradiotherapy versus altered fractionation radiotherapy in the radiotherapeutic management of locoregionally advanced head and neck squamous cell carcinoma: an adjusted indirect comparison meta-analysis. Head Neck. 2015;37:670–6.
32. Ghadjar P, Simcock M, Studer G, et al. Concomitant cisplatin and Hyperfractionated radiotherapy in locally advanced head-and-neck Cancer: 10-year follow-up of a randomized phase iii trial (Sakk 10/94). Int J Radiat Oncol. 2012;82:524–31.
33. Budach V, Stromberger C, Poettgen C, et al. Hyperfractionated accelerated radiation therapy (HART) of 70.6 Gy with concurrent 5-FU/Mitomycin C is superior to HART of 77.6 Gy alone in locally advanced head and neck Cancer: long-term results of the ARO 95-06 randomized phase III trial. Int J Radiat Oncol. 2015;91:916–24.
34. Nutting CM, Morden JP, Harrington KJ, et al. Parotid-sparing intensity modulated versus conventional radiotherapy in head and neck cancer (PARSPORT): a phase 3 multicentre randomised controlled trial. Lancet Oncol. 2011;12:127–36.
35. Spiotto MT, Weichselbaum RR. Comparison of 3D confromal radiotherapy and intensity modulated radiotherapy with or without simultaneous integrated boost during concurrent chemoradiation for locally advanced head and neck cancers. PLoS One. 2014;9:e94456.
36. Lertbutsayanukul C, Prayongrat A, Kannarunimit D, Chakkabat C, Netsawang B, Kitpanit S. A randomized phase III study between sequential versus simultaneous integrated boost intensity-modulated radiation therapy in nasopharyngeal carcinoma. Strahlenther Onkol. 2018;194:375–85.

14

Radiation-induced parotid changes in oropharyngeal cancer patients: the role of early functional imaging and patient –/treatment-related factors

Simona Marzi[1*], Alessia Farneti[2], Antonello Vidiri[3], Francesca Di Giuliano[3,4], Laura Marucci [2], Filomena Spasiano[2], Irene Terrenato[5] and Giuseppe Sanguineti[2]

Abstract

Background: Functional magnetic resonance imaging may provide several quantitative indices strictly related to distinctive tissue signatures with radiobiological relevance, such as tissue cellular density and vascular perfusion. The role of Intravoxel Incoherent Motion Diffusion Weighted Imaging (IVIM-DWI) and Dynamic Contrast-Enhanced (DCE) MRI in detecting/predicting radiation-induced volumetric changes of parotids both during and shortly after (chemo) radiotherapy of oropharyngeal squamous cell carcinoma (SCC) was explored.

Methods: Patients with locally advanced oropharyngeal SCC were accrued within a prospective study offering both IVIM-DWI and DCE-MRI at baseline; IVIM-DWI was repeated at the 10th fraction of treatment. Apparent diffusion coefficient (ADC), tissue diffusion coefficient D_t, perfusion fraction f and perfusion-related diffusion coefficient D^* were estimated both at baseline and during RT. Semi-quantitative and quantitative parameters, including the transfer constant K^{trans}, were calculated from DCE-MRI. Parotids were contoured on T2-weighted images at baseline, 10th fraction and 8th weeks after treatment end and the percent change of parotid volume between baseline/10th fr (ΔVol_{10fr}) and baseline/8th wk. (ΔVol_{post}) computed.
Correlations among volumetric changes and patient-, treatment- and imaging-related features were investigated at univariate analysis (Spearman's Rho).

Results: Eighty parotids (40 patients) were analyzed. Percent changes were 18.2 ± 10.7% and 31.3 ± 15.8% for ΔVol_{10fr} and ΔVol_{post}, respectively. Among baseline characteristics, ΔVol_{10fr} was correlated to body mass index, patient weight as well as the initial parotid volume. A weak correlation was present between parotid shrinkage after the first 2 weeks of treatment and dosimetric variables, while no association was found after radiotherapy. Percent changes of both ADC and D_t at the 10th fraction were also correlated to ΔVol_{10fr}. Significant relationships were found between ΔVol_{post} and baseline DCE-MRI parameters.

Conclusions: Both IVIM-DWI and DCE-MRI can help to detect/predict early (during treatment) and shortly after treatment completion the parotid shrinkage. They may contribute to clarify the correlations between volumetric changes of parotid glands and patient–/treatment-related variables by assessing individual microcapillary perfusion and tissue diffusivity.

Keywords: Diffusion magnetic resonance imaging, Perfusion magnetic resonance imaging, Radiotherapy, Parotid gland, Oropharyngeal Cancer

* Correspondence: simona.marzi@ifo.gov.it
[1]Medical Physics Laboratory, IRCCS Regina Elena National Cancer Institute, Via Elio Chianesi 53, 00144 Rome, Italy
Full list of author information is available at the end of the article

Background

Radiotherapy is involved in the treatment of the majority of patients with non-metastatic head and neck squamous cell carcinoma [1]. Despite intensity modulated radiotherapy (IMRT), xerostomia is still a frequent radiation-induced complication with implications on patients quality of life [2, 3]. More importantly, there is some degree of inconsistency between dosimetric data of the parotids at planning and long-term patient reported outcomes [4]. Among possible explanations, variations in intrinsic radiosensitivity among individuals [5], discrepancies between objective outcome and patient perception [6] and variations in parotid gland (PG) dosage during the course of IMRT due to shrinkage have been advocated [7, 8].

Thought the pathophysiology of parotid shrinkage during radiotherapy remains unclear [9], image-based scoring of toxicity based on early changes of irradiated organs can provide a timely, objective and consistent endpoint for patient counseling and treatment strategy adaptation [5, 10–12]. In this regard, functional magnetic resonance imaging (MRI) techniques, such as diffusion- and perfusion- MRI, may have an important role, as they provide several quantitative indices strictly related to distinctive tissue signatures with radiobiological relevance, such as tissue cellular density and vascular perfusion [12, 13].

Dynamic contrast-enhanced (DCE) MRI is a well-established technique to evaluate the hemodynamic properties of several tissues, such as vessel leakiness and permeability, by means of serial MRI scans taken before and after the intravenous injection of a contrast agent [13, 14]. Moreover, diffusion-weighted imaging (DWI) provides insights into cellular architecture, being sensitive to the thermally driven motion of water molecules in tissues [15]. Therefore, DWI indirectly assesses cell depopulation due to radiation-induced changes. Intravoxel Incoherent Motion (IVIM) imaging is a further evolution of DWI potentially able to provide both diffusion and perfusion imaging results with the additional advantage of being completely non-invasive, as it does not require contrast injection [16, 17]. IVIM-DWI assumes that the microcirculation of blood can be thought as a *pseudo-diffusion* incoherent motion, because the capillary network does not have a specific spatial orientation within a single image voxel. To separate the perfusion effects from those of thermal diffusion, IVIM-DWI requires the acquisition of images with multiple b value, where b is a factor dependent on the gradient pulse sequence (i.e. pulse duration and strength of the diffusion gradient). The perfusion effect on the signal attenuation may be significant at low b values (0–150 s/mm2) in well-vascularized tissues, while it is assumed to vanish at higher b values due to the larger drop in signal compared to the thermal diffusivity effect. By using a bi-exponential function to model the IVIM signal intensity at increasing b values [16], both perfusion-related and perfusion-free diffusion parameters may be derived, as described below in more detail.

In January 2016 we started a prospective study funded by the Italian Association for Cancer Research (AIRC, project No.17028) in locally advanced oropharyngeal SCC investigating the ability of both DCE-MRI and IVIM-DWI to predict tumor response to (chemo-)IMRT. As part of this ongoing study, we investigated also volumetric changes of parotid glands during and shortly after treatment completion. Here we report the results on 40 consecutive patients.

Methods

Patient population& treatment

To be eligible, patients had to fulfill all the following criteria: (i) age older than 18 years; (ii) Karnofsky performance status > 80; (iii) pathologically confirmed squamous cell carcinoma of the oropharynx; (iv) stage III or IV without distant metastases according to the 7th edition of the AJCC Cancer Staging Manual; (v) treatment with radiotherapy $\pm$ chemotherapy. Exclusion criteria included: any contraindication for MR examination; prior surgery, CHT (including induction chemotherapy) or radiotherapy to the primary disease and the neck. Moreover, specific informed consent was obtained from each patient before enrolling. The study protocol was approved by the local Institutional Review Board.

All patients were offered IMRT and concomitant cisplatin (CDDP), either 100 mg/m^2 for three cycles every 21 days or weekly 40 mg/m^2 for 6 cycles. If patients were not medically fit, IMRT alone was delivered. A simultaneous integrated boost technique delivering the following total doses in 35 fractions was used: 70 Gy to macroscopic disease; 63 Gy to regions at high risk of microscopic disease; 58.1 Gy to regions at intermediate risk of microscopic disease [18]. A 7-field approach with 6 MV photons was used. For each patient, the planned mean dose to the single parotid gland, D_{mean}(Gy), and the percentage of parotid volume receiving ≥30 Gy, V_{30}(%), were calculated from the treatment planning system (Eclipse version 13.5.37, Varian Medical System, Palo Alto, CA) and recorded.

MR imaging protocols

MRI scans were performed with a 1.5-T system (Optima MR 450w, GE Health-care, Milwaukee, Wisconsin) with dedicated 16-channels receive-only RF coils: a head coil, a surface neck and a spine coil. In addition to standard imaging, all patients underwent three serial MRI examinations: before treatment, after the 10th fraction of chemoradiotherapy and 8 weeks after the end of treatment. MRI scanning was avoided on the same day of chemotherapy administration.

At baseline, the MRI acquisition protocol included both IVIM-DWI and DCE-MRI examinations. However, only IVIM-DWI was repeated at the 10th fraction to reduce the use of intravenous contrast agent. Both coronal and axial fast spin echo T_2-weighted images (acquisition matrix, 288 × 256; field of view, 26–28 cm; TR/TE, 5739/100 ms; slice thickness, 4 mm; inter-slice gap, 5; acquisition time, 2 min and 40 s) were acquired in all MRI exams.

IVIM-DWI was performed using single-shot echo-planar imaging with the following parameters: acquisition matrix 128 × 128, field of view 26–28 cm, TR/TE 4500 ms/77 ms, number of slices 30–33, slice thickness 4 mm, and intersection gap 1 mm. Nine different *b* values ($b = 0$, 25, 50, 75, 100, 150, 300, 500, and 800 s/mm^2) were used, with all diffusion-sensitizing gradients applied in three orthogonal directions to obtain trace-weighted images.

To enable the perfusion-sensitive information to be accurately extracted from DWI, most of the b values (six) were chosen within the lower range 0–150 s/mm^2, while three b values in the range 300–800 s/mm^2 were considered adequate to estimate the perfusion-free tissue diffusion coefficient. The maximum b value was limited to 800 s/mm^2 as it usually provides a sufficient signal to noise ratio and a good lesion cospicuity in the head and neck region at 1.5-T.

Three signal averages were chosen for *b* values ranging from 0 to 300 s/mm^2, four for a *b* value of 500 s/mm^2, and five for a *b* value of 800 s/mm^2. Array Spatial Sensitivity Encoding Technique imaging, with a scan-time reduction factor of 2, was used, with a resulting scanning time of 6 min and 13 s.

DCE-MRI involved a 3D fast-spoiled gradient echo sequence with the following characteristics: TR/TE:3.82/1.18 ms; flip angle: 30°; acquisition matrix: 128 × 128; field of view: 28 cm; number of slices: 32; slice thickness: 4 mm; spacing between slices: 2 mm.

Sixty dynamic volumes were acquired consecutively, with a temporal resolution of 5 s and a total scanning time of 5 min. At the fourth dynamic volume, 0.1 mmol/kg body weight of gadopentetatedimeglumine contrast agent was administered intravenously, at a rate of 3 ml/s.

Parotid gland delineation

For each patient, a single observer manually outlined the entire PG on T2-weighted images acquired at each time point. 3D Slicer Software (version 4.6.2) was used for image visualization and for gland segmentation [19]. Vascular structures were meticulously excluded from the delineated PG volume. These contours were propagated onto DCE-MRI images using the 3D Slicer module *Expert Automated Registration*.

The parotid contours obtained on T2-weighted images also served as a guide to parotid gland delineation on DWI sequences with b = 800 s/mm^2. An example of parotid delineation is illustrated in Fig. 1.

Calculation of IVIM-diffusion parameters

Dedicated scripts were developed in Matlab code (Release 7.10.0, The Mathworks Inc., Natick, Massachusetts) for quantitative image analyses. The median value of the signal from all voxels within the entire gland was derived

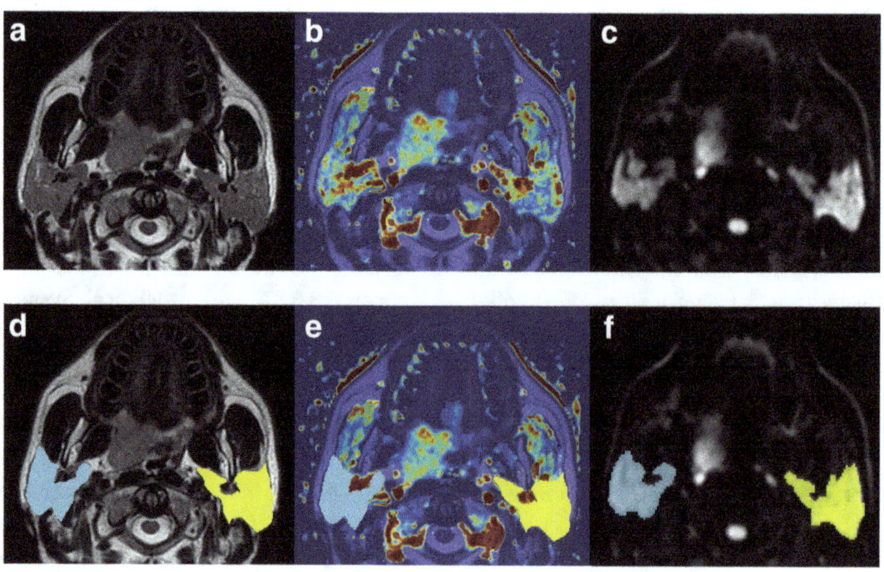

Fig. 1 Central section of parotids in a 44-year-old man affected by a tonsil carcinoma on the axial T2-weighted image (**a**), on the map of K^{trans} (**b**) and on the diffusion-weighted image obtained with b of 800 s/mm^2 (**c**) in the same anatomic location. Bottom: user-defined parotid contours overlaid on the axial T2-weighted image (**d**) and on the corresponding map of K^{trans} (**e**) and diffusion-weighted image obtained with b of 800 s/mm^2 (**f**)

for each b value and its variation at increasing b was modeled using the following bi-exponential function by a nonlinear constrained minimization algorithm [16]: $S_b / S_0 = (1-f) \cdot e^{-b \cdot D} + f \cdot e^{-b \cdot (D+D^*)}$ where S_b is the signal intensity with diffusion weighting b, S_0 is the signal intensity for a b value of 0 s/mm^2, f is the fractional volume of capillary blood, D_t is the tissue diffusion coefficient (in mm^2/s), and D* is the perfusion-related diffusion coefficient (in mm^2/s).

As described elsewhere [20], a 'two step' fitting method was implemented to avoid overfitting: firstly the D_t value was derived from data at b values of 300, 500 and 800 s/mm^2 using a mono-exponential fit; secondly fixing D_t at the value estimated above, S0, D*, and f were determined according to Eq.1. To avoid the risk of suboptimal solutions, one hundred simultaneous optimization processes were launched for each fit, starting from randomly chosen initial values of parameters between fixed bounds. The residual sum of squares value of each optimization process was recorded and the minimum value was used to assess the best solution for the parameters.

The conventional ADC was also derived from data at b values of 0, 500 and 800 s/mm^2, using a mono-exponential model [15].

Calculation of the DCE-MRI parameters

The DCE-MRI data were analyzed using a commercial software package (GenIQ General, GE Advanced Workstation, Palo Alto, CA). The pharmacokinetic analysis was performed based on the Toft model: the quantitative parameters K^{trans}, the transfer constant between plasma and the extravascular extracellular space (EES), K_{ep}, the transfer constant between EES and plasma and v_e, the fractional volume of EES were calculated [14]. A semi-quantitative parameter, the initial area under gadolinium concentration curve or IAUGC (calculated from the bolus arrival to the first 90 s) was also derived. The median of each parameter, computed from the distribution of the voxel-level values within the entire gland, was used for statistical purposes.

Statistics

The change in parotid volume was estimated as the percent volume reduction at both the 10th fraction of RT (ΔVol_{10fr}) and the 8th week after the end of IMRT (ΔVol_{post}).

The Saphiro-Wilk test was used to test the normality of the data. As some of the variables (about 49%) were not normally distributed, non-parametric analyses were performed, as they are based on distribution-free methods. The Wilcoxon test for paired samples was used to assess whether changes over time were significant. Correlations among volumetric changes at the time points and various patient-, treatment- and imaging-related features were investigated at univariate analysis with the Spearman test. We did not apply any adjustment to the *p*-values for multiple comparisons because we have only tested multiple variables within a single group and not between groups. A p level < 0.05 was considered to indicate statistical significance. SPSS software (SPSS version 21, SPSS Inc., Chicago, IL, USA) was used for the statistical analyses.

Results

Forty patients/80 parotids were accrued and analyzed. Selected patient and tumor characteristics are summarized in Table 1. All patients received the planned radiotherapy dose and all but 7 patients received concomitant chemotherapy as well. The average (±SD) patient weight loss at the 10th fraction and at the end of RT were 2.0 ± 2.7 Kg (− 2.7% ± 3.8%) and 6.8 ± 4.4 Kg (9.0% ± 5.1%), respectively. At the 10th fraction, the parotid volume decreased from a mean (±SD) value of 32.3 (±9.4) cm^3 to 26.7 (±9.0) cm^3, with a mean ΔVol_{10fr} of 18.2% (±10.7%). Eight weeks after RT, it decreased to 22.7 (±8.9) cm^3, with a mean ΔVol_{post} of 31.3% (±15.8); all but two patients were not evaluated at this time point as they died of progressive

Table 1 Selected patient and tumor characteristics

Characteristic	Parameter
Patient number	40 (80 parotids)
Sex (M/F)	30/10
Age (years)	
Mean (range)	65.5 (46–81)
Primary tumor site	
Tonsil	26 (65%)
Base of Tongue	14 (35%)
T stage	
T1	4 (10%)
T2	11 (27.5%)
T3	7 (17.5%)
T4	15 (37.5%)
T4a	3 (7.5%)
N stage	
N0	4 (10%)
N1	4 (10%)
N2a	2 (5%)
N2b	15 (37.5%)
N2c	14 (35%)
N3	1 (2.5%)
Parotid Radiation Dose	
D_{mean} (Gy)	35.8 ± 8.9
V_{30}(%)	53.6 ± 19.9

Abbreviations: D_{mean} Planned mean dose to the parotid gland, $V_{30}(\%)$ Percentage of parotid volume receiving a dose ≥30 Gy disease. No correlation was found between $\Delta Vol_{10fr}/\Delta Vol_{post}$ and the patient weight loss at the 10th fraction and at the end of RT.

At baseline, the average (±SD) values for K^{trans}, K_{ep}, v_e and IAUGC were 0.546 (±0.290) min^{-1}, 2.728 (±1.146) min^{-1}, 0.178 (± 0.061) (fractional units) and 0.287 (±0.095) (arbitrary units), respectively. Summary statistics of the diffusion parameters and their variations during treatment are shown in Table 2. Only the changes of ADC and D_t over time were significant ($p < 0.001$ for both).

Correlation between parotid shrinkage and variables at baseline

Table 3 reports the relationships between percent parotid shrinkage and various covariates at baseline. A significant correlation was found between ΔVol_{10fr} and initial parotid volume, patient weight, BMI, D_{mean} and V_{30}. Scatter plots of parotid shrinkage versus D_{mean} and $V_{30}(\%)$ are depicted in Fig. 2. Among image-related parameters, only K_{ep} was weakly associated to parotid shrinkage (Rho = 0.239, $p = 0.038$) while K^{trans} showed only a trend towards statistical significance (Rho = 0.210, $p = 0.069$).

Interestingly, none of the selected patient- and treatment-related variables was correlated to percent shrinkage at 8 weeks after treatment completion while several DCE-MRI-related parameters showed a moderate correlation at this time point, with stronger evidence (smaller significant p values) than at the 10th fraction (Table 3).

Correlation between parotid shrinkage and diffusion parameters during treatment

The correlation between parotid shrinkage and DWI-IVIM parameters at the 10th fraction are reported in Table 4. ΔVol_{10fr} significantly correlated with D_t and the percent change of both ADC and D_t between baseline and the 10th fraction.

Table 2 Summary statistics of the diffusion parameters and their variations during treatment

Parameter[a]	before RT	at the 10th	Variation from baseline (%)	p
ADC (10^{-3} mm^2/s)	1.275 ± 0.158	1.434 ± 0.205	13.6 ± 18.2	**< 0.0001**
D_t (10^{-3} mm^2/s)	0.949 ± 0.153	1.072 ± 0.184	14.5 ± 20.8	**< 0.0001**
f(%)	15.8 ± 4.7	16.3 ± 5.1	8.8 ± 41.1	0.420
D* (10^{-3} mm^2/s)	28.4 ± 18.1	31.7 ± 2.1	57.9 ± 156.5	0.185
D* × f (10^{-3} mm^2/s)	424 ± 305	466 ± 227	51.0 ± 129.1	0.076

[a]Average ± standard deviation. P values refer to Wilcoxon test. Statistically significant *p*-values are bold. Abbreviations: *ADC* Apparent diffusion coefficient, *D_t* Tissue diffusion coefficient, *D** Perfusion-related diffusion coefficient, *f(%)* Perfusion fraction, *D* × f* Product of D* by *f*

Table 3 Results of Spearman's correlation tests between parotid shrinkage and imaging/ anthropometric parameters at baseline

Variable at baseline	$\Delta Vol_{10fr}(\%)$		$\Delta Vol_{post}(\%)$	
	Spearman's Rho	p-value	Spearman's Rho	p-value
ADC	− 0.185	0.100	−0.010	0.932
D_t	−0.099	0.385	−0.061	0.609
f	−0.056	0.620	−0.002	0.986
D*	−0.019	0.865	−0.188	0.109
D* × f	−0.007	0.950	−0.167	0.154
K^{trans}	0.210	0.069	0.434	**< 0.001**
K_{ep}	0.239	**0.038**	0.349	**0.003**
v_e	0.025	0.832	0.174	0.143
IAUGC	0.139	0.231	0.375	**0.001**
Parotid volume	−0.242	**0.031**	−0.056	0.636
Age	−0.108	0.341	0.045	0.702
Weight	−0.396	**< 0.001**	−0.135	0.253
BMI	−0.368	**0.001**	−0.127	0.281
D_{mean}(Gy)	0.226	**0.044**	−0.007	0.951
V_{30}(%)	0.266	**0.017**	0.086	0.468

Statistically significant p-values are bold. Abbreviations: *ΔVol_{10fr}* Parotid shrinkage(%) at the 10th fraction, *ΔVol_{post}* Parotid shrinkage(%) 8 weeks after RT, *ADC* Apparent diffusion coefficient, *D_t* Tissue diffusion coefficient, *D** Perfusion-related diffusion coefficient, *f(%)* Perfusion fraction, *D* × f* Product of D* by *f*, *ΔADC* ADC variation (%) relative to the pretreatment value (analogously for the other imaging variables), *K^{trans}* Transfer constant between plasma and EES (extravascular extracellular space), *K_{ep}* Transfer constant between EES and plasma, *v_e* Fractional volume of EES, *IAUGC* Initial area under gadolinium concentration curve, *BMI* Body mass index, *D_{mean}* Planned mean dose to the parotid gland, *$V_{30}(\%)$* Percentage of parotid volume receiving a dose ≥30 Gy

A significant relationship was found between the final parotid shrinkage ΔVol_{post} and D_t, f and the changes in D_t and f. Moreover, ΔVol_{post} was strongly related to ΔVol_{10fr} (Rho = 0.471, $p < 0.001$).

Finally, changes in ADC/D_t were significantly related to D_{mean} ($p = 0.001$, $p = 0.011$, respectively) and $V_{30}(\%)$ (p < 0.001, $p = 0.001$, respectively) (Additional file 1: Table S3).

Illustrative cases

Two illustrative cases are presented in Figs. 3 and 4. In Fig. 3, the case of a 68-year-old man affected by a tonsil carcinoma is shown, whose initial weight and BMI were 65.5 Kg and 21.1 (Kg/m^2), respectively. The three serial MR scans documented a substantial gland shrinkage, while the corresponding perfusion maps indicated well perfused parotids at baseline (the average K^{trans} and IAUGC of parotids were 0.868 min^{-1} and 0.404, respectively). Curves of DW-signal attenuation of parotids at baseline and during RT demonstrated a noticeable increase in tissue water diffusivity, suggesting a considerable decrease in cell density as a consequence of the radiation damage (the average increase in ADC and D_t of parotids

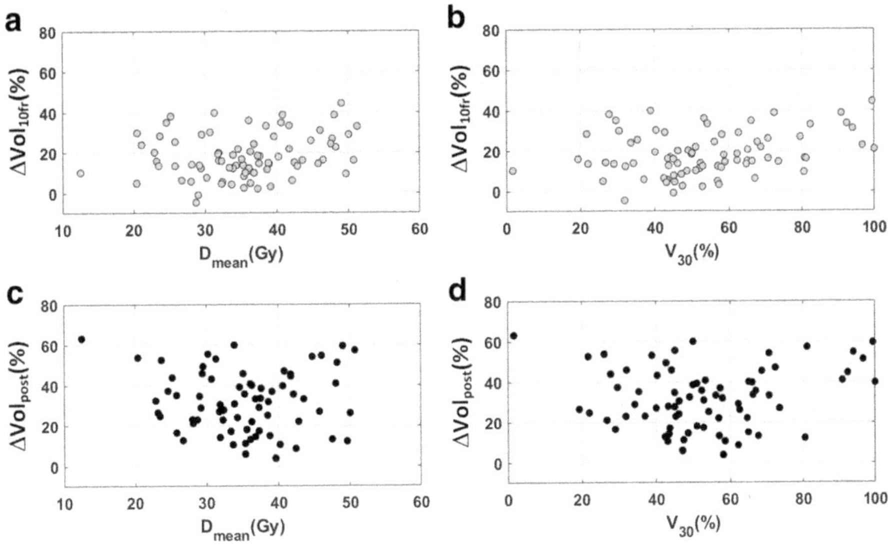

Fig. 2 Scatter plots of parotid shrinkage(%) at the 10th fraction (ΔVol_{10fr}) versus planned mean dose to the parotid gland D_{mean} (**a**) and percentage of parotid volume receiving a dose ≥30 Gy, $V_{30}(\%)$ (**b**). Analogously, scatter plots of parotid shrinkage(%) 8 weeks after RT (ΔVol_{post}) versus D_{mean} (**c**) and $V_{30}(\%)$ (**d**)

were 17% and 33%, respectively). In Fig. 4, the case of a 48-year-old man affected by a base of the tongue carcinoma is illustrated, whose initial weight and BMI were 97 Kg and 28.3 (Kg/m^2), respectively. The three serial MR scans showed only a small final parotid shrinkage, while the perfusion maps indicated moderately perfused glands at baseline (the average K^{trans} and IAUGC of parotids were 0.276 min^{-1} and 0.191, respectively). Correspondingly, a slight difference was observed between the rates at which the DW-signal attenuation of the parotids decreases during RT, suggesting a limited radiation-induced decrease in cell density (the average increase in ADC and D_t of parotids were 9% and 6%, respectively).

Table 4 Results of Spearman's correlation tests between parotid shrinkage and diffusion parameters during treatment

Variable at the 10th fraction	$\Delta Vol_{10fr}(\%)$		$\Delta Vol_{post}(\%)$	
	Spearman's Rho	*p*-value	Spearman's Rho	*p*-value
ADC	0.121	0.285	0.103	0.383
D_t	0.286	**0.011**	0.289	**0.013**
F	−0.057	0.614	−0.232	**0.047**
D*	−0.114	0.314	0.122	0.299
D* × *f*	−0.153	0.176	−0.013	0.910
ΔADC	0.228	**0.042**	0.173	0.141
ΔD_t	0.319	**0.004**	0.372	**0.001**
Δ*f*	0.022	0.844	−0.242	**0.038**
ΔD*	−0.117	0.301	0.192	0.101
ΔD* × *f*	−0.119	0.293	0.096	0.416

Statistically significant p-values are bold. Abbreviations: ΔVol_{10fr} Parotid shrinkage(%) at the 10th fraction, ΔVol_{post} Parotid shrinkage(%) 8 weeks after RT, *ADC* Apparent diffusion coefficient, D_t Tissue diffusion coefficient, *D** Perfusion-related diffusion coefficient, *f(%)* Perfusion fraction, *D* × f* Product of D* by *f*, *ΔADC* ADC variation (%) relative to the pretreatment value (analogously for the other imaging variables)

Discussion

Image-based parameters evaluating early changes of irradiated organs have shown the potential to guide both treatment optimization and personalization, as supported by the increasing number of data published in the last few years [5, 21–26]. In the present study we investigated whether either IVIM-DWI or DCE-MRI can provide quantitative indices with radiobiological relevance, as tissue cellular density and vascular perfusion, to timely detect and predict parotid gland shrinkage during/after (chemo)radiotherapy for oropharyngeal cancer. In order to maximize the potential benefits of adaptive re-planning for those patients who undergo significant parotid shrinkage, early evaluation of radiation-induced parotid gland modifications, possibly during the first 2 weeks of treatment [8, 27], is advised.

Anatomical change of parotid glands during radiotherapy may have dosimetric as well as clinical implications. The former is related to the higher dose received during treatment by the glands that show the larger variations [7, 8]; the latter to some extent that early anatomical modifications of parotids are associated with a reduction in salivary output, both acute and late [4, 26–28]. However, further investigation is underway to corroborate this point.

We found mean parotid shrinkages, ΔVol_{10fr} and ΔVol_{post}, in satisfactory agreement with those reported by other investigators [7, 8]. Interestingly, we observed relatively similar values for both ADC and D_t across patients at baseline, suggesting that the glandular tissue is

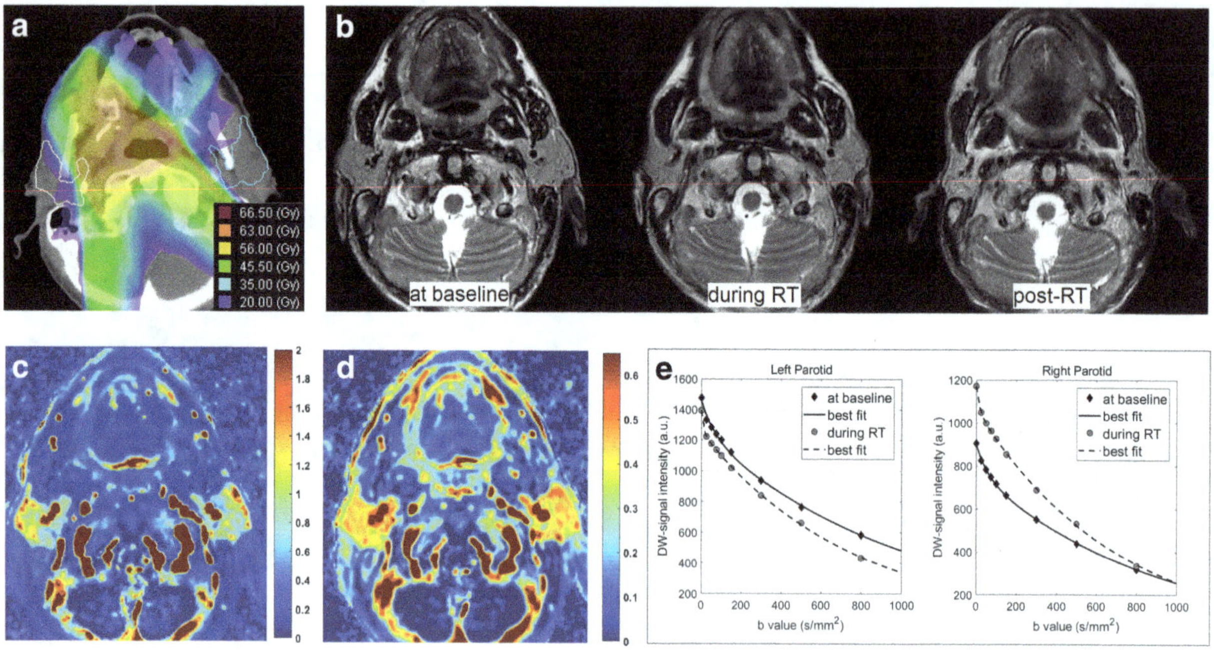

Fig. 3 A 68-year-old man affected by a tonsil carcinoma: dose distribution overlaid on the central section of the parotid glands on axial CT (**a**); T2-weighted images before, at 2 weeks of radiotherapy and 8 weeks after radiotherapy (**b**) documenting a substantial gland shrinkage; the corresponding maps of K^{trans} in min^{-1} (**c**) and IAUGC in a.u. (**d**), at baseline, indicating well perfused parotids. Curves of DW-signal attenuation of parotids at baseline and during RT (**e**): the modification of the DW-signal attenuation curves during RT documents a noticeable increase in tissue water diffusivity, suggesting a considerable decrease in cell density as a consequence of the radiation damage

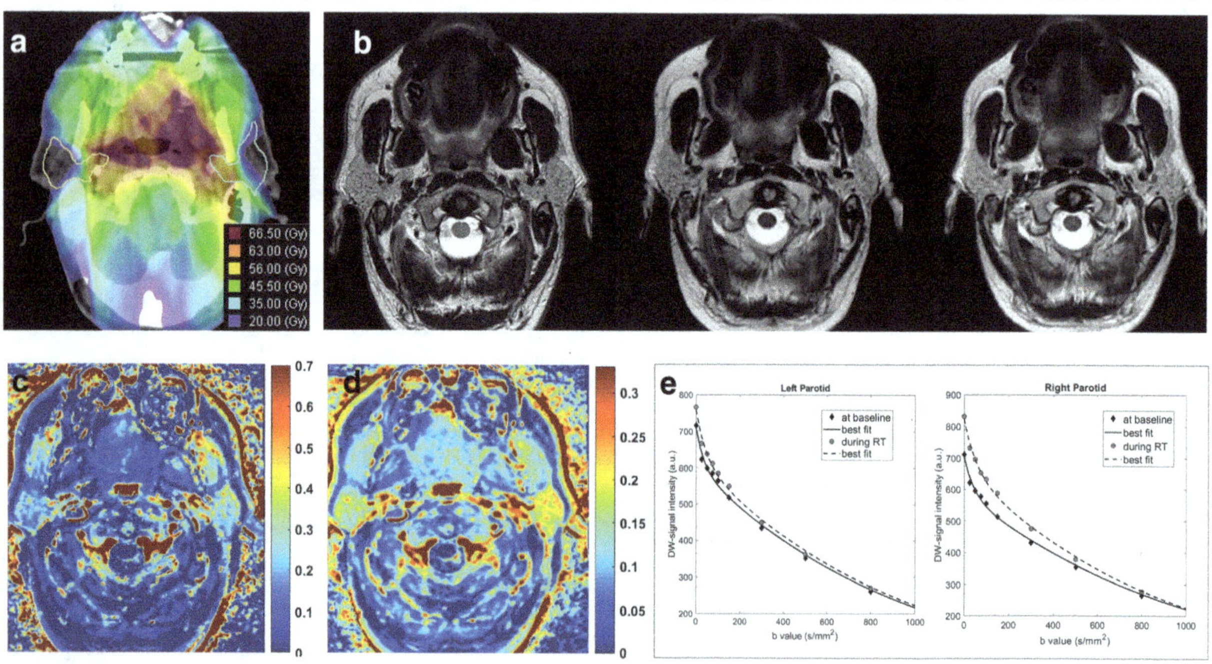

Fig. 4 A 48-year-old man affected by a base of the tongue carcinoma: dose distribution overlaid on the central section of the parotid glands on axial CT (**a**); T2-weighted images before, at 2 weeks of radiotherapy and 8 weeks after radiotherapy (**b**) showing a small final parotid shrinkage; the corresponding maps of K^{trans} in min^{-1} (**c**) and IAUGC in a.u. (**d**), at baseline, indicating moderately perfused glands. Correspondingly, a slight difference was observed between the rates at which the DW-signal attenuation of the parotids decreases during RT (**e**)

remarkably similar in diffusion coefficients in different patients, even if a small but statistically significant positive correlation was found between ADC and age (Additional file 1: Table S1 and Additional file 2: Figure S1). Such limited variability may have contributed to the lack of association between these parameters and parotid shrinkage, both during and after RT. Conversely, DCE-MRI features were highly different across patients at baseline, suggesting highly individual perfusion patterns. Moreover, the inverse relationship between BMI and DCE-MRI parameters (Additional file 1: Table S1 and Additional file 2: Figure S2) suggests a reduced proportional volume of vascular tissue in overweight patients. We also found that hypo-perfused parotids tend to show reduced ADC and D_t values, thus a reduced water molecule mobility (Additional file 1: Table S2). One may argue that this is indirectly related to the fact that the adipose tissue limits the mobility of water molecules as shown by Chang et al. [29], though no direct correlation was found between diffusion and BMI in our data. This suggests that the diffusion parameters, especially ADC and D_t, are not just a simple expression of cellularity but seem to be dependent upon the characteristics of the glandular tissue (i.e. the proportion of glandular versus fatty components). To this end, we show that both diffusion and perfusion imaging may be useful to individually assess/monitor structural and functional properties of parotids.

Selected DCE-MRI parameters, such as K^{trans} and K_{ep}, showed potential to detect parotid shrinkage both during and early after IMRT: patients with more vascularized parotid glands exhibited a greater volume reduction, possibly due to a higher tissue oxygenation and thus an increased radiosensitivity [5] (see also Figs. 3 and 4). On the other hand, Lee et al. [30] reported an inverse association between parotid shrinkage 3 months after RT for nasopharyngeal cancer and plasma volume derived from DCE-MRI. According to the Authors a higher plasma volume translates into a better perfusion thought it remains unclear how this would lead to an improved protection to radiation damage.

A previous study of Houweling et al. [21] also investigated the role of MRI to quantify the early radiation-induced modifications of the salivary glands in a population of patients with oropharyngeal carcinoma. The Authors documented a strong correlation between the increase in T2-weighted signal from baseline to 6 weeks after RT and the planned mean dose to parotid and submandibular glands. After treatment, they also found a decrease in k_{ep} and an increase in v_e which have been explained by a presumed rise in water content due to vascular edema. Similarly, we found an increase in ADC and D_t, suggesting a larger extra-cellular/extra-vascular space allowing a higher tissue water mobility.

Initial BMI and patient weight were significantly correlated to ΔVol_{10fr} consistent with a greater fatty component resulting in a smaller gland shrinkage, suggesting that in the first few weeks of treatment the glandular tissue is targeted preferentially over the adipose one [22]. The inverse relationship between parotid volume at baseline and ΔVol_{10fr} likely reflects the strong positive correlation between the PG volume at baseline and both BMI and patient weight.

Parotid shrinkage at 2 weeks was found to be weakly related to both PG D_{mean} and V_{30}, suggesting that the radiation-induced loss of acinar cells is a dose-dependent effect as previously shown [8, 23]. Accordingly, we found D_{mean} and V_{30} to be correlated to changes of ADC/D_t during the first 2 weeks of treatment that are presumed to reflect variations of cellular density (Additional file 1: Table S3). Moreover, at 2 weeks, the perfusion-free diffusion coefficient, D_t, was found to be more predictive of PG shrinkage than ADC at either checkpoint (Table 4) suggesting a higher sensitivity in variations in cellular microstructure/depopulation than ADC [23] which is susceptible to the effects of both perfusion and diffusion [15]. The present data are also in agreement with the association between parotid shrinkage and parotid density reduction (acinar cell depopulation and relative increase in fibrofatty tissue) observed in CT-based studies [22].

Similarly to others [9], we could not find an association between parotid shrinkage after radiotherapy and both D_{mean} and V_{30}, while a correlation was present after the first 2 weeks of treatment. There are multiple possible explanations for this change in predictive power of dose: progressive deterioration of the dose distribution throughout the course of treatment; delivery of a threshold dose above which parotid shrinkage is minimal; other confounding factors, such as weight loss or variability in parotid gland composition [7–9, 21, 27]. Conversely, earlier during treatment, shrinkage is likely to reflect more closely the depopulation of acinar cells, and thus, dose may play a more prominent and detectable role [8, 27]. Moreover, the limited variance in dose values and the small sample size may have contributed to mask an effect of dose on parotid shrinkage after treatment.

It is unclear why ΔVol_{post} was related to in-treatment f values and changes in f, as no significant association was observed between initial perfusion-related diffusion coefficients (D^*, f and $D^* \times f$) and any DCE-MRI perfusion parameters. However, contradictory results on the ability of IVIM-DWI in assessing tissue perfusion have been reported in the literature to date [17]. This may reflect either the presence of confounding sources of incoherent motion in biological tissues and/or the difficulty to obtain an optimal image quality with minimal motion and susceptibility artifacts, particularly in patients with head and neck cancer [15, 17].

The study has some limitations. We extracted the median value of the signal from all the voxels within the entire gland as opposed to the punctual 'local' signal from discrete sub-regions of the PG. We also did not investigate the ability of MRI to detect a different local effect of radiation dose, as suggested by others [21]; this may help to identify sub-regions with different radiosensitivity within the gland [31]. On the other hand, we believe that our approach allows the extraction of data less susceptible to motion artifacts and image co-registration issues and ultimately more consistent. Future investigations from this on-going study will include both patient-reported xerostomia as an endpoint as soon as clinical data mature and a multivariable model on selected quantitative image analyses, in addition to patient- and treatment-related covariates.

Conclusions

Both IVIM-DWI and DCE-MRI can help to detect early (during treatment) as well as late (after treatment completion) PG shrinkage. Moreover, they shed light upon the complex correlation between the volumetric change of PG and patient–/treatment-related variables by assessing individual microcapillary perfusion and tissue diffusivity.

Abbreviations

ADC: Apparent diffusion coefficient; BMI: Body mass index; $D^* \times f$: Product of D^* by f; D^*: Perfusion-related diffusion coefficient; D_{mean}: Planned mean dose to the parotid gland; D_t: Tissue diffusion coefficient; EES: Extravascular extracellular space; f(%): Perfusion fraction; IAUGC: Initial area under gadolinium concentration curve; IMRT: Intensity modulated radiotherapy; K_{ep}: Transfer constant between EES and plasma; K^{trans}: Transfer constant between plasma and EES; PG: Parotid gland; V_{30}(%): Percentage of parotid volume receiving a dose ≥30 Gy; v_e: Fractional volume of EES; ΔVol_{10fr}: Parotid shrinkage(%) at the 10th fraction; ΔADC: ADC variation (%) relative to the pretreatment value (analogously for the other imaging variables); ΔVol_{post}: Parotid shrinkage(%) 8 weeks after RT

Acknowledgements

The authors are indebted to Michele Farella and to Pierfrancesco Rinaldi for their continued technical assistance.

Funding

This work was supported by the Italian Association for Cancer Research (AIRC, project No.17028).

Authors' contributions

SM and GS conceived of the study and drafted the manuscript. LM and AF contributed to the patient enrollment and data gathering. AV was responsible for the MRI scans and participated in the design of the study. FD carried out the image delineation and participated in the image analysis. FS carried out the responsibility of collecting and maintaining the data. IT performed the statistical analysis. All authors read and approved the final manuscript.

Competing interests

The authors declare that they have no competing interests.

Author details

[1]Medical Physics Laboratory, IRCCS Regina Elena National Cancer Institute, Via Elio Chianesi 53, 00144 Rome, Italy. [2]Department of Radiotherapy, IRCCS Regina Elena National Cancer Institute, Via Elio Chianesi 53, 00144 Rome, Italy. [3]Radiology and Diagnostic Imaging Department, IRCCS Regina Elena National Cancer Institute, Via Elio Chianesi 53, 00144 Rome, Italy. [4]Department of Biomedicine and Prevention, University of Rome "Tor Vergata", Viale Oxford 81, 00133 Rome, Italy. [5]Biostatistics-Scientific Direction, IRCCS Regina Elena National Cancer Institute, Via Elio Chianesi 53, 00144 Rome, Italy.

References

1. Pfister DG, Ang KK, Brizel DM, Burtness BA, Cmelak AJ, Colevas AD, Dunphy F, Eisele DW, Gilbert J, Gillison ML, Haddad RI, Haughey BH, Hicks WL Jr, Hitchcock YJ, Kies MS, Lydiatt WM, Maghami E, Martins R, McCaffrey T, Mittal BB, Pinto HA, Ridge JA, Samant S, Sanguineti G, Schuller DE, Shah JP, Spencer S, Trotti A 3rd, Weber RS, Wolf GT, Worden F, National Comprehensive Concer Network. Head and neck cancers. J Natl Compr Cancer Netw. 2011;9:596–650.
2. Hawkins PG, Kadam AS, Jackson WC, Eisbruch A. Organ-sparing in radiotherapy for head-and-neck Cancer: improving quality of life. Semin Radiat Oncol. 2018;28:46–52.
3. Langendijk JA, Doornaert P, Verdonck-de Leeuw IM, Leemans CR, Aaronson NK, Slotman BJ. Impact of late treatment-related toxicity on quality of life among patients with head and neck cancer treated with radiotherapy. J Clin Oncol. 2008;26:3770–6.
4. van Dijk LV, Brouwer CL, van der Laan HP, Burgerhof JGM, Langendijk JA, Steenbakkers RJHM, Sijtsema NM. Geometric image biomarker changes of the parotid gland are associated with late Xerostomia. Int J Radiat Oncol Biol Phys. 2017;99:1101–10.
5. van Dijk LV, Brouwer CL, van der Schaaf A, Burgerhof JGM, Beukinga RJ, Langendijk JA, Sijtsema NM, Steenbakkers RJHM. CT image biomarkers to improve patient-specific prediction of radiation-induced xerostomia and sticky saliva. Radiother Oncol. 2017;122:185–91.
6. Meirovitz A, Murdoch-Kinch CA, Schipper M, Pan C, Eisbruch A. Grading xerostomia by physicians or by patients after intensity-modulated radiotherapy of head-and-neck cancer. Int J Radiat Oncol Biol Phys. 2006;66:445–53.
7. Barker JL Jr, Garden AS, Ang KK, O'Daniel JC, Wang H, Court LE, Morrison WH, Rosenthal DI, Chao KS, Tucker SL, Mohan R, Dong L. Quantification of volumetric and geometric changes occurring during fractionated radiotherapy for head-and-neck cancer using an integrated CT/linear accelerator system. Int J Radiat Oncol Biol Phys. 2004;59:960–70.
8. Zhang Y, Lin C, Wu J, Jiang X, Lee SWY, Tam SY, Wu VWC. A longitudinal evaluation of early anatomical changes of parotid gland in intensity modulated radiotherapy of nasopharyngeal carcinoma patients with parapharyngeal space involvement. J Med Radiat Sci. 2017;64:188–94.
9. Sanguineti G, Ricchetti F, Thomas O, Wu B, McNutt T. Pattern and predictors of volumetric change of parotid glands during intensity modulated radiotherapy. Br J Radiol. 2013;86:20130363.
10. Wang W, Lang J. Strategies to optimize radiotherapy based on biological responses of tumor and normal tissue. Exp Ther Med. 2012;4:175–80.
11. Caudell JJ, Torres-Roca JF, Gillies RJ, Enderling H, Kim S, Rishi A, Moros EG, Harrison LB. The future of personalised radiotherapy for head and neck cancer. Lancet Oncol. 2017;18:e266–73.
12. Wong KH, Panek R, Bhide SA, Nutting CM, Harrington KJ, Newbold KL. The emerging potential of magnetic resonance imaging in personalizing radiotherapy for head and neck cancer: an oncologist's perspective. Br J Radiol. 2017;90:20160768.
13. Cao Y. The promise of dynamic contrast-enhanced imaging in radiation therapy. Semin Radiat Oncol. 2011;21:147–56.
14. Tofts PS, Brix G, Buckley DL, Evelhoch JL, Henderson E, Knopp MV, Larsson HB, Lee TY, Mayr NA, Parker GJ, Port RE, Taylor J, Weisskoff RM. Estimating kinetic parameters from dynamic contrast-enhanced T(1)-weighted MRI of a diffusable tracer: standardized quantities and symbols. J Magn Reson Imaging. 1999;10:223–32.
15. Taouli B, Beer AJ, Chenevert T, Collins D, Lehman C, Matos C, Padhani AR, Rosenkrantz AB, Shukla-Dave A, Sigmund E, Tanenbaum L, Thoeny H, Thomassin-Naggara I, Barbieri S, Corcuera-Solano I, Orton M, Partridge SC,

Koh DM. Diffusion-weighted imaging outside the brain: consensus statement from an ISMRM-sponsored workshop. J Magn Reson Imaging. 2016;44:521–40.

16. Le Bihan D, Breton E, Lallemand D, Aubin ML, Vignaud J, Laval-Jeantet M. Separation of diffusion and perfusion in intravoxel incoherent motion MR imaging. Radiology. 1988;168:497–505.
17. Federau C. Intravoxel incoherent motion MRI as a means to measure in vivo perfusion: a review of the evidence. NMR Biomed. 2017;30. https://doi.org/10.1002/nbm.3780 Epub 2017 Sep 8.
18. Sanguineti G, Gunn GB, Endres EJ, Chaljub G, Cheruvu P, Parker B. Patterns of locoregional failure after exclusive IMRT for oropharyngeal carcinoma. Int J Radiat Oncol Biol Phys. 2008;72:737–46.
19. Fedorov A, Beichel R, Kalpathy-Cramer J, Finet J, Fillion-Robin JC, Pujol S, Bauer C, Jennings D, Fennessy F, Sonka M, Buatti J, Aylward S, Miller JV, Pieper S, Kikinis R. 3D slicer as an image computing platform for the quantitative imaging network. Magn Reson Imaging. 2012;30:1323–41.
20. Marzi S, Piludu F, Vidiri A. Assessment of diffusion parameters by intravoxel incoherent motion MRI in head and neck squamous cell carcinoma. NMR Biomed. 2013;26:1806–14.
21. Houweling AC, Schakel T, van den Berg CA, Philippens ME, Roesink JM, Terhaard CH, Raaijmakers CP. MRI to quantify early radiation-induced changes in the salivary glands. Radiother Oncol. 2011;100:386–9.
22. Fiorino C, Rizzo G, Scalco E, Broggi S, Belli ML, Dell'Oca I, Dinapoli N, Ricchetti F, Rodriguez AM, Di Muzio N, Calandrino R, Sanguineti G, Valentini V, Cattaneo GM. Density variation of parotid glands during IMRT for head-neck cancer: correlation with treatment and anatomical parameters. Radiother Oncol. 2012;104:224–9.
23. Marzi S, Forina C, Marucci L, Giovinazzo G, Giordano C, Piludu F, Landoni V, Spriano G, Vidiri A. Early radiation-induced changes evaluated by intravoxel incoherent motion in the major salivary glands. J Magn Reson Imaging. 2015;41:974–82.
24. Joint Head and Neck Radiotherapy-MRI Development Cooperative. Dynamic contrast-enhanced MRI detects acute radiotherapy-induced alterations in mandibular microvasculature: prospective assessment of imaging biomarkers of normal tissue injury. Sci Rep. 2016;6:29864.
25. Zhou N, Chu C, Dou X, Li M, Liu S, Zhu L, Liu B, Guo T, Chen W, He J, Yan J, Zhou Z, Yang X, Liu T. Early evaluation of irradiated parotid glands with intravoxel incoherent motion MR imaging: correlation with dynamic contrast-enhanced MR imaging. BMC Cancer. 2016;16:865-016–2900-2.
26. Zhou N, Guo T, Zheng H, Pan X, Chu C, Dou X, Li M, Liu S, Zhu L, Liu B, Chen W, He J, Yan J, Zhou Z, Yang X. Apparent diffusion coefficient histogram analysis can evaluate radiation-induced parotid damage and predict late xerostomia degree in nasopharyngeal carcinoma. Oncotarget. 2017;8:70226–38.
27. Belli ML, Scalco E, Sanguineti G, Fiorino C, Broggi S, Dinapoli N, Ricchetti F, Valentini V, Rizzo G, Cattaneo GM. Early changes of parotid density and volume predict modifications at the end of therapy and intensity of acute xerostomia. Strahlenther Onkol. 2014;190:1001–7.
28. Teshima K, Murakami R, Tomitaka E, Nomura T, Toya R, Hiraki A, Nakayama H, Hirai T, Shinohara M, Oya N, Yamashita Y. Radiation-induced parotid gland changes in oral cancer patients: correlation between parotid volume and saliva production. Jpn J Clin Oncol. 2010;40:42–6.
29. Chang HC, Juan CJ, Chiu HC, Cheng CC, Chiu SC, Liu YJ, Chung HW, Hsu HH. Effects of gender, age, and body mass index on fat contents and apparent diffusion coefficients in healthy parotid glands: an MRI evaluation. Eur Radiol. 2014;24:2069–76.
30. Lee FK, King AD, Kam MK, Ma BB, Yeung DK. Radiation injury of the parotid glands during treatment for head and neck cancer: assessment using dynamic contrast-enhanced MR imaging. Radiat Res. 2011;175:291–6.
31. van Luijk P, Pringle S, Deasy JO, Moiseenko VV, Faber H, Hovan A, Baanstra M, van der Laan HP, Kierkels RG, van der Schaaf A, Witjes MJ, Schippers JM, Brandenburg S, Langendijk JA, Wu J, Coppes RP. Sparing the region of the salivary gland containing stem cells preserves saliva production after radiotherapy for head and neck cancer. Sci Transl Med. 2015;7:305ra147.

15

Predictive value of pediatric respiratory-induced diaphragm motion quantified using pre-treatment 4DCT and CBCTs

Sophie C. Huijskens*, Irma W. E. M. van Dijk, Jorrit Visser, Brian V. Balgobind, Coen R. N. Rasch, Tanja Alderliesten and Arjan Bel

Abstract

Background: In adults, a single pre-treatment four-dimensional CT (4D-CT) acquisition is often used to account for respiratory-induced target motion during radiotherapy. However, studies have indicated that a 4D-CT is not always representative for respiratory motion. Our aim was to investigate whether respiratory-induced diaphragm motion in children on a single pre-treatment 4DCT can accurately predict respiratory-induced diaphragm motion as observed on cone beam CTs (CBCTs).

Methods: Twelve patients (mean age 14.5 yrs.; range 8.6–17.9 yrs) were retrospectively included based on visibility of the diaphragm on abdominal or thoracic imaging data acquired during free breathing. A 4DCT for planning purposes and daily/weekly CBCTs (total 125; range 4–29 per patient) acquired prior to dose delivery were available. The amplitude, corresponding to the difference in position of the diaphragm in cranial-caudal direction in end-inspiration and end-expiration phases, was extracted from the 4DCT (A_{4DCT}). The amplitude in CBCTs (A_{CBCT}) was defined as displacement between averaged in- and expiration diaphragm positions on corresponding projection images, and the distribution of A_{CBCT} was compared to A_{4DCT} (one-sample t-test, significance level $p < 0.05$).

Results: Over all patients, the mean A_{4DCT} was 10.4 mm and the mean A_{CBCT} 11.6 mm. For 9/12 patients, A_{4DCT} differed significantly ($p < 0.05$) from A_{CBCT}. Differences > 3 mm were found in 69/125 CBCTs (55%), with A_{4DCT} mostly underestimating A_{CBCT}. For 7/12 patients, diaphragm positions differed significantly from the baseline position.

Conclusion: Respiratory-induced diaphragm motion determined on 4DCT does not accurately predict the daily respiratory-induced diaphragm motion observed on CBCTs, as the amplitude and baseline position differed statistically significantly in the majority of patients. Regular monitoring of respiratory motion during the treatment course using CBCTs could yield a higher accuracy when a daily adaptation to the actual breathing amplitude takes place.

Keywords: Respiratory-induced motion, Pediatric RT, IGRT, 4DCT

Background

Respiratory motion during radiotherapy may lead to uncertainties in radiation dose delivery, and accounting for it is challenging. Continuous efforts in the field have led to innovative methods to deal with respiratory motion, such as breath holding, beam gating or tracking, or online visualizing of respiratory motion (e.g., magnetic resonance (MR) guidance) [1]. These techniques increase treatment time and clinical workload, and often require patient training which might lead to additional patient distress and anxiety. Although children could also benefit from these techniques [2, 3], it is known that they experience radiotherapy already as a stressful procedure [4–6], and therefore the use of these techniques remains limited in pediatric radiotherapy.

Respiratory motion is more commonly accounted for by the use of an internal margin (IM) that encompasses the clinical target volume (CTV), defining an internal

* Correspondence: s.c.huijskens@amc.uva.nl
Department of Radiation Oncology, Cancer Center Amsterdam, Amsterdam UMC, University of Amsterdam, Office Z1-217, Meibergdreef 9, 1105, AZ, Amsterdam, The Netherlands

target volume (ITV) [7]. This leads to unfavourable large margins, thereby increasing dose to surrounding healthy tissues. The mid-ventilation based planning target volume (PTV) approach accounts for both respiratory motion and day-to-day geometrical variations and achieves smaller margins [8–10]. No matter which approach is used, in order to assess respiratory motion, a pre-treatment respiratory-correlated four-dimensional computed tomography (4DCT) is essential.

In adults, a single pre-treatment 4DCT is used extensively to assess respiratory motion [11–13]. Our previous study showed that respiratory-induced diaphragm motion throughout the treatment course was more stable in children than previously reported by others in adults [14]. This implies that a single measurement could be more representative in children than in adults and suggests that a pre-treatment 4DCT in children could be at least equally beneficial as it is in adults [14]. To our knowledge, only few institutes have clinically introduced 4DCT for pediatric radiotherapy planning purposes and reported on this [15–17]. Generally, the conclusion was that 4DCT is an effective tool to accurately determine respiratory-induced organ motion (e.g., liver, spleen, kidneys) for pediatric specific cases, providing the data on respiratory motion needed to define margins, thereby stressing the need for individualized margins [15–17]. However, studies on adult patients have also indicated that respiratory motion, as measured on 4DCT, is not always representative for respiratory motion during the subsequent treatment course [11–13, 18]. Therefore, a single pre-treatment measurement for planning purposes might be a misrepresentation and could lead to under- or overestimating respiratory motion, yielding insufficient target coverage or undesired dose to organs at risk (OARs) [19]. In previous pediatric studies, respiratory-induced organ motion was only measured within a single 4DCT per patient [15–17], without assessing how representative the 4DCT is for respiratory-induced motion during the treatment course. To assess the daily respiratory-induced motion during the treatment course in children, cone beam CT (CBCT) scans acquired for position verification can be used [14]. With increasing use of 4DCT in pediatric radiotherapy, assessment of the predictive value of the measurements on 4DCT is essential to take full advantage of this technique.

Therefore, the aim of this study was to investigate if respiratory-induced diaphragm motion during radiotherapy in children, as a surrogate for respiratory-induced abdominal motion, can be accurately predicted by a single measurement based on a pre-treatment 4DCT. We also analyzed possible time trends in respiratory-induced diaphragm motion over the complete treatment course. Finally, to investigate if measurements on CBCTs could be predictive for respiratory-induced diaphragm motion that continues post-acquisition (i.e., the actual respiratory motion during dose delivery), we quantified and compared respiratory-induced diaphragm motion on two CBCTs acquired within one treatment session with an interval of minutes.

Methods

Patient data

From November 2014 to December 2017, fourteen patients (mean age 14.5 years, range 8.6–17.9 years) had a 4DCT scan during free breathing for treatment planning purposes and multiple CBCT scans acquired for position verification during the treatment course. Patients were included when the complete diaphragm was visible on the 4DCT and CBCTs. Two of the fourteen eligible patients were excluded

Table 1 Patient characteristics

No.	Sex	Tumor type	Age at 4DCT (years)	Height (cm)	Weight (kg)	No. of CBCTs
1	M	Ewingsarcoma	10.7	137	28.0	7
2	F	Ewingsarcoma	16.3	162	66.5	8
3[a]	F	Ewingsarcoma	17.9	163	52.6	12
4[a]	M	Osteosarcoma	14.9	186	71.6	5
5[b]	F	Ewingsarcoma	12.5	151	70.0	29
6[b]	M	ERMS	16.1	182	57.6	19
7[b]	M	Ewingsarcoma	14.3	182	55.6	6
8	M	CCS	8.6	125	23.0	5
9	F	Non Hodgkin	17.1	178	86.0	11
10	F	Ewingsarcoma	14.8	153	57.0	7
11[b]	M	RMS prostate	16.7	186	64.0	4
12	M	Non-RMS	14.4	172	59.0	12

Abbreviations: *M* male, *F* female, *4DCT* four-dimensional computed tomography, *CBCT* cone beam CT, *(E)RMS* embryonal rhabdomyosarcoma, *CCS* clear cell sarcoma

[a]Patients had within multiple treatment sessions repetitive CBCTs (only the 1st and 2nd were included in the analysis)

[b]Patients had two CBCTs within one treatment session

from this retrospective study; one patient received general anaesthesia (GA) and the imaging data of another patient showed severe motion artefacts. Patient characteristics are listed in Table 1.

4DCT

The 4DCTs (LightSpeed RT16 system, General Electric Company, Waukesha WI, USA) were acquired during free breathing (using the Varian RPM system v1.7.3). The respiratory cycle was divided into ten phase bins, resulting in ten phase scans (slice thickness 2.5 mm). Velocity (Velocity, version 3.1, Varian Medical Systems, Palo Alto, CA, USA) was used to perform a two-step rigid registration. The end-inspiration phase scan (i.e., the 0% phase scan) was used as a reference and was registered to the other nine phase scans. In one patient (no. 7), the 90% phase scan served as the reference, due to motion artefacts on the 0% phase scan. For all other patients and phase scans, no (severe) motion artefacts were seen that could have hampered the registrations. The right diaphragm domes were matched manually in the cranial-caudal (CC) direction, using translations only. The obtained translations resulted in the excursion of the right diaphragm dome throughout the respiratory cycle in the CC direction. The difference between the most extreme translations, typically the 0% to the 50% or 60% phase scan, was defined as the amplitude (A_{4DCT}) (Fig. 1a).

CBCT

For each patient, CBCT scans during free breathing (Synergy, Elekta Oncology systems, Crawly, UK) for position verification were daily and/or weekly acquired according to a customized extended no-action level (eNAL) protocol [20], totalling 125 CBCT scans (range 4–29 per patient). Six of the 12 patients had multiple CBCTs within one treatment session (total 13, range 2–5, not included in the 125), depending on their treatment protocol (e.g., stereotactic or spinal cord irradiation), or in one case a second CBCT was necessary due to artefacts. These artefacts, however, still allowed sufficient number of useable projection images for evaluation of respiratory-induced diaphragm motion. For all CBCTs, a single projection was acquired in 180 ms and the energy was 120 kV, tube current 10 mA and 10 or 40 ms exposure time per projection. The circumferential rotation varied from 200 to 360 degrees and the acquisition time varied between 35 s and 120 s, resulting in a variation in number of projection images per CBCT (180 to 760).

The methodology to extract the respiratory-induced diaphragm motion has been described previously [14]. In short, for each CBCT, an adapted version of the Amsterdam Shroud (AS) method was used to create an AS image [21], allowing for manual selection of the projection images corresponding to the end-inspiration and end-expiration positions of the right diaphragm dome.

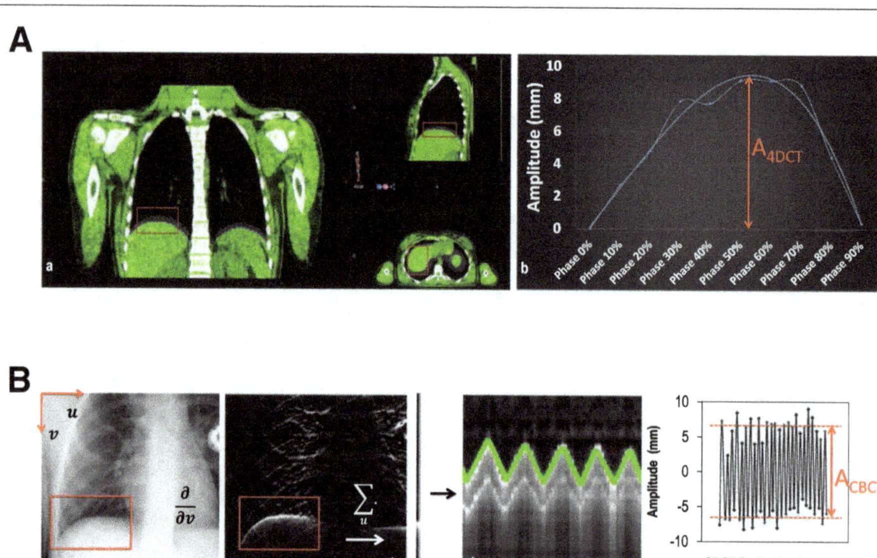

Fig. 1 **a** Left) Rigid registration of the cranial-caudal position of the right diaphragm (inside the red box) in all breathing phases. Right) The difference between the most extreme translations was defined as the amplitude (A_{4DCT}). **b** Amsterdam Shroud (AS) method to manually track the CC diaphragm position in CBCT projection images. a) Region of interest (red box). b) CC gradient filter applied and sum of all pixels creates a 1D image. C) This is repeated for all projection images, creating a 2D image. d) Detection of diaphragm positions in inhale and exhale breathing phases. e) Pixel coordinates translated to CC position. The amplitude was defined as the displacement between averaged end-inspiration and end-expiration diaphragm positions (A_{CBCT})

In each of those selected projection images, we then manually determined the CC position of the top of the right diaphragm dome. Pixel coordinates were corrected for the scanner geometry and translated relative to the patients' isocenter [22]. This resulted in a patient- and CBCT-dependent timeframe describing the CC position of the diaphragm in end-inspiration and end-expiration phases (peaks) over the course of CBCT acquisition. The amplitude was defined as the displacement between averaged end-inspiration and averaged end-expiration diaphragm positions (A_{CBCT}) (Fig. 1b).

Statistical analysis

In order to determine whether respiratory-induced diaphragm motion observed in a single pre-treatment 4DCT accurately predicted respiratory-induced diaphragm motion during the treatment course, we tested for each patient separately whether A_{CBCT} over all CBCTs differed from A_{4DCT} using a one-sample t-test (significance level $p < 0.05$). For each patient, we calculated the absolute differences between A_{4DCT} and each A_{CBCT}, and determined for which fractions the difference was larger than 3 mm (4DCT slice thickness is 2.5 mm).

To investigate possible time trends for each patient, we applied a linear regression analysis on A_{CBCT} over the course of treatment. We also calculated the inter-fractional variability of A_{CBCT} per patient (i.e., the SD over A_{CBCT}). The diaphragm position on the averaged pre-treatment 4DCT (this is the averaged scan, based on all phases of the 4DCT) was considered as a reference (i.e., baseline), for which a rigid registration on bony anatomy was taken into account. We then calculated for each patient separately shifts of the diaphragm position in CC direction (i.e., the average position of the diaphragm during one CBCT) over the course of treatment. We used a one-sample t-test to test whether diaphragm positions on CBCT significantly differed from the baseline diaphragm position on the averaged 4DCT.

Additionally, six patients received multiple CBCTs during one fraction. For above mentioned analysis, only the first CBCT was included in the analysis. To validate if respiratory-induced diaphragm motion measurements on CBCTs could be predictive for respiratory-induced motion that continues post-acquisition (i.e., the actual respiratory motion during dose delivery), we compared the amplitude measured on the first and second CBCT ($A_{CBCT(1)}$ to $A_{CBCT(2)}$; paired t-test, significance level $p < 0.05$). These are acquired within 4–10 min, which is a representative time interval between CBCT acquisition and start of dose delivery.

R Software package version 3.2.1. (R foundation for statistical Computing, Austria) was used for all statistical analysis.

Results

Over all patients, the mean A_{4DCT} was 10.4 mm (SD = 4.3 mm) and the mean A_{CBCT} was 11.6 mm (SD = 5.7 mm). For 9 out of 12 patients, A_{4DCT} differed statistically significantly ($p < 0.05$) from A_{CBCT} (Fig. 2). Underestimation of A_{4DCT} compared to A_{CBCT} was found in 76% of the measurements (95/125 CBCTs), and was observed in 11 out of 12 patients. Hence, overestimation was found in 24% of the measurements (30/125 CBCTs), and was observed in 3 out of 12 patients. Differences > 3 mm were found in 69 of the 125 CBCTs (55%).

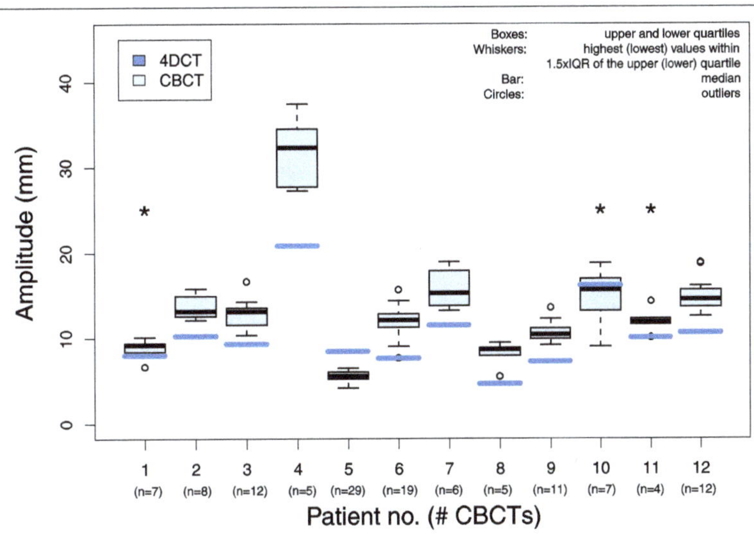

Fig. 2 Respiratory-induced diaphragm motion on 4DCT (blue solid lines) and CBCT data (boxplots) of 12 children during image-guided radiotherapy. Patients with * showed no significant differences (*p* > *0.05*)

For each patient, we plotted A_{CBCT} over time of the treatment course (Additional file 1: Figure S1) where day 0 is the day of 4DCT acquisition. We found that 8 of the 12 trend lines had a negative slope. Absolute slopes larger than 0.1 mm/day were observed in 4 patients with only few data points (4 to 6 points for patients 4, 7, 8, and 11). For the other patients, with more data points, we observed by both visual inspection and linear fits, no obvious time trend (absolute slopes ranged from 0.00–0.09 mm/day).

Overall, interfractional variability of A_{CBCT} was 2.2 mm (range 0.7–4.4 mm; individual values shown in Fig. 3). For 7 out of 12 patients, averaged diaphragm positions in CC direction observed on CBCTs differed statistically significantly (mean 7.4 mm, SD = 5.9 mm; $p < 0.05$) from the baseline diaphragm position as measured on the averaged 4DCT (Fig. 3).

Patients 3 and 4 had on multiple days additional CBCT scans. Patients 5, 6, 7, and 11 had only on one day an additional CBCT. The subsequent CBCTs were acquired within a time interval of 4–10 min. Over all six patients, $A_{CBCT(2)}$ was significantly different from $A_{CBCT(1)}$ (mean difference 2.9 mm, SD = 2.5 mm, $p = 0.002$) (Fig. 4). However, patient 4 (in Fig. 4 indicated by the green cross symbol) showed significant deviations from the group measurements. We performed a sensitivity analysis by

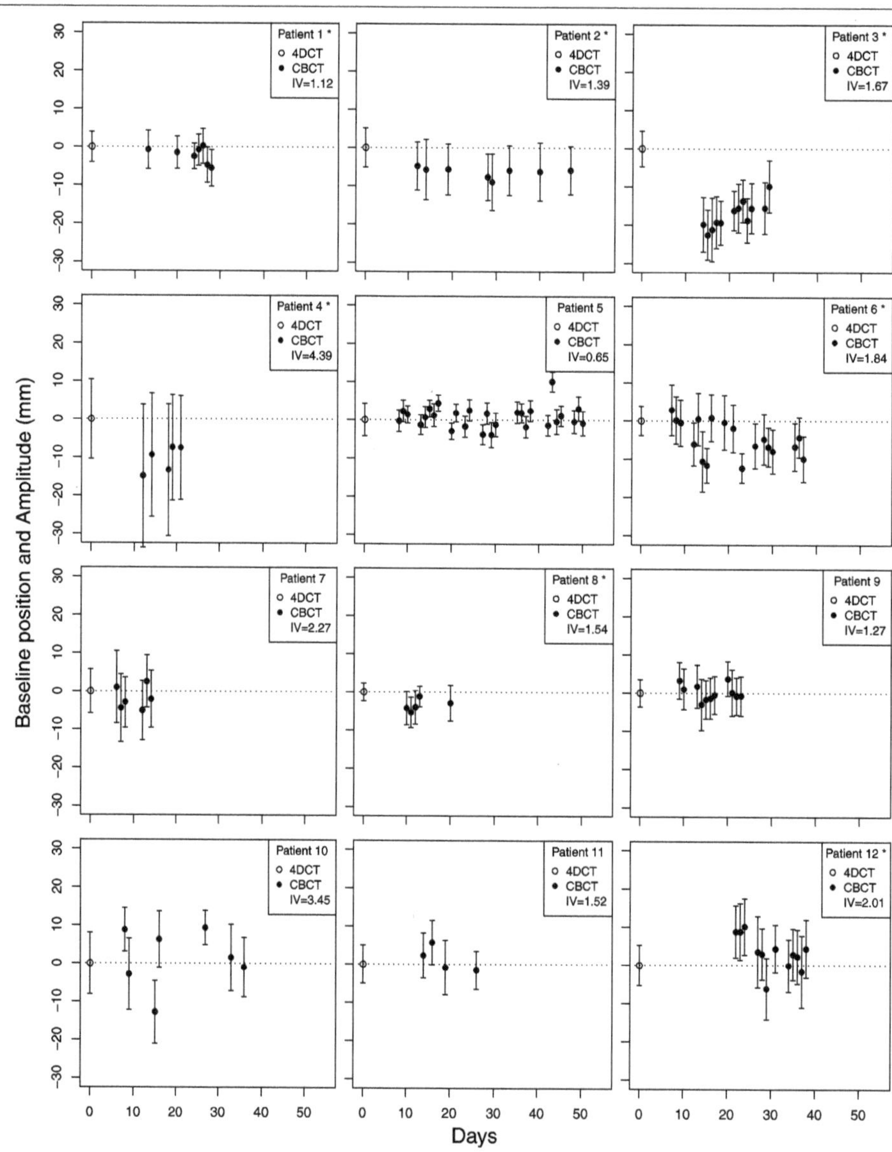

Fig. 3 Open dots and dashed lines represent the baseline diaphragm position on the planning 4DCT (averaged 4DCT). Black dots represent the average positions of the diaphragm on each CBCT. Whiskers represent measured end-inspiration and end-expiration positions on 4DCT and CBCTs for each patient plotted as function of days. Day 0 is the day of 4DCT acquisition (open dots), IV = interfractional variability, * indicates a significant difference from baseline ($p < 0.05$)

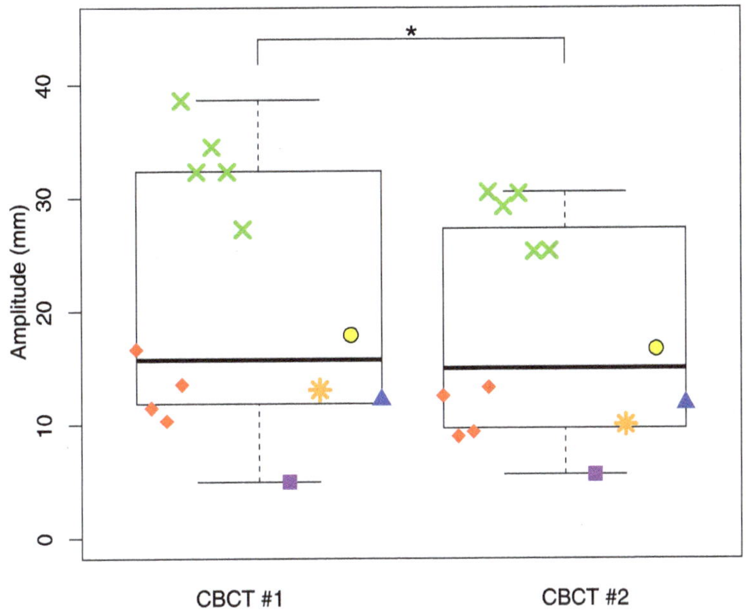

Fig. 4 Significant difference (indicated by *) between amplitudes measured on the first and second CBCT acquired within one treatment session. Each different color and symbol represent different patients

excluding this patient from the analysis. Although the average difference was now 1.7 mm (SD = 1.4 mm), $A_{BCT(2)}$ remained significantly different from $A_{CBCT(1)}$ ($p = 0.033$).

Discussion

In this study we investigated if respiratory-induced diaphragm motion in children during radiotherapy could be accurately predicted based on a 4DCT scan acquired prior to the start of radiotherapy. We compared the amplitude of the diaphragm displacement on 4DCT and daily/weekly CBCTs, enabling an encompassing analysis of pre-treatment respiratory-induced motion and during complete radiotherapy courses in children. This also enabled to investigate possible time trends and day-to-day variations. Our study showed that for the majority of patients (9/12 patients) respiratory-induced diaphragm motion on 4DCT differed significantly from measurements on CBCTs. Also, respiratory-induced diaphragm motion derived from CBCTs acquired within an interval of minutes was statistically significantly different. No obvious time trends in respiratory-induced diaphragm motion over the course of treatment were found, but significant baseline shifts of the diaphragm position were seen in 7/12 patients. These findings suggest that respiratory-induced diaphragm motion as measured on 4DCT was not representative for respiratory motion during the treatment course.

Although acquisition of 4DCT and CBCT scans differs, the amplitude was quantified in a similar way. During 4DCT acquisition, one breathing cycle is included per table position. This represents only a short time period, and amplitude between consecutive breathing cycles varies [14]. This uncertainty would be of a similar size (2.2 mm) as measured during the consecutive CBCTs. Additionally, a 4DCT scan is binned into 10 3D-breathing-phase scans corresponding to 10 phases of the respiratory cycle using phase binning, which already underestimates the diaphragm motion slightly [23]. For 4DCT, we quantified the amplitude as the maximal displacement between the most extreme diaphragm positions. On the other hand, CBCT acquisition time varied between 35 and 120 s and thus included more breathing cycles compared to the 4DCT. In the amplitude calculations for both types of CT scans, we averaged the diaphragm positions on the CBCT scan for in- and exhale phases and the difference between these averaged inhale and exhale diaphragm position defined the amplitude on CBCT. This is a slightly different approach as used by others [13, 24], who binned projection images corresponding to in- and exhale phases for (4D-) CBCT reconstructions, thereby averaging (e.g. blurring) the actual diaphragm positions on the reconstructed image. While different approaches have their advantages and limitations, for the comparison of 4DCT and CBCT data, in this study we chose to average the actual diaphragm positions at end-inspiration and end-expiration as measured on the corresponding projection image. This guarantees that all projection images are taken into account, and represents a realistic view of the actual motion happened.

Since we used respiratory-induced diaphragm motion as a surrogate for respiratory-induced abdominal motion, our outcomes cannot be directly applied for calculating safety margins. This was shown by Panandiker et al. who assessed intrafractional renal and diaphragm motion on free-breathing 4DCTs in 20 children, and concluded that measuring diaphragm motion alone does not reliably quantify renal motion [15]. Adult studies reported both positive and negative on using the diaphragm as a reliable surrogate for tumor or organ motion [25–27]. Two other pediatric studies have reported on intrafractional abdominal organ and tumor motion using 4DCT scans and concluded that 4DCT is an effective tool to accurately determine respiratory-induced organ motion for pediatric specific cases, leading to the desired more individualized treatment approach [16, 17]. However, in these studies, correlations of respiratory-induced organ motion with diaphragm motion were not investigated. Since respiratory-induced diaphragm motion does not necessarily correlate with tumor motion, using the diaphragm as a surrogate for abdominal and thoracic organ motion could induce some inaccuracies and uncertainties that need to be taken into account for treatment planning purposes.

A 4DCT involves a slightly higher imaging dose compared to a 3DCT and due to the ALARA principle (keeping doses as low as reasonably achievable) and previously reported radiation risks in children from CT scans [28–30], reluctance remains to use 4DCT in the pediatric population. It would be interesting to investigate the possible correlation between external thorax vertical displacement and the internal longitudinal diaphragm motion in children. In case of a strong and clear correlation, which was found for adults [31], the possibility of using an external reliable surrogate for internal respiratory-induced organ motion could decrease additional imaging dose. Since daily imaging dose adds to the total treatment dose, minimizing additional dose has to be carefully considered. Ultimately, the additional imaging dose in the pediatric population should be balanced with better treatment planning and delivery, in order to minimize dose to the healthy surrounding tissues. Especially, 4DMRI shows to be a promising tool for future image- and MR-guided pediatric radiotherapy, providing superior soft tissue contrast and higher resolution in CC direction, while avoiding ionizing radiation doses [32, 33].

The measured amplitude of respiratory-induced diaphragm motion on 4DCT was on average larger than the 6–17 mm range reported in literature [15, 16, 32]. However, patients in our cohort had an older age at treatment (mean 14.5 years, range 8.6–17.9 years) than those in other studies (ranges 1–20 years), and we excluded a patient treated under GA. Two studies divided their cohort into 2 groups based on age (> 9 years); when we compared our results to their older age groups ($n = 9$; mean 12.3 years [15] and $n = 18$; mean 15.3 years [32]), we saw a similar range of diaphragm motion. Although different ranges of diaphragm motion have been found for younger versus older children [15, 32], no clinically significant correlation has been found in studies investigating possible relationships between respiratory-induced diaphragm motion and age [14, 15]. The same holds for patients treated under GA; differences in amplitude of respiratory-induced diaphragm motion in patients treated with- or without GA were insignificant [14, 32].

Outcomes reported in adult studies that investigated the predictive value of measurements done in the 4DCT are not consistent; some studies found that measurements in 4DCT did not accurately predict respiratory-induced motion as seen on daily/weekly CBCT images [11–13, 18], while others concluded that respiratory-induced motion as measured in 4DCT was representative for the daily motion during the treatment course [24, 34]. These differences mostly depended on the tumor location, considering that abdominally located tumors could also be affected by abdominal processes, while thoracically located tumors are situated closer to the mediastinum. Interestingly, in those adult studies where respiratory-induced motion measured in the 4DCT was not representative, measurements overestimated daily respiratory-induced motion [11, 13], while in our pediatric cohort, the 4DCT mostly underestimated the daily respiratory-induced diaphragm motion. To account for respiratory-induced motion using such a single measurement could possibly lead to insufficient target coverage. Therefore, our results suggest monitoring of respiratory motion with CBCT on a more regular basis, and adapt treatment plans to the actual breathing amplitude when necessary.

For 7 out of 12 patients, the averaged CC positions of the diaphragm during the treatment course differed significantly from the baseline diaphragm position as measured on the 4DCT, introducing a systematic interfractional position variation. The patient number in the present study is low and some patients only had a few CBCTs. This means that measurements regarding baseline-shifts could have been random. However, these results emphasize the benefit and need for daily imaging and monitoring to enable baseline positioning correction.

Nevertheless, present and previous results also confirm that respiratory motion in children varies from day-to-day and even within consecutive breathing cycles [14, 17]. The measured respiratory-induced diaphragm motion on CBCTs acquired within a 4–10 min interval showed significant differences, meaning that the actual respiratory-induced motion during dose delivery can again be different than measured on the CBCT. However, this analysis was only based on a small number of repetitive CBCTs ($n = 13$) evaluated in six patients. Future studies should involve larger imaging datasets for evaluation of measurements on CBCTs for predicting respiratory-induced motion in children. In addition, as mentioned above, it would be interesting to asses respiratory-induced motion online using CBCTs acquired at, for example, the first three treatment fractions. This would enable to identify which patients deviate from their pre-treatment measurements on 4DCT and might benefit from an adaptive approach in order to maintain appropriate tumor dose coverage.

Conclusions

In conclusion, respiratory-induced diaphragm motion in children determined on 4DCT does not accurately predict the daily respiratory motion observed on CBCTs, as the amplitude differed statistically significantly in the majority of patients. Our results show the limitations of using a single pre-treatment 4DCT to take the patient-specific respiratory-induced diaphragm motion for treatment planning purposes into account. Regular monitoring of respiratory motion during the treatment course using CBCTs could yield a higher accuracy when a daily adaptation to the actual breathing amplitude takes place.

Abbreviations

3DCT: 3-Dimensional computed tomography; 4DCT: 4-Dimensional computed tomography; 4DMRI: 4-Dimensional magnetic resonance Imaging; A: Amplitude; ALARA: As low as reasonably achievable; AS: Amsterdam Shroud; CBCT: Cone beam computed tomography; CC: Cranial-caudal; CT: Computed tomography; CTV: Clinical target volume; eNAL: extended no-action level; GA: General anaesthesia; IM: Internal margin; ITV: Internal target volume; MR: Magnetic resonance; OAR: Organ at risk; PTV: Planning target volume; SD: Standard deviation

Funding

This work was supported by the Dutch Cancer Society (KWF Kankerbestrijding) project no. 2016-10113.

Conflict of interest statement

Dr. Alderliesten and Dr. Bel are project leaders of several Elekta-sponsored projects outside of this work. Elekta had no involvement in study design, data collection and analysis, or writing of the manuscript.

Authors' contributions

SCH has performed the data analysis and carried out writing of the manuscript. ID, JV, BVB, TA and AB contributed to the critical interpretation of the results. CRR and AB provided general supervision. All authors participated in the drafting and revising of the manuscript. All authors read and approved the final manuscript.

Competing interests

The authors declare that they have no competing interests.

References

1. Keall PJ, Mageras GS, Balter JM, Emery RS, Forster KM, Jiang SB, et al. The management of respiratory motion in radiation oncology report of AAPM task group 76. Med Phys. 2006;33:3874–900.
2. Claude L, Malet C, Pommier P, Thiesse P, Chabaud S, Carrie C. Active breathing control for Hodgkin's disease in childhood and adolescence: feasibility, advantages, and limits. Int J Radiat Oncol Biol Phys. 2007;67:1470–5.
3. Demoor-Goldschmidt C, Chiavassa S, Josset S, Mahe MA, Supiot S. Respiratory-gated bilateral pulmonary radiotherapy for Ewing's sarcoma and nephroblastoma in children and young adults: Dosimetric and clinical feasibility studies. Cancer Radiother. 2017;21:124–9.
4. Filin A, Treisman S, Peles Bortz A. Radiation therapy preparation by a multidisciplinary team for childhood cancer patients aged 31/2 to 6 years. J Pediatr Oncol Nurs. 2009;26:81–5.
5. Bucholtz JD. Comforting children during radiotherapy. Oncol Nurs Forum. 1994;21:987–94.
6. Tyc VL, Klosky JL, Kronenberg M, de Armendi AJ, Merchant TE. Children's distress in anticipation of radiation therapy procedures. Child Health Care. 2002;31:11–27.
7. Prescribing, recording and reporting photon beam therapy (supplement to ICRU report 50). ICRU report 62: International Commission on Radiation Units and Measurements; 1999. https://icru.org/home/reports/prescribing-recording-and-reporting-photon-beam-therapy-report-62.
8. Wolthaus JW, Schneider C, Sonke JJ, van Herk M, Belderbos JS, Rossi MM, et al. Mid-ventilation CT scan construction from four-dimensional respiration-correlated CT scans for radiotherapy planning of lung cancer patients. Int J Radiat Oncol Biol Phys. 2006;65:1560–71.
9. Lens E, van der Horst A, Versteijne E, van Tienhoven G, Bel A. Dosimetric advantages of Midventilation compared with internal target volume for radiation therapy of pancreatic Cancer. Int J Radiat Oncol Biol Phys. 2015;92:675–82.
10. Wolthaus JW, Sonke JJ, van Herk M, Belderbos JS, Rossi MM, Lebesque JV, et al. Comparison of different strategies to use four-dimensional computed tomography in treatment planning for lung cancer patients. Int J Radiat Oncol Biol Phys. 2008;70:1229–38.
11. Britton KR, Starkschall G, Tucker SL, Pan T, Nelson C, Chang JY, et al. Assessment of gross tumor volume regression and motion changes during radiotherapy for non-small-cell lung cancer as measured by four-dimensional computed tomography. Int J Radiat Oncol Biol Phys. 2007;68:1036–46.
12. Ge J, Santanam L, Noel C, Parikh PJ. Planning 4-dimensional computed tomography (4DCT) cannot adequately represent daily intrafractional motion of abdominal tumors. Int J Radiat Oncol Biol Phys. 2013;85:999–1005.
13. Lens E, van der Horst A, Kroon PS, van Hooft JE, Davila Fajardo R, Fockens P, et al. Differences in respiratory-induced pancreatic tumor motion between 4D treatment planning CT and daily cone beam CT, measured using intratumoral fiducials. Acta Oncol. 2014;53:1257–64.
14. Huijskens SC, van Dijk IW, Visser J, Rasch CR, Alderliesten T, Bel A. Magnitude and variability of respiratory-induced diaphragm motion in children during image-guided radiotherapy. Radiother Oncol. 2017;123:263–9.
15. Pai Panandiker AS, Sharma S, Naik MH, Wu S, Hua C, Beltran C, et al. Novel assessment of renal motion in children as measured via four-dimensional computed tomography. Int J Radiat Oncol Biol Phys. 2012;82:1771–6.
16. Kannan S, Teo BK, Solberg T, Hill-Kayser C. Organ motion in pediatric high-risk neuroblastoma patients using four-dimensional computed tomography. J Appl Clin Med Phys. 2017;18:107–14.
17. Guerreiro F, Seravalli E, Janssens GO, van de Ven CP, van den Heuvel-Eibrink MM, Raaymakers BW. Intra- and inter-fraction uncertainties during IGRT for Wilms' tumor. Acta Oncol. 2018;57(7):1–9. https://doi.org/10.1080/0284186X.2018.1438655.
18. Rankine L, Wan H, Parikh P, Maughan N, Poulsen P, DeWees T, et al. Cone-beam computed tomography internal motion tracking should be used to validate 4-dimensional computed tomography for abdominal radiation therapy patients. Int J Radiat Oncol Biol Phys. 2016;95:818–26.
19. Gierga DP, Chen GT, Kung JH, Betke M, Lombardi J, Willett CG. Quantification of respiration-induced abdominal tumor motion and its impact on IMRT dose distributions. Int J Radiat Oncol Biol Phys. 2004;58:1584–95.
20. de Boer HC, Heijmen BJ. eNAL: an extension of the NAL setup correction protocol for effective use of weekly follow-up measurements. Int J Radiat Oncol Biol Phys. 2007;67:1586–95.
21. Rit S, van Herk M, Zijp L, Sonke JJ. Quantification of the variability of diaphragm motion and implications for treatment margin construction. Int J Radiat Oncol Biol Phys. 2012;82:e399–407.

22. Marchant TE, Amer AM, Moore CJ. Measurement of inter and intra fraction organ motion in radiotherapy using cone beam CT projection images. Phys Med Biol. 2008;53:1087–98.
23. Wink N, Panknin C, Solberg TD. Phase versus amplitude sorting of 4D-CT data. J Appl Clin Med Phys. 2006;7:77–85.
24. Jin P, Hulshof M, van Wieringen N, Bel A, Alderliesten T. Interfractional variability of respiration-induced esophageal tumor motion quantified using fiducial markers and four-dimensional cone-beam computed tomography. Radiother Oncol. 2017;124:147–54.
25. Yang J, Cai J, Wang H, Chang Z, Czito BG, Bashir MR, et al. Is diaphragm motion a good surrogate for liver tumor motion? Int J Radiat Oncol Biol Phys. 2014;90:952–8.
26. Xi M, Liu MZ, Li QQ, Cai L, Zhang L, Hu YH. Analysis of abdominal organ motion using four-dimensional CT. Ai Zheng. 2009;28:989–93.
27. Siva S, Pham D, Gill S, Bressel M, Dang K, Devereux T, et al. An analysis of respiratory induced kidney motion on four-dimensional computed tomography and its implications for stereotactic kidney radiotherapy. Radiat Oncol. 2013;8:248.
28. Brody AS, Frush DP, Huda W, Brent RL, American Academy of Pediatrics Section on R. Radiation risk to children from computed tomography. Pediatrics. 2007;120:677–82.
29. Slovis TL. Children, computed tomography radiation dose, and the as low as reasonably achievable (ALARA) concept. Pediatrics. 2003;112:971–2.
30. Miglioretti DL, Johnson E, Williams A, Greenlee RT, Weinmann S, Solberg LI, et al. The use of computed tomography in pediatrics and the associated radiation exposure and estimated cancer risk. JAMA Pediatr. 2013;167:700–7.
31. Vedam SS, Kini VR, Keall PJ, Ramakrishnan V, Mostafavi H, Mohan R. Quantifying the predictability of diaphragm motion during respiration with a noninvasive external marker. Med Phys. 2003;30(4):505–13.
32. Uh J, Krasin MJ, Li Y, Li X, Tinkle C, Lucas JT Jr, et al. Quantification of pediatric abdominal organ motion with a 4-dimensional magnetic resonance imaging method. Int J Radiat Oncol Biol Phys. 2017;99:227–37.
33. Panandiker AS, Winchell A, Loeffler R, Song R, Rolen M, Hillenbrand C. 4DMRI provides more accurate renal motion estimation in IMRT in young children. Pract Radiat Oncol. 2013;3:S1.
34. Guckenberger M, Wilbert J, Meyer J, Baier K, Richter A, Flentje M. Is a single respiratory correlated 4D-CT study sufficient for evaluation of breathing motion? Int J Radiat Oncol Biol Phys. 2007;67:1352–9.

16

Auto- versus human-driven plan in mediastinal Hodgkin lymphoma radiation treatment

Stefania Clemente[1†], Caterina Oliviero[1†], Giuseppe Palma[2], Vittoria D'Avino[2], Raffaele Liuzzi[2], Manuel Conson[3], Roberto Pacelli[3] and Laura Cella[2*]

Abstract

Background: Technological advances in Hodgkin lymphoma (HL) radiation therapy (RT) by high conformal treatments potentially increase control over organs-at-risk (OARs) dose distribution. However, plan optimization remains a time-consuming task with great operator dependent variability. Purpose of the present study was to devise a fully automated pipeline based on the Pinnacle[3] Auto-Planning (AP) algorithm for treating female supradiaphragmatic HL (SHL) patients.

Methods: CT-scans of 10 female patients with SHL were considered. A "butterfly" (BF) volumetric modulated arc therapy was optimized using SmartArc module integrated in Pinnacle[3] v. 9.10 using Collapsed Cone Convolution Superposition algorithm (30 Gy in 20 fractions). Human-driven (Manual-BF) and AP-BF optimization plans were generated. For AP, an optimization objective list of Planning Target Volume (PTV)/OAR clinical goals was first implemented, starting from a subset of 5 patients used for algorithm training. This list was then tested on the remaining 5 patients (validation set). In addition to the BF technique, the AP engine was applied to a 2 coplanar disjointed arc (AP-ARC) technique using the same objective list. For plan evaluation, dose-volume-histograms of PTVs and OARs were extracted; homogeneity and conformity indices (HI and CI), OARs dose-volume metrics and odds for different toxicity endpoints were computed. Non-parametric Friedman and Dunn tests were used to identify significant differences between groups.

Results: A single AP objective list for SHL was obtained. Compared to the manual plan, both AP-plans offer comparable CIs while AP-ARC also achieved comparable HIs. All plans fulfilled the clinical dose criteria set for OARs: both AP solutions performed at least as good as Manual-BF plan. In particular, AP-ARC outperformed AP-BF in terms of heart sparing involving a lower risk of coronary events and radiation-induced lung fibrosis. Hands-on planning time decreased by a factor of 10 using AP on average.

Conclusions: Despite the high interpatient PTV (size and position) variability, it was possible to set a standard SHL AP optimization list with a high level of generalizability. Using the implemented list, the AP module was able to limit OAR doses, producing clinically acceptable plans with stable quality without additional user input. Overall, the AP engine associated to the arc technique represents the best option for SHL.

Keywords: Volumetric modulated arc therapy, Automated planning optimization, Hodgkin lymphoma, Normal tissue sparing, NTCP

* Correspondence: laura.cella@cnr.it
[†]Stefania Clemente and Caterina Oliviero contributed equally to this work.
[2]National Research Council, Institute of Biostructures and Bioimaging, Naples, Italy
Full list of author information is available at the end of the article

Background

Modern radiation therapy (RT) approaches in Hodgkin lymphoma (HL), with lower prescribed doses (20–30 Gy) and smaller irradiated volumes (involved site or involved node), lead to a reduction of organs-at-risk (OARs) exposure [1]. Accordingly, the rates of radiation-induced late toxicity are expected to be lower [2, 3] when compared with older series of successfully treated long term surviving HL patients [4, 5]. In parallel, a considerable effort has been made to identify those HL radiation delivery modalities that increased control over target as well as OAR dose distributions [6–10].

Several, widely available, intensity-modulated radiation therapy (IMRT) planning solutions have been proposed in the literature. Among the different IMRT techniques, the dosimetric advantages of the "butterfly" (BF) technique for female patients with mediastinal HL has been reported [11, 12]. In particular, BF volumetric modulated arc therapy (VMAT) showed high levels of conformation permitting to achieve the most balanced compromise between higher conformation around the target and OAR sparing [11].

Dose-volume histogram (DVH) predictors and Normal Tissue Complication Probability (NTCP) models developed for HL patient population have supported the planning optimization procedures intended to limit OAR complications. NTCP models have been reported for late side effects such as radiation induced lung damage [13–15], hypothyroidism [16, 17], and cardiovascular diseases [2, 18–20].

However, plan optimization remains a very time-consuming and operator dependent task. This issue has been addressed by the recent introduction of automated engines in treatment planning (TP) systems in order to create an optimized plan with minimal user interaction. They have proved able to generate IMRT plans of non-inferior or even higher clinical quality compared to human driven plans for many different tumour sites, such as head and neck [21], prostate [22, 23]and lung [24]. To the best of our knowledge, however, no study investigated the Auto-Planning (AP) algorithm applied to VMAT for supradiaphragmatic HL (SHL) patients.

Given this background, the current study was designed to devise a fully automated pipeline, based on the Pinnacle^3 (Philips Radiation Oncology Systems, Fitchburg, WI, USA) AP algorithm, for treating female SHL patients. For 10 female patients AP plans were compared with treatment plans generated by experienced human planners. The different TP solutions were evaluated by quantitative risk estimates based on published models for different toxicity endpoints.

Methods

Patient data

Planning CT-scans of 10 consecutive female patients with SHL (Table 1) in standard supine position were extracted from our clinical database. Involved site clinical target volume (CTV) was defined according to ILROG guidelines [1] for early stage HL. Planning Target Volume (PTV) was obtained by CTV uniform 10-mm expansion. Target and OARs structures were contoured on free-breathing CT images (voxel size = 0.94 × 0.94 × 5 mm^3). The following OARs were contoured: lungs, heart, left ventricle, left anterior descending (LAD) artery, esophagus, spinal cord, breasts and thyroid. Heart and its substructures were contoured according to heart contouring guidelines [25]. All contours were reviewed and approved by one of the authors (M.C.).

A total dose of 30 Gy was prescribed in 1.5 Gy daily fractions for all patients.

Treatment plan optimization

Each patient was purposely planned with an antero-posterior/postero-anterior weighted BF 6 MV photon beams VMAT technique by Pinnacle^3 v. 9.10. SmartArc module and Collapsed Cone Convolution Superposition dose calculation algorithm (grid resolution 3 mm) were used. The BF VMAT technique consists of 3 arcs: 2 coplanar arcs, one anterior and one posterior (width ranging from 60° to 100°) and one anterior no-coplanar (couch angle 90°) arc (width ranging from 45° to 60°). Arc width was customized to provide tumour coverage according to patient anatomy. All plans were optimized for a Varian True Beam STx Linac (Varian Medical System, Palo Alto, CA) equipped with a High Definition 120 multileaf collimator (HD120MLC).

For each patient, two different optimization approaches were used: the human-driven optimization (Manual-BF) and the AP optimization (AP-BF), both generated using the same required clinical constraints (Table 2). No constraints were used on the left ventricle and LAD artery.

The Manual-BF plan was generated using planner-dependent definitions of additional guidance contours (inner and outer rings structures for PTV), avoidance structures and associated optimization objectives. The plan was validated by 2 experienced clinical physicists (S.C., C.O.) in consensus.

The AP-BF plan was optimized using Pinnacle^3 AP algorithm. In summary, it is a fully integrated module in the TP system which uses a progressive optimization algorithm to continually adjust the optimization objective list set by the user to meet or further decrease OARs doses and related DVH parameters with minimal compromise to PTV coverage, thus simulating the decision-making process of an experienced human planner [21]. Indeed, the AP algorithm iteratively fine-tunes the target coverage and OAR sparing by creating multiple additional structures based both on the relative geometry of originally segmented ROIs and on transient dose distributions. The algorithm automatically assigns dose-volume objectives to

Table 1 Nodal disease localization and Planning Target Volume (PTV) size for each patient

Patient	Nodal disease localization	PTV size (cc)
Training		
1	VI level, upper mediastinal	252.0
2	supraclavicular right, upper mediastinal	503.2
3	supraclavicular left and right, III level right, upper mediastinal	350.7
4	supraclavicular left and right, upper mediastinal, diaphragmatic	480.3
5	supraclavicular right, upper mediastinal	247.6
Validation		
6	supraclavicular left, III level left, upper mediastinal	496.8
7	supraclavicular left, upper mediastinal	559.5
8	supraclavicular left and right, III level right, upper mediastinal	423.0
9	II and III level left, supraclavicular left, upper mediastinal	199.3
10	supraclavicular left, upper mediastinal	309.6

the additional ROIs which are added to the standard optimization list [26].

In addition to the BF technique, the AP engine was applied to a 2 coplanar disjointed arcs (AP-ARC) technique which consists of 2 full co-planar arcs moving clockwise and counter clockwise respectively avoiding the arms.

In the present study, each AP plan was obtained running a single optimization cycle.

AP optimization objective list

The starting point of Pinnacle^3 AP optimization procedure is setting a user dependent optimization list of PTV/OAR clinical goals. In order to set a single AP-BF list for SHL with a high level of generalizability, we selected 5 out of 10 patients to be used as a training set. The patient selection criterion was based on nodal disease localization and target size heterogeneity (Table 1). The remaining 5 patients were instead used as a validation set to test the obtained optimization list. In Table 1, PTV characteristics for training and validation patient sets are reported.

For all training set patients, the list was iteratively refined using the algorithm described in Fig. 1 (learning phase). The algorithm was designed to satisfy, first, the tumour-coverage criteria (at least 95% of PTV received at least 95% of prescription dose) and, secondly, the constraints on the OARs of Table 2. To this end, in the algorithm we introduced the concept of "admitted violations", intended as the maximum number of required objectives not satisfied at the end of an optimization cycle. The admitted violations for the algorithm were PTV $V_{107\%} > 1\%$ and only one OAR not

Table 2 Planning Target Volume (PTV) and Organ-At-Risk dose-volume constraints for plan optimization and patients violating the required constraints when the Auto Plan best optimization objective list was applied

Structure	Parameter	Required Objective	Patient violating the requirements		
			AP-BF Training	AP-BF Validation	AP-ARC Validation
PTV					
	D_{mean} (Gy)	30	–	–	–
	$V_{95\%}$ (%)	95	–	–	–
	$V_{107\%}$ (%)	1	3,4	6,7,8	6,7
Breast					
	V_{4Gy} (%)	50	–	–	–
	V_{10Gy} (%)	33	–	–	–
Lung-PTV					
	V_{5Gy} (%)	50	–	–	–
	V_{10Gy} (%)	33	–	–	–
Thyroid-PTV					
	D_{mean} (Gy)	20	3	–	–
	V_{18Gy} (%)	50	3	–	–
	V_{25Gy} (%)	33	–	–	–
Heart-PTV					
	D_{mean} (Gy)	3	2	6,8	6,8
	$V_{7.7Gy}$(%)	50	–	–	–
	V_{15Gy}(%)	33	–	–	–
Spinal Cord					
	D_{max} (Gy)	30	–	–	–
Esophagus-PTV					
	D_{max} (Gy)	32	–	–	–

fulfilling the required dose-volume constrains reported in Table 2.

The list thus obtained was then tested on the validation set for both AP-BF and AP-ARC configurations.

Plan analysis

For plan comparison, DVHs of PTVs and OARs were extracted. For each patient, relevant PTV/OAR DVH metrics were analyzed: the percentage volume receiving at least X dose (Vx), near maximum dose ($D_{2\%}$), near minimum dose ($D_{98\%}$), mean (D_{mean}) and median dose ($D_{50\%}$).

The target coverage was assessed via the conformity index ($CI=V_{95\%}/PTV_{vol}$) and the homogeneity index ($HI = [D_{2\%}-D_{98\%}]/ D_{50\%}$).

Toxicity risks were calculated according to several NTCP models available in the literature [2, 3, 13, 16, 18–20, 27, 28]. NTCP models specifically extrapolated from HL patients' cohorts were used.

In addition, the number of planned monitor units (MU) and the hands-on planning time were recorded.

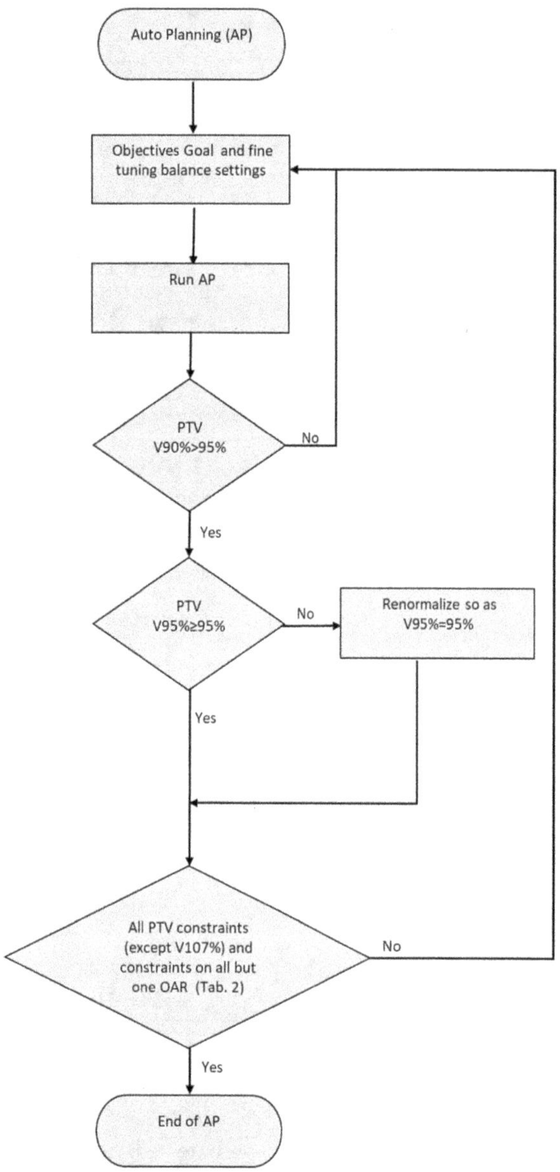

Fig. 1 The flow of the algorithm used for setting the Auto Planning optimization objective list (learning phase)

The hands-on planning time was defined as the time of human interaction with the TP system.

The median and the range were employed to describe all continuous variables and the non-parametric ANOVA (Friedman matched-pairs signed-rank test) was used to determine statistically significant differences ($p < 0.05$). A posthoc procedure was performed in order to identify significant differences between groups (Dunn's test).

Results

AP optimization objective list

At the end of the learning phase, we succeeded in implementing a single AP optimization objective list for SHL patients (details in Table 3). This list was subsequently applied, with no further refinement, to the validation set. Each AP plan of the validation set (patients 6–10) fulfilled all PTV/OAR constraints within the admitted violations of the required constraints, i.e. all PTV constraints (except $V_{107\%}$) and constraints on all but one OAR were fulfilled (Table 2 and Fig. 2).

Target volume

Median target size was 386.9 cc (199.3–559.5 cc). Figure 3 illustrates dose distributions in one representative patient for the three treatment techniques.

Median PTV DVH from the 3 plans were largely overlapping (Fig. 4.A). AP offers comparable coverage of the PTV with the manual plan. CI indices for AP plans were comparable to that of the Manual-BF plan, while AP-BF showed a higher HI compared to both Manual-BF and AP-ARC (Table 4).

Organs at risk

All AP plans fulfilled the clinical dose criteria set for OARs within the admitted violation. Data in Table 4 show that the AP solutions were never outperformed by the manual plans and the AP engine also leads to a general reduction of OARs dose metrics. In particular, AP-ARC was never outperformed by AP-BF, except for lungs V_{5Gy} and breast D_{mean}, which show a slightly higher sparing provided by AP-BF.

In terms of NTCP, AP engine was always at least as safe as manual planning (Table 5), with the exception of radiation-induced lung fibrosis where AP-BF involved a higher risk compared with manual plan. In particular, comparing AP-ARC and AP-BF, AP –ARC resulted in a lower risk of radiation-induced coronary events and lung fibrosis compared to AP-BF.

The median number of MU were 287.7 (239.6–378.9) for Manual-BF, 267.7 (214.9–382.5) for AP-BF and 375.6 (339.9–456.7) for AP-ARC ($p < 0.001$; AP-ARC > Manual-BF and AP-BF).

Hands-on planning time by AP decreased by an order of magnitude. The mean computation time (performed on a Server Expert hardware platform 32 GB RAM –http://incenter.medical.philips.com/doclib/getdoc.aspx?func=l-l&objid=10925579&objaction=open) for the automated procedures was 25 min (AP-BF) and 40 min (AP-ARC).

Discussion

The most up-to-date and optimized RT techniques applied to mediastinal HL have demonstrated a significant dose reduction to various sensitive critical structures [10–12]. Modern TP systems automate many beam parameters, in particular the beam modulation, via inverse planning computations which create IMRT or VMAT plans so that each treatment plan will result highly customized for

Table 3 Auto Planning setting list

Auto-planning Settings					
Max Itaration	60				
Engine Type	Biological				
Tuning Balance	5%				
Dose Fall-Off Margin	1.8 cm				
Hot-Spot Maximum Goal	102%				
Use Cold-Spot ROIs	YES				
Target Optimization Goals					
PTV	30 Gy				
CTV	30 Gy				
OARs Optimization Goals					
ROI	Type	Dose (Gy)	Volume (%)	Priority	Compromise
Heart	Mean dose	3		Medium	Yes
Heart	Max DVH	7.7	50	Medium	Yes
Heart	Max DVH	15	33	Medium	Yes
Left Lung	Mean dose	5		Medium	Yes
Left Lung	Max DVH	5	15	Medium	Yes
Left Lung	Max DVH	10	12	Medium	Yes
Left Lung	Max DVH	20	10	Medium	Yes
Right Lung	Mean dose	5		Medium	Yes
Right Lung	Max DVH	5	15	Medium	Yes
Right Lung	Max DVH	10	12	Medium	Yes
Right Lung	Max DVH	20	10	Medium	Yes
Esophagus	Max DVH	28	50	Medium	Yes
Esophagus	Max DVH	30	50	Medium	Yes
Thyroid	Mean dose	20		Medium	Yes
Thyroid	Max DVH	18	50	Medium	Yes
Thyroid	Max DVH	25	33	Medium	Yes
Left Breast	Mean dose	0.3		High	No
Left Breast	Max DVH	2	4	High	No
Left Breast	Max DVH	5	2	High	No
Right Breast	Mean dose	0.3		High	No
Right Breast	Max DVH	2	4	High	No
Right Breast	Max DVH	5	2	High	No
Spinal Cord	Max dose	25		High	Yes
PRV Spinal Cord	Max dose	26		High	Yes
Ring PTV (+ 1.5 cm)	Max dose	15		High	Yes
Body-PTV-Ring PTV	Max dose	10		High	Yes

Abbreviations: *ROI* Region of Interest, *PTV* planning Target Volume, *CTV* Clinical Target Volume, *OARs* Organs At Risk, *DVH* Dose Volume Histogram

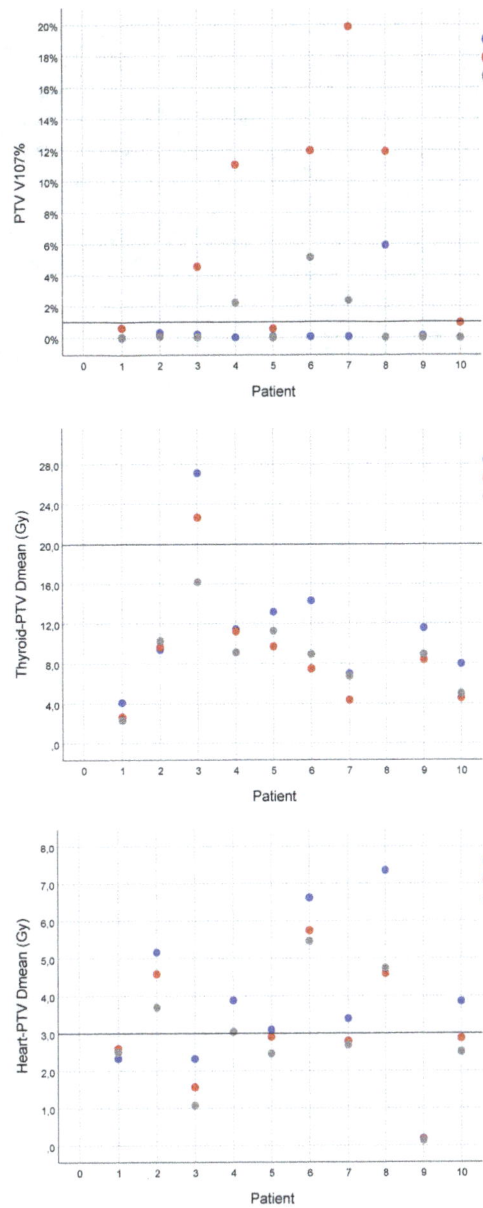

Fig. 2 Comparison of Planning Target Volume (PTV) percentage volume receiving at least 107% of the prescribed dose ($V_{107\%}$), of Thyroid-PTV mean dose (D_{mean}) and Heart-PTV mean dose (D_{mean}) values for Manual-BF, AP-BF, AP-ARC

each patient. However, the mediastinum remains a critical and complicated target area in HL, due to the heterogeneity of tumour volumes and their position relative to many different important OARs, such as the heart and its substructure or the lungs. As a consequence, HL planning optimization entails a high level of complexity with a wide variation in plan quality that strongly depends on planner skills, as demonstrated for other disease sites by [29]. This issue calls for an additional level of automation in HL RT in order to reduce the inter-operator variability of plan

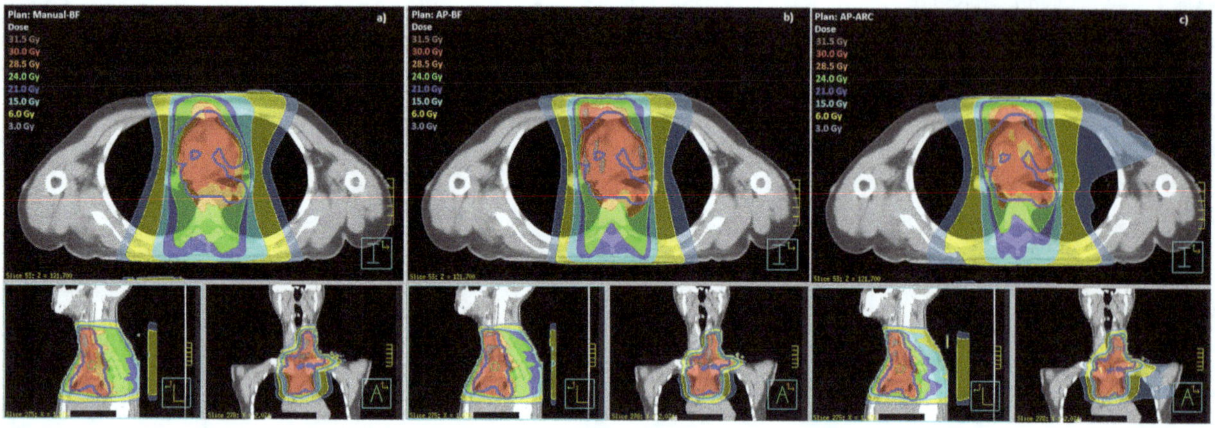

Fig. 3 Dose distributions in one representative patient for the three treatment plans: **a**) Manual-BF, **b**) AP-BF, **c**) AP-ARC

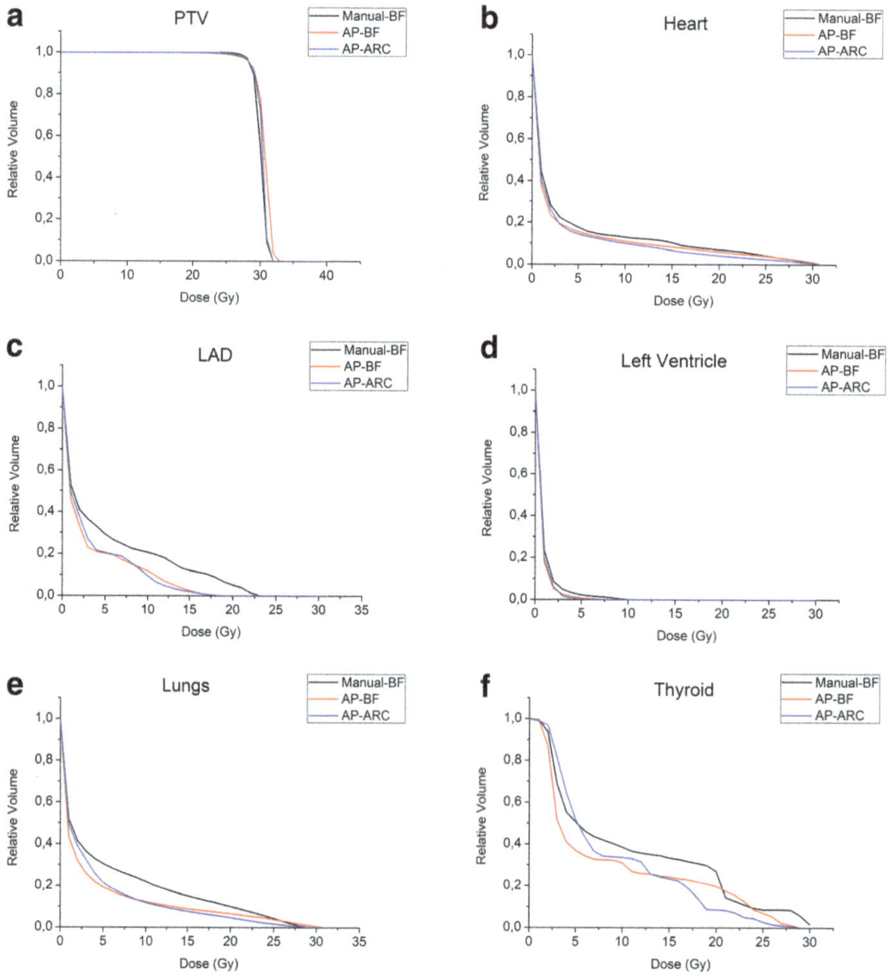

Fig. 4 Median cumulative patient dose-volume histograms (DVHs) for the Planning Target Volume-PTV (A) and the organs-at-risk (B–F) for the three treatment plans: Manual-BF, AP-BF, AP-ARC

Table 4 Dosimetric indices and comparative analysis for Planning Target Volume (PTV) and different organs at risk for manual and automated plans

Structure	Dose Index	Median (range)			p-value< 0.05[a]	
		Manual-BF	Pinnacle³Auto-Planning			
		1	AP-BF 2	AP-ARC 3	1vs.2,3	2vs.3
PTV	HI	0.12 (0.09–0.16)	0.16 (0.1–0.22)	0.13 (0.09–0.18)	1 < 2	2 > 3
	CI	0.95 (0.94–0.96)	0.95 (0.94–0.95)	0.95 (0.95–0.97)	–	–
Heart	D_{mean} (Gy)	3.8 (0.2–8.7)	3.3 (0.2–7.2)	3 (0.1–6.3)	1 > 2,3	2 > 3
	$D_{2\%}$ (Gy)	28.4 (0.4–31.5)	28.3 (0.4–31.3)	26.8 (0.3–30.2)	1 > 3	2 > 3
Left Ventricle	D_{mean} (Gy)	1 (0.1–3.1)	0.7 (0.1–1.6)	0.8 (0.1–1.7)	1 > 2,3	–
LAD	$D_{50\%}$ (Gy)	1.3 (0.0–25.7)	0.8 (0.0–11.9)	1 (0.0–13.7)	1 > 2	–
Lungs	D_{mean} (Gy)	6.3 (1.6–9.2)	4.5 (1.4–5.9)	4.6 (1.4–6.0)	1 > 2,3	–
	V_{5Gy} (%)	32.0 (7.5–52.4)	20.9 (6.3–29.0)	23.7 (7.7–35.0)	1 > 2	2 < 3
	V_{20Gy} (%)	11.6 (2.6–18.5)	8.4 (2.0–12.3)	7.2 (1.0–9.7)	1 > 3	2 > 3
Thyroid	D_{mean} (Gy)	16.8 (11.9–28.4)	15.4 (10.1–25.7)	15.5 (9.6–21.2)	1 > 2,3	–
	V_{30Gy} (%)	19.6 (7.9–51.3)	19.2 (8.7–27.9)	14.0 (3.7–22.5)	–	–
Breast	D_{mean} (Gy)	1.1 (0.1–2.3)	0.4 (0.1–1.2)	0.6 (0.1–1.6)	1 > 2,3	2 < 3
Normal Tissue	D_{mean} (Gy)	2.9 (1.5–5.4)	2.4 (1.4–3.8)	2.4 (1.2–3.7)	1 > 2	

Abbreviations: PTV planning Target Volume, *HI* Homogeneity Index, Conformity Index, D_{mean} mean dose, $D_{2\%}$ near maximum dose, $D_{50\%}$ median dose, V_X percentage volume exceeding X, *LAD* Left Anterior Descending artery
[a]Friedman and Dunn tests

quality. In recent years, different automated treatment planning approaches have been proposed and are commercially available. They show that it is possible to almost fully automate and accelerate this task, improving speed, consistency and quality of RT plans [30].

One proposed knowledge-based solution relies on the concepts of machine learning and uses a library of historical plans for a given disease site to build a model that can predict achievable DVHs for new patients and guide plan optimization [31]. Another approach instead is based on a multicriteria optimization algorithm which provides a database of Pareto-optimal plans [32]. Pinnacle³ AP algorithm uses an iterative approach of progressive optimization without requiring any prior database of successful plans [26].

In this study we devised a fully automated pipeline for treating female SHL patients using Pinnacle³ AP. First, we designed a learning phase based on a trial-and-error approach to fit an optimization list that could satisfy a number of dosimetric acceptability criteria on the training set patients (as illustrated in the flowchart of Fig. 1).

Table 5 Risk analysis for different organs and endpoints for manual and automated plans

Structure	Clinical endpoint	Reference	Median (range)			p-value< 0.05[d]	
			Manual-BF	Pinnacle³Auto-Planning			
			1	AP-BF 2	AP-ARC 3	1vs.2,3	2vs.3
			NTCP (%)				
Heart	Valvular defects	Cella et al. (2013)	26.71 (0.96–82.63)	21.14 (0.96–84.21)	16.09 (0.94–81.36)	–	–
Lungs	Radiation fibrosis[a]	Cella et al. (2015)[b]	5.85 (2.72–8.39)	6.41 (2.19–8.03)	5.53 (1.30–7.51)	1 < 2	2 > 3
		Cella et al. (2015)[c]	6.05 (3.33–16.79)	3.88 (3.21–7.87)	4.80 (3.22–7.94)	1 > 2,3	2 < 3
Thyroid	Hypothyroidism	Cella et al. (2012)	3.22 (2.08–9.98)	3.16 (2.15–4.36)	2.62 (1.78–3.58)	–	–
			RRR				
Heart	Major coronary events	van Nimwegen et al. (2015)	1.28 (1.01–1.64)	1.24 (1.01–1.53)	1.22 (1.01–1.47)	1 > 2,3	2 > 3
			OR				
LAD	Coronary stenosis	Moignier et al. (2015)	1.06 (1.00–3.43)	1.04 (1.00–1.77)	1.05 (1.00–1.93)	1 > 2	

Abbreviations: LAD Left Anterior Descending artery, *NTCP* Normal Tissue Complication Probability, *RRR* Relative Risk Ratio, *OR* Odds Ratio
[a]Computed assuming an age of 30 years at time of irradiation; [b]Model including lungs $D_{2\%}$; [c]Model including left lung V_{5Gy}; [d]Friedman and Dunn test

Then, we applied the obtained optimization list as an input for the AP algorithm on an independent validation set of patients.

On the whole, the analysis of the results on the validation set confirmed the behaviours observed in the training phase (Table 2 and Fig. 2). Namely, AP techniques seemed to favour sparing of healthy tissues over target coverage, in agreement with [26]. In particular, the requirement on PTV $V_{107\%} \leq 1\%$ was violated when AP was applied to patients 6, 7 and 8 in the validation set. Indeed, in several patients a plan renormalization was necessary to fulfil the requirement of PTV $V_{95\%} = 95\%$ at the expense of the target high dose region.

Nonetheless, with AP-ARC technique the $V_{107\%}$ was always no more than 5% while higher $V_{107\%}$ values ($\geq$ 12%) were obtained with the AP-BF technique. In this regard, AP-ARC proved able to largely reduce the gap between the manually optimized and AP-BF plans, as also reflected by the HIs (Table 4). On the other hand, AP plans naturally succeeded in satisfying OAR requirements, with the exception of the heart mean dose for one training and two validation patients, and thyroid D_{mean} and V_{18Gy} for one training patient. However, even in those cases AP engine was able to outperform manual optimization.

The quantitative assessment of DVH (Fig. 4 and Table 4) revealed that, as a general rule, AP schemes performed at least as well as the manual approach. For lungs and heart, the dosimetric advantages translated into a significant reduction of morbidity risk estimates (Fig.5 and Table 5). In addition, even when non statistically significant differences were found, the observed trends held for all the evaluated variables.

We have to remark that further refinements of the AP plans could be expected by running more than one AP optimization cycle.

Analogously, a general trend suggested that AP-ARC outperforms AP-BF, with the only exception of lungs V_{5Gy} and breast D_{mean} which shows a slightly higher sparing provided by AP-BF. The out of phase behavior

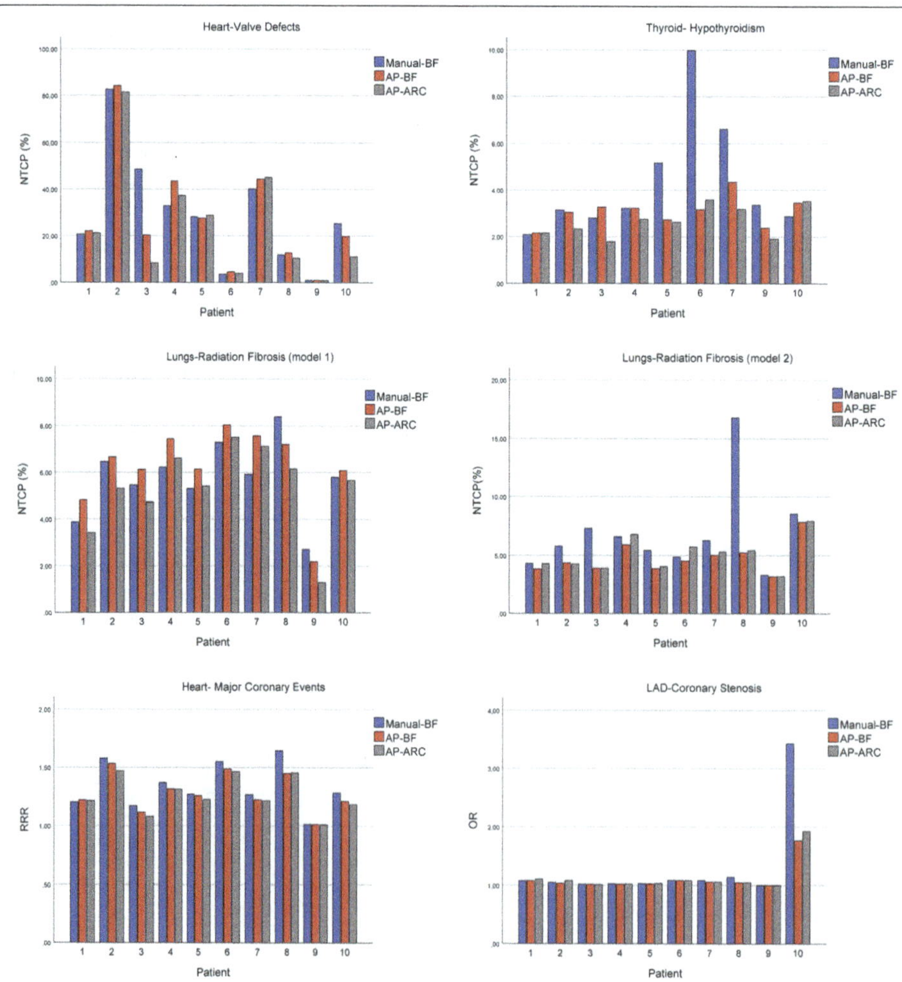

Fig. 5 Comparison of morbidity risk parameters for heart, lungs and thyroid for Manual-BF, AP-BF and AP-ARC (please note that patient number 8 underwent a thyroidectomy)

of the two considered lungs metrics (namely V_{5Gy} and V_{20Gy}) translates into a similar result for estimating the radiation fibrosis risk and reflects the famous conundrum "a lot to a little or a little to a lot" inherent to lungs radiobiology.

The better performances of AP applied to the arc beam settings compared to the well-established "butterfly" technique can be explained by the increased number of beam entries resulting in an augmented number of degrees of freedom that the optimization algorithm can exploit to satisfy the objective list. This point is best demonstrated by the higher homogeneity of the target coverage and by the lower heart doses. In addition, the longer beam-on time for AP-ARC plans (by a factor of about 1.5) is overbalanced by reduced in room times compared to AP-BF plans, which involve a non-coplanar beam. This potentially reduces the immobilization errors and facilitates more comfortable treatments. Of note, no difference between AP-ARC and AP-BF was observed in the non-target tissue mean doses.

Besides, the adoption of the AP algorithm obviously leads to a huge decrease of the hands-on time on the TP system which can be easily quantified in terms of an order of magnitude.

Summing up, the above results prove that we have succeeded in defining a procedure that leads to a fully automation of the TP process for obtaining clinically acceptable SHL plans, despite the high inter-patient target variability (size and position) inherent to the considered disease. The standardization of the treatment is a direct consequence of the automation, thus guaranteeing the quality of treatment delivered in an arbitrary institution independently from the planner's skills.

Finally, the flowchart devised for setting a single optimization objective list is not tied to the considered disease and, as such, can be applied to any tumour site in order to remove the only operator dependent task left by the Pinnacle[3] AP optimization tool.

Conclusions

In this study, we demonstrated the feasibility of a completely automated pipeline based on Pinnacle[3] AP for SHL plan optimization. The AP module was able to limit OAR doses, thus producing clinically acceptable plans of high quality without additional user interaction. On the whole, the AP engine associated to the arc technique represented the best option for SHL.

Abbreviations

AP: Auto-Planning; BF: Butterfly; CI: Conformity index; CT: Computed Tomography; CTV: Clinical target volume; DVH: Dose-volume histogram; HI: Homogeneity index; HL: Hodgkin lymphoma; IMRT: Intensity-modulated radiation therapy; LAD: Left anterior descending; MU: Monitor units; NTCP: Normal Tissue Complication Probability; OAR: Organs-at-risk; PTV: Planning Target Volume; RT: Radiation therapy; SHL: Supradiaphragmatic Hodgkin lymphoma; TP: Treatment planning; VMAT: Volumetric modulated arc therapy

Acknowledgements

We acknowledge Philips for providing the Pinnacle[3] Auto-Planning system for evaluation.

Authors' contributions

LC, GP and RP conceived and designed the study. SC and CO performed planning simulations. RL, MC reviewed patient clinical and dosimetric data. LC, RL, VDA performed modelling and analysed the data. All authors participated in drafting and revising the manuscript. All authors have given their final approval of the manuscript.

Competing interests

The authors declare that they have no competing interests.

Author details

[1]Azienda Ospedaliera Universitaria Federico II, Naples, Italy. [2]National Research Council, Institute of Biostructures and Bioimaging, Naples, Italy. [3]Department of Advanced Biomedical Sciences, Federico II University School of Medicine, Naples, Italy.

References

1. Specht L, Yahalom J, Illidge T, Berthelsen AK, Constine LS, Eich HT, et al. Modern radiation therapy for Hodgkin lymphoma: field and dose guidelines from the international lymphoma radiation oncology group (ILROG). Int J Radiat Oncol Biol Phys. 2014;89(4):854–62.
2. Cella L, Liuzzi R, Conson M, D'Avino V, Salvatore M, Pacelli R. Multivariate normal tissue complication probability modeling of heart valve dysfunction in Hodgkin lymphoma survivors. Int J Radiat Oncol Biol Phys. 2013;87(2): 304–10.
3. Cella L, Liuzzi R, Conson M, Torre G, Caterino M, De Rosa N, et al. Dosimetric predictors of asymptomatic heart valvular dysfunction following mediastinal irradiation for Hodgkin's lymphoma. Radiother Oncol. 2011;101(2):316–21.
4. Ng AK, LaCasce A, Travis LB. Long-term complications of lymphoma and its treatment. J Clin Oncol. 2011;29(14):1885–92.
5. Hodgson DC. Late effects in the era of modern therapy for Hodgkin lymphoma. Hematology Am Soc Hematol Educ Program. 2011;2011:323–9.
6. Cella L, Conson M, Pressello MC, Molinelli S, Schneider U, Donato V, Orecchia R, Salvatore M, Pacelli R. Hodgkin's lymphoma emerging radiation treatment techniques: trade-offs between late radio-induced toxicities and secondary malignant neoplasms. Radiat Oncol. 2013;8(1):22.
7. Hoppe BS, Flampouri S, Lynch J, Slayton W, Zaiden R, Li Z, Mendenhall NP. Improving the therapeutic ratio in Hodgkin lymphoma through the use of proton therapy. Oncology (Williston Park). 2012;26(5):456–9 462-455.
8. Aznar MC, Maraldo MV, Schut DA, Lundemann M, Brodin NP, Vogelius IR, Berthelsen AK, Specht L, Petersen PM. Minimizing late effects for patients with mediastinal Hodgkin lymphoma: deep inspiration breath-hold, IMRT, or both? Int J Radiat Oncol Biol Phys. 2015;92(1):169–74.
9. Rechner LA, Maraldo MV, Vogelius IR, Zhu XR, Dabaja BS, Brodin NP, Petersen PM, Specht L, Aznar MC. Life years lost attributable to late effects after radiotherapy for early stage Hodgkin lymphoma: the impact of proton therapy and/or deep inspiration breath hold. Radiother Oncol. 2017;125(1):41–7.

10. Baues C, Marnitz S, Engert A, Baus W, Jablonska K, Fogliata A, Vasquez-Torres A, Scorsetti M, Cozzi L. Proton versus photon DEEP inspiration breath hold technique in patients with hodgkin lymphoma and mediastinal radiation : a PLANNING COMPARISON OF DEEP INSPIRATION BREATH HOLD INTENSITY MODULATION RADIOTHERAPY AND INTENSITY MODULATED PROTON THERAPY. Radiat Oncol. 2018;13(1):122.
11. Fiandra C, Filippi AR, Catuzzo P, Botticella A, Ciammella P, Franco P, et al. Different IMRT solutions vs. 3D-conformal radiotherapy in early stage Hodgkin's lymphoma: dosimetric comparison and clinical considerations. Radiat Oncol. 2012;7:186.
12. Voong KR, McSpadden K, Pinnix CC, Shihadeh F, Reed V, Salehpour MR, et al. Dosimetric advantages of a "butterfly" technique for intensity-modulated radiation therapy for young female patients with mediastinal Hodgkin's lymphoma. Radiat Oncol. 2014;9:94.
13. Cella L, D'Avino V, Palma G, Conson M, Liuzzi R, Picardi M, et al. Modeling the risk of radiation-induced lung fibrosis: irradiated heart tissue is as important as irradiated lung. Radiother Oncol. 2015;117(1):36–43.
14. Pinnix CC, Smith GL, Milgrom S, Osborne EM, Reddy JP, Akhtari M, et al. Predictors of radiation pneumonitis in patients receiving intensity modulated radiation therapy for Hodgkin and non-Hodgkin lymphoma. Int J Radiat Oncol Biol Phys. 2015;92(1):175–82.
15. Palma G, Monti S, D'Avino V, Conson M, Liuzzi R, Pressello MC, et al. A voxel-based approach to explore local dose differences associated with radiation-induced lung damage. Int J Radiat Oncol Biol Phys. 2016;96(1):127–33.
16. Cella L, Liuzzi R, Conson M, DA V, Salvatore M, Pacelli R. Development of multivariate NTCP models for radiation-induced hypothyroidism: a comparative analysis. Radiat Oncol. 2012;7(1):224.
17. Pinnix CC, Cella L, Andraos TY, Ayoub Z, Milgrom SA, Gunther J, et al. Predictors of hypothyroidism in Hodgkin lymphoma survivors after intensity modulated versus 3-dimensional radiation therapy. Int J Radiat Oncol Biol Phys. 2018;101(3):530–40.
18. Cella L, Oh JH, Deasy JO, Palma G, Liuzzi R, D'Avino V, et al. Predicting radiation-induced valvular heart damage. Acta Oncol. 2015;54(10):1796–804.
19. Moignier A, Broggio D, Derreumaux S, Beaudre A, Girinsky T, Paul JF, et al. Coronary stenosis risk analysis following Hodgkin lymphoma radiotherapy: a study based on patient specific artery segments dose calculation. Radiother Oncol. 2015;117(3):467–72.
20. van Nimwegen FA, Schaapveld M, Cutter DJ, Janus CP, Krol AD, Hauptmann M, et al. Radiation dose-response relationship for risk of coronary heart disease in survivors of Hodgkin lymphoma. J Clin Oncol. 2016;34(3):235–43.
21. Kusters J, Bzdusek K, Kumar P, van Kollenburg PGM, Kunze-Busch MC, Wendling M, Dijkema T, Kaanders J: Automated IMRT planning in pinnacle : a study in head-and-neck cancer. Strahlenther Onkol 2017, 193(12):1031–1038.
22. Voet PW, Dirkx ML, Breedveld S, Al-Mamgani A, Incrocci L, Heijmen BJ. Fully automated volumetric modulated arc therapy plan generation for prostate cancer patients. Int J Radiat Oncol Biol Phys. 2014;88(5):1175–9.
23. Sharfo AWM, Dirkx MLP, Bijman RG, Schillemans W, Breedveld S, Aluwini S, Pos F, Incrocci L, Heijmen BJM. Late toxicity in the randomized multicenter HYPRO trial for prostate cancer analyzed with automated treatment planning. Radiother Oncol. 2018;128(2):349–56.
24. Della Gala G, Dirkx MLP, Hoekstra N, Fransen D, Lanconelli N, van de Pol M, Heijmen BJM, Petit SF. Fully automated VMAT treatment planning for advanced-stage NSCLC patients. Strahlenther Onkol. 2017;193(5):402–9.
25. Feng M, Moran JM, Koelling T, Chughtai A, Chan JL, Freedman L, et al. Development and validation of a heart atlas to study cardiac exposure to radiation following treatment for breast cancer. Int J Radiat Oncol Biol Phys. 2011;79(1):10–8.
26. Gintz D, Latifi K, Caudell J, Nelms B, Zhang G, Moros E, Feygelman V. Initial evaluation of automated treatment planning software. J Appl Clin Med Phys. 2016;17(3):331–46.
27. Cella L, Liuzzi R, D'Avino V, Conson M, Di Biase A, Picardi M, et al. Pulmonary damage in Hodgkin's lymphoma patients treated with sequential chemo-radiotherapy: predictors of radiation-induced lung injury. Acta Oncol. 2014; 53(5):613–9.
28. Cella L, Palma G, Deasy JO, Oh JH, Liuzzi R, D'Avino V, et al. Complication probability models for radiation-induced heart valvular dysfunction: do heart-lung interactions play a role? PLoS One. 2014;9(10):e111753.
29. Nelms BE, Robinson G, Markham J, Velasco K, Boyd S, Narayan S, Wheeler J, Sobczak ML. Variation in external beam treatment plan quality: an inter-institutional study of planners and planning systems. Pract Radiat Oncol. 2012;2(4):296–305.
30. Moore KL, Kagadis GC, McNutt TR, Moiseenko V, Mutic S. Vision 20/20: automation and advanced computing in clinical radiation oncology. Med Phys. 2014;41(1):010901.
31. Fogliata A, Belosi F, Clivio A, Navarria P, Nicolini G, Scorsetti M, Vanetti E, Cozzi L. On the pre-clinical validation of a commercial model-based optimisation engine: application to volumetric modulated arc therapy for patients with lung or prostate cancer. Radiother Oncol. 2014;113(3):385–91.
32. Ghandour S, Matzinger O, Pachoud M. Volumetric-modulated arc therapy planning using multicriteria optimization for localized prostate cancer. J Appl Clin Med Phys. 2015;16(3):5410.

17

Radiation-induced muscle fibrosis rat model: establishment and valuation

Yue Zhou[1,5], Xiaowu Sheng[3,7], Feiyan Deng[2,6], Hui Wang[1], Liangfang Shen[4], Yong Zeng[3], Qianxi Ni[1], Shibin Zhan[2] and Xiao Zhou[2,3*]

Abstract

Background: Lack of animal model of radiation induced muscle fibrosis, this study aimed to establish such a model by using 90 Gy single dose irradiation to mimic clinical relevance and also to explore the potential post-irradiation regenerative mechanism.

Methods: SD rats were randomly divided into dose investigation groups and time gradient groups. Group1–6 were irradiated with a single dose of 65Gy, 70Gy, 75Gy, 80Gy, 85Gy and 90Gy respectively, and the degree of rectus femoris fibrosis in the irradiated area was detected at 4 weeks after irradiation. Group 7–9 were irradiated with a single dose of 90Gy, and the results were detected 1, 2, 4, and 8 weeks after irradiation. Then the general condition of rats was recorded. Masson staining was used to detect muscle fibrosis. The ultrastructure of muscles was observed by electron microscope, and the expression changes of satellite cell proliferation and differentiation related genes were detected by quantitative real-time-PCR.

Results: A single dose of 90Gy irradiation could cause muscle fibrosis in rats. As time goes on, the severity of muscle fibrosis and the expression of TGF- β1 increased. Significant swelling of mitochondria, myofilament disarrangement and dissolution, obvious endothelial cell swelling, increased vascular permeability, decrease of blood cell, deposition of fibrosis tissue around the vessel could be found compared with the control group. At around the 4th week, the expressions of Pax7, Myf5, MyoD, MyoG, Mrf4 increased.

Conclusion: Irradiation of 90Gy can successfully establish the rat model of radiation-induced muscle fibrosis. This model demonstrated that regenerative process was initiated by the irradiation only at an early stage, which can serve a suitable model for investigating regenerative therapy for post-radiation muscle fibrosis.

Keywords: Radiotherapy, Radiation damage, Muscle fibrosis, Rat model, Satellite cell

Background

Radiotherapy is an effective treatment for cancer, and more than 50% of tumor patients need it for radical or palliative treatment [1], for which can be used to treat various tumors, such as nasopharyngeal carcinoma (recommended as the preferred treatment), lung cancer, breast cancer, rectal cancer, etc. Radiation-induced fibrosis (RIF) is a long-term side effect of radiation therapy, and it results in a multitude of symptoms that significantly impact quality of life or even endangers patients' life [2]. Li Jian observed 267 cases of nasopharyngeal carcinoma after radiotherapy and found that all patients presented neck radiation fibrosis, and about 24.34% patients were of heavy degree. Their post irradiation symptoms included cervical muscle fibrosis, trismus, torticollis, neck muscle weakness, muscle dystonia, shoulder pain and shoulder functional disorder [3]. Many years of our clinical records demonstrate that radiation-induced fibrosis could cause local tissue scar and contracture, leading to difficulty in re-operation for cancer recurrence, while hypoxia in local tissues can result in poor efficacy of re-irradiation. The molecular mechanism of fibrosis induced by RIF is similar to that caused by other damages, such as sports, chemical stimulation, trauma and surgery

* Correspondence: cccdon@163.com
[2]Department of Head and Neck Surgery, Hunan Cancer Hospital and The Affiliated Cancer Hospital of Xiangya School of Medicine, Changsha, Hunan Province, China
[3]Translational Medical Center, Hunan Cancer Hospital and The Affiliated Cancer Hospital of Xiangya School of Medicine, Central South University, Changsha, Hunan Province, China
Full list of author information is available at the end of the article

[4–6]. The main mechanisms are: cellular DNA damage caused by radiation [7, 8], tissue cell or stem cell injury and loss [9], cellular signal pathway alterations such as the activation of TGF-β1 signaling pathway [4, 8], and genetic or epigenetic changes [7, 10, 11]. After injury, muscle tissue undergoes four stages: degeneration, inflammation, muscle regeneration and fibrosis formation. After irradiation, DNA damage, cell apoptosis and cell necrosis occur in tissue cells. And a series of inflammatory mediators are released during inflammatory reactions, including fibrosis promoting factors such as TNFα, IL-1, IL-6 [12], TGF-β1 [13–18], CTGF [19]; and the fibrosis inhibitory factors such as HGF [20], IFN-γ [21] release etc.. This process is also correlated to the activation of skeletal satellite cells(SCs) [22, 23]. SCs are the self-renewal myogenic stem cells in muscles, and can differentiate into new tissue cells.

Normally, SCs are in resting state expressing paired box gene 7 (Pax7). They are activated when the muscle is damaged. Those activated SCs migrate towards the injured site, enter the myogenic differentiation pathway, and express myogenic factor 5 (Myf5) immediately [24]. SCs proliferate furtherly, and some continue to undergo myogenic differentiation and express myogenic determining factor(MyoD). Then the expression of myogenin (MyoG) is followed, which promotes the fusion of myoblasts, and the combination with damaged fibers to repair them [25]. The release of inflammatory cytokines and mediators, and the changes of intracellular signal pathway, induce fibroblast activation and epithelial mesenchymal transition of other precursor cells (vascular endothelial cells) to form myofibroblast [6, 26, 27]. Sustained activation and proliferation of myofibroblasts, promotes collagen secretion and extracellular matrix local deposition [28], eventually leading to the formation of fibrosis [29], and fibrosis also inhibits muscle repair [28].

It can be seen from the above, proliferation and myogenic differentiation of SCs are the key factors for the repair of muscle injury. Therefore, we hypothesize that radiation could damage SCs and cause the difficulty of their activation and proliferation, affect muscle regeneration and repair, and thus change the process of fibrosis formation. And so far, no standardized therapy prevents RIF in muscle, and animal models for therapeutic tests are poorly established [30]. Thus, we establish a rat model of radiation induced muscle fibrosis, and study the proliferation and differentiation of SCs at different stages after irradiation. This provides new ideas and foundation for the treatment of RIF in the future.

Methods

Experimental animals

The SD rats used in this experiment were all 6-month-old, weighing about 220–250 g. They were divided into 9 groups (10 mice per group, half male and half female). Researchers involved have received the Central South University animal experiment training and obtained the certificates. The animal tests, housing and environmental conditions were in line with "the Guide for the Care and Use of Laboratory Animals" [31]. Rats were divided into cages (4 rats per cage). To reduce pressure of transportation, checking and adaptation for the new environment, a week of recovery time was given. Meanwhile, their diet, feces, urine and activities were observed every day. The rats were in good health after this adaptation period.

Establishment of the rat model for radiation-induced muscle fibrosis

Five percent pentobarbital sodium was injected intraperitoneally into the anesthetized rat (0.1 mL/100 g), and the surface of the medial rectus femoris on the left thigh was marked by a marker. And 10 min later, radiation was given by Nucletron Microselectron-HDR Ir-192 afterloading System (Nucletron Company / Nederland), with the applicator tube fixed at the mark on the left thigh. The dose normalization point was 0.5 cm below the source center, and the irradiation area was 0.5 cm radius around the mark point. Group 1 to 6 were respectively given 65Gy, 70Gy, 75Gy, 80Gy, 85Gy, 90Gy single dose of irradiation, and the fibrosis degree on the rectus femoris at the irradiated site was detected 4 weeks after irradiation. Group 7 to 9 were given 90Gy single dose of irradiation, and the results were detected at the 1st, 2nd, 4th and 8th week after irradiation respectively.

General conditions

The diet, feces, urine, activity and skin condition of rats were observed, and the number of dead rats was recorded.

Masson staining

The irradiated rectus femoris muscle was fixed by 4% formaldehyde for 24 h, and then slices of paraffin-embedded biopsy were produced. Masson trichrome staining (Baso, BA-40798) was used after slice dewaxing. The inverted microscope (Zeiss, Axio Scope A1) was used for observation. All visual fields in each slice were selected, and the percentage of collagen fibrosis area was analyzed by Image-Pro Plus 6 software (Media Cybernetics, Bethesda, USA).

Electron microscopy

The rectus femoris at irradiated site was embedded in chenodeoxycholic acid, and 24 h later tissue sections were carried out. The ultrastructure of vascular endothelial cells, muscle fibers and mitochondria were observed by Tecnai G2 Spirit and electron microscopy (FEI, Oregon, Hillsboro, USA). GATAN ORIUS CCD CAMERA (GATAN,

Coronado Lane, Pleasanton, CA, USA) was used to collect images.

Real time RT-PCR

The primers were designed by NCBI Primer-Blast and synthesized by Shanghai biological engineering company. The rectus femoris of group 7–9 were irradiated, then the RNA was extracted. First-strand cDNA was synthesized from 1 mg total RNA with a First Strand cDNA Synthesis Kit (Thermo Scientific, Massachusetts, USA). Total cDNA was amplified for over 45 cycles in a system, which contained SYBR Green I TaqMan probes (Roche, Basel, Switzerland). Relative gene expression was calculated with $2^{-\Delta\Delta CT}$ method, and GAPDH was used as housekeeping gene reference for normalization. The expression of PAX7, MyoD, MyoG, Mrf4, Myf5 were detected. The primer sequence was as follows (Table 1).

Western blot

The total protein was extracted from the cell lysate of the rats' rectus femoris. 10%SDS polyacrylamide gel was configured and 20 μg protein was added before electrophoresis. After electrophoresis, the protein was transferred to the PVDF membrane. 5% of the skimmed milk was closed for 1 h, and the first antibody (TGF-β1, GAPDH, 1:1000 dilution) was incubated overnight at 4 °C, then the membrane was washed. Then it incubated with the second antibody (The sheep anti-rabbit IgG conjugated to horseradish peroxidase; 1: 3000 dilution) at room temperature for 1 h, and the enhanced chemiluminescence(ECL) was performed after the membrane was washed.

Statistical analysis

All data are represented by mean ± standard error (mean ± SEM). The experimental data was processed by SPSS 13.0 software (SPSS, Chicago, IL, USA). The difference between groups was analyzed by t-test, and $p < 0.05$ means statistically significant.

Results

Masson staining of each dose group

To determine the appropriate radiation dose for the establishment of the rat model for radiation-induced muscle fibrosis, the Ir-192 high-dose-rate afterloading unit was used. Single dose was performed on the thigh rectus femoris of SD adult rats in the following dose groups: group 65Gy, group 70Gy, group 75Gy, group 80Gy, group 85Gy, group 90Gy. Muscle fibrosis was characterized by the increased secretion of collagen fibers and the deposition of extracellular matrix [28]. TGF- β1 is an important fibrosis promoting factor [13–18]. Muscle fibrosis usually occurs 2–4 weeks after injury, and becomes more serious as time goes on [28]. To confirm whether the muscle fibrosis model was formed after radiation exposure and to identify the effect of the model, masson staining was used to detect the fibrosis degree at the irradiated site 4 weeks after radiation.

The rats were divided into 6 dose groups: 65Gy, 70Gy, 75Gy, 80Gy, 85Gy, 90Gy. Four weeks after single irradiation of each dose on left rectus femoris, the muscle tissue biopsies were made and stained with Masson. Collagen fibers were blue, and muscle fibers were red. The percentage of fibrosis area increased with increasing dose. In control group, the percentage of fibrosis area was 4.43±0.46 ($n = 10$, Fig. 1a). In 65Gy group, it was 17.03±2.06($n = 10$, Fig. 1b). In 70Gy group, it was 19.48 ±2.88($n = 10$, Fig. 1c). In 75Gy group, it was 23.85 ±2.80($n = 10$, Fig. 1d). In 80Gy group, it was 25.45 ±3.29($n = 10$, Fig. 1e). In 85Gy group, it was 25.31 ±3.30($n = 10$, Fig. 1f). In 90Gy group, it was 30.15 ±3.13($n = 10$, Fig. 1g). The fibrosis area of 65Gy–90Gy group was higher than that of control group ($p < 0.001$, Fig. 1h).

General performance of rats after 90Gy single dose irradiation

To achieve stable effect, a single dose of 90Gy was selected for the model according to the Masson staining results. After irradiation with 90Gy radiation on the rectus femoris of SD adult rats, intermittent claudication occurred in very few rats (non-statistical data). No death was found, the feces and urine were normal, and no significant weight loss or hair loss occurred.

Muscle fibrosis increased with time after 90Gy single dose irradiation

One week, 2 weeks, 4 weeks and 8 weeks after 90Gy irradiation, the rectus femoris paraffin sections of the irradiated area were taken and stained with Masson.

Table 1 Primer sequence of the marker genes

Gene name	Upstream primers	Downstream primers
GAPDH	AGGTCGGTGTGAACGGATTTG	TGTAGACCATGTAGTTGAGGTCA
PAX7	GAGTATAAGAGGGAGAACCCCG	TTGATTCTGAGCACTCGGCTAA
MyoD	GCTCTGATGGCATGATGGATTAC	CTATGCTGGACAGGCAGTCG
MyoG	ACTACCTTCCTGTCCACCTTCA	AGGCCTCATTCACTTTCTTGAG
Mrf4	ACAGCTACAAACCCAAGCAAGA	CTTGCTCCTCCTTCCTTAGCAG
Myf5	TCTGATGGCATGCCTGAATGTAA	AAGGAGCTCTTATCTGAAGCACA

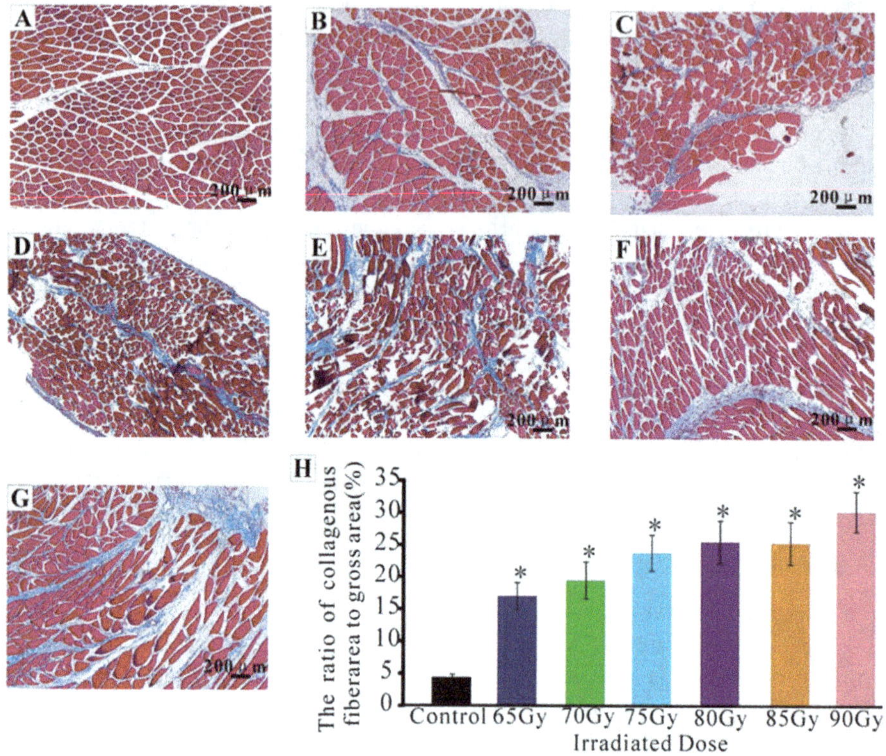

Fig. 1 Four weeks after irradiation, the Masson staining of rectus femoris muscle in each dose group. The collagen fibers were blue and the muscle fibers were red. **a** Control; **b** 65Gy; **c** 70Gy; **d** 75Gy; **e** 80Gy; **f** 85Gy; **g** 90Gy; **h**. analysis of collagen fiber area percentage in each dose group, $*p < 0.05$, compared with the control group. The area and percentage of muscular fibrosis increased with dose

Collagen fibers were almost invisible in the control group (no radiation exposure) (4.43±0.46, $n = 10$, Fig. 2a). Fibrosis area percentage in 90Gy-1w group increased comparing with the control group, but the amount was less (13.25±2.22, $n = 10$, Fig. 2b). Fibrosis area percentage in 90Gy-2w group increased comparing with the control group (20.73±2.53, $n = 10$, Fig. 2c). Fibrosis area percentage in 90Gy-4w group increased comparing with the control group (30.15±3.13, $n = 10$, Fig. 2d). Fibrosis area percentage in 90Gy-8w group increased comparing with the control group (36.36±2.73, $n = 10$, Fig. 2e).

TGF-β1 increased with time in the process of irradiation induced fibrosis

As an important fibrosis promoting factor, TGF-β1 mRNA expression level increased during the pathological process of fibrosis. The mRNA expression level of TGF-β1 was measured 1 week, 2 weeks and 4 weeks after 90Gy irradiation. No significant differences of TGF-β1 mRNA expression were found between 90Gy-1w group and the control group (1.53±0.58, $n = 6$, $p > 0.05$). Comparing with the control group, there was a growing trend of TGF-β1 mRNA expression in 90Gy-2w group, but with no statistical significance (3.34±1.22, $n = 6$, $p > 0.05$). TGF-β1 mRNA expression in 90Gy-4w group was more than that of control group (6.97±1.53, $n = 9$, $p < 0.05$) (Fig. 3a). TGF-β1 mRNA expression in 90Gy-8w group was more than that of control group (7.25±2.45, $n = 9$, $p < 0.05$) (Fig. 3a). Comparing with the control group there was an increasing tendency of TGF-β1 protein expression (Fig. 3b and c).

Ultrastructure of muscle tissue

Four weeks after the 90Gy radiation, the rectus femoris tissue of irradiated area was examined by electron microscopy. In the control group, the muscle filaments were arranged neatly (Fig. 4a and b), and the vascular endothelial shape was regular (Fig. 4c yellow arrows). Clear and obvious undamaged mitochondrial crista structures could be seen (Fig. 4d yellow circle, and Fig. 4e red stars). The shape of skeletal muscle nuclei was regular (Fig. 4f letter "N"). In 90Gy-4w group, the arrangement of muscle filaments was disordered, and the filament dissolved (Fig. 4g and h). Swollen skeletal muscle nuclei could be found (Fig. 4f letter "N"). The vascular endothelium swelled and was irregularly shaped (Fig. 4j green arrow). The linear structures were mitochondrial crista (Fig. 4l blue arrows), and the white area around (Fig. 4k and l green stars) was

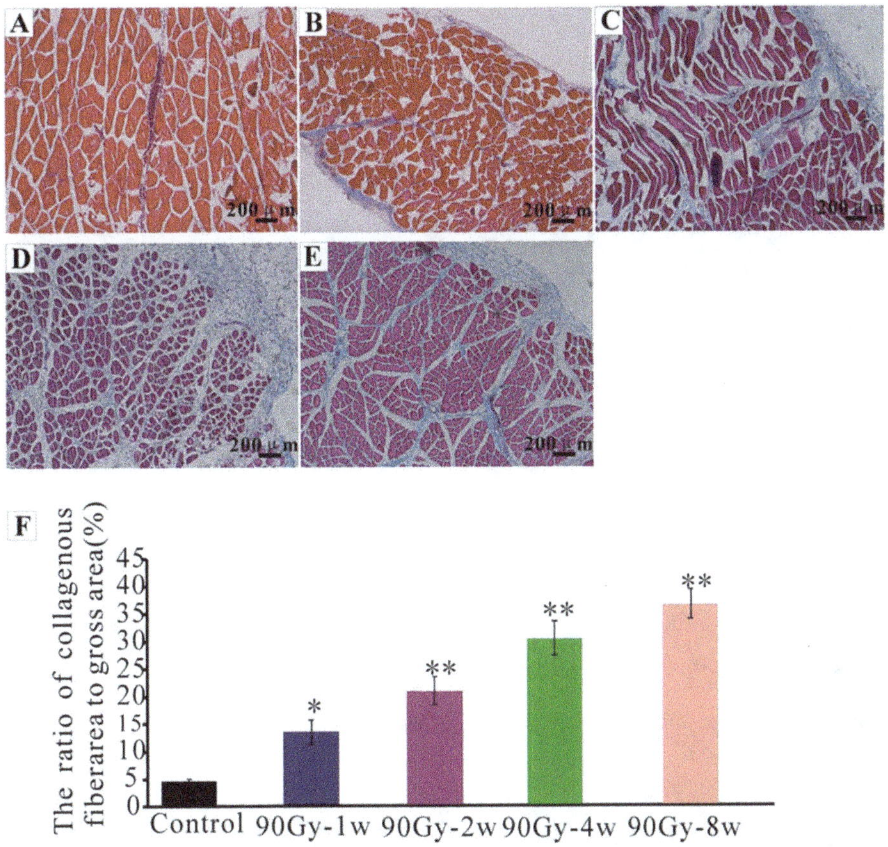

Fig. 2 Masson staining at different time points after 90Gy irradiation. The collagen fibers were blue and the muscle fibers were red. **a** control group; **b** 90Gy-1w group; **c** 90Gy-2w group; **d** 90Gy-4w group; **e** 90Gy-8w group; **f**. analysis of the collagen fiber area percentage in each group, $^*p < 0.05$, $^{**}p < 0.01$, compared with the control group. Muscle fibrosis aggravated with time

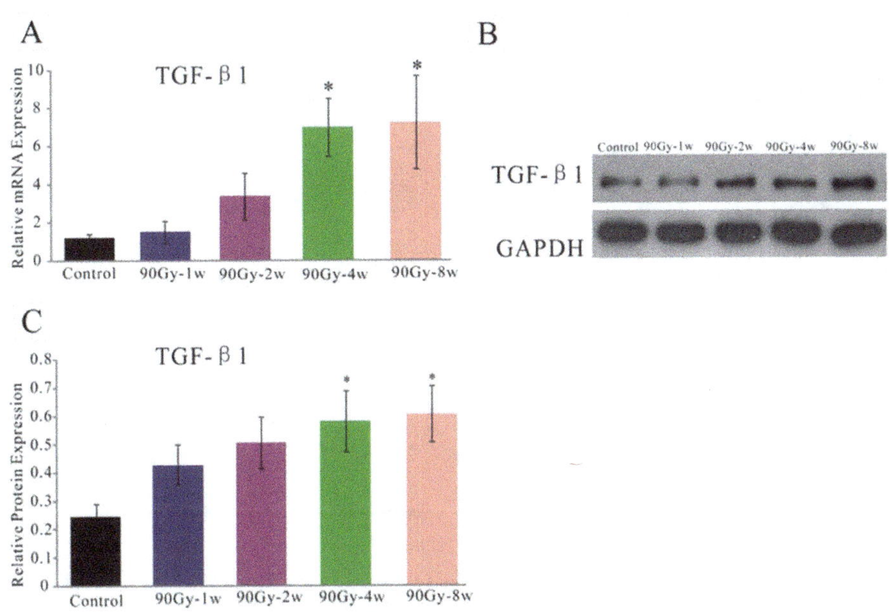

Fig. 3 a TGF-β1 mRNA expression level on 1 week, 2 weeks, 4 weeks and 8 weeks after 90Gy radiation($^*p < 0.05$). **b** Expression level of TGF-β1 protein on 1 week, 2 weeks, 4 weeks and 8 weeks after 90Gy radiation. **c** Expression level of TGF-β1 protein on 1 week, 2 weeks, 4 weeks and 8 weeks after 90Gy radiation($^*p < 0.05$). The expression of TGF- β 1 increased with time

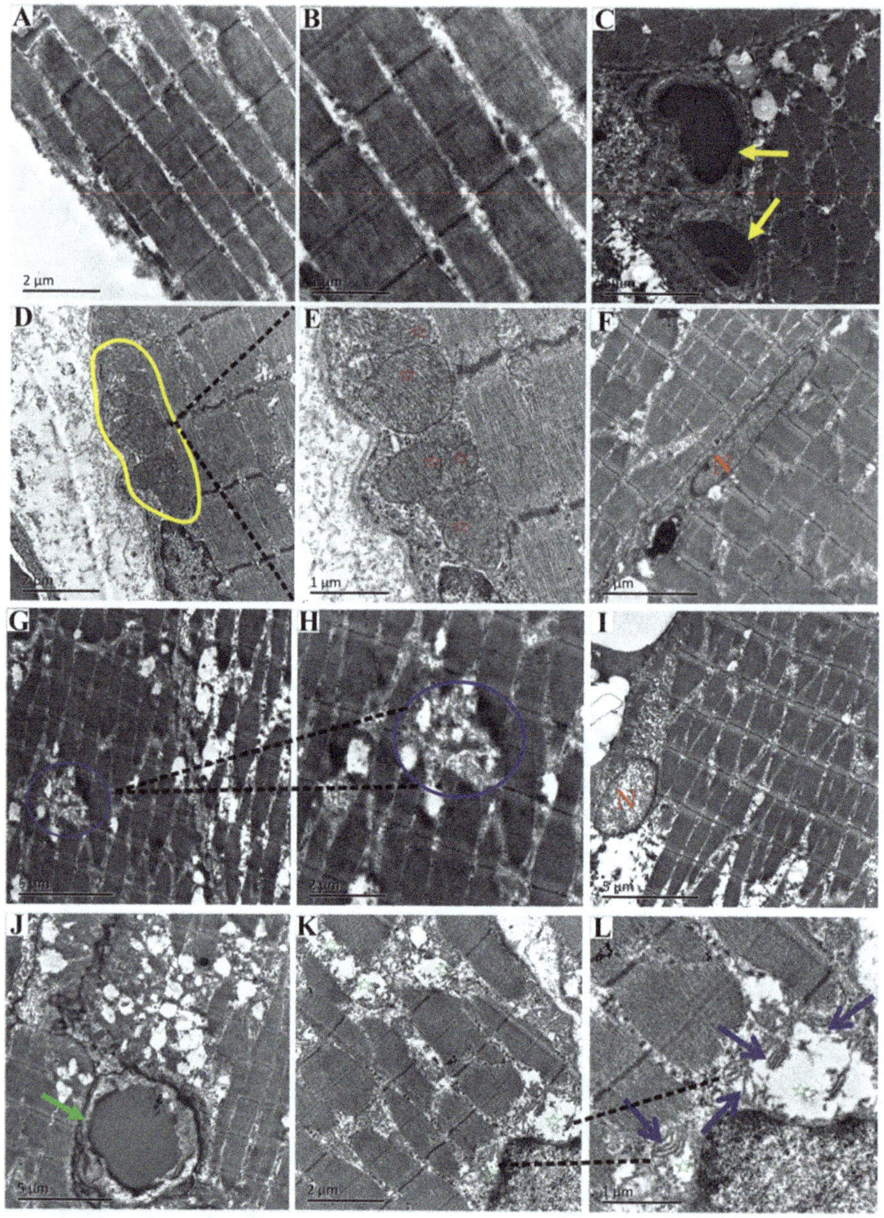

Fig. 4 Ultrastructure of muscle tissue detected by electron microscopy. **a-f**. Control group. **a-b**. Myofilaments. **c** Vascular endothelium. **d-e**. Mitochondrion. **f** Nuclei of myofilament. **g-l** 90Gy-4w group. **g-h** myofilament dissolving. **i** Swollen nuclei of myofilament. **j** Vascular endothelium. **l** Mitochondrial vacuolization

due to loss of it. Vacuolization of damaged mitochondria could be seen (Fig. 4k and l green stars).

Vascular injury

Four weeks after 90Gy radiation, Masson staining was performed on the rectus femoris tissue at the irradiated site. In the normal group, many blood cells could be seen in the lumen of the vessel (Fig. 5 A partly enlarged sectional view). In 90Gy-4w group, the blood cells decreased and even disappeared from the vessel lumen, with collagen fiber hyperplasia around the blood vessels (Fig. 5b partly enlarged sectional view).

Gene expression involved in muscle regeneration

Skeletal SCs are the myoblast stem cells in the muscle, playing an important role in the repair of muscle damage [32].

The genetic expression related to skeletal muscle satellite cells was detected at different time points after 90Gy radiation.

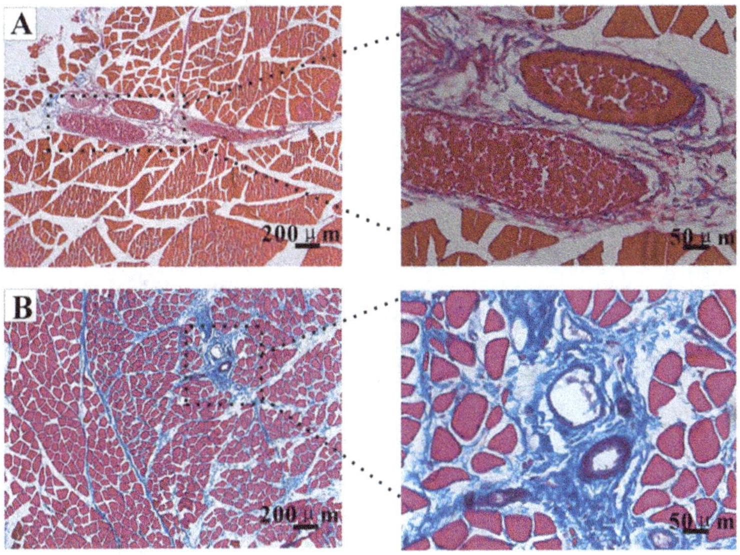

Fig. 5 Four weeks after 90 Gy irradiation, Masson staining was used to detect vascular injury. **a** Normal group. The vessel had a regular shape with lots of blood cells in the lumen; **b** 90Gy-4w group. In the arterial lumen, blood cells reduced, and tube wall was thickened. In the venous lumen, blood cells disappeared. A large amount of collagen fibers proliferated around the vessels

Pax7: 1 week after irradiation, Pax7 mRNA expression was higher than the control group, with no statistical significance (2.14±0.57, $n = 7$, $p > 0.05$). Two weeks after irradiation, its expression was higher than the control group, with no statistical significance (2.39±0.74, $n = 5$, $p > 0.05$). Four weeks after irradiation, its expression was higher than the control group, with statistically significance (3.96±0.90, $n = 10$, $p < 0.05$). Eight weeks after irradiation, there was no difference in its expression compared with the control group (0.67±0.24, $n = 8$, $p > 0.05$);

Mrf5: 1 week after irradiation, Myf5 mRNA expression was lower than the control group, with statistical significance (0.42±0.10, $n = 8$, $p < 0.05$). Two weeks after irradiation, its expression was lower than the control group, with statistical significance (2.82±0.64, $n = 6$, $p < 0.05$). Four weeks after irradiation, its expression was higher than the control group, with statistical significance (3.61 ±0.87, $n = 8$, $p < 0.05$). Eight weeks after irradiation, there was no difference in its expression compared with the control group (1.38±0.34, $n = 8$, $p > 0.05$);

MyoD: 1 week after irradiation, there was a decreasing trend of MyoD mRNA expression comparing with the control group, with no statistical significance (0.74±0.25, $n = 7$, $p > 0.05$). Two weeks after irradiation, its expression was lower than the control group, with statistical significance (2.45±0.30, $n = 6$, $p < 0.05$). Four weeks after irradiation, its expression was higher than the control group, with statistical significance (5.06±1.30, $n = 11$, $p < 0.05$). Eight weeks after irradiation, there was no difference in its expression compared with the control group (0.61±0.17, $n = 8$, $p > 0.05$);

MyoG: 1 week after irradiation, MyoG mRNA expression was lower than the control group, with statistical significance (0.45±0.10, $n = 7$, $p < 0.05$). Two weeks after irradiation, its expression was not different from the control group (1.49±0.32, $n = 6$, $p > 0.05$). Four weeks after irradiation, there was an increasing trend in the expression compared with the control group, with no statistical difference (2.91±1.14, $n = 7$, $p > 0.05$). Eight weeks after irradiation, there was no difference in its expression compared with the control group (1.24±0.33, $n = 8$, $p > 0.05$);

Mrf4: 1 week after irradiation, Mrf4 mRNA expression was lower than the control group, with statistical significance (0.55±0.12, $n = 7$, $p < 0.05$). Two weeks after irradiation, Mrf4 mRNA expression was lower than the control group, with statistical significance (2.82±0.56, $n = 6$, $p < 0.05$). Four weeks after irradiation, Mrf4 mRNA expression was higher than the control group, with statistical significance (5.73±1.39, $n = 9$, $p < 0.05$). Eight weeks after irradiation, Mrf4 mRNA expression was higher than the control group, with statistical significance (2.48±0.53, $n = 8$, $p < 0.05$).

Discussion

Commonly seen months or years after radiotherapy of head and neck tumors, radiation-induced fibrosis (RIF), a late complication of radiotherapy, is irreversible. Clinically, RIF is usually caused by high doses of fractionated radiotherapy, and its symptoms include skin ulcers, scarring, muscle atrophy and limited joint activity. Chen et al. [33] found radiation induced trismus for nasopharyngeal carcinoma patients progressed over time. Safora

Johansen [34] reported that radiotherapy for breast cancer patients may lead to arm/shoulder pain, restricted arm/shoulder mobility, fibrosis and breast cancer-related lymphedema. However, some previous studies showed that single high dose could induce similar effect on animal models. Gallet P reported 30Gy cobalt 60 irradiation could cause radiation-induced skin and muscle fibrosis in rats [35]. Xinchu Ni reported that a single dose of radiation (80Gy) from a linear accelerator was sufficient in establishing a rabbit model of skeletal muscle injury [36]. HSU et al. indicated that the Wistar rats, when exposed to 80Gy X-rays from a linear accelerator, displayed muscle cell injury [37]. But these experiments of animal models rarely described the RIF symptoms, and the reported doses deviated from clinical ones. Moreover, different radiotherapy equipments also resulted in variations of fibrosis forming efficiency. In addition, radiation-induced fibrosis is characterized by fibroblasts proliferation, myofibroblast differentiation, and synthesis of collagen, proteoglycans and extracellular matrix [29, 38]. In previous studies, those reported animal models could not reach a similar level. In clinics, radiation induced tissue fibrosis process includes skin induration and thickening, muscle shortening and atrophy, and so on [39]. To build an effective and clinical relevant animal model, we explored different doses and found that 90Gy was appropriate, because this dose caused typical pathological findings in accordance with human's, including inflammation, fibroblast recruitment and extracellular matrix deposition [2]. In addition to muscle fibrosis, we also observed that that a few days after the radiotherapy, severe skin ulcers occurred in rats. Then skin scarring appeared, and intermittent claudication happened, conforming to clinical manifestation. Therefore, 90Gy irradiation was chosen to construct the skeletal fibrosis model. Although irradiation as low as 65Gy could induce skeletal muscle fibrosis, the dosage below 90Gy failed to represent clinical relevant pathological process.

In a previous study, Wei Sun [40], reported that collagen fibers gradually increased in skeletal muscles with the time extension after irradiation. Fibrosis occurred 2–3 weeks after injury, and its area enlarged over time [28]. Our data showed that fibrosis began to appear 1 week after 90Gy irradiation, and its percentage increased over time. TGF-β1 has been considered a key profibrotic cytokine. As two features of radiation-induced fibrosis, DNA damage and inflammation lead to the activation of TGF-β1 and canonical WNT/β-catenin pathway [41]. TGF-β1 is essential for the differentiation of fibroblasts into myofibroblasts [42]. As non-muscle cells, myofibroblasts can contract and relax, and induce an active retraction of granulation tissue, leading to fibrosis [43–45]. Critical for cellular fibrosis in wound as well as numerous organs like kidney, heart, lung, and liver, myofibroblasts play an important role in the phenomenon of contraction-retraction that lasts without relaxation, with an irreversible retraction favored by the synthesis of collagen [41]. Besides, in injured skeletal muscle, TGF-β1 can also induce differentiation of myoblasts into fibrotic cells [46]. TGF-β1 expression gradually increases in a dose-dependent manner and peaks 4 weeks after irradiation [47]. In our study, fibrosis percentage ((Fig. 2) and TGF-β1 expression (Fig. 3) increased with time after irradiation. It is known that TGF-β1 promotes myofibroblast differentiation contributing to RIF, so TGF-β1 may to be proposed as a major target for antifibrotic agents [41, 48, 49].

In addition to TGF- β1, energy metabolism system may also be affected by radiation damage, as it plays an important role in the contraction and relaxation of skeletal muscle [50]. The mitochondria of skeletal muscle are closely related to energy metabolism and muscular function, as they are both the sites of oxidative phosphorylation to synthesis ATP providing energy, and the important organelles regulating intracellular calcium concentration [51]. Recent studies suggest mitochondria may be susceptible to radiation, and could be a source of radiation-induced oxidative stress [52, 53]. The results of the ultrastructure of the experiment (Fig. 4) showed that, there were vacuolated changes of mitochondria in the skeletal muscle cells after irradiation, indicating cell damage and the energy metabolism disorder caused by mitochondria damage. Damage to blood vessels and subsequent hypoxia and ischemia are known to contribute to severe tissue injury such as fibrosis and necrosis [54]. Vascular fibrosis after radiotherapy contributes to severe normal tissue damage and, in some cases, may be a vital prognosis in patients [55]. Irradiation could cause vasculature injury, which is a clinical problem, and endothelial cell damage, which is characterized by increased vascular permeability and endothelial cell apoptosis [56–58]. A few hours and weeks after irradiation, it was observed that endothelial cells would swell with edema, lymphocyte adhesion and infiltration, and endothelial cell apoptosis, which caused vasculature barrier function to lose, integrity to change and permeability to increase [58]. In our study, 4 weeks after irradiation we found endothelium cells swelling (Fig. 4) and vascular permeability changes induced by radiation, with fibrosis formation and fibrins deposition around the vasculature (Fig. 5) in this process. These phenomena indicated that vasculature injury may play a role in muscular fibrosis formation.

Enhancing muscle regeneration maybe a good strategy to overcome the fibrosis caused by radiotherapy. For this reason, we have carried out a detailed study on the genes related to muscle regeneration. Muscle satellite cells are an important cell source for muscle regeneration, and they differentiate into muscle cells through upregulating Pax7 and myogenic regulatory factors (MRFs). Quiescent Skeletal muscle satellite cells are in G0 phase, implying their resistance to radiation [59]. Pax7 is specifically expressed in proliferating myoblasts, controlling the activation and migration of satellite cell precursors [60]. Pax7 act as master regulators of early lineage specification and are expressed genetically upstream of MRFs during early muscle development [61]. And the expression of MRFs consisting of MyoD, Myf5, MyoG and Mrf4 characterizes various phases of skeletal muscle development including myoblast proliferation, cell-cycle exit, cell fusion and the maturation of myotubes to form myofibers [62]. Our data (Fig. 6) showed that 1 week after 90Gy irradiation, the expression of Pax7 were up regulated, indicating satellite cell enrichment. And the decrease in expression of MRFs may due to the radiation damage to myoblasts, causing myoblasts to decrease. At the 2nd and 4th week after irradiation, myogenic gene expressions were upregulated, indicating muscle regeneration enhancement. It is known that the Pax7 expressed in satellite cells are downregulated during muscle cell differentiation [63]. The primary MRFs including Myf5 and MyoD commit cells to a myogenic program, and the secondary MRFs consisting of MyoG and Mrf4 are terminal differentiation genes that are important for fusion of myocytes and formation of myotubes [64]. In our study (Fig. 6), 8 weeks after radiotherapy, Pax7 and MRFs except for Mrf4 fell to a state similar to that of normal muscles. And this may be that some myoblasts continue to differentiate, fuse and mature. A part of myoblast or activated skeletal muscle satellite cells return to resting state, then muscle regeneration stopped. This data indicated that satellite cells can be activated and differentiate for muscle regeneration after irradiation. But muscle regeneration after radiation was not enough to counteract the fibrosis caused by it. It showed that 8 weeks of 90gy can effectively organize the intrinsic regenerative ability of the muscles, so the model is established successfully. In the future, muscle regeneration can be explored from this model, such as local or systemic injection of stem cells, growth factors, and so on. We also suggest that these actions should be taken immediately after irradiation. This may be an effective prevention for radiation-induced fibrosis, by enhancing muscle regeneration, and inducing powerful satellite cell activation and differentiation.

Conclusions

This study established a rat model of irradiation induced muscle fibrosis with 90Gy dosage. The severity of muscle fibrosis and the expression of TGF-β1 increased with the time after radiation was demonstrated. And it was found that radiation damaged vascular endothelial cells, and deposition of fibrosis tissue around the vessel was found. Therefore, vascular endothelial injury may play an important role in the formation of fibrosis. Activation and

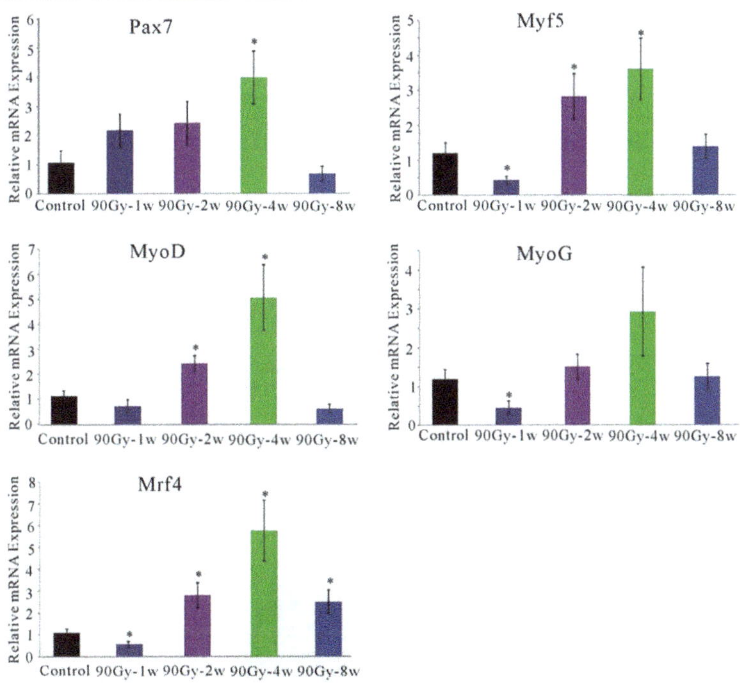

Fig. 6 At different time points after 90Gy irradiation, gene expressions (Pax7, Myf5, MyoD, MyoG and Mrf4) related to skeletal muscle satellite cell proliferation and myogenic differentiation in the rectus femoris. (*$p < 0.05$ compared with the control group.) The expression of Pax7 increased in first week, peaked the fourth week, and fell to a normal level at the eighth week. Mrf5, MyoD, MyoG dropped in the first week, then increased peaking on the fourth week, and fell to a normal level at the eighth week. Mrf4 dropped in the first week, then increased peaking on fourth week, and fell to a level higher than normal at the eighth week

myogenic differentiation of skeletal muscle satellite cells occurred after radiation, leading to muscle regeneration, though not enough to counterbalance the formation of fibrosis. In the future, we would research the relationship between vascular endothelial injury and the formation of radiation-induced muscle fibrosis, and look for a way to promote the activation, proliferation, migration and differentiation of skeletal muscle satellite cells, enhancing muscle regeneration.

Abbreviations

CSs: Satellite cells; CTGF: Connective tissue growth factor; GAPDH: Glyceraldehyde 3-phosphate dehydrogenase; HGF: Hepatocyte growth factor; IFN-γ: Interferon γ; IL-1: Interleukin 1; IL-6: Interleukin 6; Mrf5: Myogenic factor 5; MRFs: Myogenic regulatory factors; MyoD: Myogenic determining factor; MyoG: Myogenin; Pax-7: Paired box protein 7; PVDF: Polyvinylidene difluoride; RIF: Radiation-induced fibrosis; SDS: Sodium dodecyl sulfate; TGF-β1: Transforming growth factor beta 1

Acknowledgements

The authors acknowledge Lei Xue, Nina Gao, Zichao Ma, Bo Liang, Chenhui Luo for their valuable advices and help.

Funding

1. The National Health and Family Planning Commission, the national key specialist construction project of the oncology department, research and development of tissue engineering bone and cartilage and its clinical application transformation project, Health office medical letter [2013] 544.
2. Key project of Hunan Natural Science Foundation, effect observation and mechanism discussion of adipose stem cell in the treatment of radiation induced muscle fibrosis, 12JJ2047.
3. Hunan Medical Center for clinical medicine of Oncoplastic Surgery, 2013TP4087.
4. Youth Fund of Hunan Natural Science Fund, Study on the effect of chemotherapy drugs commonly used in hematological malignancies on human adipose stem cells, 2017JJ3193.
5. Hunan Natural Science Foundation, Joint project on science and health, 2018JJ6025.
6. Fund of Key Laboratory of Translational Radiation Oncology, Hunan Province, 2015TP1009.
7. National Natural Science Foundation of China, 81472802.

Authors' contributions

YZ: study design, experiment performing, data analysis, manuscript preparation and manuscript editing, manuscript review. XWS: study design, literature research, definition of intellectual content, data analysis, data interpretation, manuscript preparation. FYD: experiment performing, data acquisition, literature research. All authors made substantial intellectual contributions to drafting the article, revising the article. All authors have read and approved the final manuscript.

Competing interests

The authors declare that they have no competing interests.

Author details

[1]Department of Radiation Oncology, Key Laboratory of Translational Radiation Oncology, Hunan Province. Department of Radiation Oncology, Hunan Cancer Hospital and The Affiliated Cancer Hospital of Xiangya School of Medicine, Central South University, Changsha, Hunan Province, China. [2]Department of Head and Neck Surgery, Hunan Cancer Hospital and The Affiliated Cancer Hospital of Xiangya School of Medicine, Changsha, Hunan Province, China. [3]Translational Medical Center, Hunan Cancer Hospital and The Affiliated Cancer Hospital of Xiangya School of Medicine, Central South University, Changsha, Hunan Province, China. [4]Department of Tumor, Xiangya Hospital of Central South University, Changsha, Hunan Province, China. [5]Xiangya School of Medicine, Central South University, Changsha, Hunan Province, China. [6]University of South China, Hengyang, Hunan Province, China. [7]Central Laboratory, Hunan Cancer Hospital and The Affiliated Cancer Hospital of Xiangya School of Medicine, Central South University, Changsha, Hunan Province, China.

References

1. Shukla L, Morrison WA, Shayan R. Adipose-derived stem cells in radiotherapy injury: a new frontier. Front Surg. 2015;2:1.
2. Straub JM, New J, Hamilton CD, Lominska C, Shnayder Y, Thomas SM. Radiation-induced fibrosis: mechanisms and implications for therapy. J Cancer Res Clin Oncol. 2015;141(11):1985–94.
3. Jian LI, Wang RS, Gan LG. Radiation-induced neck fibrosis in patients with nasopharyngeal carcinoma. Chin J Radiat Mediation Prot. 2005;03:253–55.
4. Yarnold J, Brotons MC. Pathogenetic mechanisms in radiation fibrosis. Radiother Oncol. 2010;97(1):149–61.
5. Cheresh P, Kim SJ, Tulasiram S, Kamp DW. Oxidative stress and pulmonary fibrosis. Biochim Biophys Acta. 2013;1832(7):1028–40.
6. Zvaifler NJ. Relevance of the stroma and epithelial-mesenchymal transition (EMT) for the rheumatic diseases. Arthritis Res Ther. 2006;8(3):210.
7. Koturbash I, Rugo RE, Hendricks CA, Loree J, Thibault B, Kutanzi K, Pogribny I, Yanch JC, Engelward BP, Kovalchuk O. Irradiation induces DNA damage and modulates epigenetic effectors in distant bystander tissue in vivo. Oncogene. 2006;25(31):4267–75.
8. Dickey JS, Baird BJ, Redon CE, Sokolov MV, Sedelnikova OA, Bonner WM. Intercellular communication of cellular stress monitored by gamma-H2AX induction. Carcinogenesis. 2009;30(10):1686–95.
9. Coppes RP, van der Goot A, Lombaert IM. Stem cell therapy to reduce radiation-induced normal tissue damage. Semin Radiat Oncol. 2009; 19(2):112–21.
10. Mothersill C, Seymour C. Are epigenetic mechanisms involved in radiation-induced bystander effects? Front Genet. 2012;3:74.
11. Kuhmann C, Weichenhan D, Rehli M, Plass C, Schmezer P, Popanda O. DNA methylation changes in cells regrowing after fractioned ionizing radiation. Radiother Oncol. 2011;101(1):116–21.
12. Gaugler MH, Vereycken-Holler V, Squiban C, Vandamme M, Vozenin-Brotons MC, Benderitter M. Pravastatin limits endothelial activation after irradiation and decreases the resulting inflammatory and thrombotic responses. Radiat Res. 2005;163(5):479–87.
13. Pohlers D, Brenmoehl J, Loffler I, Muller CK, Leipner C, Schultze-Mosgau S, Stallmach A, Kinne RW, Wolf G. TGF-beta and fibrosis in different organs - molecular pathway imprints. Biochim Biophys Acta. 2009; 1792(8):746–56.
14. Kruse JJ, Floot BG, te Poele JA, Russell NS, Stewart FA. Radiation-induced activation of TGF-beta signaling pathways in relation to vascular damage in mouse kidneys. Radiat Res. 2009;171(2):188–97.
15. Ruiz-Ortega M, Rodriguez-Vita J, Sanchez-Lopez E, Carvajal G, Egido J. TGF-beta signaling in vascular fibrosis. Cardiovasc Res. 2007;74(2):196–206.
16. Fujii H, Kawada N. Inflammation and fibrogenesis in steatohepatitis. J Gastroenterol. 2012;47(3):215–25.
17. Westbury CB, Yarnold JR. Radiation fibrosis--current clinical and therapeutic perspectives. Clin Oncol (R Coll Radiol). 2012;24(10):657–72.
18. Li C, Wilson PB, Levine E, Barber J, Stewart AL, Kumar S. TGF-beta1 levels in pre-treatment plasma identify breast cancer patients at risk of developing post-radiotherapy fibrosis. Int J Cancer. 1999;84(2):155–9.

19. Haydont V, Riser BL, Aigueperse J, Vozenin-Brotons MC. Specific signals involved in the long-term maintenance of radiation-induced fibrogenic differentiation: a role for CCN2 and low concentration of TGF-beta1. Am J Phys Cell Physiol. 2008; 294(6):C1332–41.
20. Hu S, Chen Y, Li L, Chen J, Wu B, Zhou X, Zhi G, Li Q, Wang R, Duan H, et al. Effects of adenovirus-mediated delivery of the human hepatocyte growth factor gene in experimental radiation-induced heart disease. Int J Radiat Oncol Biol Phys. 2009;75(5):1537–44.
21. Gottlober P, Steinert M, Bahren W, Weber L, Gerngross H, Peter RU. Interferon-gamma in 5 patients with cutaneous radiation syndrome after radiation therapy. Int J Radiat Oncol Biol Phys. 2001;50(1):159–66.
22. Best TM, Hunter KD. Muscle injury and repair. Phys Med Rehabil Clin N Am. 2000;11(2):251–66.
23. Russell B, Dix DJ, Haller DL, Jacobs-El J. Repair of injured skeletal muscle: a molecular approach. Med Sci Sports Exerc. 1992;24(2):189–96.
24. Pownall ME, Gustafsson MK, Emerson CP Jr. Myogenic regulatory factors and the specification of muscle progenitors in vertebrate embryos. Annu Rev Cell Dev Biol. 2002;18:747–83.
25. Wang YX, Rudnicki MA. Satellite cells, the engines of muscle repair. Nat Rev Mol Cell Biol. 2011;13(2):127–33.
26. Krenning G, Zeisberg EM, Kalluri R. The origin of fibroblasts and mechanism of cardiac fibrosis. J Cell Physiol. 2010;225(3):631–7.
27. Hinz B, Phan SH, Thannickal VJ, Galli A, Bochaton-Piallat ML, Gabbiani G. The myofibroblast: one function, multiple origins. Am J Pathol. 2007;170(6):1807–16.
28. Huard J, Li Y, Fu FH. Muscle injuries and repair: current trends in research. J Bone Joint Surg Am. 2002;84-a(5):822–32.
29. Wynn TA. Cellular and molecular mechanisms of fibrosis. J Pathol. 2008; 214(2):199–210.
30. Bracey D, Willey JS, Tallant EA, Gallagher PD, Smith TL, Callahan MF, Emory CL. The endogenous peptide angiotensin-(1-7) prevents radiation-induced muscle fibrosis: an in vivo murine model. Int J Radiat Oncol Biol Phys. 2013;87(2):S167.
31. Care NRCCftUotGft, Animals UoL. Guide for the care and use of laboratory animals. Astronomy Astrophysics. 2011;327(3):963–5.
32. Endo T. Molecular mechanisms of skeletal muscle development, regeneration, and osteogenic conversion. Bone. 2015;80:2–13.
33. Yuan-Yuan Chen MD, Chong ZM, Jin WM, Hong-Lian Ma MD, Shu-Zheng Lai MD, Yuan LM, Fei HM, Li-Xia Lu MD, Yong BM, Ming CM. Intensity-modulated radiation therapy reduces radiation-induced trismus in patients with nasopharyngeal carcinoma. Cancer. 2011;117(13):2910–6.
34. Johansen S, Fosså K, Nesvold IL, Malinen E, Fosså SD. Arm and shoulder morbidity following surgery and radiotherapy for breast cancer. Acta Oncol. 2014;53(4):521.
35. Gallet P, Phulpin B, Merlin JL, Leroux A, Bravetti P, Mecellem H, Tran N, Dolivet G. Long-term alterations of cytokines and growth factors expression in irradiated tissues and relation with histological severity scoring. PLoS One. 2011;6(12):e29399.
36. Ni X, Sun W, Sun S, Yu J, Wang J, Nie B, Sun Z, Ni X, Cai L, Cao X. Therapeutic potential of adipose stem cells in tissue repair of irradiated skeletal muscle in a rabbit model. Cell Reprogram. 2014;16(2):140–50.
37. Hsu HY, Chai CY, Lee MS. Radiation-induced muscle damage in rats after fractionated high-dose irradiation. Radiat Res. 1998;149(5):482–6.
38. Wynn TA. Fibrotic disease and the T(H)1/T(H)2 paradigm. Nat Rev Immunol. 2004;4(8):583–94.
39. Dörr W, Hendry JH. Consequential late effects in normal tissues. Radiother Oncol. 2001;61(3):223–31.
40. Sun W, Ni X, Sun S, Cai L, Yu J, Wang J, Nie B, Sun Z, Ni X, Cao X. Adipose-derived stem cells alleviate radiation-induced muscular fibrosis by suppressing the expression of TGF-beta1. Stem Cells Int. 2016;2016:5638204.
41. Vallee A, Lecarpentier Y, Guillevin R, Vallee JN. Interactions between TGF-beta1, canonical WNT/beta-catenin pathway and PPAR gamma in radiation-induced fibrosis. Oncotarget. 2017;8(52):90579–604.
42. Wei J, Bhattacharyya S, Jain M, Varga J. Regulation of matrix remodeling by peroxisome proliferator-activated receptor-gamma: a novel link between metabolism and Fibrogenesis. Open Rheumatol J. 2012;6:103–15.
43. Gabbiani G, Hirschel BJ, Ryan GB, Statkov PR, Majno G. Granulation tissue as a contractile organ. A study of structure and function. J Exp Med. 1972; 135(4):719–34.
44. Hasan HF, Abdel-Rafei MK, Galal SM. Diosmin attenuates radiation-induced hepatic fibrosis by boosting PPAR-gamma expression and hampering miR-17-5p-activated canonical Wnt-beta-catenin signaling. Biochem Cell Biol. 2017;95(3):400–14.
45. Zampieri F, Coen M, Gabbiani G. The prehistory of the cytoskeleton concept. Cytoskeleton (Hoboken, NJ). 2014;71(8):464–71.
46. Li Y, Foster W, Deasy BM, Chan Y, Prisk V, Tang Y, Cummins J, Huard J. Transforming growth factor-beta1 induces the differentiation of myogenic cells into fibrotic cells in injured skeletal muscle: a key event in muscle fibrogenesis. Am J Pathol. 2004;164(3):1007–19.
47. Imaeda M, Ishikawa H, Yoshida Y, Takahashi T, Ohkubo Y, Musha A, Komachi M, Nakazato Y, Nakano T. Long-term pathological and immunohistochemical features in the liver after intraoperative whole-liver irradiation in rats. J Radiat Res. 2014;55(4):665–73.
48. Martin M, Lefaix J, Delanian S. TGF-beta1 and radiation fibrosis: a master switch and a specific therapeutic target? Int J Radiat Oncol Biol Phys. 2000; 47(2):277–90.
49. Citrin DE, Prasanna PGS, Walker AJ, Freeman ML, Eke I, Barcellos-Hoff MH, Arankalayil MJ, Cohen EP, Wilkins RC, Ahmed MM, et al. Radiation-induced fibrosis: mechanisms and opportunities to mitigate. Report of an NCI workshop, September 19, 2016. Radiat Res. 2017;188(1):1–20.
50. Soboll S, Conrad A, Eistert A, Herick K, Kramer R. Uptake of creatine phosphate into heart mitochondria: a leak in the creatine shuttle. Biochim Biophys Acta. 1997;1320(1):27–33.
51. Alexander KC, Aiyar AS, Sreenivasan A. Site of impairment of oxidative phosphorylation in irradiated rats. Biochim Biophys Acta. 1972;283(2):206–16.
52. Barjaktarovic Z, Schmaltz D, Shyla A, Azimzadeh O, Schulz S, Haagen J, Dorr W, Sarioglu H, Schafer A, Atkinson MJ, et al. Radiation-induced signaling results in mitochondrial impairment in mouse heart at 4 weeks after exposure to X-rays. PLoS One. 2011;6(12):e27811.
53. Barjaktarovic Z, Shyla A, Azimzadeh O, Schulz S, Haagen J, Dorr W, Sarioglu H, Atkinson MJ, Zischka H, Tapio S. Ionising radiation induces persistent alterations in the cardiac mitochondrial function of C57BL/6 mice 40 weeks after local heart exposure. Radiother Oncol. 2013;106(3):404–10.
54. Milliat F, Francois A, Isoir M, Deutsch E, Tamarat R, Tarlet G, Atfi A, Validire P, Bourhis J, Sabourin JC, et al. Influence of endothelial cells on vascular smooth muscle cells phenotype after irradiation: implication in radiation-induced vascular damages. Am J Pathol. 2006;169(4):1484–95.
55. Dorresteijn LD, Kappelle AC, Boogerd W, Klokman WJ, Balm AJ, Keus RB, van Leeuwen FE, Bartelink H. Increased risk of ischemic stroke after radiotherapy on the neck in patients younger than 60 years. J Clin Oncol. 2002;20(1):282–8.
56. Heckmann M, Douwes K, Peter R, Degitz K. Vascular activation of adhesion molecule mRNA and cell surface expression by ionizing radiation. Exp Cell Res. 1998;238(1):148–54.
57. Langley RE, Bump EA, Quartuccio SG, Medeiros D, Braunhut SJ. Radiation-induced apoptosis in microvascular endothelial cells. Br J Cancer. 1997;75(5): 666–72.
58. Paris F, Fuks Z, Kang A, Capodieci P, Juan G, Ehleiter D, Haimovitz-Friedman A, Cordon-Cardo C, Kolesnick R. Endothelial apoptosis as the primary lesion initiating intestinal radiation damage in mice. Science (New York, NY). 2001; 293(5528):293–7.
59. Hubenak JR, Zhang Q, Branch CD, Kronowitz SJ. Mechanisms of injury to normal tissue after radiotherapy: a review. Plast Reconstr Surg. 2014;133(1):49e–56e.
60. Seale P, Sabourin LA, Girgis-Gabardo A, Mansouri A, Gruss P, Rudnicki MA. Pax7 is required for the specification of myogenic satellite cells. Cell. 2000;102(6):777–86.
61. Collins CA, Gnocchi VF, White RB, Boldrin L, Perez-Ruiz A, Relaix F, Morgan JE, Zammit PS. Integrated functions of Pax3 and Pax7 in the regulation of proliferation, cell size and myogenic differentiation. PLoS One. 2009;4(2):e4475.
62. Lee EJ, Malik A, Pokharel S, Ahmad S, Mir BA, Cho KH, Kim J, Kong JC, Lee DM, Chung KY, et al. Identification of genes differentially expressed in myogenin knock-down bovine muscle satellite cells during differentiation through RNA sequencing analysis. PLoS One. 2014;9(3):e92447.
63. Kuang S, Rudnicki MA. The emerging biology of satellite cells and their therapeutic potential. Trends Mol Med. 2008;14(2):82–91.
64. Yin H, Zhang S, Gilbert ER, Siegel PB, Zhu Q, Wong EA. Expression profiles of muscle genes in postnatal skeletal muscle in lines of chickens divergently selected for high and low body weight. Poult Sci. 2014;93(1):147–54.

18

Estimation of the risk for radiation-induced liver disease following photon- or proton-beam radiosurgery of liver metastases

Gracinda Mondlane[1,2*], Ana Ureba[3], Michael Gubanski[4], P A Lind[3,5] and Albert Siegbahn[3,5]

Abstract

Background: Radiotherapy of liver metastases is commonly being performed with photon-beam based stereotactic body radiation therapy (SBRT). The high risk for radiation-induced liver disease (RILD) is a limiting factor in these treatments. The use of proton-beam based SBRT could potentially improve the sparing of the healthy part of the liver. The aim of this study was to use estimations of normal tissue complication probability (NTCP) to identify liver-metastases patients that could benefit from being treated with intensity-modulated proton therapy (IMPT), based on the reduction of the risk for RILD.

Methods: Ten liver metastases patients, previously treated with photon-beam based SBRT, were retrospectively planned with IMPT. A CTV-based robust optimisation (accounting for setup and range uncertainties), combined with a PTV-based conventional optimisation, was performed. A robustness criterion was defined for the CTV ($V_{95\%} >$ 98% for at least 10 of the 12 simulated scenarios). The NTCP was estimated for different endpoints using the Lyman-Kutcher-Burman model. The ΔNTCP ($NTCP_{IMPT} - NTCP_{SBRT}$) for RILD was registered for each patient. The patients for which the NTCP (RILD) < 5% were also identified. A generic relative biological effectiveness of 1.1 was assumed for the proton beams.

Results: For all patients, the objectives set for the PTV and the robustness criterion set for the CTV were fulfilled with the IMPT plans. An improved sparing of the healthy part of the liver, right kidney, lungs, spinal cord and the skin was achieved with the IMPT plans, compared to the SBRT plans. Mean liver doses larger than the threshold value of 32 Gy led to NTCP values for RILD exceeding 5% (7 patients with SBRT and 3 patients with the IMPT plans). ΔNTCP values (RILD) ranging between − 98% and − 17% (7 patients) and between 0 and 2% (3 patients), were calculated.

Conclusions: In this study, liver metastases patients that could benefit from being treated with IMPT, based on the NTCP reductions, were identified. The clinical implementation of such a model-based approach to select liver metastases patients to proton therapy needs to be made with caution while considering the uncertainties involved in the NTCP estimations.

Keywords: RILD, Liver metastases, SBRT, IMPT, Patient selection

* Correspondence: gracinda.mondlane@ki.se
[1]Department of Physics – Medical Radiation Physics, Stockholm University, Stockholm, Sweden
[2]Department of Physics, Universidade Eduardo Mondlane, Maputo, Mozambique
Full list of author information is available at the end of the article

Background

Radiotherapy of liver metastases is commonly performed using photon-beam based extracranial radiosurgery, also known as stereotactic body radiation therapy (SBRT) [1]. The radiosensitivity of the liver sets a limit for how high doses that can be delivered. If the recommended threshold doses are exceeded, there will be an increased risk for the development of radiation-induced liver disease (RILD). RILD occurs between 2 weeks and 4 months after the completion of the liver irradiation and is a clinical syndrome of anicteric hepatomegaly, ascites and elevated liver enzymes [2]. However, it has been observed clinically that it is possible to deliver high hypofractionated doses to limited volumes of the liver, while only producing low levels of toxicity [1, 3], owing to the parallel functional organization of the liver [4].

Research and technological progress in recent years have led to the introduction of new radiation treatment techniques, e.g., scanned proton-beam therapy (PBT). The physical characteristics of proton-beam dose deposition allow highly conformal dose distributions to be delivered to the tumour volumes with reduced integral doses given to the healthy tissues, compared to when photon-beams are used [5]. For instance, if PBT is used for the treatment of liver malignancies, the improved dosimetric sparing of the healthy part of the liver could potentially lead to a reduction of the occurrence of RILD. However, the achievable sparing of the healthy part of the liver can be expected to vary from patient to patient depending on the individual anatomy, diagnosis and underlying liver disease/function.

The selection of liver metastases patients for treatment with PBT should be clinically justified in terms of improvements in the dose sparing of the healthy non-targeted part of the liver and a reduction of the corresponding risks for treatment-induced liver toxicity, compared to what can be achieved with photon-beam based SBRT. In addition, treatment decisions are based on different aspects, such as cost-effectiveness. When identifying patients suitable for treatment with either photon or proton therapy, the relatively high cost of proton therapy has to be balanced against the clinical gain in terms of sparing of the OARs [6]. In this context, a method for patient selection, based on comparisons of dosimetric values and of normal-tissue complication probabilities (NTCPs), has been proposed [7]. In a previous study by Mondlane et al. of radiosurgery of liver metastases [8], the potential to reduce the integral doses given to the organs at risk (OARs) with intensity-modulated proton therapy (IMPT) was demonstrated. In the present study, a comparison of the NTCPs calculated for SBRT- or IMPT-based radiosurgery of liver metastases was performed. The aim of this study was to identify patients, for which IMPT could provide a reduction of the risk for RILD, compared to photon-based SBRT.

Methods

Patients and delineation of the structures

Ten patients (aged between 66 and 89 years) diagnosed with liver metastases from colorectal-cancer were included in this study. These patients had previously been treated with photon-based SBRT at the Karolinska University Hospital. Information about the patient setup, fractionation schedule, photon dose-delivery mode, tumour location and abdominal compression are shown in Table 1.

The delineation of the relevant structures was performed on the planning computed tomography (CT) image sets with the Eclipse treatment planning system (TPS) (Varian Medical Systems, Palo Alto, California, Version 13.0, Build 13.0.33). These CT image sets contained 3.0 mm thick slices. The planning target volume (PTV) was created by expansion of the clinical target volume (CTV) with 10 mm in the cranio-caudal direction and 5 mm in the axial plane. Four-dimensional CT (4D-CT) image sets were used to assess the amplitude of the CTV motion. Abdominal compression was used to

Table 1 Patient setup and treatment description

Patient	*SBRT*	*Fractionation*	*Abdominal compression*	*PTV (cm^3)*	*CTV (cm^3)*	*Tumour location (liver segment)*
1	3D-CRT	15 Gy × 3	Yes	59.6	21.3	7
2	3D-CRT	17 Gy × 3	Yes	73.1	21.6	4a
3	VMAT	8 Gy × 7	No	332.3	157.0	7
4	3D-CRT	8 Gy × 5	Yes	302.6	142.3	5
5	3D-CRT	7 Gy × 8	No	66.4	19.8	1
6	VMAT	7 Gy × 8	No	294.1	145.1	8
7	3D-CRT	15 Gy × 3	No	18.6	3.5	4b
8	VMAT	7 Gy × 8	Yes	78.6	23.8	4a
9	3D-CRT	17 Gy × 3	No	30.2	4.7	5
10	3D-CRT	15 Gy × 3	No	72.3	24.8	5

reduce the target volume motion if the motion amplitude was larger than the CTV-to-PTV margin. The median values of the CTV and PTV were 22.7 cm^3 (range 3.5–157.0 cm^3) and 72.7 cm^3 (range 18.6–332.3 cm^3), respectively. The OARs considered in this study were the healthy part of the liver, skin, lungs, spinal cord and right kidney. The heathy part of the liver was considered to be the whole liver volume, subtracted with the CTV. The skin and spinal cord structures were delineated in the irradiated region of the body structure. To obtain the skin structure, a 3-mm layer was extracted from the body structure. The lungs and the right kidney were also contoured.

Treatment planning

The Eclipse TPS was used to prepare both the SBRT and IMPT plans. The SBRT treatments were delivered with 6-MV photon beams generated by a Varian linear accelerator (Varian Medical Systems, Palo Alto, California). The proton beam data used in the IMPT planning was obtained from a facility with an IBA cyclotron (Ion Beam Applications S.A., Louvain-La-Neuve, Belgium), with which proton kinetic energies between 60 and 230 MeV can be used for treatment. A range shifter of water-equivalent thickness of 3.5 g/cm^2 was used when necessary to ensure target dose-coverage at shallow depths. A generic relative biological effectiveness (RBE) value of 1.1 was assumed for the proton beams.

The SBRT plans, used for the actual treatments, were set as reference plans in the comparison. These SBRT plans had been prepared for three-dimensional conformal radiotherapy (3D-CRT), implemented with co-planar static fields (7 patients) or volumetric-modulated arc therapy (VMAT) performed with two full arcs (3 patients). The VMAT method was used for the patient cases for which the target volume was large, of a more complex shape, and a satisfactory sparing of the healthy part of the liver could otherwise not be achieved. The planning objective for SBRT was set to cover the entire PTV with at least 100% of the prescribed dose. An inhomogeneous dose distribution was allowed inside of the PTV, with maximum doses in the range from 145 to 150% of the prescribed dose. The doses given to the periphery of the CTV in the SBRT plans were registered and used to define the objectives in the IMPT planning.

The IMPT plans were prepared using the selective robust optimisation approach, as described by Li et al. [9], in which a CTV-based robust optimisation is performed, taking both the range and setup uncertainties into consideration. A conventional optimisation for the PTV is also considered in this method, using the same objectives as in the SBRT planning. This approach was chosen to allow for the inhomogeneous target doses typically used in SBRT treatments. A setup uncertainty of 10 mm (cranio-caudal direction) and 5 mm (axial plane), which corresponds to the CTV-to-PTV expansion margins used in the planning for SBRT, was considered as perturbation parameter values in the robust optimisation of the IMPT plans. In addition, a proton range uncertainty of 3.5% was also assumed. In the IMPT planning, an irradiation configuration with two fields was chosen in order to obtain a high degree of target-dose conformity, while sparing as much as possible the surrounding healthy tissues, mainly the healthy part of the liver. When selecting the angles of incidence of the proton beams, the direct irradiation through one of the kidneys and the spinal cord was avoided. The same fixation and immobilisation of the patients were assumed in the planning for IMPT, as for photon-beam SBRT. The stereotactic body frame, which was used for patient fixation during the acquisition of the planning CT image sets and during treatment with SBRT, was assigned the Hounsfield unit value of air in the IMPT planning. This step was taken to avoid introducing additional uncertainties in the proton dose calculation related to the partly unknown material composition of the frame. The normal tissue optimisation constraints used in the SBRT- and IMPT-planning were set as follows (the doses are shown for equivalent 2-Gy per fraction treatments): $D_{40} < 24$ Gy (IsoE) for the right kidney, $D_{max} < 45$ Gy (IsoE) for the spinal cord and $V_{20} < 20\%$ for the lungs. Efforts were also made to minimise the mean dose given to the healthy part of the liver.

Dosimetric evaluation

For each patient, a robustness analysis of the IMPT plans was performed based on the robustness criterion defined for the CTV, i.e., $D_{98} > 95\%$, for at least 10 of the 12 simulated scenarios. The target dose coverage in the SBRT and IMPT treatment plans was then evaluated by comparing pairwise the D_2 and D_{98} values for the CTV and the conformity index (CI) [10] for the PTV. The dosimetric evaluation of the IMPT plans was performed on the nominal plans. The dose volume histograms (DVHs) obtained for the OARs with the two treatment modalities were compared and the liver mean dose was also registered.

Assessment of NTCP

The assessment of NTCP was done using the Lyman-Kutcher-Burman (LKB) model [11, 12]. The physical doses in the extracted DVHs were converted to equivalent DVHs for 1.5 Gy per-fraction (for the healthy part of the liver) and 2 Gy per-fraction (for the remaining OARs). The LKB-model parameters used and the biological endpoints considered are shown in Table 2. These parameters are the most updated published NTCP

Table 2 Values of the LKB-model parameters, the corresponding biological-endpoints and the LQ-model parameter for all OARs

OAR	n	m	TD_{50} (Gy)	Endpoint	α/β (Gy)	Sources
Skin	0.38	0.14	39	Radiation-induced skin toxicity	3[a]	Pastore et al. (2016) [31]
Lung	1	0.41	29.9	Symptomatic radiation pneumonitis	3	Semenenko & Li (2008) [32]
Liver	0.97	0.12	45.8	Radiation-induced liver disease (RILD)	2	Dawson et al. (2002) [2]
Spinal cord	0.05	0.175	66.5	Radiation myelitis	0.87[b]	Burman et al. (1991) [33]
Right kidney	0.70	0.10	28	Clinical nephritis	3[a]	Burman et al. (1991) [33]

[a]Values of the assumed α/β parameter for these OARs; [b]the value of the α/β parameter for the spinal cord was taken from Schultheiss (2008) [34]

parameters and the most clinically relevant for the respective OARs considered. The values of the linear-quadratic (LQ) model parameter α/β for the different OARs used are also presented in Table 2.

To identify patients who would benefit from being treated with IMPT, two different approaches were considered. The first approach consisted in determining the difference in the estimated NTCP for RILD for the SBRT and IMPT plans, i.e., the ΔNTCP ($NTCP_{IMPT} - NTCP_{SBRT}$) [13]. The second approach was based on accepting patients for IMPT if the NTCP for RILD was lower than SBRT and also below 5%. This threshold NTCP value corresponds to a liver mean dose of 32 Gy for 2 Gy per fraction treatments [4]. It is also the commonly used dosimetric constraint for the liver [14]. The NTCPs obtained for the remaining OARs with the two treatment modalities were also compared.

Statistical analysis

The obtained dosimetric and NTCP values with the SBRT and IMPT plans, were compared pairwise using a two-sided Wilcoxon signed-rank test. A p-value of < 0.05 was considered statistically significant.

Results

Typical dose distributions obtained with the SBRT and IMPT plans are presented in Fig. 1 for patient #3. The SBRT treatment for this patient was performed with VMAT.

The robustness criterion set for the CTV was achieved for all patients with the IMPT plans. For the CTV, the median values of the IMPT-to-SBRT ratios of D_2 and of D_{98} were 1.0 (range 1.0–1.0), $p > 0.05$. For the PTV, a median value of the CI of 1.2 (range 1.0–1.4) was obtained with the SBRT plans and 1.5 (range 1.1–2.3) with the IMPT plans, $p < 0.05$. In general, an improved dosimetric sparing of the OARs was obtained with the IMPT plans, compared to the SBRT plans (Fig. 2). For the particular case of the healthy part of the liver, significantly lower mean doses were registered with IMPT (Table 3).

The IMPT plans resulted in a significant reduction of the calculated NTCP for RILD, compared to the SBRT

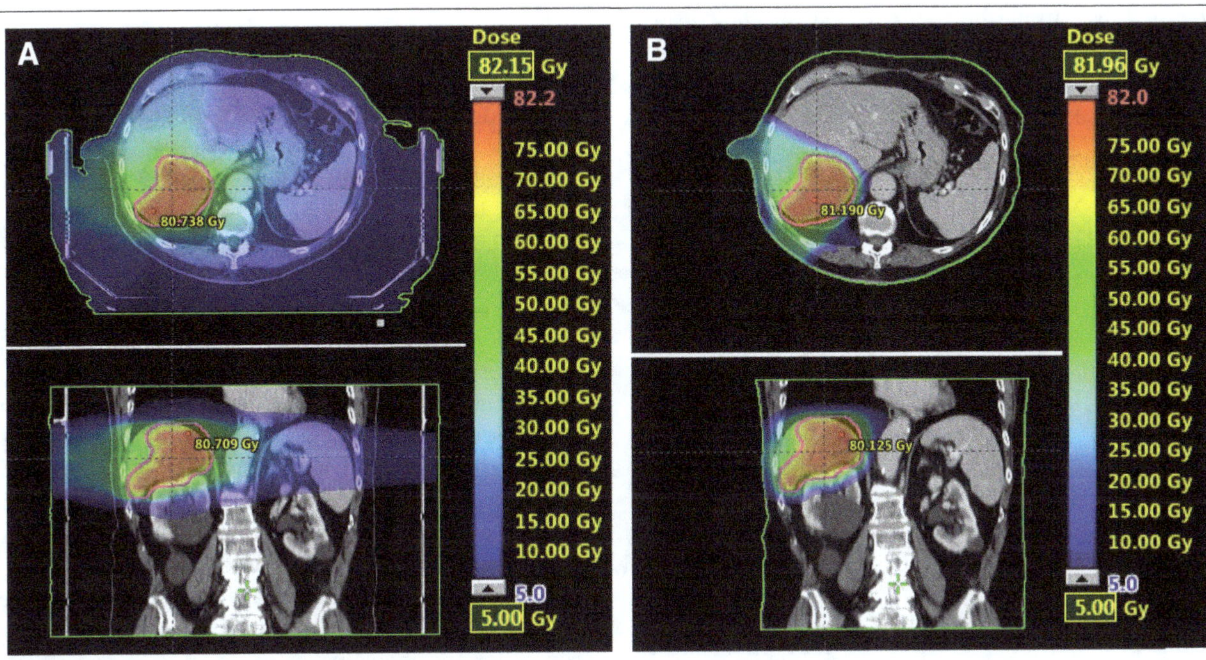

Fig. 1 Dose distributions on axial and coronal CT-slices for patient #3 for (**a**) VMAT and (**b**) IMPT

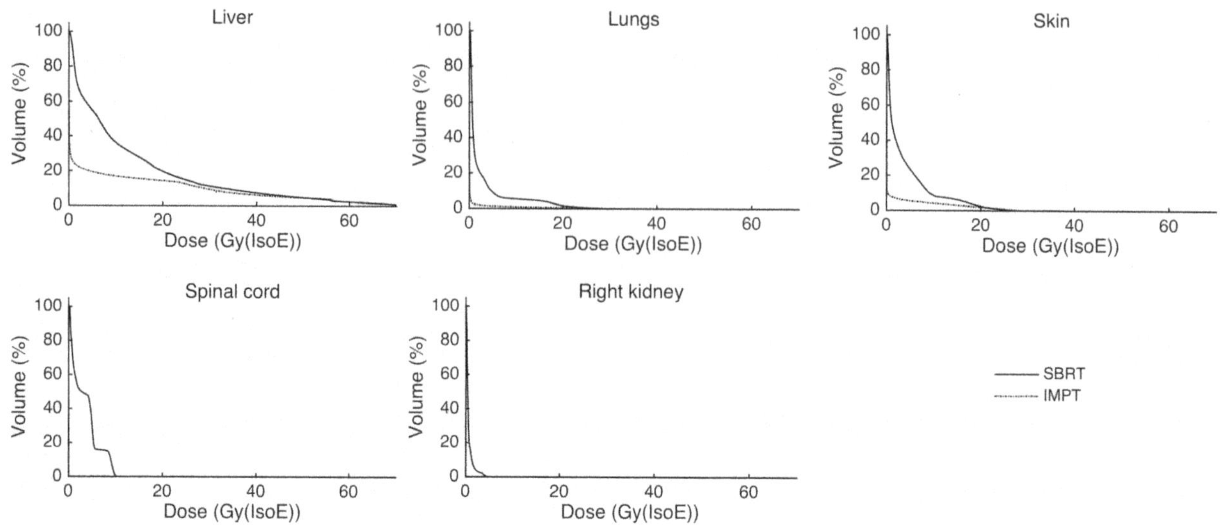

Fig. 2 Median DVHs for the OARs with the SBRT- (full lines) and the nominal IMPT-plans (dashed lines)

plans (Table 3). The median NTCP for RILD was 41% (range 0 - 100%) with SBRT and 1% (0 - 59%) with IMPT ($p < 0.05$). In the assessment of ΔNTCP for the healthy part of the liver, negative ΔNTCP values (ranging from – 97% to – 17%) were obtained for 7 patients, who would benefit from being treated with IMPT (Table 3). For the remaining 3 patients, ΔNTCP values of 0% and 2% were determined, which indicated that improved plans could not be achieved with IMPT for these patients. Furthermore, NTCP (RILD) values below 5%, which were also lower with IMPT compared to SBRT, were obtained for 4 patients (Table 3). For the remaining patients, SBRT would be the treatment of choice since comparable NTCPs for RILD were obtained with both the SBRT and the IMPT plans (3 patients) and because the NTCPs determined with either the SBRT or IMPT plans were greater than 5% (3 patients).

Table 3 Mean doses (2 Gy per-fraction), NTCPs and ΔNTCP for the healthy part of the liver

Patient #	Liver mean dose (Gy (IsoE))		NTCP for RILD (%)		ΔNTCP (%)
	SBRT	IMPT[a]	SBRT	IMPT[a]	
1	38	18 (15–21)	38	0 (0–0)	- 38
2	49	26 (21–30)	98	1 (0–5)	–97
3	60	39 (31–45)	100	53 (5–91)	–47
4	51	33 (30–35)	99	10 (4–16)	- 89
5	30	31 (29–33)	3	5 (1–5)	2
6	39	22 (17–25)	44	0 (0–0)	- 44
7	26	19 (17–20)	0	0 (0–0)	0
8	18	14 (9–18)	0	0 (0–0)	0
9	34	15 (14–16)	17	0 (0–0)	- 17
10	56	40 (36–41)	100	59 (27–73)	- 41

[a]The values in parentheses represent the range of values of the mean doses and NTCPs obtained for the simulated uncertainty scenarios in the IMPT plans

A significant decrease in the NTCP values was also registered for the lungs with the IMPT plans ($p < 0.05$). However, for the remaining OARs (right kidney, spinal cord and skin), there was no significant difference between the NTCP values obtained with the SBRT and IMPT plans ($p > 0.05$). A summary of the results obtained in the NTCP assessment is presented in Fig. 3, for all OARs. For the particular case of the healthy part of the liver, the NTCP results obtained with the SBRT and IMPT plans are also shown in Fig. 4.

Discussions

In the present study, an NTCP-model based approach for selecting liver metastases patients to radiosurgery performed with SBRT or IMPT was evaluated. Patients who would benefit from being treated with IMPT were identified based on the reduction of the NTCP for RILD. We found that the probability of observing RILD was reduced with IMPT for the majority of the patients included in this study. The improved sparing of the surrounding healthy tissue, which was achieved with IMPT also led to a reduction of the NTCP for the lungs, while similar NTCP values were obtained for the remaining OARs, compared to the SBRT plans. These results indicate that the main advantage of IMPT in the treatment of liver tumours is connected to the improved sparing of the healthy part of the liver, which is also known to be the limiting OAR in these treatments.

The advent of new radiotherapy modalities introduces new considerations in the optimal treatment selection process for the individual patients. NTCP-model based approaches for patient selection to photon- or

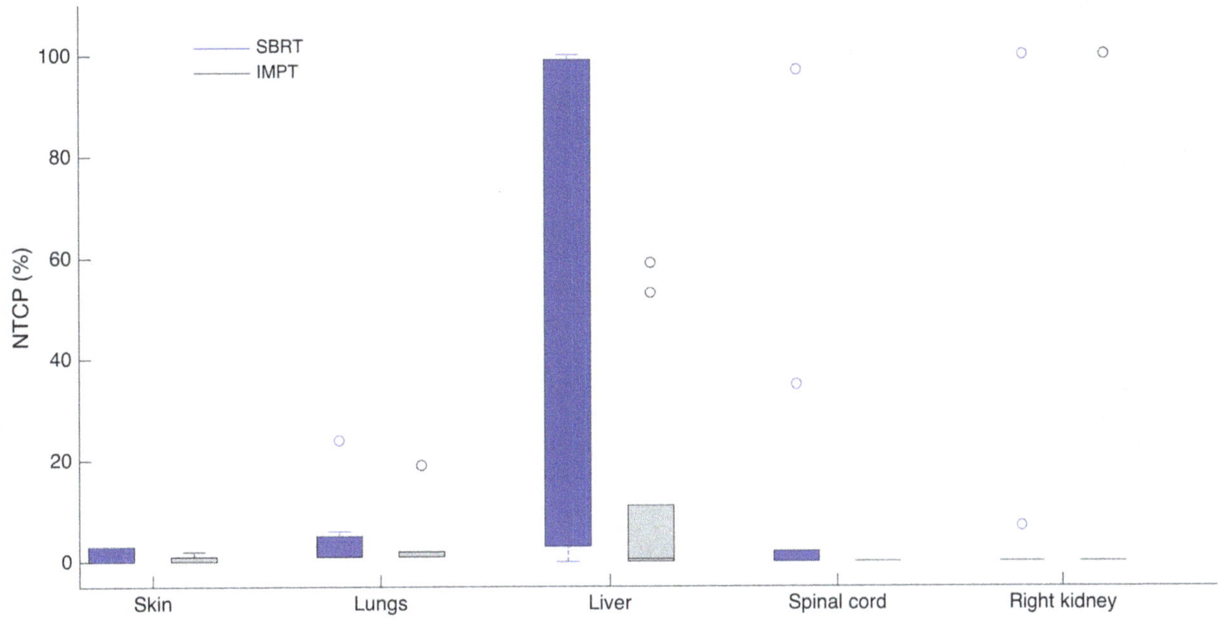

Fig. 3 Boxplot showing the calculated NTCPs for all OARs for the SBRT- (blue) and IMPT-plans (grey)

proton-beam therapy, have also been suggested [7, 13]. These models are based on the potential reduction of normal tissue toxicity with PBT, compared to what is achievable with photon beams. In this study, we considered two selection criteria. The first of these was based on the difference in the estimated NTCPs calculated for the IMPT and SBRT plans. According to this criterion, a patient should be selected to be treated with the technique which provided the lowest NTCP. According to the second criterion, patients should only be selected to IMPT if the estimated NTCP for RILD was lower than for SBRT and also below 5%. Based on the first criterion, 70% of the patients included in this study would be selected for IMPT, while with the second criterion, only 40% of the patients would be selected for IMPT. The use of the ΔNTCP approach requires that a threshold value, which is clinically meaningful, is set. However, the reduction of toxicity achievable with proton therapy, which can be translated into a level of clinical gain, is still to be determined for specific tumour sites and their corresponding OARs. Moreover, as proposed by Widder et al. [13], the NTCP-model based estimations should also be validated against the observed toxicity following proton therapy.

The advantages of PBT, compared to photon-beam RT, are in general more enhanced for larger tumour

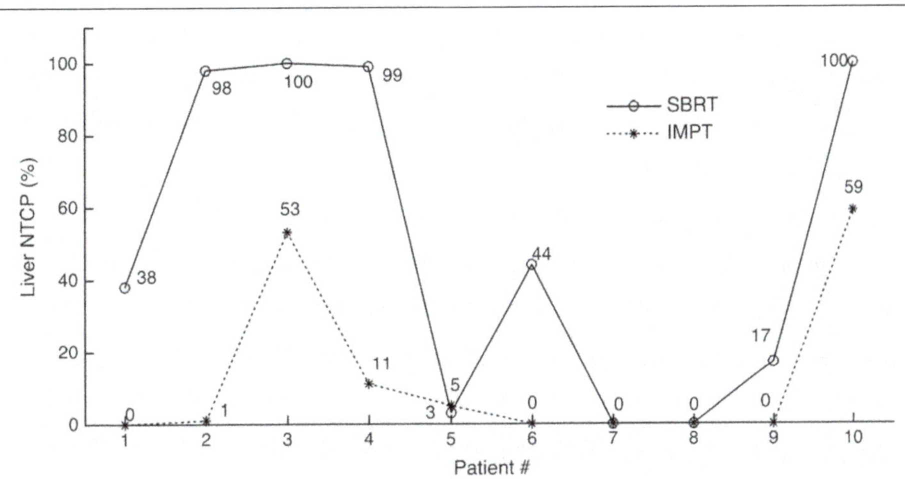

Fig. 4 Risk for radiation-induced liver disease obtained with the SBRT and IMPT plans for all patients

volumes. Photon RT of large tumour volumes involves the irradiation of large volumes of healthy tissue surrounding the target volume. These large irradiated volumes can potentially be reduced with the use of PBT. For smaller tumour volumes, on the other hand, the use of PBT does not lead to considerable improvements. This fact was observed in the present study for three patients (patients #5, 7 and 8) with small PTVs (between 18.6 and 78.6 cm^3), located in the liver segments 1, 4b and 4a, respectively (Table 1). For these patients, comparable values of the liver mean dose and of the estimated NTCP were obtained for the healthy part of the liver with the SBRT and IMPT plans.

Studies of partial liver irradiation [4], have shown that the tolerance of the healthy part of the liver is correlated with the liver mean dose. The risk of RILD has been shown to increase rapidly with increasing mean liver dose above the threshold value of 32 Gy. In this study, for all patient cases whose liver mean dose was above this threshold value (7 patients for SBRT and 3 patients for IMPT) the estimated risk for RILD was higher than 5% (Table 3). Because the liver is an organ with parallel organization, high doses given to a limited volume can be tolerated and the risk of toxicity is dominated by the average dose given to the whole organ. Therefore, the liver could benefit from the reduction of the integral dose, which is possible with IMPT.

The sparing of the healthy part of the liver is of utmost importance for patients with primary liver cancer, which in most of the cases have liver cirrhosis of different grades. For these patients, radiotherapy often leads to migration to higher grades of cirrhosis [15], which ultimately can lead to liver failure and death [2]. Proton therapy could appear to be the treatment of choice for patients with a reduced liver function and for postoperative treatment of patients with a reduced total liver volume. In order to fully exploit the potential of PBT for this patient group, functional imaging techniques, e.g., magnetic resonance imaging, can be used to evaluate the liver function prior to the treatment planning. Based on the information obtained in the functional imaging, IMPT plans can be designed in which the beams pass through the parts of the liver which were found to have a reduced liver function.

Clinical follow-up studies have shown that the frequency of RILD occurring after photon beam therapy of liver tumours is low, but that the consequences can be severe. In a follow-up study (median follow-up time of 12.9 months) by Romero et al. [16], it was reported that none of the 34 liver metastases patients developed RILD after being treated with SBRT. In another study conducted by Liu et al. [17], which involved 62 patients with primary and metastatic liver tumours (median follow-up time of 18 months) treated with SBRT, none of the patients with metastatic disease developed RILD, but RILD was diagnosed in one patient with primary liver cancer (Child-Pugh B). One case of death due to liver failure was registered in a follow-up study of colorectal liver-metastases patients (median follow-up time of 4.3 years) who received SBRT [18].

The use of IMPT in the management of tumour sites influenced by organ motion, e.g., the liver, is currently challenging. In IMPT, the individual fields are optimised separately resulting in inhomogeneous dose distributions, which are combined among all the fields included to reach a certain overall dose distribution across the target volume. For SBRT treatments, this overall dose distribution presents large dose gradients. The delivery of high target doses with IMPT, while sparing the OARs, demands that planning and treatment-delivery strategies are adopted to account for the proton-specific and patient-related uncertainties. If not accounted for, these uncertainties may cause changes in the dose distributions produced by the proton beams which may result in a loss of the potential advantages of IMPT. In photon-beam based SBRT of liver tumours, the impact of organ motion are generally minimized by using adequate CTV to PTV margins combined with adequate means of motion mitigation, such as abdominal compression, which was used if required for the patient group included in this study. For IMPT, however, the conventional PTV-based plan optimisation has been shown inappropriate. The use of CTV-based robust optimization allows for a safer delivery of PBT in the presence of proton-specific uncertainties [19]. However, for IMPT-based radiosurgery, there is still no generally accepted standard method for performing a robust optimisation. To create the inhomogeneous dose distribution used in extra-cranial radiosurgery treatments, a robust optimisation which includes nominal objectives for the PTV should be performed. This strategy augmented the CI for the PTV in the present study, as discussed in the study on selective robust optimisation conducted by Li et al. [9]. Despite this fact, the potential of IMPT to reduce the mean doses given to the healthy part of the liver and the estimated NTCP for RILD was still observed.

Another issue of concern in IMPT of moving targets is the so-called interplay effect. In the present study, the planning for IMPT was performed on static CT sets, in which organ motion amplitude was reduced by means of abdominal compression. Even though the impact of organ motion on the dose distributions produced in IMPT are partly reduced with the use of robust optimisation [20, 21], a more thorough analysis of its importance would be valuable. A review of the effects of intra-fraction organ motion and their mitigation strategies have been published by Bert and Durante [22]. The uncertainties introduced by organ motion can be reduced in the clinic by using different motion-mitigation strategies, which include among others, the use of abdominal compression, tumour tracking, gated delivery, re-scanning and the use of larger spot sizes.

In most of the reports presenting comparative studies of photon- and proton-beam therapy, which have been based on the use of radiobiological models [23–25], it has been assumed that the biological-model parameters, obtained in follow-up studies of photon-beam treatments, are also valid for the proton-beam treatments. The same assumption was made in the present work. The NTCP-model parameters used will be updated at a later stage with the clinically observed outcomes following proton therapy. Other sources of uncertainties should also be considered prior to the clinical implementation of the NTCP model-based approach for patient selection. These include the uncertainties in the radiobiological model parameters [26], the inter-patient variation in radiosensitivity [26, 27] and the reduction of the actual three-dimensional dose distributions to DVHs [26]. Furthermore, the DVHs are calculated without taking into account the daily spatial variation in the dose distribution delivered to the patient [28]. A dependence of the estimated NTCP values on the algorithms used for the dose calculations has also been reported [28]. Therefore, the calculated NTCP values must at this point be used with caution for predicting the outcome of radiation treatments.

The patients included in this study have been indicated for palliative treatment with photon-beam based SBRT. The advances in the search of predictive markers for liver metastases [29] could create the possibility to treat curatively patients that were previously considered only for palliative treatment. Moreover, the underlying biological processes at the cellular level, such as enhanced anti-tumour immune response, triggered by the high-dose of SBRT treatments have recently attracted interest [30].

Conclusions

In this work we found that IMPT could provide a significant reduction of the risk for RILD for most of the patients studied. The successful clinical implementation of an NTCP-model based approach for selection of liver metastases patients requires that a patient data base with follow-up information on the occurrence of side effects, following photon- and proton-beam radiosurgery, is gathered and continuously updated.

Abbreviations

3D-CRT: Three-dimensional conformal radiation therapy; 4D-CT: Four-dimensional computed tomography; CI: Conformity index; CT: Computed tomography; CTV: Clinical target volume; DVH: Dose volume histogram; IBA: Ion Beam Applications; IMPT: Intensity-modulated proton therapy; LKB: Lyman-Kutcher-Burman; LQ: Linear-quadratic; NTCP: Normal tissue complication probability; OAR: Organ at risk; PBT: Proton beam therapy; PTV: Planning target volume; RBE: Relative biological effectiveness; RILD: Radiation-induced liver disease; SBRT: Stereotactic body radiation therapy; TPS: Treatment planning system; VMAT: Volumetric-modulated arc therapy

Acknowledgements

The authors would like to acknowledge the Swedish International Development Cooperation Agency (SIDA), the International Science Programme (ISP) and the Cancer Research Funds of Radiumhemmet, Karolinska Institutet, Stockholm, Sweden.

Authors' contributions

GM participated in the conception and design of the study. GM evaluated the approach to be used in the preparation of the plans for IMPT-based radiosurgery, performed the treatment planning for IMPT, performed the calculations of the NTCPs and the statistical analyses of the obtained results. GM, AU and AS participated in the writing of the manuscript. AU participated actively in the analysis and interpretation of the results and critically reviewed the manuscript. MG and PL evaluated the obtained results and critically reviewed the manuscript, in particular the medical/clinical parts. AS participated in the analyses of the results and critically reviewed the manuscript. All authors read and approved the final version of the manuscript.

Competing interests

The authors declare that they have no competing interests.

Author details

[1]Department of Physics – Medical Radiation Physics, Stockholm University, Stockholm, Sweden. [2]Department of Physics, Universidade Eduardo Mondlane, Maputo, Mozambique. [3]Department of Oncology and Pathology, Karolinska Institutet, Stockholm, Sweden. [4]Department of Oncology and Pathology, Karolinska University Hospital, Stockholm, Sweden. [5]Department of Oncology, Södersjukhuset, Stockholm, Sweden.

References

1. Lax I, Blomgren H, Näslund I, Svanström R. Stereotactic radiotherapy of malignancies in the abdomen. Methodological aspects. Acta Oncol. 1994;33: 677.
2. Dawson LA, Normolle D, Balter JM, McGinn CJ, Lawrence TS, Ten Haken RK. Analysis of radiation-induced liver disease using the Lyman NTCP model. Int J Radiat Oncol. 2002;53:810–21. https://doi.org/10.1016/S0360-3016(02)02846-8.
3. Blomgren H, Lax I, Näslund I, Svanström R. Stereotactic high dose fraction radiation therapy of extracranial tumors using an accelerator: clinical experience of the first thirty-one patients. Acta Oncol (Madr). 1995;34:861–70. https://doi.org/10.3109/02841869509127197.
4. Dawson LA, Ten Haken RK. Partial volume tolerance of the liver to radiation. Semin Radiat Oncol. 2005;15:279–83.
5. Dionisi F, Ben-Josef E. The use of proton therapy in the treatment of gastrointestinal cancers. Liver Cancer Journal. 2014;20:371–7.
6. Lundkvist J, Ekman M, Ericsson SR, Jönsson B, Glimelius B. Proton therapy of cancer: potential clinical advantages and cost-effectiveness. Acta Oncol. 2005;44:850–61. https://doi.org/10.1080/02841860500341157

7. Langendijk JA, Lambin P, De Ruysscher D, Widder J, Bos M, Verheij M. Selection of patients for radiotherapy with protons aiming at reduction of side effects: the model-based approach. Radiother Oncol. 2013;107:267–73.
8. Mondlane G, Gubanski M, Lind P, Henry T, Ureba A, Siegbahn A. Dosimetric comparison of plans for photon- or proton-beam based radiosurgery of liver metastases. Int J Part Ther. 2016;3:277–84.
9. Li Y, Niemela P, Liao L, Jiang S, Li H, Poenisch F, et al. Selective robust optimization: a new intensity-modulated proton therapy optimization strategy. Med Phys. 2015;42:4840–7. https://doi.org/10.1118/1.4923171.
10. ICRU. ICRU report 62. Prescribing, recording, and reporting photon beam therapy (supplement to ICRU report 50). Bethesda, Maryland: Oxford University Press; 1999.
11. Lyman JT. Complication probability as assessed from dose-volume histograms. Radiat Res. 1985;104:S13. https://doi.org/10.2307/3576626.
12. Kutcher GJ, Burman C. Calculation of complication probability factors for non-uniform normal tissue irradiation: the effective volume method. Int J Radiat Oncol Biol Phys. 1989;16:1623–30. https://doi.org/10.1016/0360-3016(89)90972-3.
13. Widder J, van Der Schaaf A, Lambin P, Marijnen CAM, Pignol J-P, Rasch CR, et al. The quest for evidence for proton therapy: model-based approach and precision medicine. Int J Radiat Oncol Biol Phys. 2016;95:30–6.
14. Marks LB, Yorke ED, Jackson A, Ten Haken RK, Constine LS, Eisbruch A, et al. Use of Normal tissue complication probability models in the clinic. Int J Radiat Oncol Biol Phys. 2010;76:S10–9.
15. Schulz RA, Huntzinger C, Blacksbburg S, Rosenzweig K. Stereotactic body radiation therapy (SBRT) for early-stage primary liver cancer (HCC). Appl Rad Oncol. 2013:12–8.
16. Méndez Romero A, Wunderink W, Hussain SM, De Pooter JA, Heijmen BJM, Nowak PCJM, et al. Stereotactic body radiation therapy for primary and metastatic liver tumors: a single institution phase i-ii study. Acta Oncol (Madr). 2006;45:831–7. https://doi.org/10.1080/02841860600897934.
17. Liu E, Stenmark MH, Schipper MJ, Balter JM, Kessler ML, Caoili EM, et al. Stereotactic body radiation therapy for primary and metastatic liver tumors. Transl Oncol. 2013;6:442–6.
18. Hoyer M, Roed H, Traberg Hansen A, Ohlhuis L, Petersen J, Nellemann H, et al. Phase II study on stereotactic body radiotherapy of colorectal metastases. Acta Oncol (Madr). 2006;45:823–30. https://doi.org/10.1080/02841860600904854.
19. Fredriksson A, Forsgren A, Hårdemark B. Minimax optimization for handling range and setup uncertainties in proton therapy. Med Phys. 2011;38:1672–84. https://doi.org/10.1118/1.3556559.
20. Li H, Zhang X, Park P, Liu W, Chang J, Liao Z, et al. Robust optimization in intensity-modulated proton therapy to account for anatomy changes in lung cancer patients. Radiother Oncol. 2015;114:367–72.
21. Liu W, Liao Z, Schild SE, Liu Z, Li H, Li Y, et al. Impact of respiratory motion on worst-case scenario optimized intensity modulated proton therapy for lung cancers. Pract Radiat Oncol. 2015;5:e77–86. https://doi.org/10.1016/j.prro.2014.08.002.
22. Bert C, Durante M. Motion in radiotherapy: particle therapy. Phys Med Biol. 2011;56:R113–44.
23. Tommasino F, Durante M, D'Avino V, Liuzzi R, Conson M, Farace P, et al. Model-based approach for quantitative estimates of skin, heart, and lung toxicity risk for left-side photon and proton irradiation after breast-conserving surgery. Acta Oncol (Madr). 2017;:1–7.
24. Widesott L, Pierelli A, Fiorino C, Lomax AJ, Amichetti M, Cozzarini C, et al. Helical Tomotherapy vs. intensity-modulated proton therapy for whole pelvis irradiation in high-risk prostate Cancer patients: Dosimetric, Normal tissue complication probability, and generalized equivalent uniform dose analysis. Int J Radiat Oncol Biol Phys. 2011;80:1589–600.
25. Jakobi A, Bandurska-Luque A, Stützer K, Haase R, Löck S, Wack L-J, et al. Identification of patient benefit from proton therapy for advanced head and neck Cancer patients based on individual and subgroup Normal tissue complication probability analysis. Int J Radiat Oncol Biol Phys. 2015;92:1165–74.
26. Yorke ED. Modeling the effects of inhomogeneous dose distributions in normal tissues. Semin Radiat Oncol. 2001;11:197–209. https://doi.org/10.1053/srao.2001.23478.
27. Tsougos I, Nilsson P, Theodorou K, Kjellén E, Ewers S-B, Jarlman O, et al. NTCP modelling and pulmonary function tests evaluation for the prediction of radiation induced pneumonitis in non-small-cell lung cancer radiotherapy. Phys Med Biol. 2007;52:1055–73. https://doi.org/10.1088/0031-9155/52/4/013.
28. Hedin E, Bäck A. Influence of different dose calculation algorithms on the estimate of NTCP for lung complications. J Appl Clin Med Phys. 2013;14:127–39. https://doi.org/10.1120/jacmp.v14i5.4316.
29. Gustafson MP, Bornschlegl S, Park SS, Gastineau DA, Roberts LR, Dietz AB, et al. Comprehensive assessment of circulating immune cell populations in response to stereotactic body radiation therapy in patients with liver cancer. Adv Radiat Oncol. 2017;2:540–7. https://doi.org/10.1016/j.adro.2017.08.003.
30. Herrera FG, Bourhis J, Coukos G. Radiotherapy combination opportunities leveraging immunity for the next oncology practice. CA Cancer J Clin. 2017;67:65–85. https://doi.org/10.3322/caac.21358.
31. Pastore F, Conson M, D'Avino V, Palma G, Liuzzi R, Solla R, et al. Dose-surface analysis for prediction of severe acute radio-induced skin toxicity in breast cancer patients. Acta Oncol (Madr). 2016;55:466–73. https://doi.org/10.3109/0284186X.2015.1110253.
32. Semenenko VA, Li XA. Lyman–Kutcher–Burman NTCP model parameters for radiation pneumonitis and xerostomia based on combined analysis of published clinical data. Phys Med Biol. 2008;53:737–55. https://doi.org/10.1088/0031-9155/53/3/014.
33. Burman C, Kutcher GJ, Emami B, Goitein M. Fitting of normal tissue tolerance data to an analytic function. Int J Radiat Oncol Biol Phys. 1991;21:123–35.
34. Schultheiss TE. The radiation dose–response of the human spinal cord. Int J Radiat Oncol. 2008;71:1455–9. https://doi.org/10.1016/J.IJROBP.2007.11.075.

19

Short-term outcomes and clinical efficacy of stereotactic body radiation therapy (SBRT) in treatment of adrenal gland metastases from lung cancer

Xianzhi Zhao[1†], Xiaofei Zhu[1†], Jianfeng Fei[2†], Haipeng Ren[3], Yangsen Cao[1], Xiaoping Ju[1], Zhiyong Yuan[4] and Huojun Zhang[1*]

Abstract

Background: To assess the efficacy and safety of stereotactic body radiation therapy (SBRT) in the management of adrenal gland metastases (AGMs) from lung cancer. Moreover, it is the first two-institutional experience and the largest-to-date study to report the safety and efficacy of SBRT for inoperable AGM from lung cancer.

Methods: In this retrospective study, 30 patients (27 males, 3 females) with 32 AGMs were treated by SBRT from October 2006 to June 2016. Of these, 11 patients were treated with the intent of controlling all known metastatic sites and 19 for palliation of bulky AGMs. Follow-up was performed every 3 months for evaluations of efficacy and safety. Factors predictive of overall survival (OS) and local control (LC) were identified with univariate and then multivariate analysis.

Results: Median follow-up time was 10.7 months (2.9–96.4 months). The complete response (CR), partial response (PR), stable disease (SD) and progressive disease (PD) rates were 23.3%, 33.3%, 33.3% and 16.7% respectively. The 6-month, 1, and 2-year LC rates were 96.9%, 96.9%, and 72.7% respectively. Additionally, the 6-month, 1, and 2-year OS rates were 85.6%, 58.1%, and 54.0% respectively while 6-month, 1, and 2-year progression free survival (PFS) rates were 39.5%, 24.6%, and 8.2%, respectively. All the patients with cancer-induced pain (8 with abdominal pain and 6 with lumbar back pain) had significant alleviations after SBRT. The treatment was well tolerated with only 1 patient reporting grade-3 diarrhoea. No predictors of OS and LC were found after multivariate analysis, while it was demonstrated that biologic equivalent dose (BED_{10}, $\alpha/\beta = 10$) ≥85.5Gy ($P = 0.007$) and gross tumor volume < 30 ml ($P = 0.003$) correlated with LC only after univariate analysis.

Conclusion: SBRT is a safe and effective treatment modality in the management of AGMs from lung cancer with high LC rates and acceptable toxicity.

Keywords: Adrenal gland metastases, Stereotactic body radiotherapy (SBRT), Lung cancer, Local control, Response

* Correspondence: chyyzhj@163.com
†Xianzhi Zhao, Xiaofei Zhu and Jianfeng Fei contributed equally to this work.
[1]Department of Radiation Oncology, Shanghai Changhai Hospital, the Second Military Medical University, Shanghai 200433, China
Full list of author information is available at the end of the article

Background

The adrenal gland is one of the most frequently involved sites of metastases in lung cancer. Adrenal gland metastases (AGMs) from lung cancer are usually characterized by insidious onset and patients only occasionally have back or abdominal pain due to a large or rapidly growing tumor. Rarely, in the case of bilateral adrenal involvement, patients may develop adrenal insufficiency, which may result in attenuation of quality of life (QOL) and often worse survival [1]. A new radiographically evidence of tumor in the adrenal gland contributed to early diagnosis of AGM during follow-up [2].

An obvious increase in tumor burden may prompt systemic aggressive treatment. However, for those with AGMs who may have already received first-line chemotherapy and have disease progressions thereafter, alternative regimens might not provide survival benefits, as well as probably contribute to high incidences of toxicity. Furthermore, though the adverse effects of targeted therapy for patients with EGFR mutation are mild, drug resistance remains the biggest problem. Surgery is considered as a curative option for some isolated metastases, but the adrenalectomy sometimes may result in adrenal insufficiency and perioperative complications [3]. Percutaneous image-guided radiofrequency ablation (RFA) is a safe and well-tolerated modality for unresectable primary or metastatic adrenal gland tumor, which greatly contributes to short-term local control, especially for the tumors with diameters less than 5 cm [4]. Nevertheless, RFA is still micro-invasive option. Hence, a non-invasive, safe and effective alternative is required.

Recently, due to the advantages of stereotactic body radiation therapy (SBRT), including precise delivery and abrupt dose fall-off outside targets and high local dose conformation, it has been commonly used in selected patients with and without metastatic lesions, with high local control (LC) rates and acceptable toxicity, especially when surgery is declined or contraindicated [5–7]. High doses could be precisely delivered to an extracranial target within the body, either as a single dose or a small limited number of radiation fractions [8]. It can be performed either with a traditional linear accelerator or a robotic arm (CyberKnife®). CyberKnife was developed in the 1990s at Stanford (Accuray Inc., Sunnyvale, CA, USA) [9], which represented an innovations of traditional stereotactic surgery. Given the real-time tracking, beam angles could be simultaneously corrected intra-fractionally via pre-identified patient's breathing patterns [10]. Despite the previous employment of SBRT in the lung cancer, pancreatic cancer, prostate cancer and liver cancer [11–14], few studies investigated the management of AGMs from lung cancer with SBRT. The aim of this retrospective study was to assess the efficacy and safety of SBRT for AGMs from lung cancer.

Methods

Patient characteristics

SBRT was delivered for 30 patients with AGMs from lung cancer (total 32 lesions) from October 2006 to June 2016 at Tianjin Medical University Cancer Institute and Hospital, and Changhai Hospital of the Second Military Medical University. All patients were examined by an oncologist before the study. Patients with AGMs diagnosed by biopsy or at least imaging examinations. Besides, those with a Karnofsky performance score ≥ 70, a life expectancy of > 3 months and who declined or were not amenable to surgical resections due to comorbidities were included in the study. Informed consent was obtained from all patients prior to the enrolment and the study was conducted according to the Declaration of Helsinki. The review and use of medical records of patients for analysis were approved by the ethical committee.

Treatments

Of the 30 patients, 11 were treated with the intent of controlling all known metastatic lesions, and 19 underwent SBRT for palliation of bulky adrenal metastases. SBRT was delivered by CyberKnife (Accuray Corporation, Sunnyvale, CA, USA). All patients were immobilized in supine position with arms by their sides using thermoplastic body mask. Computed tomography (CT) scan was performed with a slice thickness of 1.5 mm, with the scan range of at least 10 cm below and above the tumor. According to the adrenal gland motions during radiotherapy reported by Wang et al. [15], for patients with X-sight spine tracking, the gross tumor volume (GTV) was defines as a radiographically lesion in the adrenal gland. Planning target volume (PTV) was delineated with a 3–5 mm margin expansion in the lateral direction and anteroposterior direction, a 5–7 mm margin expansion in the cephalo-caudal direction from GTV. When Synchrony™ Respiratory Tracking System was used, PTV was determined by a 3 mm margin expansion in the lateral direction and anteroposterior direction, a 3–5 mm margin expansion in the cephalo-caudal direction. Synchrony™ Respiratory Tracking System was performed in 9 patients with 11 lesions, while X-sight spine tracking was employed in 21 patients with 21 lesions. The treatment parameters were presented in Table 1. The dose-volume constraints for organs at risk were referred to the American Association of Physicists in Medicine guidelines in TG-101 [16], which was as follows: renal hilum/vascular trunk, V_{23} < 2/3 volume; renal cortex (right and left), $V_{17.5} < 200$ mL; duodenum, $D_{5mL} < 18$ Gy, $D_{10mL} < 12.5$ Gy and $D_{max} <$ 32 Gy; liver $V_{21} < 700$ mL; spinal cord, $D_{0.35mL} < 23$ Gy, $D_{1.2mL} < 14.5$ Gy and $D_{max} < 30$ Gy; medulla spinal cord (5-6 mm above and below level treated per Ryu), $V_{23} < 10\%$ of subvolume and $D_{max} < 30$ Gy; stomach, $D_{10mL} < 18$ Gy

Table 1 Patient demography and clinical presentation

Characteristics	Values		
Age (years)	63(range 42–85)		
Gender (male/female)	27/3 (90%/10.0%)		
Karnofsky performance score ≥ 70	30 (100%)		
Pathology of primary tumor		Lesions per patient	
▪ Squamous cell carcinoma	7(23.3%)	▪ 1	28 (93.3%)
▪ Adenocarcinoma	12 (40.0%)	▪ > 1	2 (6.7%)
▪ Small cell lung cancer	5 (16.7%)	Systemic therapy after SBRT	
▪ Adenosquamous carcinoma	3 (10.0%)		
▪ Unknown	3 (10.0%)	▪ Yes	18 (60%)
Location of AGMs		▪ None	12 (40%)
▪ Left	16 (53.3%)	Metastases in other sites	
▪ Right	12 (40%)	▪ Yes	15 (50%)
▪ Left and right	2 (6.7%)	▪ No	15 (50%)
Symptoms		SBRT for other sites	
▪ Presented	14 (46.7%)	▪ Yes	9 (30%)
▪ None	16 (53.3%)	▪ No	21 (70%)

and $D_{max} < 32$ Gy; duodenum, $D_{5mL} < 18$ Gy, $D_{10mL} < 12.5$ Gy and $D_{max} < 32$ Gy.

Response evaluation and follow-up

Patients were re-evaluated every 3 months after radiotherapy with contrast-enhanced CT scans, PET-CT scans or contrast-enhanced MRI. Adverse events, amelioration of symptoms and sequential treatment were recorded. Acute and late toxicity was scored according to the Common Terminology Criteria for Adverse Events (CTCAE) version 4.0 [17]. Tumor response was defined as complete response (CR), partial response (PR) and stable disease (SD), which was determined using the Response Evaluation Criteria in Solid Tumors (RECIST), version 1.1 [18]. Therefore, the local control (LC) rate was the ratio of the number of lesions with the effective response from the completion of SBRT to a determined time point to the total number of lesions. OS was defined as the time from the date of the receipt of SBRT to death from any cause or the last follow-up for included patients. PFS was defined as the time from the date of the receipt of SBRT to the confirmation of disease progressions at any sites or death by any cause.

Statistical analysis

LC, OS and PFS curves were calculated by the Kaplan-Meier method. Potential factors associated with LC, OS and PFS were identified with univariate log-rank comparisons and then multivariate proportional hazards regression model. Statistical analyses were performed using SPSS 18.0 (IBM Corporation, Armonk, NY, USA). Two-sided P values < 0.05 were considered statistically significant.

Results

Patient characteristics

Patient characteristics were shown in Table 1. A total of 30 patients with a median age of 63 years (range: 42–85), including 27 males and 3 females, were treated with CyberKnife® (Accuray Incorporated, Sunnyvale, CA, USA),. Of all patients, 16 and 12 lesions were in the left and right adrenal gland while 2 patients had bilateral AGMs without adrenal insufficiency due to quite small lesions. The patlatehological types of lung cancer included squamous cell carcinoma ($n = 7$, 23.3%), adenocarcinoma ($n = 12$, 40.0%), small cell lung cancer ($n = 5$, 16.7%), adenosquamous carcinoma ($n = 3$, 10.0%), and unknown type (n = 3, 10.0%). Among all the patients, 15 (50.0%) had other site metastases in addition to AGMs. Eighteen patients (60.0%) had received chemotherapy after SBRT, and 9 (30.0%) had more than one lesions treated. Furthermore, 16 patients (53.3%) were symptom-free, while 14 (46.7%) suffered from abdominal pain or lumbar back pain.

The median dose was 44.4 Gy (range 32–50 Gy), which was delivered in 5 fractions (3–8 fractions), with a corresponding biologic effective dose ($\alpha/\beta = 10$, BED_{10}) of 85.5 Gy (range: 44.8–112.5 Gy). The median prescription dose for control and palliation intent was 45Gy (range: 42-50Gy) and 42Gy (range: 32-50Gy), respectively. The median GTV was 23.9 ml (range: 2.5–115.3 ml). Treatment planning parameters were demonstrated in Table 2. Additionally, an illustrative case was shown in Fig. 1.

Table 2 Treatment parameters used for SBRT

	All lesions	Lesions with local control	Lesions without local control
GTV (ml)	23.9 (2.5–115.3)	17.8 (2.5–75)	60.7 (26.4–115.3)
Maximum dose (Gy)	58 (43.2–70.4)	57.7 (43.2–70.4)	58.6 (44.9–66.2)
Total prescribed dose (Gy)	44.4 (32–50)	45 (32–50)	41.6 (35–45)
Number of fractions	5 (3–8)	5 (3–8)	5 (3–8)
Dose per fraction (Gy)	9 (4–15)	9 (4–15)	7 (5.2–15)
BED_{10} (Gy)	85.5 (44.8–112.5)	85.5 (44.8–112.5)	67.2 (59.5–112.5)
Prescription isodose line (%)	73 (66–82)	74 (66–82)	71 (66–79)

All data were shown as median values (range)

Efficacy outcomes

All patients were followed up until death or June 2018. By the last follow-up, 19 patients (63.3%) died while 11 were alive. One patient died of heart disease, whereas 18 patients died of distant metastasis. Hence, local failure and radiation-induced toxicity did not contribute to the death. The median follow-up was 10.7 months (2.9–96.4 months), and median OS and PFS was 24.4 months (95% CI: 4.4–44.4 months) and 3.5 months (95% CI: 1.3–5.7), respectively. The 6-month, 1-year, and 2-year LC rates were 96.9%, 96.9%, and 72.7%, respectively (Fig. 2a). Furthermore, the 6-month, 1-year, and 2-year OS rates were 85.6%, 58.1%, and 54.0%, respectively (Fig. 2b), And the 6-month, 1-year, and 2-year PFS rates were 39.5%, 24.6%, and 8.2%, respectively (Fig. 2c). Tumor response of each lesion of the adrenal gland was evaluated. Therefore, based on the RECIST criteria, the CR, PR and SD rates were 21.9% ($n = 7$), 31.2% ($n = 10$), and 31.2% ($n = 10$) respectively, while 5 (15.7%) foci showed disease progression (PD).

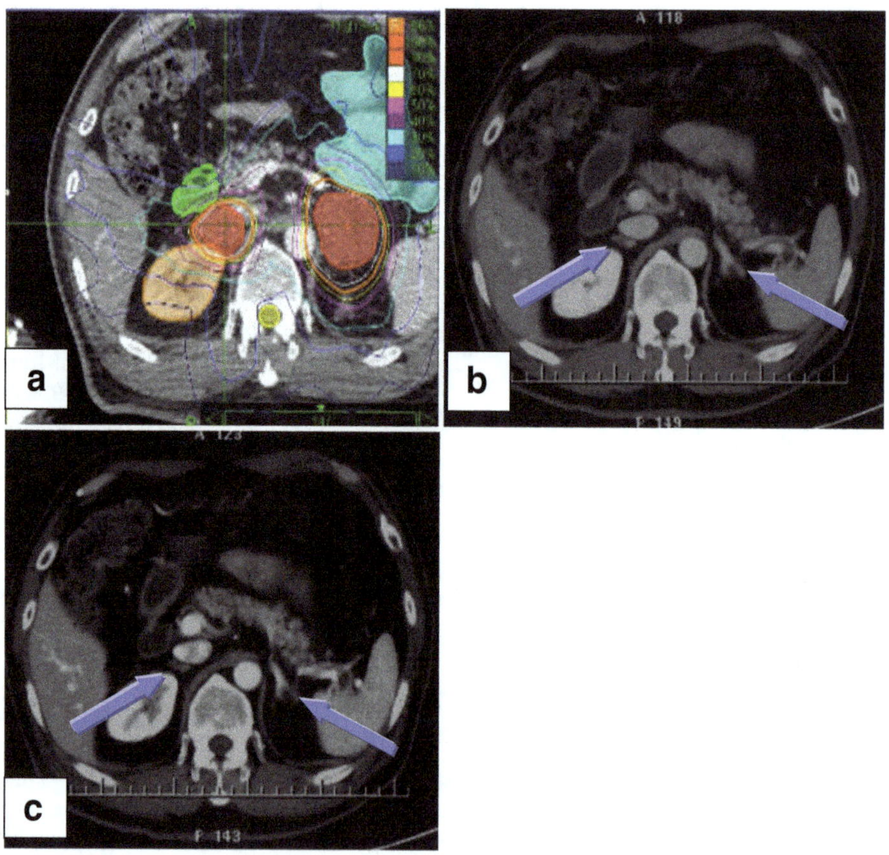

Fig. 1 An illustrative case of successful SBRT for 51-year-old man with two AGMs from NSCLC. **a** CT scan before SBRT and 45 Gy in 5 fractions was prescribed for each AGMs. Red shadow areas represented bilateral GTV. **b** Enhanced CT scan one month after SBRT. **c** Enhanced CT scan three months after SBRT.GTV: gross tumor volume; AGMs: adrenal gland metastases; SBRT: stereotactic body radiation therapy; CT: computed tomography. Note: The arrows indicate AGMs after SBRT

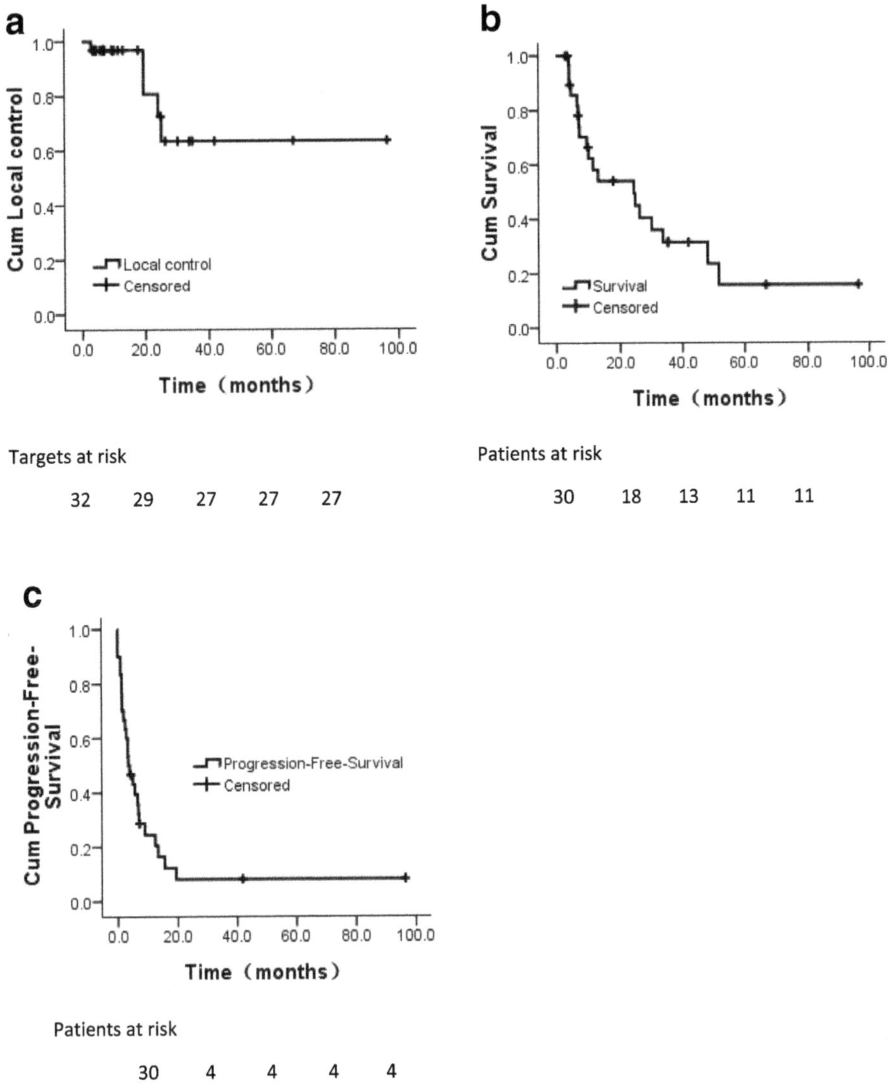

Fig. 2 Actuarial survival analysis of patients. **a** Overall local control. **b** Overall survival in general. **c** Overall progression-free-survival. Cum, cumulative

Nineteen of thirty patients (21/32 targets) were treated for palliation purpose. The 6-month, 1, and 2-year LC rates of these targets were 95.2%, 95.2%, and 47.6% respectively, whereas the 6-month, 1, and 2-year OS rates of these patients were 76.0%, 54.9%, and 54.9% respectively. Elven of thirty patients (11/32 targets) were treated for radical purpose. The 6-month, 1, and 2-year LC rates of these targets were all 100%, whereas the 6-month, 1, and 2-year OS rates of these patients were 100%, 63.6%, and 54.5% respectively.

In the univariate analysis, patients with GTV < 30 ml had a high LC rate than those with GTV ≥ 30 ml ($P = 0.003$, Table 3). Moreover, $BED_{10} \geq 85.5$Gy was predictive of better LC ($P = 0.007$, Table 3). However, no factors were found to be correlated with LC after the multivariate analysis.

Similarly, no predictors were associated with OS after univariate and multivariate analysis (Table 4).

Among the patients who had tumor-induced symptoms prior to the treatment (including 8 with abdominal pain and 6 with lumbar back pain), all of them (100.0%) had alleviations of symptoms after SBRT.

Treatment toxicity

The treatment was well-tolerated. No grade 4 or higher acute toxicity was observed and only 1 patient had grade 3 diarrhea. Fatigue, poor appetite, nausea, thrombocytopenia, leucopenia, vomiting and pain were the most common side effects during treatment. There were no grade 3 or higher late gastrointestinal toxicities. Furthermore, even grade 1 or 2 late gastrointestinal toxicity was not recorded during follow-up.. All the adverse effects were temporary, reversible

Table 3 Univariate analysis for LC rate

	1-year LC rate (%)	2-year LC rate (%)	*P* Value
BED (Gy)			
<85.5	92.3	23.1	0.007
≥ 85.5	100	100	
Prescription dose (Gy)			
<42	100	25.0	0.072
≥ 42	95.5	95.5	
GTV (ml)			
<30	100	100	0.003
≥ 30	92.9	23.2	
Systemic therapy after SBRT			
Yes	100	70.0	0.913
No	92.9	92.9	
Tracking method			
X-sight spine	95.2	81.6	0.869
synchrony respiratory motion	100	60.0	

and ameliorated by medication, which did not prevent patients from completing the treatment (Table 5). Additionally, three patients and one patient received tyrosine-kinase inhibitors and anti-vascular endothelial growth factor agent. and only mild toxicities, including skin rash or diarrhea, were found and alleviated by supportive care.

Discussion

The study investigated the efficacy of SBRT for AGMs from lung cancer. Overall, SBRT may provide high LC rates, survival benefits with the median OS of 24.4 months and symptom relief without serious toxicities. Additionally, no grade 4 or above acute toxicities were reported. Therefore, it may be implied that SBRT was a promising modality in the management of AGMs from lung cancer, especially for a palliative purpose to relieve various symptoms caused by the metastases.

Table 4 Univariate analysis for OS rate

	1-year OS rate (%)	2-year OS rate (%)	*P* Value
Concurrence of metastasis in other sites			
Yes	59.4	59.4	0.740
No	57.1	50.0	
Systemic therapy after SBRT			
Yes	71.4	71.4	0.119
No	41.0	30.8	
Local control			
Yes	50.4	45.3	0.320
No	100	100	
Metastasis in other sites after SBRT			
Yes	56.7	52.0	0.164
No	66.7	66.7	
Age (years)			
<60	56.2	46.9	0.674
≥ 60	58.7	58.7	

Surgery was considered as a standard curative-intent strategy for isolated adrenal metastasis from non-small cell lung cancer (NSCLC). In the analysis of 13 retrospective studies, the median OS of patients with NSCLC and isolated adrenal metastasis treated with segmentectomy, lobectomy or pneumonectomy, and adrenalectomy was 18 months, and the 1-, 2- and 5-year survival rates were 66.5, 40.5 and 28.2%, respectively [19]. Another efficacious local-regional treatment was image-guided RFA. A retrospective study evaluated 35 patients with 41 AGMs with the mean size of 3.3 cm from various types of primary tumors. At the last follow-up, 27 patients (77%) achieved local control. The 1-, 3-, and 5-year OS rates were 75%, 34%, and 30% respectively, with a median survival time of 26.0 months [20]. Nevertheless, in our study, 15 patients had metastases in other sites in addition to AGMs. Moreover, there were 8 AGMs with the diameter more than 5 cm, 14 AGMs with the volume more than 30 ml. Hence, those patients may not be amenable to surgical resections and RFA. Due to quick dose fall-off and fewer low dose areas outside targets compared with conventional radiotherapy, SBRT may be beneficial for them, especially when they had failed in adjuvant chemotherapy, molecular targeted drug therapy, and conventional radiotherapy.

Recently, SBRT has been an alternative for patients with AGMs from different types of tumor [21–24]. In a Florence study [21], 48 patients, most of whom had AGMs from lung cancer, received SBRT. The median follow-up was 16.2 months. Both of the actuarial 1-year and 2-year LC rate were 90%, and the1-year and 2-year OS rates were 39.7% and 14.5%, respectively. The

Table 5 Adverse effects reported/observed

AE	Grade 1–2	Grade3 or more	Total *N* (%)
Nausea	10 (33.3%)	0 (–)	10 (33.3%)
Vomiting	2 (6.7%)	0 (–)	2 (6.7%)
Poor appetite	11 (36.7%)	0 (–)	11 (36.7%)
Diarrhea	2 (6.7%)	1 (3.3%)	3 (10.0%)
Hepatic injury	1 (3.3%)	0 (–)	1 (3.3%)
Renal injury	2 (6.7%)	0 (–)	2 (6.7%)
Leucopenia	5 (16.7%)	0 (–)	5 (16.7%)
Thrombocytopenia	6 (20.0%)	0 (–)	6 (20.0%)
Fatigue	14 (46.7%)	0 (–)	14 (46.7%)
Myalgia	2 (6.7%)	0 (–)	2 (6.7%)
Abdominal pain	11 (36.7%)	0 (–)	11 (36.7%)

actuarial 1-year disease control rate was 9%. In another study, 30 patients with AGMs underwent SBRT. The 1-year OS, LC, and distant control rate was 44%, 55%, and 13%, respectively. No patients developed grade 2 or greater toxicity [22]. However, few studies focused on AGMs exclusively from lung cancer. In a relevant report, SBRT was performed in 18 patients with AGMs from NSCLC. The median follow-up was 12 months. Ten out of thirteen patients (77%) with an isolated lesion in the adrenal gland achieved local control with a median OS and PFS of 21 and 4.2 months, respectively [25]. Besides, another study reported the 1-year and 2-year local control rates of 15 patients after SBRT were 60% and 46.6%, respectively. The median OS was 17.3 months. One- and two-year disease free survival rate was 60% and 46.6%, respectively, while the median disease-free survival was 10.5 months [26]. Similar outcomes were also found in Franzese et al. with the median OS of 28.5 months and 1-year and 2-year LC rates of 65.5% and 40.7%, respectively [27]. Nevertheless, the median OS was inferior than those in the above studies when patients received SBRT or conventional radiotherapy [28], which might be attributable to lower BED_{10} compared with those of SBRT. The findings in current study were consistent with previous studies. The 0.5, 1, and 2-year LC rates were 96.9%, 96.9% and 72.7% respectively. The 0.5, 1, and 2-year OS rates were 85.6%, 58.1%, and 54.0% respectively, and similarly the corresponding PFS rates were 39.5%, 24.6%, and 8.2% respectively. Moreover, it was the first multicenter study to report the safety and efficacy of SBRT for inoperable AGMs from lung cancer.

A dose-response relationship has been observed in several studies about SBRT for AGMs. Previous studies demonstrated that $BED_{10} < 60Gy$ was predictive of lower 1-year LC rates [22, 29, 30] while other reports identified that $BED_{10} > 85Gy$ correlated with better LC [21, 31, 32]. In our study, patients with $BED_{10} \geq 85.5Gy$ had higher 1- and 2-year LC rates compared with those with $BED_{10} < 85.5Gy$ ($P = 0.007$).

In our study, no late gastrointestinal or renal toxicities were found, which was consistent with the previous studies [25–28]. Only two patients developed multiple gastric or duodenal ulcer [25]. The low incidence of late toxicity may be attributable to the smaller tumor volume compared with that in Holy, Celik and Scorsetti et al. [25, 26, 28], though the radiation doses in our study were higher than those prescribed in all those studies.

In Zishan' s study, they evaluated and examined the influence of tumor size on outcomes for medically inoperable early-stage non-small cell lung cancer after SBRT. As a result, tumor size was not associated with local failure but regional failure and distant failure [33]. However, in Doré's study, they evaluated local control after postoperative hypofractionated stereotactic radiosurgery in patients with brain metastasis. On univariate analysis, initial tumour volume less than 9.5 cm^3 ($P = 0.05$) and PTV less than 12 cm^3 ($P = 0.005$) were associated with improved LC [34]. In our study, tumor size was an important predictor of local control. We observed patients who had smaller AGMs (GTV < 30 ml) had a better LC rate ($P = 0.003$) than those who had bigger ones (GTV ≥ 30 ml). Notably, it must be noted that high LC rates cannot be achieved with the compromise of protections of organs at risk. Therefore, high radiation doses may not be prescribed in the case of large tumors due to dose constraints of surrounding normal tissues, while smaller lesions may receive higher doses. Hence, a prospective trial is needed to confirm these preliminary observations.

Typically, abdominal pain and lumbar back pain were the two most common symptoms in patients with AGMs. We found that all of the patients had symptomatic relief after SBRT. A previous study reported that all 3 patients with AGMs rated their score as 0 on a 10-point scale, which were 4–5 before SBRT [22]. The results were consistent with our study. What is interesting and worth investigating is that since SBRT is effective in symptoms ameliorations, it might be indicated that SBRT could be employed soon after AGMs are found to prevent potential tumor-induced symptoms.

There were some limitations of this study. It was retrospective, and with a limited number of patients or targets. In addition, the treatment schedules were heterogeneous: there was a wide range of doses prescribed with various fractionations. Furthermore, a longer follow-up is warranted to examine the impact of LC on regional or distant disease control and survival.

Conclusion

SBRT is an effective modality with fast symptom relief, and acceptable toxicity for lung cancer patients with AGMs. Patients with $BED_{10} \geq 85.5$ Gy and GTV < 30 ml had a better LC rate. Because most patients died of or were at high risk of distant metastasis, local treatment combined with systemic treatment may contribute to a better outcome. Moreover, the efficacy and safety of SBRT for patients with AGMs from lung cancer needed to be validated in the prospective studies.

Abbreviations

AGM: Adrenal gland metastase; BED: Biologic equivalent dose; CR: Complete response; CT: Computed tomography; CTCAE: Common terminology criteria for adverse events; DVH: Dose-volume histogram; GTV: Gross tumor volume; LC: Local control; NSCLC: Non-small cell lung cancer; OS: Overall survival; PD: Progressive disease; PFS: Progression free survival; PR: Partial response; PTV: Planning target volume; QOL: Quality of life; RECIST: Response evaluation criteria in solid tumors; RFA: Radiofrequency ablation; SBRT: Stereotactic body radiation therapy; SD: Stable disease

Funding
This study is sponsored by China Health Promotion Foundation THC2015001.

Authors' contributions
X.Z.Z., X.F.Z. and J.F.F. conceived, designed the experiments and wrote the paper. Y.S.C. helped to analyze the treatment planning. H.P.R. and X.P.J. helped to collect and analyze the data. Z.Y.Y. and H.J.Z revised the paper. All authors read and approved the final manuscript.

Competing interests
The authors declare that they have no competing interests.

Author details
[1]Department of Radiation Oncology, Shanghai Changhai Hospital, the Second Military Medical University, Shanghai 200433, China. [2]Department of Radiology, Shanghai Changhai Hospital, the Second Military Medical University, Shanghai 200433, China. [3]Department of Oncology, Weifang People's Hospital, Weifang 261041, China. [4]Department of Radiation Oncology and CyberKnife Center, Key Laboratory of Cancer Prevention and Therapy, Tianjin's Clinical Research Center for Cancer, Tianjin Medical University Cancer Institute and Hospital, National Clinical Research Center for Cancer, Tianjin 300060, China.

References

1. Brunt LM, Moley JF. Adrenal incidentaloma. World J Surg. 2001;25:905–13.
2. Yun M, Kim W, Alnafisi N, Lacorte L, Jang S, Alavi A. 18F-FDG PET in characterizing adrenal lesions detected on CT or MRI. J Nucl Med. 2001;42: 1795–9.
3. Tanvetyanon T, Robinson LA, Schell MJ, Strong VE, Kapoor R, Coit DG, et al. Outcomes of adrenalectomy for isolated synchronous versus metachronous adrenal metastases in non-small-cell lung cancer: a systematic review and pooled analysis. J Clin Oncol. 2008;26:1142–7.
4. Ng AW, Tung SY, Wong VY. Hypofractionated stereotactic radiotherapy for medically inoperable stage I non-small cell lung cancer – report on clinical outcome and dose to critical organs. Radiother Oncol. 2008;87:24–8.
5. Scorsetti M, Franceschini D, De Rose F, Comito T, Villa E, Iftode C, et al. Stereotactic body radiation therapy: a promising chance for oligometastatic breast cancer. Breast. 2016;26:11–7.
6. Su T-S, Liang P, Lu H-Z, Liang JN, Liu JM, Zhou Y, et al. Stereotactic body radiotherapy using CyberKnife for locally advanced unresectable and metastatic pancreatic cancer. World J Gastroenterol. 2015;21:8156–62.
7. Meng M, Wang H, Zeng X, Zhao L, Yuan Z, Wang P, et al. Stereotactic body radiation therapy: a novel treatment modality for inoperable hepatocellular carcinoma. Drug Discov Ther. 2015;9:372–9.
8. Potters L, Kavanagh B, Galvin JM, Hevezi JM, Janjan NA, Larson DA, et al. American Society for Therapeutic Radiology and Oncology (ASTRO) and American College of Radiology (ACR) practice guideline for the performance of stereotactic body radiation therapy. Int J Radiat Oncol Biol Phys. 2010;76:326–32.
9. Martin A, Gaya A. Stereotactic body radiotherapy: a review. Clin Oncol (R Coll Radiol). 2010;22:157–72.
10. Dieterich S, Gibbs IC. The CyberKnife in clinical use: current roles, future expectations. Front Radiat Ther Oncol. 2011;43:181–94.
11. Chang JY, Senan S, Paul MA, Mehran RJ, Louie AV, Balter P, et al. Stereotactic ablative radiotherapy versus lobectomy for operable stage I non-small-cell lung cancer: a pooled analysis of two randomised trials. Lancet Oncol. 2015;16:630–7.
12. Kato H, Yoshida H, Taniguch H, Nomura R, Sato K, Suzuki I, et al. Cyberknife treatment for advanced or terminal stage hepatocellular carcinoma. World J Gastroenterol. 2015;21:13101–12.
13. Fan C-Y, Chao H-L, Huang W-Y, Lin CS, Chen CM, Lo CH. Stereotactic ablative radiotherapy with CyberKnife in the treatment of locally advanced prostate cancer: preliminary results. Tumori J. 2015;101:684–91.
14. Zhu X, Li F, Ju X, Cao F, Cao Y, Fang F, et al. Prognostic role of stereotactic body radiation therapy for elderly patients with advanced and medically inoperable pancreatic cancer. Cancer Med. 2017;6:2263–70.
15. Wang J, Fengtong L, Yang D, Song Y, Yuan Z. Clinical study on the influence of motion and other factors on stereotactic radiotherapy in the treatment of adrenal gland tumor. Onco Targets Ther. 2016;15:4295–9.
16. Benedict SH, Yenice KM, Followill D, Galvin JM, Hinson W, Kavanagh B, et al. Stereotactic body radiation therapy: the report of AAPM task group 101. Med Phys. 2010;37:4078–101.
17. Cancer Institute N. Common Terminology Criteria for Adverse Events (CTCAE) Common Terminology Criteria for Adverse Events v4.0 (CTCAE): Publish; 2009. https://doi.org/10.1080/00140139.2010.489653.
18. Bogaerts J, Ford R, Sargent D, Schwartz LH, Rubinstein L, Lacombe D, et al. Individual patient data analysis to assess modifications to the RECIST criteria. Eur J Cancer. 2009;45:248–60.
19. Gao XL, Zhang KW, Tang MB, Zhang KJ, Fang LN, Liu W. Pooled analysis forsurgical treatment for isolated adrenal metastasis and non-small cell lung cancer. Interact Cardiovasc Thorac Surg. 2017;24:1–7.
20. Hasegawa T, Yamakado K, Nakatsuka A, Uraki J, Yamanaka T, Fujimori M, et al. Unresectable adrenal metastases: clinical outcomes of radiofrequency ablation. Radiology. 2015;277:584–93.
21. Casamassima F, Livi L, Masciullo S, Menichelli C, Masi L, Meattini I, et al. Stereotactic radiotherapy for adrenal gland metastases: University of Florence experience. Int J Radiat Oncol. 2012;82:919–23.
22. Chawla S, Chen Y, Katz AW, Muhs AG, Philip A, Okunieff P, et al. Stereotactic body radiotherapy for treatment of adrenal metastases. Int J Radiat Oncol Biol Phys. 2009;75:71–5.
23. Ippolito E, D'Angelillo RM, Fiore M, Molfese E, Trodella L, Ramella S. SBRT: a viable option for treating adrenal gland metastases. Reports Pract Oncol Radiother. 2015;20:484–90.
24. Plichta K, Camden N, Furqan M, Hejleh TA, Clamon GH, Zhang J, et al. SBRT to adrenal metastases provides high local control with minimal toxicity. Adv Radiat Oncol. 2017;2:581-7.
25. Holy R, Piroth M, Pinkawa M, Eble MJ. Stereotactic body radiation therapy (SBRT) for treatment of adrenal gland metastases from non-small cell lung cancer. Strahlenther Onkol. 2011;187:245–51.
26. Celik E, Semrau R, Baues C, Trommer-Nestler M, Baus W, Marnitz S, et al. Robot-assisted extracranial stereotactic radiotherapy of adrenal metastases in Oligometastatic non-small cell lung Cancer. Anticancer Res. 2017;37:5285–91.
27. Franzese C, Franceschini D, Cozzi L, D'Agostino G, Comito T, De Rose F, et al. Minimally invasive Stereotactical Radio-ablation of Adrenal Metastases as an alternative to surgery. Cancer Res Treat. 2017;49:20–8.
28. Buergy D, Rabe L, Siebenlist K, Stieler F, Fleckenstein J, Giordano FA, et al. Treatment of adrenal metastases with conventional or Hypofractionated image-guided radiation therapy - patterns and outcomes. Anticancer Res. 2018;38:4789–96.
29. Scorsetti M, Alongi F, Filippi AR, Pentimalli S, Navarria P, Clerici E, et al. Long-term local control achieved afterhypofractionated stereotactic body radiotherapy for adrenalgland metastases: a retrospective analysis of 34 patients. Acta Oncol. 2012;51:618–23.
30. Guiou M, Mayr NA, Kim EY, Williams T, Lo SS. Stereotactic body radiotherapy for adrenal metastases from lung cancer. J Radiat Oncol. 2012;1:155–63.
31. Ahmed KA, Barney BM, Macdonald OK, Miller RC, Garces YI, Laack NN, et al. Stereotactic body radiotherapy in the treatment of adrenal metastases. Am J Clin Oncol. 2013;36:509–13.
32. Oshiro Y, Takeda Y, Hirano S, Ito H, Aruga T. Role of radiotherapy for local control ofasymptomatic adrenal metastasis from lung cancer. Am J Clin Oncol. 2011;34:249–53.
33. Allibhai Z, Taremi M, Bezjak A, Brade A, Hope AJ, Sun A, et al. The impact of tumor size on outcomes after stereotactic body radiation therapy for medically inoperable early-stage non-small cell lung cancer. Int J Radiat Oncol Biol Phys. 2013;87:1064–70.
34. Doré M, Martin S, Delpon G, Clément K, Campion L, Thillays F. Stereotactic radiotherapy following surgery for brain metastasis: predictive factors for localcontrol and radionecrosis. Cancer radiother. 2017;21:4-9.

Does baseline [18F] FDG-PET/CT correlate with tumor staging, response after neoadjuvant chemoradiotherapy, and prognosis in patients with rectal cancer?

Letizia Deantonio[1,2], Angela Caroli[1], Erinda Puta[3], Daniela Ferrante[4], Francesco Apicella[1], Lucia Turri[1], Gianmauro Sacchetti[3], Marco Brambilla[5] and Marco Krengli[1,2*]

Abstract

Background: [18F] fluorodeoxyglucose positron emission tomography/computed tomography ([18F] FDG-PET/CT) may be used for tumor staging and prognosis in several tumors but its role in rectal cancer is still debated. The aim of the present study was to assess the correlation of baseline [18F] FDG-PET parameters with tumor staging, tumor response (tumor regression grade (TRG)), and outcome in a series of patients affected by locally advanced rectal cancer (LARC) treated with neoadjuvant chemoradiotherapy (CRT).

Methods: One hundred patients treated with neoadjuvant CRT and radical surgery were enrolled in the present study. Maximum standardized uptake value (SUVmax), SUVmean, metabolic tumor volume (MTV), and total lesion glycolysis (TLG) at the baseline [18F] FDG-PET were calculated. These PET parameters were correlated with tumor staging, histopathological data (TRG1 vs. TRG2–5 and TRG1–2 vs. TRG3–5), disease-free survival, and overall survival.

Results: SUVmax and SUVmean of primary tumor were statistically associated with T4-stage. SUVmax, SUVmean, and TLG did not result statistically associated with TRG (TRG1 or TRG1–2). MTV resulted statistically associated with TRG1–2 group (OR 2.9; 95% CI 1.2–7.1). Finally, no PET parameter was significantly associated with disease-free or overall survival.

Conclusion: Our results showed that baseline [18F] FDG-PET parameters correlated with tumor staging, and only MTV correlated with TRG 1–2. PET parameters failed to predict disease-free and overall survival after treatment completion. The results leave open to further studies the issue of identifying patients suitable for conservative approaches.

Keywords: Rectal cancer, [18F] fluorodeoxyglucose positron emission tomography, Standardized uptake value, Metabolic tumor volume, Total lesion glycolysis, Predictive value

Background

Treatment approach to rectal cancer has greatly evolved over the past years. In locally advanced rectal cancer (LARC), neoadjuvant chemoradiotherapy (CRT) followed by surgical resection with total mesorectal excision is the current standard treatment approach [1, 2].

According to literature data, 50 to 60% of the patients can reach a down-staging following CRT with about 20% of complete pathological response [3]. This rate of pathological response has raised the issue of organ preservation. Notably, Habr-Gama et al. [4] pioneered this innovative concept by avoiding surgery when a complete response was achieved at restaging after CRT. The study reported 49% of complete clinical response after CRT in a series of 183 patients with T2–4 N0–2 distal rectal tumors. Subsequently, the "watch and wait" strategy or the local excision after CRT has been explored as organ-preserving

* Correspondence: marco.krengli@med.uniupo.it
[1]Radiotherapy, University Hospital "Maggiore della Carità", Novara, Italy
[2]Department of Translational Medicine, University of "Piemonte Orientale", Novara, Italy
Full list of author information is available at the end of the article

alternatives in selected patients' cohorts with encouraging results [5, 6].

Tumor response after CRT is usually assessed by the tumor regression grade (TRG) as proposed by Mandard et al. [7], based on the pathological exam of the surgical specimen. Nowadays, the diagnostic challenge for an organ preservation approach is to find an adequate surrogate of histology able to discriminate responders from non-responders. The attention on morphological (i.e. magnetic resonance imaging, MRI) and even more on metabolic imaging suitable for predicting CRT response is constantly increasing [8, 9]. In this regard, the role that [18F] -fluorodeoxyglucose positron emission tomography/computed tomography ([18F] FDG-PET/CT) has in staging and treatment planning of rectal cancer is still quite debatable [10–12] as well as in measuring treatment response [13–18].

The primary aim of the present study was to evaluate whether in LARC metabolic characteristics detected by [18F] FDG-PET/CT, prior to neoadjuvant CRT, could correlate with clinical tumor stage, with tumor regression after surgery, and with MRI findings. A secondary endpoint was to determine the prognostic value of [18F] FDG-PET/CT in terms of disease-free survival (DFS) and overall survival (OS).

Methods

Patients

From 2008 to 2016, one hundred patients were enrolled in the present observational study after obtaining a written informed consent following the rules of our institution. The local ethics committee approved the present study. Inclusion criteria were as follows: biopsy proven rectal adenocarcinoma, age > 18 years, cT3–4 cN0–2 disease at staging, absence of distant metastasis or other concomitant tumors, no contraindication to chemotherapy, and availability of the [18F] FDG-PET/CT images retrieved from our institutional digital archive. All cases were discussed in a multidisciplinary conference with gastroenterologists, surgeons, radiation oncologists, and medical oncologists.

Pre-treatment workup included blood chemistry, clinical examination, endoscopy with biopsy, and chest and abdomen CT. Tumor extension and lymph-nodal involvement were assessed by pelvic MRI on a 1.5 Tesla scanner (Achieva, Philips Medical System, Best, Holland) and [18F] FDG-PET/CT [8]. Final staging was defined according to the American Joint Committee on Cancer (AJCC) TNM classification [19]. The main clinical characteristics of patients are listed in Table 1.

Table 1 Patients' clinical characteristics

Characteristics	Value	(%)
Gender (No. of patients)		
Male	65	(65.0)
Female	35	(35.0)
Age (years)		
Median	67	
Range	41–83	
Tumor clinical stage (No. of patients)		
cT3	85	(85.0)
cT4	15	(15.0)
Nodal clinical stage (No. of patients)		
cN0	32	(32.0)
cN+	68	(68.0)
Rectal segment, distance to the anal verge		
Upper third	20	(20.0)
Middle third	42	(42.0)
Lower third	38	(38.0)
Pathological stage (No. of patients)		
ypT0 N0	16	(16.0)
ypT1 N0-N1	5	(5.0)
ypT2 N0-N2	19	(19.0)
ypT3 N0-N1-N2	56	(56.0)
ypT4 N0-N1-N2	4	(4.0)
TRG (No. of patients)		
TRG 1	16	(16.0)
TRG 2	15	(15.0)
TRG 3	25	(25.0)
TRG 4	22	(22.0)
TRG 5	22	(22.0)

No number, *TRG* Tumor regression grade

[18F] FDG-PET/CT imaging

The patients underwent [18F] FDG-PET/CT within five working days from CT simulation by hybrid PET/CT scanner (Biograph 16 HI-REZ, Siemens Medical Solutions, Berkeley CA), equipped with Pico-3D digital electronics and reconstruction with ordered subset expectation maximization (OSEM3D) algorithm (2 iterations × 24 subsets, and a post-reconstruction Gaussian filter with a full width at maximum of 8 mm), on a 256 × 256 image frame (voxel size 2.66 mm × 2.66 mm × 2.00 mm). Images were analyzed using a dedicated workstation Leonardo (Siemens Medical Solutions, Berkeley CA). CT images were used for both attenuation correction of PET data and localization of pathological FDG uptake. CT scan was performed without administration of intravenous contrast with a low-dose protocol for CT acquisition. Fasting time was at least 6 h prior to examination. The blood glucose levels of all patients were measured before the injection of [18F] FDG and were < 150 mg/dL. The injected activity of FDG was 3 MBq/Kg and the mean time between injection and acquisition was 70 min (range: 55–90 min). [18F] FDG-PET/CT imaging was performed from the proximal femur to the base of the skull. Emission images were acquired for 2–5 min per bed position, depending on patient's body mass index as described in a previous study [20].

The processed images were displayed in coronal, transverse, and sagittal plans and interpreted in standard clinical fashion, both separately and in fused mode. The [18F] FDG-PET/CT images were reviewed for abnormal FDG uptake of the primary tumor, lymph nodes, and distant sites. The maximum standardized uptake value (SUVmax) was calculated for each primary tumor, along with the mean standardized uptake value (SUVmean), the metabolic tumor volume (MTV) and the total lesion glycolysis (TLG) according to the European Agency of Nuclear Medicine (EANM) guidelines [21].

The SUVmax was automatically calculated to determine the [18F] FDG-PET activity and recorded using a volumetric region of interest (VOI), positioned around the pathological [18F] FDG uptake in the attenuation-corrected images. Each VOI was checked visually to exclude areas of physiological uptake as bladder. The MTV was defined as the volume of hypermetabolic tissue with a threshold greater than 41% of the maximum pixel value in the primary tumor [21]. The software calculated the SUVmean within the MTV. The TLG was defined as the SUVmean multiplied by the MTV.

Treatment

All patients were treated with neoadjuvant CRT. External beam RT was delivered by Linear accelerators (Varian Clinac 600 DBX and Varian Clinac DHX, Varian Medical Systems, Milpitas CA) to a total dose of 45 Gy, with daily fraction of 1.8 Gy. RT was given to all patients in a homogeneous way including the identification of the clinical target volume (CTV) which was defined as the gross tumor volume with the mesorectal fascia and the pelvic lymph nodes as recommended by Roels et al. [22]. An isotropic expansion of 8 mm around the CTV was applied to define the planning target volume (PTV). Treatment planning (Pinnacle, Philips, Adac Laboratories, Milpitas CA) was performed through 3-dimension-conformal RT (3D-CRT) technique in 57 patients and by "step and shot" intensity modulated radiotherapy (IMRT) in 43 patients. In the present study, ^{18}F FDG-PET/CT imaging was used for both tumor staging, and target identification as reported in a previous study [8]. Concomitant chemotherapy was administered during the five weeks of RT with daily oral capecitabine (825 mg/m^2 twice daily) or continuous infusion of 5-fluorouracil (225 mg/m^2).

After CRT, all patients were re-staged with the same imaging modality (CT/MRI) performed for baseline tumor staging, in particular 42 patients were re-staged with MRI (TSE T2 weighted and post-contrast weighted TFE T1 sequences). A total mesorectal excision with anterior or abdominoperineal resection was performed 6–11 weeks (median 8 weeks) after CRT according to the clinical presentation.

Clinical endpoints

Data was collected to evaluate metabolic parameters detected by [18F] FDG-PET/CT prior to neoadjuvant CRT in relation with pre-treatment tumor characteristics (i.e. tumor extension, distance from the anal verge, and presence of pathological lymph-nodes), treatment response, response assessment with MRI, and survival.

Post-surgical staging was assessed according to the AJCC/TNM classification (ypTNM) [19]. A pathological finding of ypT0N0 was considered a complete pathological response, while any ypT1–4 N0–2 a non-complete pathological response (Table 1). These findings were scored according to TRG classification following the criteria defined by Mandard et al. [7]: TRG1 = complete tumor response, no residual cancer cell; TRG2 = residual cancer cells scattered through fibrosis; TRG3 = increased number of residual cancer cells with predominant fibrosis; TRG4 = residual cancer outgrowing fibrosis; and TRG5 = no regressive changes within the tumor. We performed the analysis between TRG1 and TRG2–5 and between TRG1–2 and TRG3–5.

In the subset of 42 patients who repeated MRI after neoadjuvant treatment (TSE T2 weighted, post-contrast weighted TFE T1 sequences), the response assessment, scored by Response Evaluation Criteria in Solid Tumors (RECIST) [23] was compared with PET parameters.

During follow-up, patients underwent the same exams as at baseline every 6 months for the first 2 years and then every year. Diagnosis of recurrent tumor and distant metastasis was based on clinical and radiological evidence of tumor relapse, confirmed by biopsy.

Statistical analysis

All quantitative PET imaging parameters (SUVmax, SUVmean, MTV, and TLG) were expressed as mean ± standard deviation (SD). The student 2-tailed t-test after normalization using logarithmic transformation was used to compare the quantitative parameters of the clinical variables categorized as follows: cT3 vs. cT4, TRG1 vs. TRG2–5, and TRG1–2 vs. TRG3–5.

Binary logistic regression was performed to evaluate the association of SUV, MTV and TLG with TRG using the median value as cut-off. The odds ratios (OR) and the 95% confidence interval (95% CI) were calculated. The analysis of variance (ANOVA) after normalization using logarithmic transformation was performed to evaluate PET parameters differences among upper, middle and lower rectal cancer locations. Mann Whitney test was performed to analyze the time interval from the end of CRT and surgery among TRG classes.

Logistic regression was applied to analyze and compare PET and MRI images at restaging.

Follow-up time was analyzed from the last day of CRT to the date of the last follow-up, recurrence, or death. DFS and OS rates were calculated using Kaplan-Meier analysis stratified according to cut-off value (median value) and compared using the log-rank test. Recurrent and non-recurrent patients were compared with Fisher test.

The statistical power of the study was 50%. This was calculated on 100 patients enrolled, on value of alpha equal to 0.05, and on the 4-years OS for SUVmax median value as cut-off equal to 0.90 (for patients with a SUVmax < 20.6) and to 0.75 (for patients with a SUVmax > 20.6). A p value ≤0.05 was considered as statistically significant. Statistical analysis was performed using STATA v11 (Stata Corporation, College Station, TX, USA).

Results

Metabolic characteristics in relation to clinical stage and restaging

The mean values and SD of SUVmax, SUVmean, MTV, and TLG of the baseline [18F] FDG-PET/CT were reported in Table 2. The SUVmax (p = 0.01), SUVmean (p = 0.01), MTV (p = 0.003) and TLG (p = 0.0004) values were significantly higher in the cT4 than in the cT3 cases. Conversely, PET parameters were not influenced by rectal tumor origin in the upper, middle and lower rectum. By logistic regression model, primary tumors with SUVmax or SUVmean higher than median values were statistically associated with cT4-stage (both ORs 8.4; 95% CI 1.8–39.7).

Response assessment with MRI was available in 42 patients out of 100. None of the PET parameters resulted statistically associated with MRI findings (1 complete response and 20 partial responses vs. 11 stable diseases).

Pathological response evaluation

All patients underwent surgery with total mesorectal excision 6–8 weeks after CRT; anterior resection was performed in 79 patients (79%) and abdominoperineal resection in 21 patients (21%). The ypTNM classification was available for all the 100 patients (Table 1). At pathological examination, 16 patients (16%) were classified as TRG1 (ypT0 N0) and 84 (84%) as TRG2–5 (ypT1–4 N0–2). Sixty-one out of 100 patients (61%) achieved tumor downstaging. Negative margins were observed in all but two patients, classified as TRG3 and TRG5 respectively, after neoadjuvant CRT.

Table 2 [18F] FGD-PET parameters of the primary tumor

Variable	Mean (SD)	Minimum	Maximum
SUVmax	22.7 (9.7)	5.7	54.1
SUVmean	13.2 (5.7)	3.1	32.6
MTV	21.4 (21.9)	1.2	153.9
TLG	313.0 (480.0)	8.0	3331.0

SD Standard deviation, *SUVmax* Maximum standardized uptake value, *SUVmean* Mean standardized uptake value, *MTV* Metabolic tumor volume, *TLG* Total lesion glycolysis

Comparing [18F] FDG-PET parameters of TRG1 and TRG2–5 no significant difference was found, but comparing TRG1–2 and TRG3–5 MTV significantly changed (14.8 vs. 24.4, p = 0.01). Thus, only MTV resulted statistically associated with TRG1–2 group (OR 2.9; 95% CI 1.2–7.1) (Table 3).

Analyzing interval time between the last day of CRT and surgery, no significant differences were observed between TRG1 and TRG2–5 (p = 0.49) or TRG1–2 and TRG3–5 (p = 0.30).

Metabolic characteristics in relation to DFS and OS

The median follow-up time of the whole series was 32 months (range 12–116 months). Twenty-four patients (24%) developed loco-regional or at distance relapse. Although all but one of them were classified as TRG2–5 at the histological analysis, the comparison of tumor relapses between TRG1 and TRG2–5 did not achieve a statistical significance (p = 0.1). Ten patients developed a loco-regional recurrence (41.7%) and 14 liver and/or lung metastasis (58.3%). At the time of analysis, 8 patients were dead (8%), 6 out of the 8 died of metastatic progression disease. Moreover, none PET parameters significantly correlated with DFS or OS (Figs. 1 and 2).

Discussion

It is well recognized that neoadjuvant CRT for LARC has an impact on tumor downsizing and can achieve a higher percentage of long-term local control and better quality of life than adjuvant CRT [24]. Moreover, the achievement of a complete pathological response has a demonstrated positive prognostic impact on disease control [25]. Nowadays, the challenge is how to discriminate responders from non-responders to preoperative CRT, in order to tailor the treatment strategy. Less aggressive surgery or "watch and wait" policy after CRT for responders or more aggressive treatment for non-responders. In this setting, the most appropriate imaging approach to assess tumor response is a key point and it is still matter of investigation. In this regard, endorectal ultrasounds and MRI are routinely used for re-staging before surgical procedure, but these imaging modalities suffer of limited accuracy in distinguishing residual tumor from post-treatment changes such as fibrosis [26]. Of note, some authors [27–30] investigated the early prediction of tumor response based on [18F] FDG-PET/CT imaging performed during and after neoadjuvant CRT by comparing the baseline [18F] FDG-PET with that ad interim and before surgery. They observed that tumor response was predicted by metabolic changes in the first two weeks of RT, proving that [18F]

Table 3 [18F] FGD-PET/CT parameters related to clinical variables

Variables	cT stage Mean ± SD		TRG Mean ± SD		TRG Mean ± SD	
	cT3	cT4	TRG1	TRG2–5	TRG1–2	TRG3–5
SUVmax	21.6 ± 9.3	28.9 ±9.8	22.9 ±9.9	21.7 ±8.8	22.9 ±8.9	21.7 ± 10
	$p = 0.01$		$p = 0.68$		$p = 0.75$	
SUVmean	12.6 ± 5.5	16.6 ± 5.7	13.3 ± 5.9	12.5 ± 4.9	13.5 ± 5.4	13.3 ± 5.9
	$p = 0.01$		$p = 0.68$		$p = 0.6$	
MTV	18.0 ± 13.2	41.0 ± 43.2	22.4 ± 23.3	16.7 ± 11.7	14.8 ± 10.3	24.4 ± 24.9
	$p = 0.003$		$p = 0.21$		$p = 0.01$	
TLG	221.1 ± 172.6	833.5 ± 1053.0	330.1 ± 515.4	222.9 ± 200.8	210.6 ± 183.9	358.9 ± 560
	$p = 0.0004$		$p = 0.23$		$p = 0.08$	

T Tumor stage, *TRG* Tumor regression grade, *SD* Standard deviation, *SUVmax* Maximum standardized uptake value, *SUVmean* Mean standardized uptake value, *MTV* Metabolic tumor volume, *TLG* Total lesion glycolysis, *p* p- value calculated with Student T-test

FDG-PET/CT can be useful to predict pathological response for rectal cancer. A weakness of these studies [27–30] was related to the small sample size of patients that could have biased the results.

Our observational study analyzed whether the only pretreatment [18F] FDG PET/CT could be correlated with tumor stage and predict tumor response and survival in a relatively large number of patients. Because the choice of the best PET parameter to be used is still debatable, in addition to the most frequently used parameters (i.e. SUVmax and SUVmean), we decided to investigate also MTV and TLG which are be able to predict treatment response in other tumor types [31, 32].

In our study, a higher level of metabolic and volumetric parameters was significantly associated with cT4 stage, generally considered a more aggressive disease.

Although the median baseline SUV, MTV, and TLG showed higher values in TRG2–5 than TRG1, the absence of a significant difference seems to support the conclusion that the baseline [18F] FDG-PET parameters cannot predict the achievement of rectal cancer complete regression after neoadjuvant CRT. We also considered PET parameters in the light of MRI response assessment in a subset of 42 patients and we were not able to find any significant association with tumor response detected by MRI performed before surgery. In this regard, a future study could consider the use of

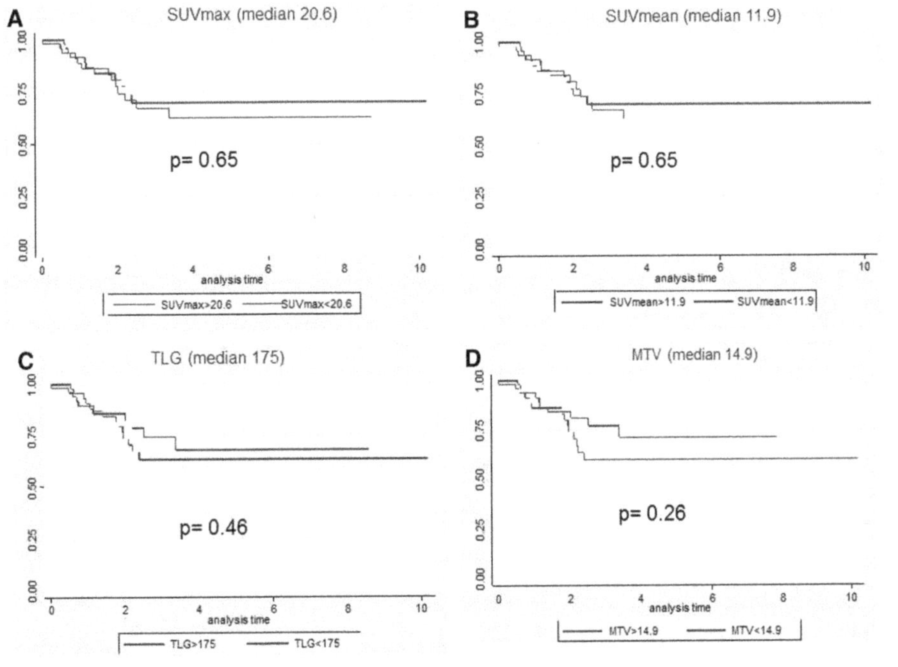

Fig. 1 4-years disease-free survival (DFS). Kaplan-Meier curves with the Log-Rank value of the PET parameters (SUVmax, SUVmean, TLG, and MTV) using the median values as cut-off. The blue lines correspond to values higher than median, the red lines correspond to values lower than the median

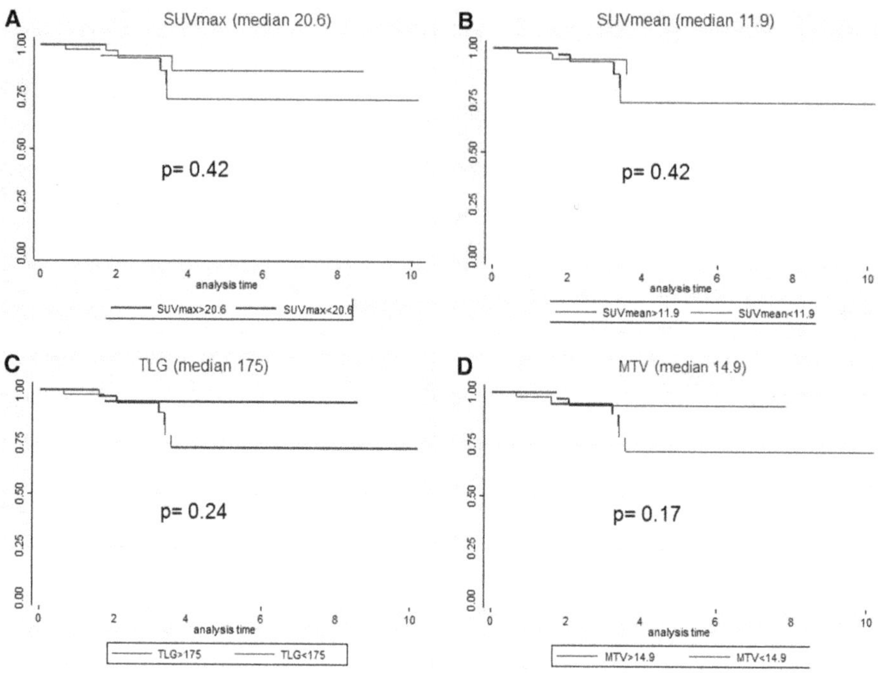

Fig. 2 4-years overall survival (OS). Kaplan-Meier curves with the Log-Rank value of the PET parameters (SUVmax, SUVmean, TLG, and MTV) using the median values as cut-off. The blue lines correspond to values higher than median, the red lines correspond to values lower than the median

PET/MRI, including also DWI sequences, in the attempt to optimize the response assessment.

Exploring the hypothesis that baseline[18F] FDG-PET parameters might be able to predict patients with a complete pathologic response, who may be treated with organ preserving strategies, we compared either TRG1 vs. TRG2–5 or TRG1–2 vs. TRG3–5. As a matter of fact, only TRG1 cases represent true complete responses in which a transanal endoscopic resection or a wait and see policy could be justified. However, MTV resulted predictive of tumor response only when TRG1–2 was compared to TRG3–5. In this regard, only few studies [26, 33–35] analyzed the predictive value of baseline [18F] FDG-PET parameters with contrasting results, leaving this issue still open for further investigation. Chennupati et al. [33] did not find any correlation between pathological response and SUVmax or MTV at baseline in 35 patients who underwent [18F] FDG-PET. Similar findings on 88 patients were reported by Park el al. [26] who found no differences of the pre-treatment [18F] FDG-PET parameters (SUV or MTV) between responder and non-responder groups. In contrast, Bang et al. [34] in a sample of 74 patients found that MTV calculated using different thresholds was significantly associated with TRG1–2, however this association was not confirmed after multivariate analysis. Moreover, Hatt et al. [35] found that response to CRT in a small sample of 28 patients was correlated with higher levels of SUVmean ($p = 0.02$) but not with TLG and MTV.

Considering the survival findings, we have not observed any significant correlation of [18F] FDG-PET parameters with DFS or OS (Figs. 1, and 2). However, all but one patient, who experienced a loco-regional or at distance progression, were observed in the non-responder group. Most likely, the low number of tumor relapses could have influenced the non-significance of the correlation of PET parameters with survival. In this regard, literature studies reported only some and contrasting data on the correlation between PET parameters and survival. Bang et al. [34] reported that baseline MTV calculated with various thresholds was significantly associated with 3-year DFS, while Leccisotti et al. [36], analyzing baseline post-treatment metabolic changes, did not find any correlation with DFS or OS because of the very low rate of tumor relapses after a median follow-up time of 68 months.

As shown by our study and by the other literature series, the predictive role of [18] FDG-PET is still unclear and deserves further investigation (Table 4). Although the present study has the limitation of a relatively low statistical power, most likely related to the low number of tumor relapses, it analyzed quite a large number of patients treated in a homogeneous way at the same institution and observed for quite a long follow-up time.

Table 4 Comparison among principal clinical series and our series

Study	Number of patients	Pathological responders % (TRG)	PET parameter	Correlation PET with pCR *p Value*	Correlation PET with DFS/OS
Martoni 2011 [15]	80	20% (TRG4 by Dworak)	SUVmax pre SUVmax post	Negative $p = 0.05$ Negative $p = 0.0003$	Disease recurrence: SUVmax post >/< 5 p = 0.0003
Calvo 2013 [16]	38	50% (TRG3–4 by Dworak)	SUVmax pre SUVmax post	Negative $p = 0.12$ Negative $p < 0.0001$	ΔSUVmax< 4 risk of Recurrence $p = 0.0007$ ΔSUVmax< 4 HR = 5.73 $p = 0.05$
Park 2014 [26]	88	19.3% (TRG1 by Mandard)	SUVmax pre SUVmax post MTV pre MTV post	NS $p < 0.001$ $p = 0.029$ $p < 0.0001$	NA
Dos Anjos 2016 [28]	90	22.2% (TRG NA)	ΔSUVmax (40%) ΔMTV (40%) ΔTLG (40%)	p < 0.0001 $p = 0.005$ $p = 0.03$	NA
Janssen 2012 [30]	26 20	42.3%(TRG1–2 by Mandard) 20% (TRG1–2 by Mandard)	RI SUVmax	48% SUVmax: Spec 100% Sens 64% Spec 93% Sens 83%	NA
Chennupati 2012 [33]	35	40% (TRG 0–1 by Ryan)	SUVmax pre MTV pre SUVmax post MTV post ΔSUVmax ΔMTV	NS NS NS NS NS NS	NA
Bang 2016 [34]	74	23% (TRG 0–1 by AJCC)	SUVmax pre SUVpeak pre SUVmean pre + 2 SDs	NS NS negative $p = 0.0045$	3-years DFS NS 3-years DFS NS 3-years DFS $p = 0.01$
Leccisotti 2015 [36]	126	24.6% (TRG1 by Mandard)	Early RI SUVmax Late RI SUVmax	Cut-off 61% $p < 0.001$ cut-off not found	10.3% local recurrences 4.8% deaths
Our series	100	16% (TRG1 by Mandard) 31% (TRG1–2 by Mandard)	SUVmax pre SUVmean pre MTV pre TLG pre SUVmax pre SUVmean pre MTV pre TLG pre	NS NS NS NS NS NS p = 0.01 NS	4-years DFS NS 4-years OS NS

pCR Pathological complete response, *TRG* Tumor regression grade, *RI* Response index, *Spec* Specificity, *Sens* sensibility, Δ indicates percent residual, *pre* Before radiochemotherapy, *post* After radiochemotherapy, *SD* Standard deviation, *SUVmax* Maximum standardized uptake value, *SUVmean* Mean standardized uptake value, *MTV* Metabolic tumor volume, *TLG* Total lesion glycolysis, *AJCC* American Joint Committee on Cancer, *NS* Not significant, *NA* Not available

Conclusions

This study describes one of the largest series analyzing baseline [18] FDG-PET parameters in LARC. The results showed that SUVmax and SUVmean correlated with tumor staging at diagnosis, and MTV was predictive of tumor response. However, no parameter was predictive of true complete response (TRG1). Moreover, none of the analyzed parameters was able to predict DFS and OS.

The issue of identifying patients suitable for conservative approaches is still open, and different schedules of imaging studies, including repeated PET after neoadjuvant CRT, should be explored more deeply in the view of a true personalized treatment modality.

Abbreviations

(SUVmean): Mean standardized uptake value; [18F] FDG-PET/CT: [18F] fluorodeoxyglucose positron emission tomography/computed tomography; 3D-CRT: 3-dimension-conformal RT; AJCC: American Joint Committee on Cancer; ANOVA: Analysis of variance; CI: Confident interval; CRT: Chemoradiotherapy; CTV: Clinical target volume; DFS: Disease-free survival; EANM: European Agency of Nuclear Medicine; IMRT: Intensity modulated radiation therapy; LARC: Locally advanced rectal cancer; MRI: Magnetic resonance imaging; MTV: Metabolic tumor volume; OR: Odd ratio; OS: Overall survival; PTV: Planning target volume; RECIST: Response evaluation criteria in solid tumors; SD: Standard deviation; SUVmax: Maximum standardized uptake value; TLG: Total lesion glycolysis; TRG: Tumor regression grade

Acknowledgements

The work of L. Deantonio was supported by the "Lega italiana per la lotta ai tumori, LILT" section of Vercelli and "Fondazione Cassa di Risparmio" of Vercelli, Italy. We thank Prof. M. Abrile for English editing.

Funding
Not applicable

Authors' contributions
Conception and design: MK and LD. Provision of study materials or patients: LD, AC, FA and LT. Collection and assembly of data: LD, EP, AC, and FA. Data analysis and interpretation: LD, DF, EP and MK. Manuscript writing: All authors. All authors read and approved the final manuscript.

Competing interests
The authors declare that they have no competing interests.

Author details
[1]Radiotherapy, University Hospital "Maggiore della Carità", Novara, Italy. [2]Department of Translational Medicine, University of "Piemonte Orientale", Novara, Italy. [3]Nuclear Medicine, University Hospital "Maggiore della Carità", Novara, Italy. [4]Department of Translational Medicine, Unit of Medical Statistics and Cancer Epidemiology, CPO Piemonte and University of "Piemonte Orientale", Novara, Italy. [5]Medical Physics, University Hospital "Maggiore della Carità", Novara, Italy.

References

1. Sauer R, Liersch T, Merkel S, Fietkau R, et al. Preoperative versus postoperative Chemoradiotherapy for locally advanced rectal Cancer: results of the German CAO/ARO/AIO-94 randomized phase III trial after a median follow-up of 11 years. J Clin Oncol. 2012;30:1926–33.
2. Ciria JP, Eguiguren M, Cafiero S, et al. Could preoperative short-course radiotherapy be the treatment of choice for localized advanced rectal carcinoma? Rep Pract Oncol Radiother. 2015;20:1–11.
3. O'Neill BD, Brown G, Heald RJ, Cunningham D, Tait DM. Nonoperative treatment after neoadjuvant chemoradiotherapy for rectal cancer. Lancet Oncol. 2007;8:625–33.
4. Habr-Gama A, Gama-Rodrigues J, Sao Juliao GP. Local recurrence after complete clinical response and watch and wait in rectal cancer after neoadjuvant chemoradiation: impact of salvage therapy on local disease control. Int J Radiat Oncol Biol Phys. 2014;88:822–8.
5. Appelt AL, Pløen J, Harling H, et al. High-dose chemoradiotherapy and watchful waiting for distal rectal cancer: a prospective observational study. Lancet Oncol. 2015;16:919–27.
6. Garcia-Aguilar J, Renfro LA, Chow OS, et al. Organ preservation for clinical T2N0 distal rectal cancer using neoadjuvant chemoradiotherapy and local excision (ACOSOG Z6041): results of an open-label, single-arm, multi-institutional, phase 2 trial. Lancet Oncol. 2015;16:1537–46.
7. Mandard AM, Dalibard F, Mandard JC, Marnay J, Henry-Amar M, Petiot JF. Pathologic assessment of tumor regression after preoperative chemoradiotherapy of esophageal carcinoma. Clinicopathologic correlations. Cancer. 1994;73:2680–6.
8. Denecke T, Rau B, Hoffmann KT, et al. Comparison of CT, MRI and FDG-PET in response prediction of patients with locally advanced rectal cancer after multimodal preoperative therapy: is there a benefit in using functional imaging? Eur Radiology. 2005;15:1658–66.
9. Lambrecht M, Deroose C, Roels S, et al. The use of FDG-PET/CT and diffusion-weighted magnetic resonance imaging for response prediction before, during and after preoperative chemoradiotherapy for rectal cancer. Acta Oncol. 2010;49:956–63.
10. Bassi MC, Turri L, Sacchetti G, et al. FDG-PET/CT imaging for staging and target volume delineation in preoperative conformal radiotherapy of rectal cancer. Int J Radiat Oncol Biol Phys. 2008;70:1423–6.
11. Krengli M, Cannillo B, Turri L, et al. Target volume delineation for preoperative radiotherapy of rectal cancer: inter-observer variability and potential impact of FDG-PET/CT imaging. Technol Cancer Res Treat. 2010;9:393–8.
12. Di Genesio Pagliuca M, Turri L, Munoz F, et al. Patterns of practice in the radiation therapy management of rectal cancer: survey of the interregional group Piedmont, Valle d'Aosta and Liguria of the "Associazione Italiana di Radioterapia Oncologica (AIRO)". Tumori. 2013;99:61–7.
13. van Stiphout RG, Lammering G, Buijsen J, et al. Development and external validation of a predictive model for pathological complete response of rectal cancer patients including sequential PET-CT imaging. Radiother Oncol. 2011;98:126–33.
14. Yeung JM, Kalff V, Hicks RJ, et al. Metabolic response of rectal cancer assessed by 18-FDG PET following chemoradiotherapy is prognostic for patient outcome. Dis Colon Rectum. 2011;54:518–25.
15. Martoni AA, Di Fabio F, Pinto C, Castellucci P, Pini S, Ceccarelli C. Prospective study on the FDG-PET/CT predictive and prognostic values in patients treated with neoadjuvant chemoradiation therapy and radical surgery for locally advanced rectal cancer. Ann Oncology. 2011; 22:650–6.
16. Calvo F, Sole CV, de la Mata D, et al. (18)F-FDG PET/CT-based treatment response evaluation in locally advanced rectal cancer: a prospective validation of long-term outcomes. Eur J Nucl Med Mol Imaging. 2013;40:657–67.
17. Deantonio L, Milia ME, Cena T, et al. Anal cancer FDG/PET standard uptake value: correlation with tumor characteristics, treatment response and survival. Radiol Med. 2016;121:54–9.
18. Alongi F, Fersino S, Mazzola R, et al. Radiation dose intensification in pre-operative chemo-radiotherapy for locally advanced rectal cancer. Clin Transl Oncol. 2017;19:189–96.
19. Edge SB, Byrd DR, Compton CC, et al., editors. AJCC cancer staging manual, 7th edn. New York: Springer; 2010.
20. Brambilla M, Matheoud R, Secco C, et al. Impact of target-to-background ratio, target size, emission scan duration, and activity on physical figures of merit for a 3D LSO-based whole body PET/CT scanner. Med Phys. 2007;34: 3854–65.
21. Boellaard R, Delgado-Bolton R, Oyen WJG, et al. FDG PET/CT: EANM procedure guidelines for tumour imaging: version 2.0. Eur J Nucl Med Mol Imaging. 2015;42:328–54.
22. Roels S, Duthoy W, Haustermans K, et al. Definition and delineation of the clinical target volume for rectal cancer. Int J Radiation Oncology Biol Phys. 2006;65:1129–42.
23. Eisenhauer E, Therasse P, Bogaerts J, et al. New response evaluation criteria in solid tumours: revised RECIST guideline (version 1.1). Eur J Cancer. 2009; 45(2):228–47.
24. Martin ST, Heneghan HM, Winter DC. Systematic review and meta-analysis of outcomes following pathological complete response to neoadjuvant chemoradiotherapy for rectal cancer. Br J Surg. 2012;99:918–28.
25. García-Aguilar J, Hernandez de Anda E, Sirivongs P, Lee SH, Madoff RD, Rothenberger DA. A pathologic complete response to preoperative chemoradiation is associated with lower local recurrence and improved survival in rectal cancer patients treated by mesorectal excision. Dis Colon Rectum. 2003;46:298–304.
26. Park J, Chang KJ, Seo YS, et al. Tumor SUVmax normalized to liver uptake on 18F-FDG PET/CT predicts the pathologic complete response after neoadjuvant chemoradiotherapy in locally advanced rectal cancer. Nucl Med Mol Imaging. 2014;48:295–302.
27. Maffione AM, Chondrogiannis S, Capirci C, et al. Early prediction of response by 18F-FDG PET/CT during preoperative therapy in locally advanced rectal cancer: a systematic review. Eur J Surg Oncol. 2014;40:1186–94.
28. Dos Anjos DA, Perez R, Habr-Gama A, et al. Semiquantitative volumetry by sequential PET/CT may improve prediction of complete response to neoadjuvant chemoradiation in patients with distal rectal cancer. Dis Colon Rectum. 2016;59:805–12.
29. Cascini GL, Avallone A, Delrio P, et al. 18F-FDG PET is an early predictor of pathologic tumor response to preoperative radiochemotherapy in locally advanced rectal cancer. J Nucl Med. 2006;47:1241–8.
30. Janssen MH, Ollers MC, Riedl RG, et al. Accurate prediction of pathological rectal tumor response after two weeks of preoperative radiochemotherapy using (18)F-fluorodeoxyglucose-positron emission tomographycomputed tomography imaging. Int J Radiat Oncol Biol Phys. 2010;77:392–9.
31. Bazan JG, Koong AC, Kapp DS, et al. Metabolic tumour volume predicts disease progression and survival in patients with squamous cell carcinoma of the anal canal. J Nucl Med. 2013;54:27–32.
32. Lee P, Bazan JG, Lavori PW, et al. Metabolic tumor volume is an independent prognostic factor in patients treated definitively for non-small-cell lung cancer. Clin Lung Cancer. 2012;13:52–8.

33. Chennupati SK, Quon A, Kamaya A, et al. Positron emission tomography for predicting pathologic response after neoadjuvant chemoradiotherapy for locally advanced rectal cancer. Am J Clin Oncol. 2012;35:334–9.
34. Bang JI, Ha S, Kang SB, et al. Prediction of neoadjuvant radiation chemotherapy response and survival using pretreatment [18F]FDG PET/CT scans in locally advanced rectal cancer. Eur J Nucl Med Mol Imaging. 2016;43:422–31.
35. Hatt M, van Stiphout R, le Pogam A, et al. Early prediction of pathological response in locally advanced rectal cancer based on sequential 18F-FDG PET. Acta Oncol. 2013;52:619–26.
36. Leccisotti L, Gambacorta MA, de Waure C, et al. The predictive value of 18F-FDG PET/CT for assessing pathological response and survival in locally advanced rectal cancer after neoadjuvant radiochemotherapy. Eur J Nucl Med Mol Imaging. 2015;42:657–66.

21

Progressive resistance training in cachectic head and neck cancer patients undergoing radiotherapy

Manuel Grote[1,2,3*], Cornelius Maihöfer[1,4], Martin Weigl[2], Patricia Davies-Knorr[2] and Claus Belka[1,4]

Abstract

Background: Cancer cachexia is a prevalent symptom of head and neck neoplasms. The reduction in skeletal muscle mass is one of the main characteristics which can lead to poor physical functioning. The purposes of this pilot randomized controlled trial were to determine the feasibility of progressive resistance training in cachectic head and neck cancer patients during radiotherapy and to explore possible risks and benefits.

Methods: Twenty cachectic participants with head and neck cancer receiving radiation were randomized to obtain either a machine supported progressive resistance training ($n = 10$) or usual care (n = 10). The training took place 3 times weekly for 30 min. Intervention included 3 exercises for major muscle groups with 8–12 repetition maximum for 3 sets each. Bioelectrical impedance analysis, hand-held dynamometry, Six-Minute Walk Test and standardized questionnaires for fatigue and quality of life were used for evaluating outcomes at baseline before radiotherapy (t1), after 7 weeks of radiotherapy (t2) and 8 weeks after the end of radiotherapy (t3).

Results: All participants ($n = 20$) completed the trial. No serious adverse events occurred. At the initial assessment the cachectic patients had already lost 7.1 ± 5.2% of their body weight. General fatigue (score 10.7 ± 3.3) and reduced quality of life (score 71.3 ± 20.6) were prevalent in cachectic head and neck cancer patients even before radiotherapy. An average improvement of weight loading for leg press (+ 19.0%), chest press (+ 29.8%) and latissimus pull-down (+ 22.8%) was possible in the intervention group. Participants had at least 13 training sessions. The outcome measures showed nonsignificant changes at t2 and t3, but a trend for a better course of general fatigue and quality of life at t2 in the intervention group.

Conclusions: Despite advanced tumor stage and burdensome treatment the intervention adherence is excellent. Progressive resistance training in cachectic head and neck cancer patients during radiotherapy seems to be safe and feasible and may have beneficial effects of general fatigue and quality of life.

Keywords: Head and neck cancer, Cachexia, Resistance training, Radiotherapy, Randomized controlled trial, Feasibility study

* Correspondence: Manuel.Grote@bw.aok.de
[1]Department of Radiation Oncology, University Hospital, LMU Munich, 81377 Munich, Germany
[2]Department of Orthopaedics, Physical Medicine and Rehabilitation, University Hospital, LMU Munich, 81377 Munich, Germany
Full list of author information is available at the end of the article

Background

Head and neck cancer (HNC) is the ninth most common cause of cancer death [1]. In 2012 an estimated 529,000 new cases of cancer of the oral cavity and pharynx occurred worldwide. In Germany data describe incidence estimates of 13,800 and relative 5-year-survival rates between 48% for men and 61% for women in 2010 [2].

Tobacco use and alcohol consumption are the most significant risk factors for the development of oral cavity neoplasms [3]. A strong multiplicative effect for alcohol interacting with smoking further increases risk [4]. In addition human papillomavirus infection has a potential role mainly in the increased incidence for oropharyngeal cancers [5].

HNC and its medical treatments can lead to a complex interacting range of adverse effects which includes fatigue [6], altered body image [7], modified nourishment [8], psychosocial distress [9], shoulder dysfunction [10], trismus [11], dysphagia [12], xerostomia [13], mucositis [14], cachexia [15, 16], all resulting in reduced quality of life [17].

Modern radiotherapy techniques can reduce acute and chronic side effects. Intensity modulation [18, 19] and image guided [20] radiotherapy allow improved dose distribution thus sparing critical organs and improving quality of life [21, 22].

Considering the above mentioned debilitating symptoms, rehabilitation for HNC patients is warranted and potentially beneficial after medical treatment. In recent years it has been shown that physical exercises after and even during treatment relieve many of the side effects experienced by patients with various neoplasms [23–25].

Cancer cachexia and its key feature of weight loss do not develop to the same extent in every cancer entity. One of the high-risk populations developing cachexia is HNC patients [26, 27]. A generalized inflammatory state with high interleukin-6 levels is seen as a critical factor for muscle wasting [28, 29]. Loss of muscle mass leads to asthenia which is responsible for poor physical functioning [30].

The primary objectives of this pilot feasibility randomized controlled trial (RCT) were to determine the practicability of recruitment and the feasibility of progressive resistance training (PRT) during radiotherapy (RT) for cachectic HNC patients. Secondary objectives were to gather preliminary results for safety and responsiveness of the training.

Methods

Trial design

This study is a pilot, 2-arm, RCT. Between June 2013 and January 2015 a total of 20 patients at the university hospital Munich, Großhadern were randomly assigned to receive PRT (intervention group) or usual care (control group) during RT. Ethical clearance was obtained from institutional ethics committee (Project-Nr. 531–12) and written informed consent obtained from all participants before initiating study activities. Participants with a cancer diagnosis of the lung, pancreas, esophagus, head and neck, colon, rectum or anus were subsequently reviewed for inclusion and exclusion criteria. Study inclusion criteria were: (1) planned inpatient or outpatient RT, (2) ≥ 18 years of age, (3) diagnosed state of cachexia (weight loss greater than 5% over the past 6 months) or pre-cachexia (unintentional weight loss of 5% or less of usual body weight during the last 6 months). Patients with (1) metastatic disease, (2) severe neurological problems or other contraindications for the PRT were excluded. The project coordinator screened potential participants for eligibility via MOSAIQ®-Software (Radiation Oncology Information System). This software manages the aspects of the radiation oncology program and collects all information of the patients and makes them accessible. Study information sheets were sent to patients in the form of invitation letters. Participants who met the diagnosed tumor localization were met at the time of computer tomography-planning to explain the study, screen again for eligibility, and obtain informed consent. Registered participants were planned for baseline assessment. Participants were allocated at random to the control or exercise group via blocked randomization in sealed envelopes.

Baseline data for all participants were ascertained via medical records and patient interview. This included demographic information, UICC-status (Union internationale contre le cancer, tumor staging system), comorbidities and the results of blood samples. One study coordinator completed all assessments to enhance patient compliance. Body weight loss percentage was calculated via the individuals' body weight 6 months before (in retrospect) and the current body weight. Participants completed two questionnaires: The Multidimensional Fatigue Inventory (MFI) [31] which consists of 20 items that measure subgroups (general, physical and mental fatigue as well as reduced motivation and reduced activity) of fatigue with a 5-point Likert scale and the Functional Assessment of Anorexia/Cachexia Therapy (FAACT) questionnaire [32, 33] which registers well-being for physical, social/family, emotional and functional aspects of quality of life and additional concerns in cachexia with 5-point Likert scale for 39 items. To measure physical performance the Six-Minute Walk Test (6MWT) [34] was applied. This assessment instrument includes walking distance as well as heart rate, pulse oximetry (Contec Medical Systems CO., Ltd., Model: CMS50E), fatigue (with a rating of perceived exertion (RPE) from 0 to 10) and dyspnea (RPE 0–10) before and after the test. To document changes in muscle force, strength of the functional muscle group for elbow flexion in supine position as well as of knee extension in sitting position (in each case right and left) was tested via hand-held dynamometry (Mecmesin Ltd., Broadbridge Heath, West Sussex, RH12 3IR, UK) for isometric maximal muscle strength [35]. Bioelectrical impedance analysis (BIA; AKERN SRL, BIA 101 New Edition) was executed to assess the adaption in body composition [36]. Patients were lying supine on a therapy table. The measurements took place at the right side of the body with the tetrapolar-technique of 4 standard electrodes on the surface of the hand and the foot. Constant frequency of 50 kHz and 400 μA constant current in electrical resistance of the body were used to measure resistance and reactance. The above mentioned assessments were carried out at baseline (t1), after 7 weeks of radiotherapy (t2) and 8 weeks after radiotherapy (t3).

Before each training session the current condition of the patient was accurately gathered. This included communication with the responsible nurse and/or physician about the ongoing state, including the results of the latest investigations such as blood pressure, temperature and laboratory investigations. As a last safety action the patient was asked if he felt able to carry out the training. Heart rate during training was monitored by a chest strap that sends the current heart rate by a radio signal to a wristwatch. It was payed attention that the participant's heart rate never exceeded the maximum heart rate measured during the 6MWT and that the heart rate became slower in the breaks during the sets and the changes to another exercise machine. After the training each inpatient was personally carried back to the ward and asked for any complaints. Furthermore, the responsible nurse and/or physician were informed about the patients return to the ward and any noticeable situations during the training.

The exercise intervention was undertaken in the hospitals department of physical and rehabilitation medicine and based on standardized but individualized training protocols. All exercises were carried out within the individuals given limb range of motion and in a dynamic way without defined execution time for the concentric and eccentric phase. Goal of the very first training was to determine the training load set for hypertrophic adaption. Because of the vulnerable patient group a submaximal step by step approach within 3 sets and 8–12 repetitions was chosen. The first two sets acted as both muscular and movement adaption. The last set served as submaximal one-repetition maximum estimation. The evaluation of the training prescription was done in real-time by a supervising physiotherapist.

The training protocol consisted of a warm up period for 5 min on a bicycle ergometer or an upper body cycle with individual selectable wattage. A leg press, a latissimus pull-down and a chest press (Kaphingst) formed the three equipment supported core exercises. All exercises were performed with 8–12 repetitions and 3 sets. After each set and during the changes to another exercise machine a break of maximum 60 s was assured. After each machine the patients rated their perceived exertion from 0 to 10. The weight loading was increased at the next workout if RPE < 7. For the two upper limbs exercise a progression of 2.5 kg weight loading and for the lower limbs exercise a progression of 5.0 kg weight loading was implemented. The exercises were supervised all the time for performance and safety reasons by physiotherapists experienced in oncology rehabilitation and certified in medical training therapy.

For exercise participants with concomitant chemotherapy to their RT protocol timing for the training intervention was organized e.g. between the changes of 24 h constant-rate infusion. In the rare cases where this was not possible the exercise intervention was adjusted in order to protect the peripheral venous catheter in the Vena mediana cubiti by limiting an exercise in the range of motion or by replacing the two upper body machine supported exercises by: low pulley seated bench cable crossover and low pulley lateral extensions because of the almost static elbow angulation.

The control group received usual care. This could include inpatient physiotherapy if prescribed by the ward physician. Muscle strengthening techniques were not part of the usual care.

Statistical analyses

Descriptive statistics were calculated to check for data normality. Normality was tested using Kolmogorov-Smirnov test. Single variables were compared using Student's t-test and dichotomous outcomes were analyzed using a Chi-squared test or Fisher's exact test as appropriate. Between group analysis was done using independent t-test or Mann-Whitney test. Statistical significance was set as $p < .05$. The statistic package IBM SPSS 23 was used for these analyses.

Sample size

Physical outcomes have been tested following exercise interventions in cancer studies. The outcome of physical function was analyzed with meta-analytic procedures and the overall weighted mean effect size for two-group comparisons was 0.52 [37]. This effect size calculated with an α-error probability of 0.05 and a power of 0.8 for a two-sided t-test resulted in a required sample size of 120 participants. For the control and intervention group 60 participants each.

Results

On review of the recruitment process in July 2014 it was noted that there were only HNC patients included (one patient with esophageal cancer). Afterwards solely HNC patients were screened for inclusion criteria to generate a homogenous analysis.

Patient recruitment (Fig. 1)

Between June 2013 and January 2015 100 eligible cancer patients scheduled for RT treatment were subsequently screened. 20 patients were included giving a recruitment rate of 20%. 80 patients were excluded for following reasons: metastases ($n = 20$), second cancer diagnosis and/or relapse ($n = 18$), no exercise therapy possible due to other comorbidities ($n = 8$), no interest ($n = 16$), no time ($n = 4$), RT at non-study site ($n = 3$) and other reasons ($n = 11$). All included patients were randomized into intervention and control groups before beginning RT. The completion rate was 100%.

Feasibility outcomes

The 10 participants from the training group achieved a total of 168 training sessions, with a mean of 16.8 training sessions (range 13–25) during the course of RT. A total of 84 h of training could be accomplished with 30 min for each session. This is a mean of 8.4 h of training for each exercising patient. A mean of 32 days of RT (range 25–33) results in 2.7 training sessions of the planned 3 sessions per week (range 1.7–3.8). Mean time between hospital admission and the first training session was 1 working day (range 0–3). Mean time between the last training session and the last RT was 3 working days (range 13–0). Explanations for not completing all planned training sessions included pain due to severe mucositis (4 patients). Change from in- to outpatient status during RT led to reduced training time slots because participants had to organize the time for training considering RT time (4 patients). Three participants reported paused progression in the exercise of a latissimus pull-down due to abdominal tension following recently placed percutaneous endoscopic gastrostomy (PEG).

None of the participants reported muscle strains to the physiotherapist. No infections of peripheral venous catheter, no chemotherapy extravasation and no other adverse events during or after the training were observed.

Inpatient physiotherapy was prescribed in 3 participants of the control group. Chest physiotherapy to facilitate expectoration and movement therapy for the shoulder girdle after neck dissection were contents of the therapy sessions. A total of 17 therapy sessions with 15–35 min were carried out.

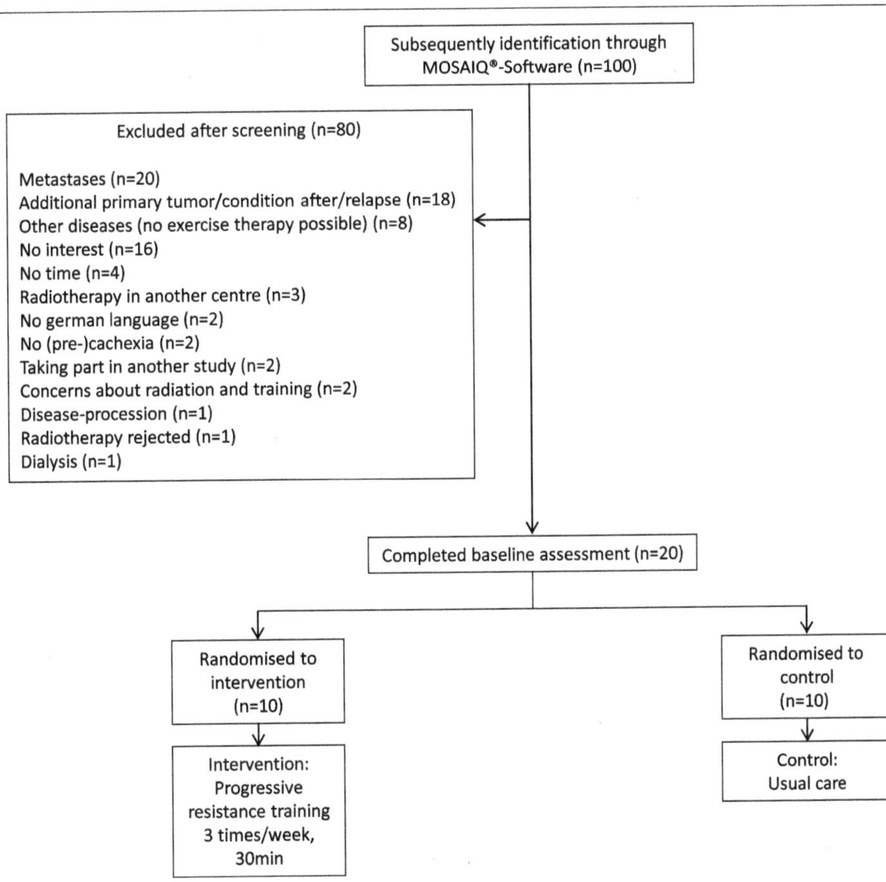

Fig. 1 Participant flow chart

Clinical characteristics

The study population ($n = 20$) consists of upper aerodigestive tract neoplasms of which 85% ($n = 9$ intervention, $n = 8$ control) are head and neck squamous cell carcinoma (HNSCC). Whereas the remaining 15% are patients with tumors of the esophagus ($n = 1$ intervention) or the salivary gland (n = 2 control).

Table 1 shows the baseline characteristics of the patients. Both of the groups were comparable at baseline with regard to age, sex, cancer stage, alcohol and smoking in the medical history, medical treatment, carried out neck dissection and PEG. Of the 20 patients 15 were men and 11 had a history of either smoking and/or alcohol abuse. 35% received RT as single medical treatment. All patients received fractionated radiotherapy with 60–70 Gy (five fractions/week). Thirteen patients received concurrent chemotherapy, most of them cisplatin 20 mg/m^2 and 5-fluoruracil 600 mg/m^2 body surface area on day 1–5 and repeated as of day 29. Neck dissection and percutaneous endoscopic gastrostomy has been performed in 11 patients each.

The comparison of baseline values for blood sample data (C-reactive protein $p = 0.922$, hemoglobin $p = 0.710$ and interleukin-6 $p = 0.620$) and bodyweight ($p = 0.094$) or weight loss ($p = 0.274$) was similar between both groups. At the time of giving consent to the study patients had lost at an average 7.1 ± 5.2% of their body weight (72.1 ± 12.7 kg) as compared to 6 months before. C-reactive protein (standard value ≤0.5 mg/dl) was only slightly increased (1.0 ± 1.5 mg/dl) and hemoglobin (standard value 13.5–17.5 g/dl) was at the lower limit (13.4 ± 1.3 g/dl). Elevated interleukin-6 levels (12.0 ± 18.2 pg/ml, standard value ≤5.9 pg/ml, $n = 18$) were also shown.

All participants ($n = 20$) were assessed for functional capacity with the 6MWT. It shows a mean of 475 ± 101 m (intervention group 500 ± 77 m, control group 450 ± 119 m, between group analyses $p = 0.284$). Hand-held dynamometry for testing maximal isometric strength demonstrated for knee extension of right lower extremity 30.2 ± 11.9 kp, left lower extremity 30.0 ± 11.9 kp (between group comparison $p = 0.254$ respectively $p = 0.077$). Isometric testing of the upper extremity via flexion of the elbow showed for the right side a mean of 18.8 ± 6.0 kp and left 19.0 ± 5.8 kp (between group comparison $p = 0.171$ respectively $p = 0.433$).

The results of the questionnaires for fatigue (Multidimensional Fatigue Inventory) and quality of life in anorexia/cachexia (Functional Assessment of Anorexia/Cachexia Therapy) are presented in Table 2. These show that both groups were balanced at baseline. Fatigue subscale scores range from 8.0–11.5 and the FACT-G score is 77.9 ± 15.2, demonstrating a moderate symptom occurrence before medical treatment.

We found comparable baseline values for muscle ($p = 0.917$) and fat ($p = 0.279$) mass between the groups. A mean of 41.8 ± 7.7% (29–59) muscle mass and 19.9 ± 8.3% (3–35) fat mass was shown ($n = 20$)

Training effects (Table 3)

The increase in general ($p = 0.879$), physical ($p = 0.478$) and mental ($p = 0.696$) fatigue is not significantly different between t1 and t3 comparing intervention and control group. Similarly, the reduced activity increased in both groups (control 8%, intervention 11%) to a non-significantly extent ($p = 0.700$). In the reduced motivation dimension, the intervention group showed a decrease of 7%,

Table 1 Clinical characteristics

Variable	All ($n = 20$)	Intervention ($n = 10$)	Control ($n = 10$)	*P* value
Age (years)	60.9 ± 11.3 (27–82)	60.2 ± 4.7 (50–66)	61.5 ± 15.7 (27–82)	0.807
Sex				0.303[b]
Men	15 (75%)	9 (90%)	6 (60%)	
Women	5 (25%)	1 (10%)	4 (40%)	
Cancer stage[a]				0.420
Stadium I/II	6 (30%)	3 (30%)	3 (30%)	
Stadium III/IV (M0)	14 (70%)	7 (70%)	7 (70%)	
Alcohol abuse, yes	5 (25%)	3 (30%)	2 (20%)	1.000[b]
Smoking, yes	6 (30%)	3 (30%)	3 (30%)	1.000[b]
Chemoradiation, yes	13 (65%)	8 (80%)	5 (50%)	0.350
Neck dissection, yes	11 (55%)	5 (50%)	6 (60%)	1.000
Feeding tube, yes	11 (55%)	7 (70%)	4 (40%)	0.370[b]

[a] *UICC* Classification
[b] Fisher's exact test

Table 2 Baseline data for fatigue and quality of life in anorexia/cachexia

Variable	All (n = 20)	Intervention (n = 10)	Control (n = 10)	P value
Fatigue				
MFI general fatigue (4–20)	10.7 ± 3.3 (5–16)	11.3 ± 3.7 (5–16)	10.1 ± 2.9 (6–14)	0.393
MFI physical fatigue (4–20)	11.0 ± 4.1 (4–20)	12.0 ± 5.0 (4–20)	10.0 ± 2.9 (6–14)	0.393
MFI reduced activity (4–20)	11.5 ± 4.0 (4–20)	11.5 ± 5.0 (4–20)	11.4 ± 2.7 (6–15)	0.912
MFI reduced motivation (4–20)	8.8 ± 3.9 (4–16)	8.6 ± 4.2 (4–16)	9.0 ± 3.9 (5–16)	0.853
MFI mental fatigue (4–20)	8.0 ± 4.1 (4–20)	7.6 ± 4.9 (4–20)	8.3 ± 3.4 (4–13)	0.436
Quality of life in anorexia/cachexia				
FACT-G total score (0–108)	77.9 ± 15.2[a] (49–104)	80.1 ± 11.2[b] (61–96)	75.7 ± 18.8[b] (49–104)	0.730

[a]n = 18, [b]n = 9 (three patients had a overall item response rate smaller than 80%)

while the control group indicated an increase of 14% between t1 and t3 (p = 0.437).

Comparing the decrease in quality of life in the control and intervention group is non-significant (p = 0.891). The relative decrease between t1 and t3 was 7% in the intervention group and 19% in the control group. In the period between t1 and t2 the quality of life of the control group decreased by 27% and in the intervention group by 18%.

The intervention group shows a 30% loss of fat mass, the control group decreased 20% of fat mass in the observation period. In the t2-t3 interval, the untreated group increased its fat mass by 2% and the intervention group decreased 16%. While the lean mass in the intervention group increased by 1% during the observation period, it decreased by 3% in the control group (p = 0.267).

Training progression

All of the 10 participants had a minimum of 13 training sessions. Figure 2 displays the mean course of the training regarding weight loading (in kg) for the 3 equipment supported exercises: leg press, chest press and latissimus pull-down in the first 13 sessions. Increases in strength can be shown for each of the equipment supported exercises. Especially during the first 5 sessions of the training it was possible to increase the load substantially (see Fig. 2). Afterwards the progression in loading tended to level off. During the whole course of 13 training sessions there was an average increase of 19.0% of weight loading for the leg press; starting from 63.2 kg in the first session and 75.2 kg in the last. Weight loading for the chest press began at 31.2 kg to 40.5 kg at last; equivalent to an improvement of 29.8%. Maximum weight loading for the latissimus pull-down was in the fifth training session (starting with 28.5 kg and ending 35.0 kg; 22.8% weight loading progression).

Discussion

The primary intention of this prospective trial was to determine the feasibility of individually tailored PRT in cachectic patients diagnosed with HNC. The main finding of the present study is that even in cachectic patients with HNC receiving RT a PRT seems to be safe and well tolerated. None of the participants reported muscle strains. No infections of the peripheral venous catheter, chemotherapy extravasation or other adverse events were reported during or after the training. Additionally, it was possible to increase the training loads within the first 5 sessions and maintain them throughout the medical treatment.

When considering physical strength as an outcome parameter it is important to be able to quantify muscle strength. Strength measurement in this trail needed to be easy to apply, mobile and inexpensive. A hand-held dynamometric device was therefore used to measure maximal isometric muscle strength. This pilot study was able to show 294 ± 117.7 Newton for knee extension at baseline. Although Knols et al. [38] found similar data (278 ± 93.6 Newton) their sample was more than 10 years younger (49.45 ± 14.85 vs. 60.9 ± 11.3) and in various types and stages of cancer chemotherapy treatment. The comparison of strength values measured via a hand-held dynamometry are not generalizable as can be seen by the fact that reliability is significantly influenced by the strength of the tester [39]. Therefore, the measurements should always be carried out by the same tester within a study (as it was done in our trial). The 6MWT is a valid measurement for physical performance in cancer patients. This was also demonstrated in this study with a mean distance of 475 ± 101 m achieved. When compared to the walking distance (652 m) in healthy population based samples [40] the discrepancy could be explained as a result of the decreased

Table 3 Training effects of fatigue dimensions, quality of life and fat and lean mass at test intervals t1, t2 and t3

Variable	Intervention $n = 10$	Control $n = 10$	*P* Value (t1-t3)
Fatigue (4–20)			
General Fatigue pre	11.3 ± 3.7	10.1 ± 2.9	0.879
General Fatigue post	12.3 ± 5.3	14.1 ± 3.5	
General Fatigue follow-up	11.8 ± 4.3	11.9 ± 4.6	
Physical Fatigue pre	12.0 ± 5.0	10.0 ± 2.9	0.478
Physical Fatigue post	13.5 ± 4.5	13.8 ± 2.8	
Physical Fatigue follow-up	13.3 ± 5.0	11.8 ± 5.1	
Mental Fatigue pre	7.6 ± 4,9	8.3 ± 3.4	0.696
Mental Fatigue post	9.6 ± 4.4	9.7 ± 4.0	
Mental Fatigue follow-up	8.3 ± 2.3	9.2 ± 2.3	
Reduced Activity pre	11.5 ± 5.0	11.4 ± 2.7	0.700
Reduced Activity post	13.1 ± 4.8	14.8 ± 2.8	
Reduced Activity follow-up	12.4 ± 4.4	12.6 ± 4.2	
Reduced Motivation pre	8.6 ± 4.2	9.0 ± 3.9	0.437
Reduced Motivation post	9.2 ± 4.1	9.9 ± 2.2	
Reduced Motivation follow-up	8.0 ± 2.5	10.3 ± 4.8	
Quality of life in anorexia/cachexia (0–104)			
Quality of Life pre	80.1 ± 11.2	75.7 ± 18.8	0.891
Quality of Life post	56.5 ± 18.4	53.4 ± 19.8	
Quality of Life follow-up	64.4 ± 18,4	59.5 ± 26.5	
Bioelectrical Impedance analysis (kg)			
Fat mass pre	14.7 ± 8.6	16.4 ± 7.0	0.545
Fat mass post	12.1 ± 7.0	12.9 ± 6.2	
Fat mass follow-up	10.2 ± 6.6	13.2 ± 5.3	
Lean mass pre	58.6 ± 4.9	54.4 ± 12.5	0.267
Lean mass post	57.8 ± 8.9	53.5 ± 11.9	
Lean mass follow-up	59.1 ± 7.1	52.7 ± 12.1	

Variables: *Fatigue* Multidimensional Fatigue Inventory (possible scoring 4–20), *Quality of life in anorexia/cachexia* Functional Assessment of Anorexia/Cachexia Therapy *FAACT* questionnaire (possible scoring 0–104), *Bioelectrical Impedance analysis* Body composition measurement (in kilogram); pre (t1): before radiotherapy, post (t2): after 7 weeks of radiotherapy and follow-up (t3): 8 weeks after radiotherapy represent the time at which the outcome was assessed. Analysis of variance for repeated measurements with the two factors Time and Group, $p < 0.05$

physical function caused by cachexia. Cachexia not only reduces physical activity which leads to noteworthy changes in performance status. It also directly impacts on quality of life which is a complex outcome measure in cancer patient trials. Both cachectic NSCLC and HNC patients seem to have a similar reduction in quality of life related to anorexia/cachexia. A FAACT score of 111 ± 17 was reported [41] for 26 patients with anorexia-cachexia syndrome in an outpatient cancer care situation. Among our patients a FAACT sore of 112 ± 23 seems to be comparable. This is surprising considering that HNC patients regularly have to cope with tracheostoma or feeding tubes that are required to bypass tumor-related complications. This often leads to changes in eating habits which also can have an effect to the adaption and change of muscles when they are used. Especially resistance training provokes an increase in the cross-sectional area of the muscle fiber types, referred to as muscle hypertrophy, which is able to gain muscle weight if factors such as age, sex, nutrition and training status have a positive basis in an individual. Strength gains during the early phases of resistance training are a common adaption of the neuro-muscular system [34, 35]. It could be shown that during the first five training sessions patients were able to progressively increase loading compared to the following sessions. Consequently the neuro-muscular-system was able to process more loading in this early phase of training. The training resistance could also be increased more easily at the beginning because no side effects such as painful mucositis had yet occurred. The performance stagnation in the further course of the training could be explained by the fear of pushing oneself additionally or to the begin of adverse side effects to the medical therapy.

BIA serves to determine the body composition. Percentage body fat was measured with BIA in our trial at baseline. Sun et al..... [42] measured BIA in 591 healthy volunteers with a mean age of 42.15 ± 10.27 (19–60) and found a body fat mass of 32.85 ± 8.00 (10.6–58.3) percent. In Isenring et al's research HNC patients were randomized before RT in a nutrition intervention (NI) group or a usual care (UC) group [43]. Both groups in Isenring et al's research were comparable at baseline with respect to fat mass in kg (19.4 ± 4.8 vs 20.5 ± 9.7; $p = 0.640$). A calculated mean of 25.1% fat mass in the NI group and 26.7% in the UC group is comparable to our analyzed fat mass of 19.9 ± 8.3%. The lower fat mass in this study could be explained with the cachectic state of our patients. Research into body composition status with respect to skeletal muscle mass in advanced esophageal cancer patients undertaken by Ida et al. 30 patients underwent BIA before neoadjuvant chemotherapy [44]. They found a mean muscle mass of 24.9 ± 0.8 kg with a mean body weight of 59.1 ± 1.7 kg which corresponds to 42.1% muscle mass proportion. With 37% Takekiyo et al. [45] found approximately equal values for muscle mass at baseline. In their analysis eighty-six patients underwent BIA before hematopoietic stem cell transplantation. When compared to our results of 41.8 ± 7.7% muscle mass in an already cachectic patient sample seems to be quite a lot. Cancer cachexia is however a heterogeneous phenomenon which can vary through the time spectrum (pre-cachexia, cachexia, and refractory cachexia), tumor type, site and mass. Metabolic change as well as reduced food intake, co-morbidity, pre-existing sarcopenia, cancer therapy and genetic predisposition can play a role in cancer cachexia [46].

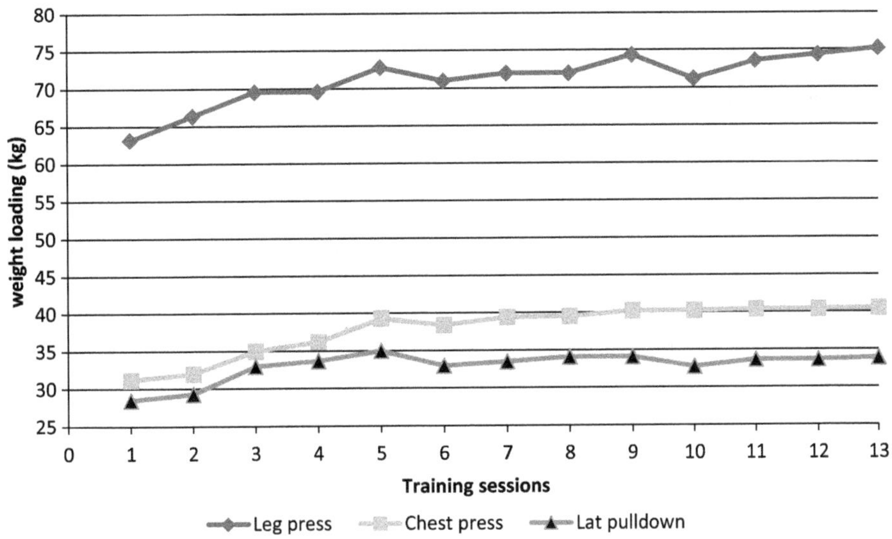

Fig. 2 Weight loading progression during the first 13 training sessions for the equipment supported exercises

Training effects

Although the results of the MFI did not show any significant differences between groups over the study period, it should be noted that in 4 out of 5 subcategories, the control group had a higher average percentage increase in fatigue scores over the interval t1 to t2. The main difference was found in the dimension general fatigue. In this dimension the fatigue score in the intervention group worsened by 9%, whereas the control group experienced a 40% worsening. This is in line with a Cochrane review that found a significant beneficial effect of tumor related fatigue in patients who performed aerobic exercise and positive, although nonsignificant, trends for resistance training and other forms of exercise therapy [47].

In the t1-t2 period the questionnaire FAACT showed a notable result for the quality of life of cachectic tumor patients. Here it is indicated that the decrease in quality of life by 18%, compared to the control group with 27%, the intervention group had less loss of quality of life over the period of medical therapy. Cancer patients often have many mental and physical side effects as a result of their cancer or treatment. Some studies have suggested that physical exercises may be helpful in reducing negative outcomes and improving the quality of life of cancer patients during their treatment [48].

The via bioelectrical impedance analysis measured lean mass essentially represents the mass of the muscles, the organs, the skeletal system and the central nervous system. The lean mass is calculated on the basis of body water (total body water / 0.73 = lean mass). A relatively constant hydrogenation of 73% is assumed. This could also basically mean that the courses of the lean mass and the total body water are similar. The control group loses 3% (intervention + 1%) lean mass over the entire study period. However, as the subjects are tumor patients who suffer from oral fluid and food intake limitations, the results are arguable. Fat mass is calculated from the weight difference of lean mass and body weight. Both groups lost a noteworthy proportion of their fat mass throughout the study period. By contrast, the decrease in muscle mass only affected the period from t1 to t2. There, both groups equally relieved muscle mass. During the same period, the intervention group lost 18% and the control group 21% of their fat mass. This result is consistent with the statement that in tumor patients fat is degraded to a greater degree than muscle mass [49]. This result allows important conclusions: Firstly, a nutritional intervention with a fatty component should be incorporated as soon as possible and in the long term in order to reduce the early and preferential breakdown of fat mass. On the other hand, the musculature necessary for the functioning of patients in their daily environment appears to be a non-primary source of supply for the maintenance of cachexia.

In our sample of cachectic HNC patients the selected assessments for the measurement of physical performance, quality of life and body composition could be implemented without difficulty.

The present pilot study has certain limitations. The small sample size and non-blinding of assessors and therapists are major limitations which reflect lack of time and budget in pilot studies. Especially in physical activity studies selection bias is ubiquitous and generates an inevitable risk for data extrapolation. Appropriately powered analyses were not sought due to the pilot character of this study. However, randomization, the presence of a control group and an approach to characterize cachectic body components as an outcome measure for resistance training are major strengths of this study.

Conclusion

In this pilot RCT a new therapy focus on the high-risk patient group of cachectic HNC patients during RT has been established. Progressive resistance training during RT for cachectic HNC patients is feasible. In our sample of patients, it was well tolerated and safe, but due to the small sample size we may have missed less frequent adverse events. In the early phase of training patients could progressively manage more resistance. This suggests that cachectic HNC patients might benefit from PRT in the early phase of RT. No significant benefits in fatigue and QOL were found, but the slightly better outcomes for general fatigue and QOL in the intervention group and the feasibility results can be used to design a future definitive clinical trial.

Abbreviations

6MWT: Six-minute walk test; BIA: Bioelectrical impedance analysis; FAACT: Functional assessment of anorexia/cachexia therapy; HNC: Head and neck cancer; HNSCC: Head and neck squamous cell carcinoma; MFI: Multidimensional fatigue inventory; NSCLC: Non-small cell lung cancer; PEG: Percutaneous endoscopic gastrostomy; PRT: Progressive resistance training; RPE: Rating of perceived exertion; RT: Radiotherapy

Acknowledgements

Not applicable.

Funding

None.

Authors' contributions

MG designed the project, performed and supervised the treatment, participated in the statistical analysis and drafted the manuscript. CM analyzed the medical data of the patients, helped with medical questions and proofread the manuscript. MW contributed to the description of the methods and the interpretation of the results. He also revised the manuscript for important content. PDK revised the manuscript critically for important content. CB supervised the study and helped to finalize the manuscript. All authors read and approved the final manuscript.

Competing interests

The authors declare that they have no competing interests.

Author details

[1]Department of Radiation Oncology, University Hospital, LMU Munich, 81377 Munich, Germany. [2]Department of Orthopaedics, Physical Medicine and Rehabilitation, University Hospital, LMU Munich, 81377 Munich, Germany. [3]Present Address: Department of Health Promotion/Occupational Health Management, AOK Baden-Württemberg, 70191 Stuttgart, Germany. [4]Clinical Cooperation Group 'Personalized Radiotherapy in Head and Neck Cancer' Helmholtz Zentrum München, German Research Center for Environmental Health GmbH, 85764 Neuherberg, Germany.

References

1. Stewart BWW, Christopher P. World Cancer Report 2014: Lyon: International Agency for Research on Cancer/world health organization; 2014. https://doi.org/10.1603/EC14197, http://publications.iarc.fr/Non-Series-Publications/World-Cancer-Reports/World-Cancer-Report-2014.
2. Kaatsch, P., et al., Krebs in Deutschland 2009/2010–9. Ausgabe, 2013. 2013, Robert Koch-Institut.
3. Radoi L, Luce D. A review of risk factors for oral cavity cancer: the importance of a standardized case definition. Community Dent Oral Epidemiol. 2013;41(2):97–109, e78-91. https://doi.org/10.1111/j.1600-0528.2012.00710.x.
4. Turati F, et al. A meta-analysis of alcohol drinking and oral and pharyngeal cancers: results from subgroup analyses. Alcohol Alcohol. 2013;48(1):107–18. https://doi.org/10.1093/alcalc/ags100.
5. Chaturvedi AK, et al. Worldwide trends in incidence rates for oral cavity and oropharyngeal cancers. J Clin Oncol. 2013;31(36):4550–9. https://doi.org/10.1200/JCO.2013.50.3870.
6. Jereczek-Fossa BA, et al. Fatigue during head-and-neck radiotherapy: prospective study on 117 consecutive patients. Int J Radiat Oncol Biol Phys. 2007;68(2):403–15. https://doi.org/10.1016/j.ijrobp.2007.01.024.
7. Fingeret MC, et al. The nature and extent of body image concerns among surgically treated patients with head and neck cancer. Psycho-Oncology. 2012;21(8):836–44. https://doi.org/10.1002/pon.1990.
8. Nugent B, Lewis S, O'Sullivan Joe M. Enteral feeding methods for nutritional management in patients with head and neck cancers being treated with radiotherapy and/or chemotherapy. Cochrane Database Syst Rev. 2013. https://doi.org/10.1002/14651858.CD007904.pub3.
9. Semple C, et al. Psychosocial interventions for patients with head and neck cancer. Cochrane Database Syst Rev. 2013. https://doi.org/10.1002/14651858.CD009441.pub2.
10. Carvalho Alan PV, Vital Flávia MR, Soares Bernardo GO. Exercise interventions for shoulder dysfunction in patients treated for head and neck cancer. Cochrane Database Syst Rev. 2012. https://doi.org/10.1002/14651858.CD008693.pub2.
11. Bensadoun RJ, et al. A systematic review of trismus induced by cancer therapies in head and neck cancer patients. Support Care Cancer. 2010;18(8):1033–8. https://doi.org/10.1007/s00520-010-0847-4.
12. Platteaux N, et al. Dysphagia in head and neck cancer patients treated with chemoradiotherapy. Dysphagia. 2010;25(2):139–52. https://doi.org/10.1007/s00455-009-9247-7.
13. Vissink A, et al. Clinical management of salivary gland hypofunction and xerostomia in head-and-neck cancer patients: successes and barriers. Int J Radiat Oncol Biol Phys. 2010;78(4):983–91. https://doi.org/10.1016/j.ijrobp.2010.06.052.
14. Rodriguez-Caballero A, et al. Cancer treatment-induced oral mucositis: a critical review. Int J Oral Maxillofac Surg. 2012;41(2):225–38. https://doi.org/10.1016/j.ijom.2011.10.011.
15. Couch M, et al. Cancer cachexia syndrome in head and neck cancer patients: part I. diagnosis, impact on quality of life and survival, and treatment. Head Neck. 2007;29(4):401–11. https://doi.org/10.1002/hed.20447.
16. George J, et al. Cancer cachexia syndrome in head and neck cancer patients: part II. Pathophysiology Head Neck. 2007;29(5):497–507. https://doi.org/10.1002/hed.20630.
17. Chandu A, Smith AC, Rogers SN. Health-related quality of life in oral cancer: a review. J Oral Maxillofac Surg. 2006;64(3):495–502. https://doi.org/10.1016/j.joms.2005.11.028.
18. Fregnani ER, et al. IMRT delivers lower radiation doses to dental structures than 3DRT in head and neck cancer patients. Radiat Oncol. 2016;11(1):116.
19. Askoxylakis V, et al. Intensity modulated radiation therapy (IMRT) for sinonasal tumors: a single center long-term clinical analysis. Radiat Oncol. 2016;11:17.
20. Straube C, et al. Reduced volume SIB-IMRT/IGRT to head and neck cancer in elderly and frail patients: outcome and toxicity. Radiat Oncol. 2016;11(1):133.

21. Kiang A, et al. Long-term disease-specific and cognitive quality of life after intensity-modulated radiation therapy: a cross-sectional survey of nasopharyngeal carcinoma survivors. Radiat Oncol. 2016;11(1):127.
22. Orth M, et al. Current concepts in clinical radiation oncology. Radiat Environ Biophys. 2014;53(1):1–29. https://doi.org/10.1007/s00411-013-0497-2.
23. Speck RM, et al. An update of controlled physical activity trials in cancer survivors: a systematic review and meta-analysis. J Cancer Surviv. 2010;4(2): 87–100. https://doi.org/10.1007/s11764-009-0110-5.
24. Pekmezi DW, Demark-Wahnefried W. Updated evidence in support of diet and exercise interventions in cancer survivors. Acta Oncol. 2011;50(2):167–78. https://doi.org/10.3109/0284186X.2010.529822.
25. Grabenbauer A, et al. Feasibility of a 12-month-exercise intervention during and after radiation and chemotherapy in cancer patients: impact on quality of life, peak oxygen consumption, and body composition. Radiat Oncol. 2016;11:42.
26. Jager-Wittenaar H, et al. Critical weight loss in head and neck cancer--prevalence and risk factors at diagnosis: an explorative study. Support Care Cancer. 2007;15(9):1045–50. https://doi.org/10.1007/s00520-006-0212-9.
27. Bozzetti F. Screening the nutritional status in oncology: a preliminary report on 1,000 outpatients. Support Care Cancer. 2009;17(3):279–84. https://doi.org/10.1007/s00520-008-0476-3.
28. Carson JA, Baltgalvis KA. Interleukin 6 as a key regulator of muscle mass during cachexia. Exerc Sport Sci Rev. 2010;38(4):168–76. https://doi.org/10.1097/JES.0b013e3181f44f11.
29. Douglas E, McMillan DC. Towards a simple objective framework for the investigation and treatment of cancer cachexia: the Glasgow prognostic score. Cancer Treat Rev. 2014;40(6):685–91. https://doi.org/10.1016/j.ctrv.2013.11.007.
30. Parmar MP, Swanson T, Jagoe RT. Weight changes correlate with alterations in subjective physical function in advanced cancer patients referred to a specialized nutrition and rehabilitation team. Support Care Cancer. 2013; 21(7):2049–57. https://doi.org/10.1007/s00520-013-1762-2.
31. Smets EM, et al. Application of the multidimensional fatigue inventory (MFI-20) in cancer patients receiving radiotherapy. Br J Cancer. 1996;73(2):241–5. https://doi.org/10.1038/bjc.1996.42.
32. Chang VT, Xia Q, Kasimis B. The functional assessment of anorexia/Cachexia therapy (FAACT) appetite scale in veteran cancer patients. J Support Oncol. 2005;3(5):377–82.
33. Ribaudo JM, et al. Re-validation and shortening of the functional assessment of anorexia/Cachexia therapy (FAACT) questionnaire. Qual Life Res. 2000;9(10):1137–46. https://doi.org/10.1023/A:1016670403148.
34. Schmidt K, et al. Validity of the six-minute walk test in cancer patients. Int J Sports Med. 2013;34(7):631–6. https://doi.org/10.1055/s-0032-1323746.
35. Knols RH, et al. Hand-held dynamometry in patients with haematological malignancies: measurement error in the clinical assessment of knee extension strength. BMC Musculoskelet Disord. 2009;10:31.
36. Kyle UG, et al. Bioelectrical impedance analysis--part I: review of principles and methods. Clin Nutr. 2004;23(5):1226–43. https://doi.org/10.1016/j.clnu.2004.06.004.
37. Conn VS, et al. A meta-analysis of exercise interventions among people treated for cancer. Support Care Cancer. 2006;14(7):699–712. https://doi.org/10.1007/s00520-005-0905-5.
38. Knols RH, et al. Isometric strength measurement for muscle weakness in cancer patients: reproducibility of isometric muscle strength measurements with a hand-held pull-gauge dynamometer in cancer patients. Support Care Cancer. 2002;10(5):430–8. https://doi.org/10.1007/s00520-002-0343-6.
39. Stone CA, et al. Hand-held dynamometry: tester strength is paramount, even in frail populations. J Rehabil Med. 2011;43(9):808–11. https://doi.org/10.2340/16501977-0860.
40. Manttari A, et al. Six-minute walk test: a tool for predicting maximal aerobic power (VO2 max) in healthy adults. Clin Physiol Funct Imaging. 2018. https://doi.org/10.1111/cpf.12525.
41. LeBlanc TW, et al. Validation and real-world assessment of the functional assessment of anorexia-Cachexia therapy (FAACT) scale in patients with advanced non-small cell lung cancer and the cancer anorexia-cachexia syndrome (CACS). Support Care Cancer. 2015;23(8):2341–7. https://doi.org/10.1007/s00520-015-2606-z.
42. Sun G, et al. Comparison of multifrequency bioelectrical impedance analysis with dual-energy X-ray absorptiometry for assessment of percentage body fat in a large, healthy population. Am J Clin Nutr. 2005;81(1):74–8. https://doi.org/10.1093/ajcn/81.1.74.
43. Isenring E, et al. The impact of nutrition support on body composition in cancer outpatients receiving radiotherapy. Acta Diabetol. 2003; 40(Suppl 1):S162–4.
44. Ida S, et al. Changes in body composition secondary to neoadjuvant chemotherapy for advanced esophageal cancer are related to the occurrence of postoperative complications after esophagectomy. Ann Surg Oncol. 2014;21(11):3675–9. https://doi.org/10.1245/s10434-014-3737-z.
45. Takekiyo T, et al. Effect of exercise therapy on muscle mass and physical functioning in patients undergoing allogeneic hematopoietic stem cell transplantation. Support Care Cancer. 2015;23(4):985–92. https://doi.org/10.1007/s00520-014-2425-7.
46. Johns N, Stephens NA, Fearon KC. Muscle wasting in cancer. Int J Biochem Cell Biol. 2013;45(10):2215–29. https://doi.org/10.1016/j.biocel.2013.05.032.
47. Cramp, F. and J. Byron-Daniel, Exercise for the management of cancer-related fatigue in adults. Cochrane Database Syst Rev, 2012. 11: p. Cd006145.
48. Mishra SI, et al. Exercise interventions on health-related quality of life for people with cancer during active treatment. Cochrane Database Syst Rev. 2012;(8):Cd008465. https://doi.org/10.1002/14651858.CD008465.pub2.
49. Locher JL, et al. Prophylactic percutaneous endoscopic gastrostomy tube placement in treatment of head and neck cancer: a comprehensive review and call for evidence-based medicine. JPEN J Parenter Enteral Nutr. 2011; 35(3):365–74. https://doi.org/10.1177/0148607110377097.

22

Dose escalation of radiation therapy with or without induction chemotherapy for unresectable locally advanced pancreatic cancer

Sung Jun Ma, Kavitha M. Prezzano, Gregory M. Hermann and Anurag K. Singh*

Abstract

Background: Dose escalation of conventionally fractionated radiation therapy (CFRT) above 45–54 Gy has an unclear survival benefit. Prior National Cancer Database (NCDB) analyses have shown improved overall survival with induction chemotherapy (iC) prior to concurrent chemoradiation (CRT) in locally advanced pancreatic cancer. Our study compared dose-escalated CFRT with and without iC.

Methods: The NCDB was queried for primary stage III, cT4 N0–1 M0 LAPC treated with CRT with or without iC (2004–2015). CFRT was stratified by < 55 Gy and ≥ 55 Gy. Cohort iC + CRT and CRT included those with and without iC, respectively. The primary endpoint was overall survival (OS). Kaplan-Meier analysis, Cox proportional hazards method, and propensity score matching were used.

Results: Among 2029 patients, cohort iC + CRT had 738 patients ($n = 601$ for 45–55 Gy and $n = 137$ for ≥55 Gy) and cohort CRT had 1291 patients ($n = 1066$ for 45–55 Gy and $n = 225$ for ≥55 Gy). Median follow-up was 24.3 months and 24.6 months for cohorts iC + CRT and CRT, respectively. Dose escalation showed improved survival in the multivariable analysis in cohort iC + CRT (HR 0.77, $p = 0.013$) but not in cohort CRT (HR 0.91, $p = 0.19$). Using 2:1 propensity score matching, a total of 387 patients for cohort iC + CRT and 549 patients for cohort CRT were matched. After matching, dose escalation remained significant for improved overall survival in cohort iC + CRT (median OS 16.2 vs 15.2 months; 2-yr OS 33.4% vs 25.4%; $p = 0.022$) but not in cohort CRT (median OS 11.8 vs 10.6 months; 2-yr OS 13.3% vs 10.1%; $p = 0.16$).

Conclusions: Patients with locally advanced pancreatic cancer who undergo iC have improved survival with radiation dose escalation above 55 Gy. For patients without iC, there is no clear association between radiation dose escalation and survival.

Keywords: Induction chemotherapy, Locally advanced pancreatic cancer, Dose escalation, Conventionally fractionated

Background

Pancreatic adenocarcinoma is the fourth leading cause of cancer death in the United States with a dismal 5 year survival of 8% [1]. Surgical resection remains the only potential curative approach in the treatment of this disease, though only 20% of patients are initially able to undergo resection [2]. For patients with unresectable pancreatic cancer, induction chemotherapy (iC), concurrent chemoradiation (CRT) and radiation therapy (RT) alone are among the combination of regimens that have been used as various treatment options.

The role of RT in the setting of locally advanced pancreatic cancer is controversial since responses are limited and the predominant cause of death in these patients is distant metastatic disease. More recent evidence from postmortem studies has shown that up to 30% of deaths from pancreatic cancer are due to locally advancing disease, pointing to the importance of local control in preventing tumor progression and potentially improving overall survival [3].

* Correspondence: Anurag.Singh@roswellpark.org
Department of Radiation Medicine, Roswell Park Comprehensive Cancer Center, Elm and Carlton Streets, Buffalo, NY 14263, USA

Radiation dose escalation has been posited as a potential strategy to improve outcomes in this challenging patient population, though results have been mixed. A phase II study of RT alone found that dose escalation to 70–72 Gy was feasible [4]. A National Cancer Database (NCDB) review of patients who received definitive CRT for unresectable pancreatic cancer did not find an overall survival (OS) benefit with the use of RT doses exceeding 45 Gy [5]. Institutional reports have found that dose escalation may provide a significant survival benefit when used in conjunction with iC [6–8].

This study used the NCDB to identify patients with non-metastatic, unresected pancreatic cancer in order to evaluate the role of dose-escalated CRT. We further sought to compare the outcomes of dose escalation in those patients who received iC prior to CRT versus those who underwent definitive CRT alone.

Methods

Patient population

The NCDB registry was used to identify pancreatic adenocarcinoma cases diagnosed between 2004 and 2015 (the most recent dataset available at the time of this study). The NCDB is a national cancer database capturing approximately 70% of cancer incidences in the United States and obtains data from over 1500 hospitals [9]. It is a de-identified dataset and this study was exempt from institutional review board review.

Our patient selection flow diagram is shown in Fig. 1. Our initial query identified patients with unresected stage III, clinical T4 N0–1 M0 pancreatic adenocarcinoma who had been treated with curative-intent CRT with or without iC. American Joint Committee on Cancer (AJCC) 6th and 7th editions were used to determine stage III disease in 2004–2015.

To address variability in dose fractionation among hospitals for LAPC, conventionally fractionated radiation therapy (CFRT) was categorized as 1.8–2.5 Gy/fractions up to a total of 45–70 Gy [6]. The radiation dose was stratified by < 55 Gy and ≥ 55 Gy based on National Comprehensive Cancer Network (NCCN) guidelines suggesting 45–54 Gy as the standard dose of radiation therapy [10]. Chemotherapy or radiation therapy delivered within 30 days of each other was considered as CRT. Chemotherapy administered within 31–180 days prior to the radiation therapy was considered as iC followed by CRT. Patients who received chemotherapy more than 180 days prior to radiation therapy were excluded from our analysis. Other exclusion criteria were: having undergone surgery, incomplete follow-up, incomplete radiation dose or fractionation, missing data on the number of days between diagnosis and treatments, and palliative-intent treatments. Those who survived less than 3 months after their diagnosis were excluded in order to omit patients who expired prior to completing their treatment course.

Baseline characteristics for analysis included: treatment facility type, age, gender, race, insurance status, household income, residential setting, Charlson-Deyo Score (CDS), year of diagnosis, the location of primary tumor within the pancreas, tumor size, clinical N stage, single- vs multi-agent chemotherapy (defined by the NCDB as the first course of therapy), radiation dose, and radiation fractionation. Cohorts iC + CRT and CRT were constructed to include patients with and without iC, respectively. Age and tumor size were stratified by ≥65 years or < 65 years and < 3.8 cm or ≥ 3.8 cm based on their median values. The household income level of residential area was based on the 2012 American Community Survey data adjusted for inflation (the most recent data at the time of this study), and it was stratified by above or below the median value of $48,000.

Pertinent prognostic factors such as a patient's performance status, or the type and duration of chemotherapy received are unavailable in the NCDB. Other important outcomes such as toxicity, local and distant recurrences are also unavailable in the NCDB. CA 19–9 factor and tumor grade were missing in 1090 (53.7%) and 1574 (77.6%) patients, respectively. Radiation techniques data for intensity-modulated radiation therapy (IMRT) or conformal 3-D therapy were only available in 457 (61.9%) patients for cohort iC + CRT and 570 (44.2%) patients for cohort CRT. The primary outcome was overall survival (OS), which was characterized as time between the diagnosis and the last follow-up or death.

Statistical analysis

Kaplan-Meier and log-rank tests were used to evaluate OS. Categorical and continuous variables between the < 55 Gy and ≥ 55 Gy groups were compared using Fisher's exact and Mann-Whitney U tests, respectively. Logistic regression univariable (UVA) and multivariable analyses (MVA) were performed to identify potential predictors for the dose escalation and were reported as odds ratio (OR). Cox proportional hazard UVA and MVA were performed to identify potential predictors for the OS and were reported as hazards ratio (HR). All statistically significant factors from UVA were used to construct the MVA model, which was finalized using a backward stepwise elimination. Potential treatment interactions with other variables were evaluated using Cox MVA by adding interaction terms. To minimize selection bias, propensity score matching was performed. Matching was based on baseline characteristics, including facility type, age, CDS, year of diagnosis, tumor size, clinical N stage, and single- vs multi-agent

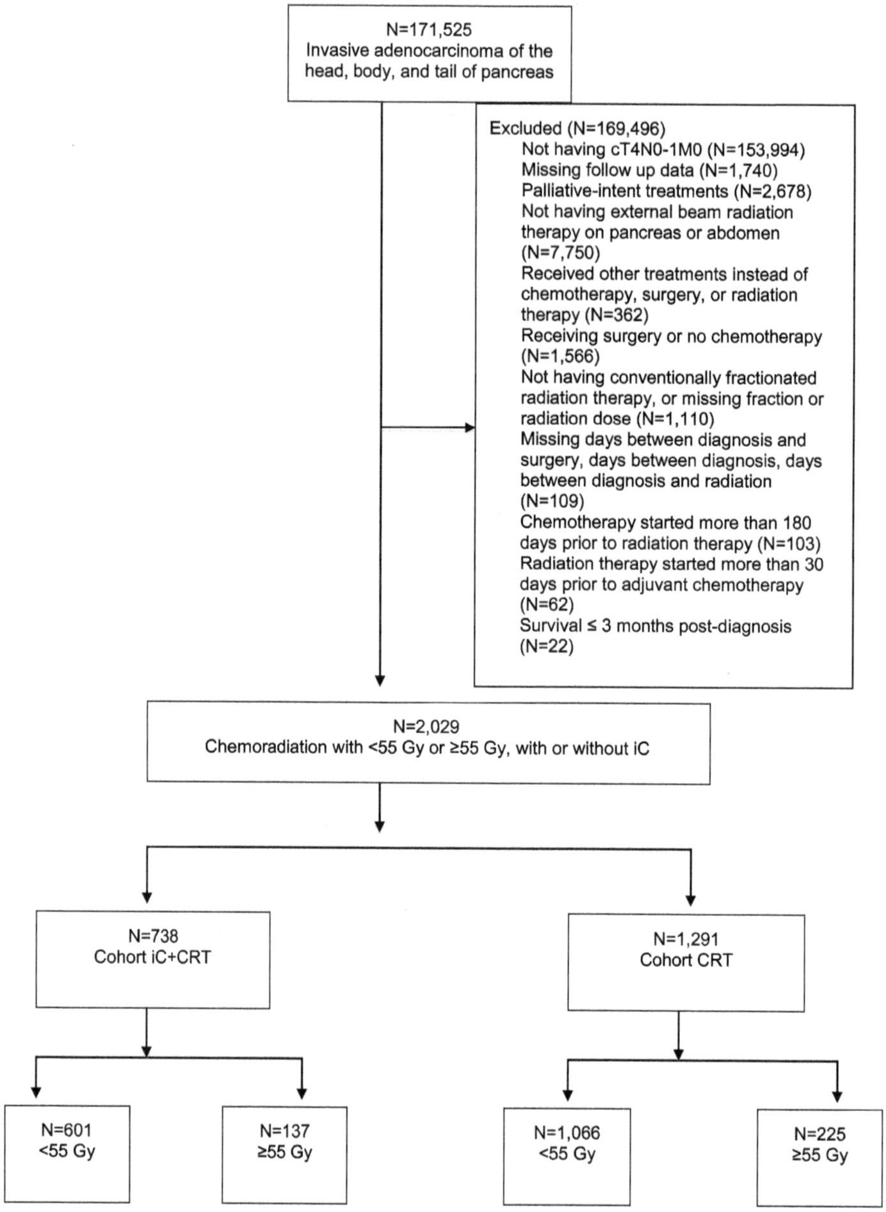

Fig. 1 CONSORT diagram for patient selection criteria. iC: induction chemotherapy; CRT: chemoradiation

chemotherapy. Additional variables were included if they were statistically significant in Cox MVA for OS. All matching was performed in a 2:1 ratio without any replacement, using nearest neighbor method with a caliper distance of 0.2 of the standard deviation of the logit of the propensity score [11]. MatchIt package (version 3.0.1) was used for matching. After matching, matched-sample Cox UVA was used to assess the effect of dose escalation on OS. R software (version 3.4.3, R Foundation for Statistical Computing, Vienna, Austria) was used to perform all aforementioned analyses. All *p* values were two-sided, and the p values less than 0.05 were deemed statistically significant.

Results

Cohort iC + CRT

A total of 2029 patients with unresected clinical stage III T4 N0–1 M0 pancreatic adenocarcinoma treated with concurrent chemoradiation were examined. Of those, 738 patients received iC and were included in cohort iC + CRT. Radiation dose of < 55 Gy was delivered to 601 patients, while that of ≥55 Gy was given to 137 patients. The majority of patients in this cohort had clinical T4N0M0 adenocarcinoma of the pancreatic head (Table 1). The patient group treated with ≥55 Gy was more likely to have female patients and fewer patients treated in 2012–2015. Other variables were well balanced.

Table 1 Baseline characteristics, before matching

	Cohort iC + CRT					Cohort CRT				
	45–55 Gy		55+ Gy			45–55 Gy		55+ Gy		
	N	%	N	%	P	N	%	N	%	P
Facility					0.39					0.0031
Nonacademic	335	56	71	52		672	63	163	72	
Academic	259	43	65	47		390	37	58	26	
NA	7	1	1	1		4	0	4	2	
Age					1					0.0081
< 65	303	50	69	50		474	44	122	54	
≥ 65	298	50	68	50		592	56	103	46	
NA	0	0	0	0		0	0	0	0	
Gender					0.047					1
Female	297	49	81	59		514	48	109	48	
Male	304	51	56	41		552	52	116	52	
NA	0	0	0	0		0	0	0	0	
Race					0.88					0.18
White	493	82	115	84		869	82	190	84	
Black	81	13	17	12		168	16	27	12	
Other	19	3	3	2		20	2	7	3	
NA	8	1	2	1		9	1	1	0	
Insurance					0.31					0.095
None	12	2	2	1		28	3	7	3	
Nonprivate	320	53	63	46		633	59	117	52	
Private	265	44	70	51		391	37	99	44	
NA	4	1	2	1		14	1	2	1	
Income					1					0.45
Above median	389	65	90	66		546	51	118	52	
Below median	207	34	47	34		503	47	97	43	
NA	5	1	0	0		17	2	10	4	
Residential setting					0.33					0.077
Metro	488	81	114	83		807	76	151	67	
Urban	77	13	16	12		189	18	53	24	
Rural	10	2	5	4		34	3	7	3	
NA	26	4	2	1		36	3	14	6	
Charlson-Deyo Score					1					0.25
0–1	575	96	131	96		1006	94	217	96	
≥ 2	26	4	6	4		60	6	8	4	
NA	0	0	0	0		0	0	0	0	
Year of diagnosis					0.016					< 0.001
2004–2007	52	9	7	5		317	30	92	41	
2008–2011	245	41	74	54		529	50	105	47	
2012–2015	304	51	56	41		220	21	28	12	
NA	0	0	0	0		0	0	0	0	
Primary tumor site					0.068					0.014
Head	411	68	94	69		764	72	140	62	

Table 1 Baseline characteristics, before matching *(Continued)*

	Cohort iC + CRT					Cohort CRT				
	45–55 Gy		55+ Gy			45–55 Gy		55+ Gy		
	N	%	N	%	P	N	%	N	%	P
Body	171	28	43	31		271	25	74	33	
Tail	19	3	0	0		31	3	11	5	
NA	0	0	0	0		0	0	0	0	
Tumor size (cm)					0.70					0.018
< 3.8	265	44	65	47		486	46	82	36	
≥ 3.8	283	47	64	47		448	42	111	49	
NA	53	9	8	6		132	12	32	14	
Clinical N stage					0.44					0.70
0	367	61	89	65		692	65	143	64	
1	234	39	48	35		374	35	82	36	
NA	0	0	0	0		0	0	0	0	
Chemotherapy					0.20					0.74
Single agent	166	28	30	22		789	74	164	73	
Multi agent	435	72	107	78		277	26	61	27	
NA	0	0	0	0		0	0	0	0	
Total radiation dose (Gy)					< 0.001					< 0.001
Median	50.4		59.4			50.4		59.4		
IQR	50.4–52.5		56.0–59.4			50.4–52.0		57.5–60.0		
Fraction					< 0.001					< 0.001
Median	28		30			28		32		
IQR	27–28		28–33			26–28		30–33		

iC induction chemotherapy, *CRT* chemoradiation, *IQR* interquartile range, *NA* not available

On logistic regression UVA, male patients were less likely to receive ≥55 Gy (OR 0.68, $p = 0.041$). No other variables were statistically significant for the receipt of dose escalation.

On Cox MVA (Table 2), having treatments at academic facilities (HR 0.79, $p = 0.0045$), diagnosis between the years 2012–2015 (HR 0.71, $p = 0.021$), the use of multi-agent chemotherapy (HR 0.77, $p = 0.0041$), and dose escalation ≥55 Gy (HR 0.77, $p = 0.013$) were associated with improved survival. After Cox MVA, there was no treatment interaction with age ≥ 65 vs < 65 ($p = 0.54$), CDS ≥2 vs 0–1 ($p = 0.90$), year of diagnosis (2008–2011, $p = 0.93$, 2012–2015, $p = 0.89$), tumor size ≥3.8 cm vs < 3.8 cm ($p = 0.37$), or pancreatic tumor site (body and tail, $p = 0.18$). The ideal period of induction chemotherapy was identified using a restricted cubic spline method, which demonstrated HR 1.0 crossing at approximately 91 days. Therefore, two patient population groups were constructed ($n = 360$ for < 90 days, $n = 378$ for ≥90 days). Longer duration of induction chemotherapy remained statistically significant for improved overall survival in multivariable analysis (HR 0.83, $p = 0.025$).

The overall median follow-up in cohort iC + CRT was 24.3 months (interquartile range [IQR] 16.2–38.0). The < 55 Gy group had a median follow-up of 22.8 months (IQR 15.5–33.6) and the ≥55 Gy group had that of 29.6 months (IQR 22.0–54.2). The median OS was 15.9 months (IQR 11.1–22.4) for the < 55 Gy group and 16.4 months (IQR 12.0–26.5) for the ≥55 Gy group (log-rank $p = 0.026$). OS at 2 years was 25.1% for the < 55 Gy group and 35.2% for the ≥55 Gy group.

A total of 387 patients were matched, with 258 patients in the < 55 Gy group and 129 patients in the ≥55 Gy group. All variables were well balanced between these groups (Table 3). The overall median follow-up for the matched patients was 24.8 months (IQR 16.5–42.7). The median OS was 15.2 months (IQR 10.4–22.3) for the < 55 Gy group and 16.2 months (IQR 12.0–25.3) for the ≥55 Gy group (log-rank $p = 0.022$). OS at 2 years was 25.4% for the < 55 Gy group and 33.4% for the ≥55 Gy group (Fig. 2).

Cohort CRT

A total of 1291 patients received no iC and were included in cohort CRT. A radiation dose of < 55 Gy was

Table 2 Cox UVA and MVA for cohort iC + CRT

Variable	Cox UVA			Cox MVA		
	HR	95% CI	P	HR	95% CI	P
Facility						
Nonacademic	1	Ref		1	Ref	
Academic	0.76	0.65–0.89	< 0.001	0.79	0.67–0.93	0.0045
Age						
< 65	1	Ref				
≥ 65	1.04	0.89–1.21	0.64			
Gender						
Female	1	Ref		1	Ref	
Male	1.19	1.02–1.39	0.031	1.09	0.93–1.29	0.29
Race						
White	1	Ref				
Black	0.86	0.68–1.10	0.23			
Other	0.86	0.54–1.36	0.52			
Insurance						
None	1	Ref				
Nonprivate	1.07	0.57–2.02	0.82			
Private	1.07	0.57–2.01	0.83			
Income						
Above median	1	Ref				
Below median	1.05	0.90–1.24	0.52			
Residential setting						
Metro	1	Ref				
Urban	1.00	0.79–1.26	0.98			
Rural	1.35	0.80–2.25	0.26			
Charlson-Deyo Score						
0–1	1	Ref				
≥ 2	1.08	0.75–1.57	0.67			
Year of diagnosis						
2004–2007	1	Ref		1	Ref	
2008–2011	0.95	0.71–1.28	0.75			
2012–2015	0.67	0.50–0.89	0.0068	0.71	0.53–0.95	0.021
Primary tumor site						
Head	1	Ref				
Body	0.87	0.73–1.04	0.12			
Tail	1.25	0.78–2.01	0.35			
Tumor size (cm)						
< 3.8	1	Ref		1	Ref	
≥ 3.8	1.20	1.02–1.41	0.027	1.16	0.98–1.37	0.082
Clinical N stage						
0	1	Ref				
1	1.15	0.98–1.34	0.091			
Chemotherapy						
Single agent	1	Ref		1	Ref	
Multi agent	0.69	0.58–0.82	< 0.001	0.77	0.64–0.92	0.0041
Dose escalation						
< 55 Gy	1	Ref		1	Ref	
≥ 55 Gy	0.80	0.65–0.97	0.027	0.77	0.63–0.95	0.013

UVA univariate analysis, *MVA* multivariable analysis, *HR* hazard ratio, *CI* confidence interval, *Ref* reference

delivered to 1066 patients, while that of ≥55 Gy was given to 225 patients. Similar to the cohort one, the majority of patients had clinical T4N0M0 adenocarcinoma of the pancreatic head (Table 1). The ≥55 Gy group was more likely to have patients treated at nonacademic facilities, age < 65, diagnosis between 2004 and 2007, body of pancreas as a primary site, and larger tumors.

Table 3 Baseline characteristics, after matching

	Cohort iC + CRT					Cohort CRT				
	45–55 Gy		55+ Gy			45–55 Gy		55+ Gy		
	N	%	N	%	P	N	%	N	%	P
Facility1										0.26
Nonacademic	129	50	65	50		273	75	128	70	
Academic	129	50	64	50		93	25	55	30	
Age					0.91					0.59
< 65	128	50	65	50		196	54	93	51	
≥ 65	130	50	64	50		170	46	90	49	
Charlson-Deyo Score					0.65					0.48
0–1	242	94	123	95		351	96	178	97	
≥ 2	16	6	6	5		15	4	5	3	
Income										0.65
Above median						205	56	107	58	
Below median						161	44	76	42	
Year of diagnosis					0.71					0.85
2004–2007	10	4	5	4		133	36	71	39	
2008–2011	131	51	71	55		177	48	86	47	
2012–2015	117	45	53	41		56	15	26	14	
Tumor size (cm)					0.67					0.78
< 3.8	137	53	65	50		161	44	78	43	
≥ 3.8	121	47	64	50		205	56	105	57	
Clinical N stage					0.58					0.51
0	160	62	84	65		224	61	118	64	
1	98	38	45	35		142	39	65	36	
Chemotherapy					0.59					0.54
Single agent	49	19	28	22		273	75	132	72	
Multi agent	209	81	101	78		93	25	51	28	

iC induction chemotherapy, *CRT* chemoradiation

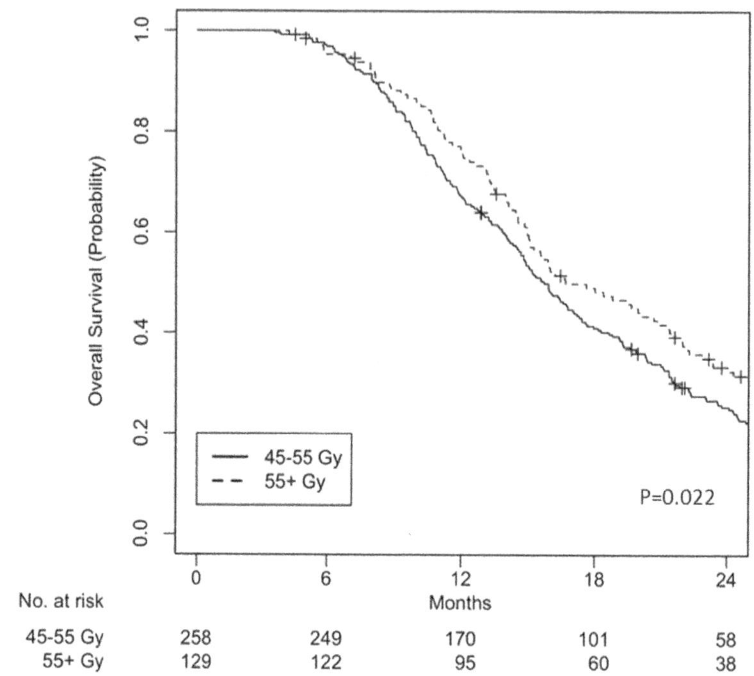

Fig. 2 Overall survival for cohort iC + CRT, after matching

On logistic MVA, patients with treatments at academic facilities (OR 0.65, $p = 0.015$) and a diagnosis between 2012 and 2015 (OR 0.49, $p = 0.0037$) were less likely to receive ≥55 Gy. In contrast, a larger tumor (OR 1.52, $p = 0.010$) was associated with the receipt of ≥55 Gy.

On Cox MVA (Table 4), age ≥ 65 (HR 1.18, $p = 0.0055$) and lower income (HR 1.21, $p < 0.001$) were associated with higher mortality. In contrast, the use of multi-agent chemotherapy was associated with improved survival (HR 0.81, $p = 0.0016$). On Cox UVA, the association between dose escalation and survival was not statistically significant (HR 0.91, $p = 0.19$) and was excluded from the Cox MVA model. After Cox MVA, no treatment interaction was observed with age ≥ 65 vs < 65 ($p = 0.27$), CDS ≥2 vs 0–1 ($p = 0.93$), year of diagnosis (2008–2011, $p = 0.99$; 2012–2015, $p = 0.73$), tumor size ≥3.8 cm vs < 3.8 cm ($p = 0.75$), or pancreatic tumor site (body and tail, $p = 0.74$).

The overall median follow-up was 24.6 months (IQR 9.8–51.4) in cohort CRT. The median follow-up was 22.5 months (IQR 8.5–47.6) for the < 55 Gy group and 30.8 months (IQR 22.6–68.1) for the ≥55 Gy group. The median OS of the < 55 Gy group was 10.8 months (IQR 7.1–16.9) and that of the ≥55 Gy group was 11.6 months (IQR 7.6–18.1, log-rank $p = 0.18$). OS at 2 years was 11.3% for the < 55 Gy group and 13.7% for the ≥55 Gy group.

A total of 549 patients were matched, with 366 patients in the < 55 Gy group and 183 patients in the ≥55 Gy group. All variables were well balanced (Table 3). The overall follow-up for the matched patients was 27.9 months (IQR 11.2–55.2). The median OS of the < 55 Gy group was 10.6 months (IQR 6.8–16.7) and that of the ≥55 Gy group was 11.8 months (IQR 7.7–18.3, log-rank $p = 0.16$). OS at 2 years was 10.1% for the < 55 Gy group and 13.3% for the ≥55 Gy group (Fig. 3).

Total cohort

3D conformal radiation therapy (3D-CRT) was delivered to 269 patients ($n = 192$ without induction chemotherapy, $n = 77$ with induction chemotherapy) and intensity-modulated radiation therapy (IMRT) was delivered to 690 patients ($n = 378$ without induction chemotherapy, $n = 312$ with induction chemotherapy). For all patients, 3D-CRT was not associated with worse mortality (HR 1.05, 95% CI 0.91–1.22, $p = 0.50$) compared to IMRT. Table 5 shows COX UVA/MVA for the total cohort and demonstrates iC improves OS (HR 0.73, $p < 0.001$) in the multivariable analysis.

Discussion

This NCDB analysis sought to examine the effect of radiation dose escalation in patients with locally advanced pancreatic cancer when given concurrently with chemotherapy. To our knowledge, this is the first study that compares the effect of dose escalation in patients who have received iC versus those who received CRT alone. We show that there is a significant OS benefit with the use of dose-escalated RT with concurrent chemotherapy in patients who have first received iC versus those who receive dose-escalated radiation with concurrent chemotherapy alone.

Table 4 Cox UVA and MVA for cohort CRT

Variable	Cox UVA			Cox MVA		
	HR	95% CI	P	HR	95% CI	P
Facility						
Nonacademic	1	Ref		1	Ref	
Academic	0.89	0.79–0.997	0.045	0.91	0.81–1.03	0.14
Age						
< 65	1	Ref		1	Ref	
≥ 65	1.18	1.06–1.32	0.0038	1.18	1.05–1.32	0.0055
Gender						
Female	1	Ref				
Male	1.05	0.94–1.17	0.44			
Race						
White	1	Ref				
Black	0.99	0.85–1.16	0.91			
Other	0.99	0.67–1.48	0.98			
Insurance						
None	1	Ref				
Nonprivate	1.33	0.94–1.88	0.11			
Private	1.09	0.77–1.55	0.63			
Income						
Above median	1	Ref		1	Ref	
Below median	1.21	1.08–1.36	< 0.001	1.21	1.08–1.36	< 0.001
Residential setting						
Metro	1	Ref				
Urban	1.02	0.88–1.17	0.83			
Rural	1.14	0.83–1.56	0.43			
Charlson-Deyo Score						
0–1	1	Ref				
≥ 2	1.01	0.78–1.30	0.94			
Year of diagnosis						
2004–2007	1	Ref				
2008–2011	0.92	0.81–1.04	0.19			
2012–2015	0.91	0.77–1.07	0.25			
Primary tumor site						
Head	1	Ref				
Body	0.96	0.85–1.09	0.57			
Tail	1.04	0.76–1.43	0.80			
Tumor size (cm)						
< 3.8	1	Ref				
≥ 3.8	1.08	0.96–1.21	0.22			
Clinical N stage						
0	1	Ref				
1	1.09	0.97–1.22	0.17			
Chemotherapy						
Single agent	1	Ref		1	Ref	
Multi agent	0.79	0.70–0.90	< 0.001	0.81	0.71–0.92	0.0016
Dose escalation						
< 55 Gy	1	Ref				
≥ 55 Gy	0.91	0.78–1.05	0.19			

UVA univariate analysis, *MVA* multivariable analysis, *HR* hazard ratio, *CI* confidence interval, *Ref* reference

The use of CRT in the setting of unresectable pancreatic cancer is still controversial. The landmark LAP-07 trial, which randomized patients to CRT compared to chemotherapy alone did not demonstrate an improvement in survival, calling into question the utility of RT in locally advanced pancreatic cancer [12]. However, this trial was criticized for its randomization of a heterogeneous cohort of patients, as well as for its use of obsolete chemotherapeutic regimens, and historical radiation techniques. Retrospective studies have reported a survival benefit for patients receiving multi-agent induction chemotherapy followed by CRT [13–15]. A recent NCDB analysis similarly showed that maximal systemic chemotherapy prior to CRT improved survival in patients with unresectable, non-metastatic pancreatic cancer [16]. Interestingly, the Johns Hopkins experience indicated that patients receiving > 2 cycles of iC had decreased progression and trended toward better OS [15]. A recent NCDB analysis similarly showed that maximal systemic chemotherapy prior to CRT improved survival in patients with unresectable, non-metastatic pancreatic cancer, which is consistent with our analysis [16]. Our study adds that in the setting of the maximal systemic chemotherapy prior to CRT, an improved local control with dose-escalated CRT may be translated to an improved OS.

Optimization of the sequencing of chemotherapy and CRT has been explored and is also controversial. A recent investigation by Chung et al. showed a survival advantage in patients receiving a total RT dose ≥61 Gy with concurrent chemotherapy followed by maintenance chemotherapy [7]. However, the FFCD/SFRO (Fédération Francophone de Cancérologie Digestive/ Société Francophone de Radiothérapie Oncologique) phase III trial compared induction chemoradiation to chemotherapy alone, followed by maintenance chemotherapy for all patients with locally advanced, unresectable pancreatic cancer [17]. They showed that patients receiving the more intensive induction chemoradiation had worse survival than those receiving chemotherapy alone [17]. This result was corroborated by the Johns Hopkins experience indicating that induction chemotherapy may sensitize tumors to subsequent chemoradiation

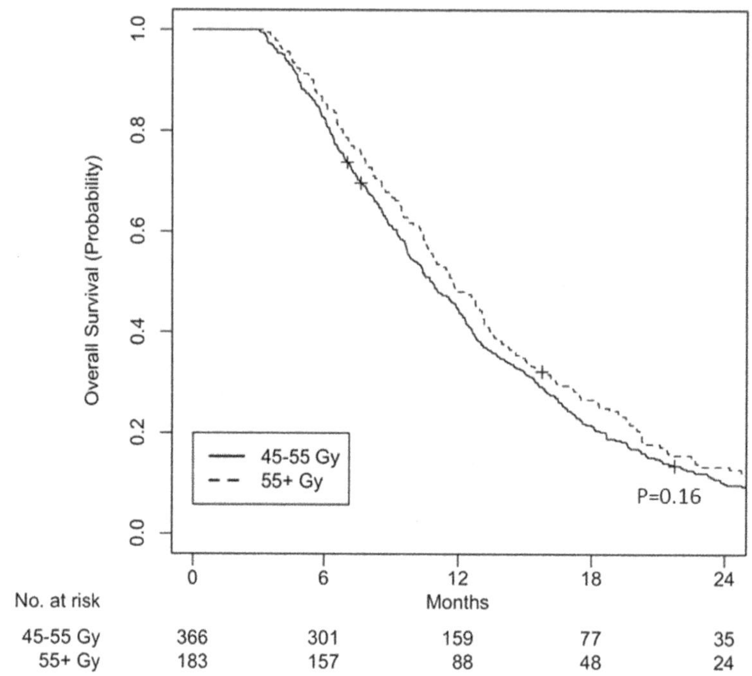

Fig. 3 Overall survival for cohort CRT, after matching

[15]. It may also be hypothesized from these data that upfront chemotherapy can affect early micrometastatic disease, allowing for increased efficacy of—and improved overall outcomes with—subsequent local therapy.

Based on the FFCD/SFRO study and the Johns Hopkins experience, our finding that patients who underwent iC had a significant survival benefit with dose escalated RT when compared to those who received CRT alone may be explained by the reduction in distant failures with the use of induction chemotherapy [15, 17]. Better local control may then translate into improved OS. Just as in the positive retrospective studies of multi-agent chemotherapy, so too did we find on Cox MVA that multi-agent chemotherapy was associated with improved survival in both cohorts [13, 14, 16]. Since distant failure remains a significant concern in this patient population, any local control benefit that dose escalation may have provided could have been negated in the cohort of patients that did not receive iC. This may explain why dose escalation was ineffective in the absence of iC, but it was effective when used along with iC in prior studies [5, 6]. This hypothesis cannot be validated in our study since the NCDB does not include data on local or distant failure rates, though it is notable that both cohorts included approximately two-thirds of patients with clinical node-negative (N0) disease, suggesting the presence of micro-metastatic disease may be effectively treated by iC. Of course, this does not account for the presumption that patients who received iC were better performers and were able to receive more aggressive therapy.

The SCALOP-2 (Systemic Therapy and Chemoradiation in Advanced Localised Pancreatic Cancer-2) trial is currently enrolling patients with locally advanced, non-metastatic pancreatic cancer on a multi-center, randomized trial evaluating iC followed by standard-dose or dose-escalated radiotherapy with concurrent chemotherapy (ClinicalTrials.gov Number NCT02024009). The results of this study will provide valuable information regarding the benefits and risks associated with intensified local therapies.

Our logistic MVA showed larger tumors were more likely treated with dose-escalated CRT, while treatments in an academic facility were less likely to involve dose escalation. These associations are consistent with a prior NCDB study [5]. Our Cox MVA showed treatments at academic facilities and recently diagnosed patients in 2012–2015 were associated with improved survival, whereas elderly age was associated with worse mortality. These are consistent with previous studies, and treatments at academic facilities with survival benefits may be due to treatment volume [6, 18, 19]. Recent diagnosis with improved survival outcomes in our cohort iC + CRT may be due to the recent adoption of FOLFIRINOX (5-fluorouracil, leucovorin, irinotecan, and oxaliplatin) as iC after the publication of the phase III trial by Conroy et al. in 2011 [18, 20].

A number of limitations, inherent to any retrospective review, are present in this study. Lack of information regarding chemotherapy regimens prevents a more nuanced stratification of patients. Further, data regarding radiation techniques (3D-CRT or IMRT) was limited in

Table 5 Cox UVA and MVA for the total cohort

Variable	Cox UVA			Cox MVA		
	HR	95% CI	P	HR	95% CI	P
Facility						
Nonacademic	1	Ref		1	Ref	
Academic	0.80	0.73–0.88	< 0.001	0.90	0.81–0.99	0.036
Age						
< 65	1	Ref		1	Ref	
≥ 65	1.15	1.05–1.26	0.0027	1.18	1.07–1.30	0.0013
Gender						
Female	1	Ref		1	Ref	
Male	1.11	1.01–1.22	0.024	1.08	0.98–1.19	0.13
Race						
White	1	Ref				
Black	0.96	0.85–1.10	0.58			
Other	0.89	0.66–1.20	0.43			
Insurance						
None	1	Ref				
Nonprivate	1.20	0.88–1.62	0.25			
Private	1.02	0.75–1.38	0.91			
Income						
Above median	1	Ref		1	Ref	
Below median	1.22	1.11–1.34	< 0.001	1.20	1.08–1.32	< 0.001
Residential setting						
Metro	1	Ref				
Urban	1.07	0.95–1.21	0.27			
Rural	1.25	0.96–1.64	0.10			
Charlson-Deyo Score						
0–1	1	Ref				
≥ 2	1.06	0.86–1.30	0.61			
Year of diagnosis						
2004–2007	1	Ref		1	Ref	
2008–2011	0.85	0.76–0.95	0.0045	0.92	0.81–1.05	0.20
2012–2015	0.62	0.55–0.71	< 0.001	0.77	0.66–0.89	< 0.001
Primary tumor site						
Head	1	Ref				
Body	0.92	0.83–1.01	0.088			
Tail	1.13	0.87–1.48	0.35			
Tumor size (cm)						
< 3.8	1	Ref		1	Ref	
≥ 3.8	1.11	1.01–1.22	0.035	1.15	1.04–1.27	0.0049
Clinical N stage						
0	1	Ref				
1	1.08	0.99–1.19	0.098			
Chemotherapy						
Single agent	1	Ref		1	Ref	
Multi agent	0.63	0.57–0.69	< 0.001	0.78	0.69–0.87	< 0.001
Induction chemotherapy						
No	1	Ref		1	Ref	
Yes	0.58	0.53–0.64	< 0.001	0.73	0.65–0.83	< 0.001
Dose escalation						
< 55 Gy	1	Ref		1	Ref	
≥ 55 Gy	0.86	0.76–0.97	0.012	0.87	0.76–0.99	0.029

UVA univariate analysis, *MVA* multivariable analysis, *HR* hazard ratio, *CI* confidence interval, *Ref* reference

many patients. Nonetheless, we included a comparison of 3D-CRT and IMRT, which showed there was no detriment in survival for the delivery of 3D-CRT. This is important, since recent evaluations have shown superior dosimetric constraints and decreased patient morbidity with the use of IMRT, suggesting that there may be an improvement in outcomes with the use of more conformal RT techniques. However our findings are not consistent with a survival advantage, which may be a result of confounding factors within the group of patients whose radiation technique was coded as "unknown" [21–23]. Performance status is not recorded by the NCDB and was therefore unable to be accounted for in this study. Performance status has been shown to be a prognostic factor for overall survival in patients with pancreatic cancer [24], though various studies have also reported that its prognostic significance may be lost in multi-variate analysis [25, 26]. Nevertheless, patients included in this study who were deemed fit enough to tolerate iC were likely to be better performers, and the lack of this information is a confounder on our interpretation. Moreover, the receipt of more aggressive therapy (such as iC and dose escalated RT) would presumably improve outcomes. As part of our methodology, we excluded patients who survived less than 3 months after their diagnosis in order to omit patients who would have been unlikely to complete their course of treatment. Of note, no patients who were excluded for survival less than 3 months, received dose-escalated RT. While this may have unintentionally excluded patients who had increased toxicities from their treatment course, our suspicion that this small number of excluded patients would have suffered acute or fatal toxicities from dose escalation was relatively low, based on several studies [6, 7].

Dose-escalated RT is limited by normal tissue dose constraints, which can result in significant acute and late toxicities. Specifically, tumors in close proximity to stomach and duodenum may limit the amount of RT that could be safely delivered, due to concerns for radiation-induced gastrointestinal toxicities. In this study, no treatment interaction was seen in patients with a tumor size or with tumors located at the body or tail of the pancreas. These variables were also statistically insignificant for survival outcomes after Cox MVA in our study, indicating that they less likely play a major role in the survival outcome of dose escalation seen in both cohorts. Specific toxicities in the two cohorts could not be assessed in this study, since this data is not collected by the NCDB.

The database was also re-examined to evaluate 848 patients who had CA 19–9 factor values, ranging from 0 to > 98. Among 398 patients with no iC, only 47 patients received escalated dose-escalated RT. The sample size of the cohorts with escalated radiation dose was felt to be too small for repeating propensity scored matching. Among 450 patients with induction chemotherapy, only 92 patients received dose-escalated RT. With 1:1 propensity score matching of baseline characteristics including CA 19–9 values, a total of 174 patients were matched. Other ratios such as 2:1 could not be performed since not all patients (55+ Gy) were matched with corresponding, control patients (45–55 Gy). Patients with dose-escalated RT were associated with improved overall survival (log--rank $p = 0.013$).

Conclusion

This novel NCDB analysis of patients with unresectable, cT4 N0–1 pancreatic cancer shows that dose-escalated RT with concurrent chemotherapy improves survival in patients who have received iC. Use of dose-escalated RT in this setting may be the favored option for definitive treatment of unresectable pancreatic cancer, and further studies may be warranted for this challenging patient population.

Abbreviations

AJCC: American Joint Committee on Cancer; CDS: Charlson-Deyo Score; CFRT: conventionally fractionated radiation therapy; CRT: concurrent chemoradiation; FFCD: Fédération Francophone de Cancérologie Digestive; FOLFIRINOX: 5-fluorouracil, leucovorin, irinotecan, and oxaliplatin; HR: hazards ratio; iC + CRT: induction chemotherapy followed by concurrent chemoradiation; iC: induction chemotherapy; IMRT: intensity-modulated radiation therapy; MVA: multivariable analyses; NCCN: National Comprehensive Cancer Network; NCDB: National Cancer Database; NCDB: National Cancer Database; OR: odds ratio; OS: overall survival; RT: radiation therapy; SFRO: Société Francophone de Radiothérapie Oncologique; UVA: univariable analysis

Acknowledgements

Not applicable.

Funding

This research received no external funding support.

Authors' contributions

Study conception and design: S.M. Data acquisition: S.M. Quality control of data: S.M., K.P., G.M.H., A.K.S. Data analysis and interpretation: S.M., K.P., G.M.H., A.K.S. Statistical analysis: S.M. Manuscript preparation and editing: S.M., K.P., G.M.H., A.K.S. Manuscript review: S.M., K.P., G.M.H., A.K.S. All authors read and approved the final manuscript.

Competing interests

The authors declare that they have no competing interests.

References

1. Siegel RL, Miller KD, Jemal A. Cancer statistics, 2018. CA Cancer J Clin. 2018; 68(1):7–30.
2. Gillen S, Schuster T, Meyer Zum Buschenfelde C, Friess H, Kleeff J. Preoperative/neoadjuvant therapy in pancreatic cancer: a systematic review and meta-analysis of response and resection percentages. PLoS Med. 2010; 7(4):e1000267.
3. Iacobuzio-Donahue CA, Fu B, Yachida S, Luo M, Abe H, Henderson CM, et al. DPC4 gene status of the primary carcinoma correlates with patterns of failure in patients with pancreatic cancer. J Clin Oncol. 2009;27(11):1806–13.
4. Ceha HM, van Tienhoven G, Gouma DJ, Veenhof CH, Schneider CJ, Rauws EA, et al. Feasibility and efficacy of high dose conformal radiotherapy for patients with locally advanced pancreatic carcinoma. Cancer. 2000;89(11):2222–9.
5. Hall WA, Colbert LE, Nickleach D, Switchenko J, Liu Y, Gillespie T, et al. The influence of radiation therapy dose escalation on overall survival in unresectable pancreatic adenocarcinoma. J Gastrointest Oncol. 2014;5(2):77–85.
6. Krishnan S, Chadha AS, Suh Y, Chen HC, Rao A, Das P, et al. Focal radiation therapy dose escalation improves overall survival in locally advanced pancreatic Cancer patients receiving induction chemotherapy and consolidative Chemoradiation. Int J Radiat Oncol Biol Phys. 2016;94(4):755–65.
7. Chung SY, Chang JS, Lee BM, Kim KH, Lee KJ, Seong J. Dose escalation in locally advanced pancreatic cancer patients receiving chemoradiotherapy. Radiother Oncol. 2017;123(3):438–45.
8. Zschaeck S, Blumke B, Wust P, Kaul D, Bahra M, Riess H, et al. Dose-escalated radiotherapy for unresectable or locally recurrent pancreatic cancer: dose volume analysis, toxicity and outcome of 28 consecutive patients. PLoS One. 2017;12(10):e0186341.
9. Bilimoria KY, Stewart AK, Winchester DP, Ko CY. The National Cancer Data Base: a powerful initiative to improve cancer care in the United States. Ann Surg Oncol. 2008;15(3):683–90.
10. National Comprehensive Cancer Network Pancreatic Adenocarcinoma (Version 1.2018) [Available from: https://www.nccn.org/professionals/physician_gls/pdf/pancreatic.pdf.
11. Austin PC. Optimal caliper widths for propensity-score matching when estimating differences in means and differences in proportions in observational studies. Pharm Stat. 2011;10(2):150–61.
12. Hammel P, Huguet F, van Laethem JL, Goldstein D, Glimelius B, Artru P, et al. Effect of Chemoradiotherapy vs chemotherapy on survival in patients with locally advanced pancreatic Cancer controlled after 4 months of gemcitabine with or without Erlotinib: the LAP07 randomized clinical trial. JAMA. 2016;315(17):1844–53.
13. Huguet F, Andre T, Hammel P, Artru P, Balosso J, Selle F, et al. Impact of chemoradiotherapy after disease control with chemotherapy in locally advanced pancreatic adenocarcinoma in GERCOR phase II and III studies. J Clin Oncol. 2007;25(3):326–31.
14. Krishnan S, Rana V, Janjan NA, Varadhachary GR, Abbruzzese JL, Das P, et al. Induction chemotherapy selects patients with locally advanced, unresectable pancreatic cancer for optimal benefit from consolidative chemoradiation therapy. Cancer. 2007;110(1):47–55.
15. Faisal F, Tsai HL, Blackford A, Olino K, Xia C, De Jesus-Acosta A, et al. longer course of induction chemotherapy followed by Chemoradiation favors better survival outcomes for patients with locally advanced pancreatic Cancer. Am J Clin Oncol. 2016;39(1):18–26.

16. Torgeson A, Lloyd S, Boothe D, Tao R, Whisenant J, Garrido-Laguna I, et al. Multiagent induction chemotherapy followed by chemoradiation is associated with improved survival in locally advanced pancreatic cancer. Cancer. 2017;123(19):3816–24.
17. Chauffert B, Mornex F, Bonnetain F, Rougier P, Mariette C, Bouche O, et al. Phase III trial comparing intensive induction chemoradiotherapy (60 Gy, infusional 5-FU and intermittent cisplatin) followed by maintenance gemcitabine with gemcitabine alone for locally advanced unresectable pancreatic cancer. Definitive results of the 2000-01 FFCD/SFRO study. Ann Oncol. 2008;19(9):1592–9.
18. Conroy T, Desseigne F, Ychou M, Bouche O, Guimbaud R, Becouarn Y, et al. FOLFIRINOX versus gemcitabine for metastatic pancreatic cancer. N Engl J Med. 2011;364(19):1817–25.
19. Haj Mohammad N, Bernards N, Besselink MG, Busch OR, Wilmink JW, Creemers GJ, et al. Volume matters in the systemic treatment of metastatic pancreatic cancer: a population-based study in the Netherlands. J Cancer Res Clin Oncol. 2016;142(6):1353–60.
20. Christians KK, Tsai S, Mahmoud A, Ritch P, Thomas JP, Wiebe L, et al. Neoadjuvant FOLFIRINOX for borderline resectable pancreas cancer: a new treatment paradigm? Oncologist. 2014;19(3):266–74.
21. Brown MW, Ning H, Arora B, Albert PS, Poggi M, Camphausen K, et al. A dosimetric analysis of dose escalation using two intensity-modulated radiation therapy techniques in locally advanced pancreatic carcinoma. Int J Radiat Oncol Biol Phys. 2006;65(1):274–83.
22. Ben-Josef E, Schipper M, Francis IR, Hadley S, Ten-Haken R, Lawrence T, et al. A phase I/II trial of intensity modulated radiation (IMRT) dose escalation with concurrent fixed-dose rate gemcitabine (FDR-G) in patients with unresectable pancreatic cancer. Int J Radiat Oncol Biol Phys. 2012;84(5):1166–71.
23. Tunceroglu A, Park JH, Balasubramanian S, Poppe M, Anker CJ, Poplin E, et al. Dose-painted intensity modulated radiation therapy improves local control for locally advanced pancreas cancer. ISRN Oncol. 2012;2012:572342.
24. Tas F, Sen F, Odabas H, Kilic L, Keskin S, Yildiz I. Performance status of patients is the major prognostic factor at all stages of pancreatic cancer. Int J Clin Oncol. 2013;18(5):839–46.
25. Park JK, Yoon YB, Kim YT, Ryu JK, Yoon WJ, Lee SH. Survival and prognostic factors of unresectable pancreatic cancer. J Clin Gastroenterol. 2008;42(1):86–91.
26. Lee KJ, Yi SW, Chung MJ, Park SW, Song SY, Chung JB, et al. Serum CA 19-9 and CEA levels as a prognostic factor in pancreatic adenocarcinoma. Yonsei Med J. 2013;54(3):643–9.

23

Transportable system enabling multiple irradiation studies under simultaneous hypoxia in vitro

Olli Metsälä[1,2†], Joose Kreutzer[3†], Heidi Högel[1,4*], Petra Miikkulainen[1,2], Pasi Kallio[3] and Panu M. Jaakkola[1,2,5]

Abstract

Background: Cells in solid tumours are variably hypoxic and hence resistant to radiotherapy - the essential role of oxygen in the efficiency of irradiation has been acknowledged for decades. However, the currently available methods for performing hypoxic experiments in vitro have several limitations, such as a limited amount of parallel experiments, incapability of keeping stable growth conditions and dependence on CO_2 incubator or a hypoxia workstation. The purpose of this study was to evaluate the usability of a novel portable system (Minihypoxy) in performing in vitro irradiation studies under hypoxia, and present supporting biological data.

Materials and methods: This study was conducted on cancer cell cultures in vitro. The cells were cultured in normoxic (~ 21% O_2) or in hypoxic (1% O_2) conditions either in conventional hypoxia workstation or in the Minihypoxy system and irradiated at dose rate 1.28 Gy/min ± 2.9%. The control samples were sham irradiated. To study the effects of hypoxia and irradiation on cell viability and DNA damage, western blotting, immunostainings and clonogenic assay were used. The oxygen level, pH, evaporation rate and osmolarity of the culturing media on cell cultures in different conditions were followed.

Results: The oxygen concentration in interest (5, 1 or 0% O_2) was maintained inside the individual culturing chambers of the Minihypoxy system also during the irradiation. The radiosensitivity of the cells cultured in Minihypoxy chambers was declined measured as lower phosphorylation rate of H2A.X and increased clonogenic capacity compared to controls (OER~ 3).

Conclusions: The Minihypoxy system allows continuous control of hypoxic environment in multiple wells and is transportable. Furthermore, the system maintains the low oxygen environment inside the individual culturing chambers during the transportation and irradiation in experiments which are typically conducted in separate facilities.

Keywords: Hypoxia, Cancer, Radiotherapy, Radiation, In vitro, Minihypoxy

Background

The lack of sufficient oxygen in tissues, i.e., hypoxia plays a central role in many physiological and pathological conditions. It is a major microenvironmental factor affecting cellular signalling in many diseases including cancer, stroke, atherosclerosis, inflammatory diseases such as rheumatoid arthritis, and neurodegenerative diseases [1, 2]. Several studies have shown that most solid tumours suffer from insufficient oxygen supply both acutely and chronically (reviewed in [3]). This is mainly caused by structurally and functionally abnormal vascularization of the tumour and limited diffusion capacity of oxygen. Hypoxia causes genome and proteome level changes in cancer cells leading to alterations in cell proliferation, cell cycle progression, metabolism, and cell survival and death (reviewed in [4]). Some of the changes restrict the tumour growth but hypoxia causes also a strong selective pressure towards a more aggressive tumour type.

Besides cancer progression, hypoxia also affects the outcome of cancer treatments including chemotherapy

* Correspondence: hhhoge@utu.fi
†Olli Metsälä and Joose Kreutzer contributed equally to this work.
[1]Turku Centre for Biotechnology, University of Turku and Åbo Akademi University, Tykistökatu 6, FIN-20520 Turku, Finland
[4]Turku PET Centre, University of Turku and Turku University Hospital, Kiinamyllynkatu 4-8, FIN-20521 Turku, Finland
Full list of author information is available at the end of the article

and radiotherapy [5]. The effect of radiotherapy relies partially on direct DNA damage but mainly on the oxygen radicals (ROS) formed by irradiation that requires molecular oxygen (reviewed in [6, 7]). Additionally, hypoxia also changes the positioning of the cells in cell cycle, which is a major factor affecting the responsiveness of the cancer cells to treatment including radiotherapy [8–10]. Many of the hypoxia responsive events are mediated by hypoxia-inducible factors (HIFs). HIFs are transcription factors governing the expression of over two hundred known genes involved in cell survival and metabolism, cell cycle progression and proliferation, motility and apoptosis (reviewed in [11]).

The conditions where in vitro studies are conducted would ideally correspond to the conditions in vivo as authentically as possible. Chemicals partially mimicking hypoxia such as cobalt chloride ($CoCl_2$) as well as desferrioxamine (DFO) and dimethyloxalylglycine (DMOG) that act as inhibitors of prolyl 4-hydroxylases regulating the activity of HIFs but fail to mimic the tumour microenvironment. Various set-ups for achieving true hypoxic conditions in vitro have been established [12, 13]. The conventional method to induce hypoxia is to incubate cells in a tri-gas incubator or a hypoxia workstation. However, this restricts the types of treatments that can be performed in a low oxygen environment. Using workstations, the effect of hypoxia on radiosensitivity can only be studied by preincubating the cells in hypoxia to induce the adaptive system to low oxygen [14, 15]. The drawback of this method is that the cells are reoxygenated prior to irradiation. Therefore, it does not represent hypoxic tumour microenvironment. In addition, reoxygenation itself induces DNA damage [16], and thus interferes the detection of DNA damage caused by reoxygenation observed in tumours after radiotherapy [17–19].

To achieve mobility in the experiments and to expose cells to simultaneous hypoxia and irradiation, the most common solution is to use commercially available hypoxia containers. Here the cells are placed in a sealed container that is purged with a desired gas mix [20–25]. Similarly, sealed containers can be utilized to create anaerobic conditions or low oxygen conditions with oxygen scavengers [26, 27]. However, there is no independent temperature or further O_2 or CO_2 control. Therefore, the entire container with the cells inside needs to be incubated inside a normal incubator, and during the transportation and treatment, the temperature drops rapidly. In addition to commercially available products, there are also other solutions including a hypoxic atmosphere generated in a plastic bag [28] or in a self-made hypoxia containers [29]. Although budget-friendly, the oxygen conditions inside these types of hypoxia containers is difficult to maintain without feedback control [30]. Furthermore, the final oxygen level in the culture medium depends on the materials placed inside the chamber [21, 31]. Additionally, the hypoxia containers require high volume of expensive ready-made gas mixtures. Most importantly, large hypoxia containers exclude the use of multiple parallel experiments.

Here we present a novel system for performing hypoxia and especially hypoxic in vitro irradiation experiments. The portable Minihypoxy system consists of 1–6 individual 1-well culture chambers. Each chamber is independent from others and equipped with its own gas supply port. This enables flexible experiment planning where several different radiation doses and time points can be used within the same experiment. In our experiments, we have used a gas mixture supplied with 1% O_2 but the partial oxygen pressure is convertible down to anoxic (< 0.1% O_2) conditions. Our results show that the Minihypoxy system is functional and easy to use. The individual chambers can be disengaged from the system at least for 10 min without losing the hypoxic conditions or the desired temperature inside the chamber. This enables hypoxic in vitro irradiation experiments with multiple radiation doses and time points within one single experiment.

Materials and methods

Minihypoxy system

The Minihypoxy system is based on our previous studies [32, 33]. Briefly, it is a portable platform that maintains the desired atmosphere while transporting cells and, for example, during microscopy or irradiation experiments. The Minihypoxy system consists of a refillable gas cylinder (Catalina Cylinders, CA, USA), an ITO heater plate and a controller (Okolab s.r.l., Italy), a custom-made 6-well flow divider and 1-well culture chambers (Minihypoxy chambers) with covers and lids (Fig. 1a and b). The refillable gas cylinder can be loaded with any desired gas mixture. In this study, we used a gas mixture of 1% O_2, 5% CO_2, and 94% N_2 (Linde gas, Riihimäki, Finland). Gas flow is regulated by adjusting the outlet pressure from the cylinder. In this study, we used a flow rate of 5 ml/min for all six supply lines (30 ml/min in total for six-wells). The operation time of the Minihypoxy systems with one fully loaded gas container for six Minihypoxy chambers is about 30 h. The gas mixture flows through the custom-made aluminium 6-well flow divider (SaloTeam Oy, Salo, Finland) to the Minihypoxy chambers. The ITO heater maintains the temperature in the desired temperature (37 °C in this study). The Minihypoxy culture chambers were fabricated as described in [32] using gas permeable polydimethylsiloxane (PDMS, Sylgard 184, Dow Corning, USA). Each chamber was sealed water-tightly using a glass lid (1 mm thick and

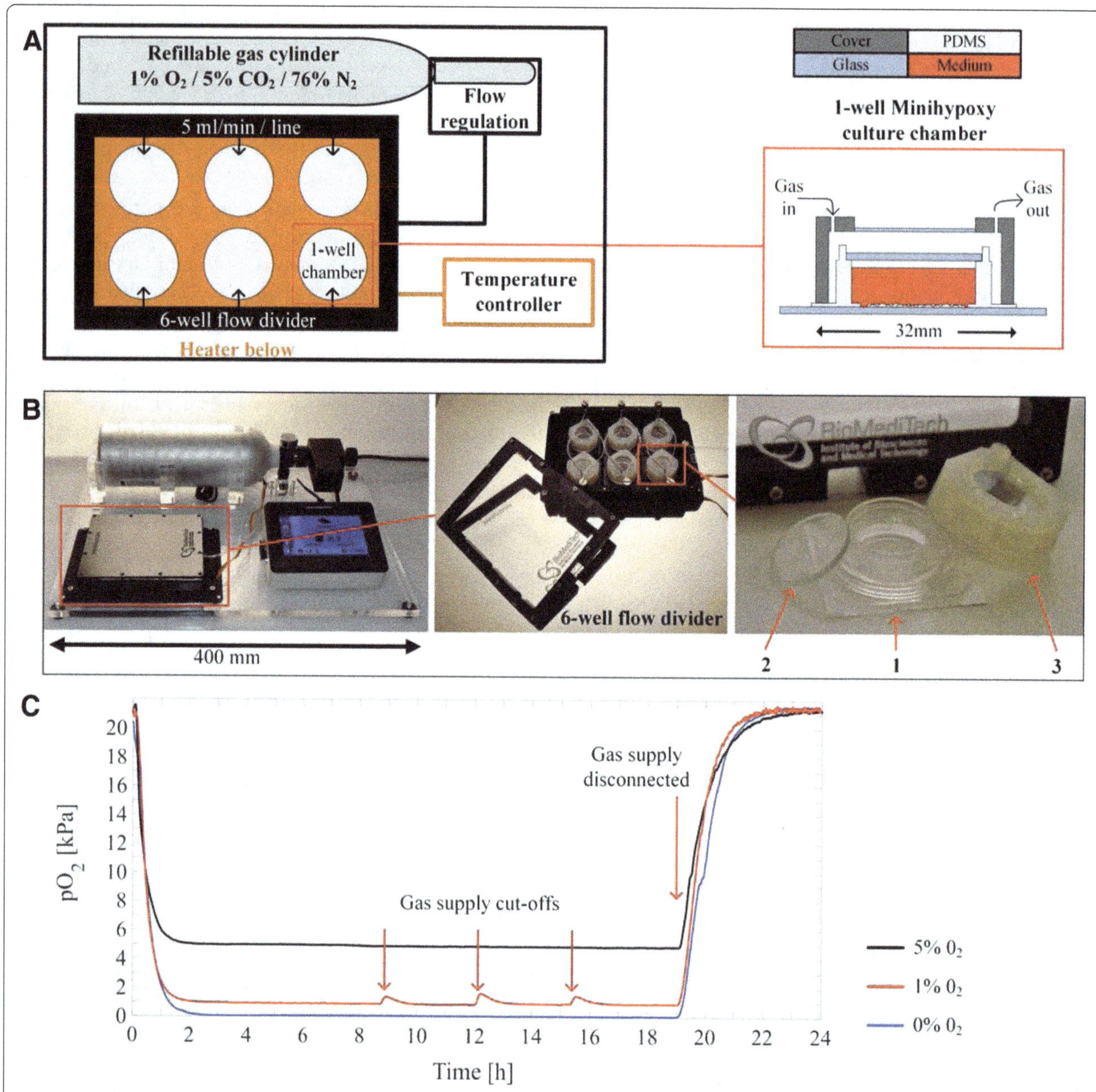

Fig. 1 Structure and functionality of the Minihypoxy system. **a** A schematic diagram of the detailed structure of the system. The system consists of a refillable gas cylinder, a 6-well flow divider, a heater and a temperature controller, and six 1-well culture chambers (Minihypoxy chambers) made from polydimethylsiloxane (PDMS). **b** A picture of the Minihypoxy system, the 6-well flow divider and the Minihypoxy culture chamber on a glass substrate (1) with a lid (2) and a cover (3). **c** Dynamic response in the Minihypoxy culture chamber to descending and ascending oxygen level. The responses were tested on three different oxygen concentrations: 5% O_2 (black line), 1% O_2 (red line) and 0% O_2 (blue line). Ascending oxygen level was reached by disconnecting the gas supply. The 1% O_2 curve shows also the response to three short gas supply cut-offs

20.5 mm in diameter) from the top. The lid prevented evaporation and contamination inside the chamber. The cover is made of polymer by 3D printing (Keijom Oy, Pirkkala, Finland). The purpose of the cover is to maintain the desired gas environment around the PDMS culture chamber. Because of high gas permeability of PDMS, the gas mixture diffuses through the Minihypoxy chamber to the cells. The weight of the Minihypoxy system is 3.3 kg.

Measuring oxygen concentration inside the Minihypoxy chamber

The oxygen concentrations inside the culture chamber were measured utilizing an in-house developed optical oxygen measurement setup [34]. Briefly, the Minihypoxy culture chamber was placed on top of a 0.5 mm thick glass substrate which contained oxygen sensitive fluorescent dyes. The chamber was filled with deionized water (1 ml), sealed using the lid and the cover, and placed on top of the ITO heater that maintained temperature at 37 °C. Optical reading of the fluorescent dyes in the Minihypoxy chamber was performed, through the ITO and glass substrates. The oxygen concentrations were measured using gas mixtures containing 0, 1 and 5% oxygen supplied from the prefilled gas cylinders. We also determined the dynamics of the oxygen concentration change in the Minihypoxy system when the gas supply was disconnected for a 5-min time period to mimic the irradiation treatment. All experiments were done with the flow rate of 5 ml/min.

pH, evaporation and osmolarity of cell culture medium

The pH was measured as an end-point measurement utilizing a microFET pH meter (SI600with microFET sensor, Sentron, The Netherlands). Evaporation was estimated by determining the mass change during the experiment by weighting the wells before and after the experiment. OsmoMat 030 osmometer (GonoTec GmbH, Germany) was used for measuring the osmolarity.

Cell culture

HeLa cervical cancer cell line and LNCaP prostate cancer cell line were obtained from ATCC (Rockville, MD, USA). UT-SCC74 primary cell line derived from human head and neck squamous cell carcinoma (HNSCC) was kindly provided by Prof Reidar Grénman. HeLa cells were cultured in Dulbecco's Modified Eagle Medium (DMEM, Sigma-Aldrich), UT-SCC74 cells in Minimun Essential Medium Eagle with alpha modification (α-MEM, Gibco) and LNCaP cells in Roswell Park Memorial Institute medium (RPMI-1640, Gibco). All media were supplied with 10% fetal calf serum (FCS), L-glutamine and antibiotics (penicillin and streptomycin). Cells were cultured in 37 °C in air/5% CO_2 and tested negative for mycoplasma once a month. The reference cells for the Minihypoxy system were cultured in 1% oxygen and 5% CO_2 in the hypoxia workstation (Invivo2 400, Ruskinn Technology). The reference cells were plated on Minihypoxy culture chambers attached to glass substrate. Chambers were covered with the glass lid and kept on Petri dishes during incubation and for convenience in handling. For live cell imaging the cells were transfected with EGFP expression vector. Transfection reagent Lipofectamine 3000 (Invitrogen) was used according to manufacturer's specifications. The images were obtained with LSM780 microscope (Carl Zeiss, Oberkochen, Germany).

Protein detection and antibodies

For protein detection, western blotting and immunofluorescence staining were used. For protein expression analysis, cells were harvested in SDS-Triton lysis buffer. Protein concentration was measured using Bio-Rad DC Protein assay and protein detection using Pierce ECL Western blotting substrate (Thermo Scientific). Antibodies used were: HIF-1α (610959, BD Transduction Laboratories), phospho-H2A.X (Ser139) (2577, Cell Signaling), H2A.X (2595, Cell Signaling), GAPDH (5G4-6C5, HyTest), and β-actin (Ac-74, Sigma-Aldrich).

For immunofluorescence staining, cells were fixed with ice cold methanol. The DNA double strand breaks were visualized using antibody against phosphorylated H2A.X (γH2A.X) (2577, Cell Signaling). The nuclei were stained using Hoechst 33342 (Invitrogen). Cells were imaged with Olympus BX60 (40X). The intensity of the phosphorylated H2A.X staining per cell (minimum 4 optical fields yielding minimum 150 cells per condition) was measured using ImageJ software (NIH, USA). Experiments were done as parallel treatments and each experiment was repeated at least three times.

Irradiation

Irradiations were performed using the Faxitron Multirad 350 (Faxitron Bioptics, LLC) located in Turku PET Centre at the Turku University Hospital and University of Turku, Finland. The voltage was set to 250 kV with a current of 14 mA (dose rate 1.28 Gy/min ± 2.9% at 50 cm distance from the radiation source). The X-ray beam was hardened with a 0.3 mm copper filter. Cells were exposed to 2 or 6 Gy doses. The control samples (0 Gy) were sham irradiated.

The cells were transported to the irradiator in protected boxes (normoxic and hypoxic preconditioned references) or in the Minihypoxy system. This minimized the possible stress caused by temperature variations. Radiation exposures were conducted at room temperature. The Minihypoxy chambers were disconnected from the flow divider and placed in the irradiator. After the irradiation, the Minihypoxy chambers were connected back to the Minihypoxy system. Reference cultures were placed into a standard incubator for 1 h before the sample collection.

Clonogenic assay

To study the radiosensitivity of the cells, clonogenicity was determined. First, to find an optimal cell amount for the assay, the plating efficiency (PE) was determined. Briefly, cells were plated at different densities on 6-well plates (100–1000 cells/ml) and cultured for seven days at standard cell culturing conditions (+ 37 °C in air/5% CO_2). The colonies were stained using crystal violet and colonies (> 50 cells) were counted using Image J. The PE was calculated by dividing the average colony count with cells plated (PE = no of colonies formed/no of cells seeded * 100). For the actual radiosensitivity experiment, density of 750 cells per well was selected.

The cells were seeded into the Minihypoxy chambers and incubated in 1% O_2 (Minihypoxy and preconditioned reference in the hypoxia workstation) or 21% oxygen (normoxic reference in a standard incubator) for 24 h. The cells were irradiated at doses of 0, 2 or 6 Gy and immediately re-plated on a 6 well plate at 375 cells/ml, 2 ml per well for clonogenic assay and cultured in standard cell culturing conditions for seven days. Staining and quantification was performed as described above. The survival fraction was calculated using formula SF = no of colonies formed after treatment/(no of cells seeded * PE) as described previously [35].

Results

Partial oxygen pressure (pO_2) inside the Minihypoxy culture chamber

The Minihypoxy system consists of a refillable gas cylinder, a heat plate and a controller, a custom-made 6-well flow divider and 1-well culture chambers (Minihypoxy chambers) (Fig. 1a and b). A gas mixture flows through the 6-well flow divider to the Minihypoxy chambers. The heat plate maintains the temperature in the desired temperature (37 °C in this study). The Minihypoxy culture chambers were sealed using glass lids and the whole chamber with the lid is covered by a polymer-made cover. A more detailed description of the system is provided in materials and methods.

To demonstrate the dynamic response of the Minihypoxy system to changes in oxygen supply, we followed the oxygen concentration at the bottom of the Minihypoxy culture chamber during the descending and ascending oxygen step response and during the gas supply cut-offs. As shown in Fig. 1c, the oxygen concentration reached the set point relatively fast. The time constants for the descending oxygen step responses from ambient oxygen level to the target concentration values of 5, 1 and 0% were 21 min, 21 min and 29 min, respectively. The oxygen concentration remained at the same level during the experiment and was maintained as long as the gas supply was connected. During the 5 min of gas supply cut-off, the oxygen concentration rose approximately 0.6 percentage points but returned to the set point after 1 h. When the Minihypoxy culture chamber was entirely disconnected from the gas supply, the time constants of the ascending oxygen concentration from 5, 1 and 0% to the ambient oxygen level was 52 min, 46 min and 56 min respectively.

pH, evaporation and osmolarity measurements

To show that the Minihypoxy culture chamber sealed with a lid and a cover maintains desired cell culturing conditions also during the irradiation treatment, we plated HeLa cells in the Minihypoxy culture chambers and incubated them either in the Minihypoxy system, in a hypoxia workstation (Invivo2, Ruskinn Technology), or a standard CO_2 incubator. The chambers were irradiated, and culture media was collected to measure the pH, evaporation and osmolarity of the culturing media after irradiation.

The measurements show that the evaporation was slightly smaller in the Minihypoxy system than inside the hypoxia workstation or in the incubator (Table 1). No change was observed in the osmolarity between the different culturing conditions. The pH increased at a relatively high level in cultures incubated in the hypoxia workstation or in the incubator, while the pH measured from media of the Minihypoxy system remained significantly lower (7.18 vs. 7.51 and 7.65). This is probably due to the continuous gas supply and the regulated constant temperature throughout incubation in the Minihypoxy system, while the chambers from hypoxia workstation and incubator are lacking a steady CO_2 supply to buffer the media during irradiation.

Hypoxia is generated and maintained inside the Minihypoxy chamber for a prolonged time

In addition to measuring the partial oxygen pressure (pO_2) inside the Minihypoxy chamber, we determined biological effects on cells cultured in a Minihypoxy chamber by using hypoxia-inducible factor 1 alpha (HIF-1α) as a marker protein since it serves as a sensitive indicator for hypoxia. HIF-1α is induced by hypoxia and is rapidly degraded in response to increased oxygen supply (> 5% O_2) [36–39]. To ensure the effective HIF-1α induction in the Minihypoxy chambers supplied with 1% O_2, HeLa and UT-SCC74 cells were cultured in the Minihypoxy chamber for 24 h. Both cell lines showed a marked induction of HIF-1α level (Fig. 2a). The magnitude of the induction was in line with the level of HIF-1α determined from cells cultured in the hypoxia workstation in 1% O_2 for 24 h.

In in vitro radiotherapy studies, the cells are disconnected from the Minihypoxy flow divider and placed into the irradiator for approximately 5 min depending on the radiation dose. To study how long the Minihypoxy chambers maintain the hypoxic microenvironment inside the chamber without the gas flow, we performed an experiment where the chambers were disconnected from the Minihypoxy flow divider. After 24-h culturing, samples were collected at four time points (5, 10, 20, and 30 min) after cut-off of the gas flow (Fig. 2b). The

Table 1 Evaporation, pH and osmolarity measured from the 1-well culture chambers on glass substrate in the Minihypoxy system, the hypoxia workstation (hypoxia WS) and the standard incubator ($n = 6$)

		Evaporation [ul]	Evaporation [ul/h]	pH	Osmolarity [mOsm]
Minihypoxy system (n = 6)	mean (std)	59 (14)	2.46 (0.57)	7.18 (0.06)	0.309 (0.004)
1-well in hypoxia WS (n = 6)	mean (std)	94 (46)	3.90 (1.91)	7.51 (0.09)	0.306 (0.002)
1-well in incubator (n = 6)	mean (std)	69 (40)	2.89 (1.67)	7.65 (0.02)	0.297 (0.002)
Fresh Medium (n = 6)	mean (std)	-	-	7.38 (0.01)	0.298 (0.001)

reference samples were cultured in hypoxia workstation (1% O_2) for 24 h and then transported to a standard incubator with ~ 21% oxygen. The level of HIF-1α was significantly higher after 5, 10 and 20 min of removing gas flow in cells cultured in the Minihypoxy chamber as compared to reoxygenated reference samples (Fig. 2b). Together with the measurements showing the changes in the partial oxygen pressure inside the chamber (Fig. 1c), this indicates that the Minihypoxy chamber sealed with the lid and the cover maintains hypoxia up to 20 min without the gas flow.

Enhancement of cellular radiation resistance under hypoxia in the Minihypoxy chambers

To test the Minihypoxy system for simultaneous hypoxia and irradiation, we determined the sensitivity of cultured cells to radiotherapy in two oxygen conditions (1 and 21%). The experiments included determining the level of DNA damage and cell growth studies (work flow presented in Fig. 3). Several previous studies have demonstrated that hypoxia causes resistance to radiation and thus shows less DNA damage as measured by serine phosphorylation (Ser139) of H2A.X histone (γH2A.X), which is commonly used as an indicator of double strand DNA breakage [10, 40]. The cells were plated on the Minihypoxy chambers and cultured in 1% O_2 for 24 h prior to irradiation. The reference samples were cultured in 21% O_2 or in the hypoxia workstation in 1% O_2 for 24 h (hypoxic preconditioning). The cells were irradiated at single doses of 0, 2 and 6 Gy, and samples for immunostaining and western blot analysis were collected one hour after irradiation (Fig. 3). As expected, immunostaining revealed a dose-dependent increase in the intensity of γH2A.X on HeLa cell nuclei 1 h after

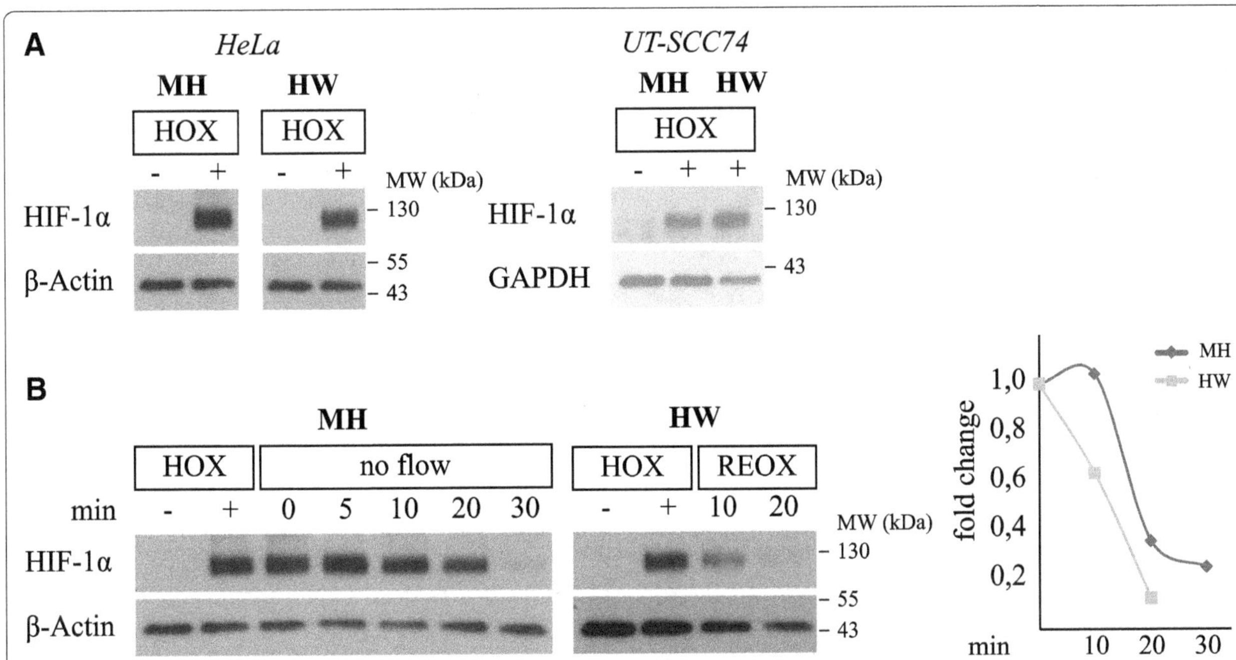

Fig. 2 Hypoxic conditions are maintained in Minihypoxy chambers. **a** Hypoxia-inducible factor HIF-1α is equally induced in Minihypoxy system (MH) and in hypoxia workstation (HW) in 1% O_2 (HOX). The hypoxic response is shown with two carcinoma cell lines (HeLa, UT-SCC74). **b** The Minihypoxy chambers (MH) were disconnected from the gas flow (no flow) and the level of HIF-1α was followed for 30 min. The control cells were cultured in hypoxia workstation (HW) for 24 h and then transferred to normal cell incubator with 21% O_2 (REOX). The samples were collected accordingly

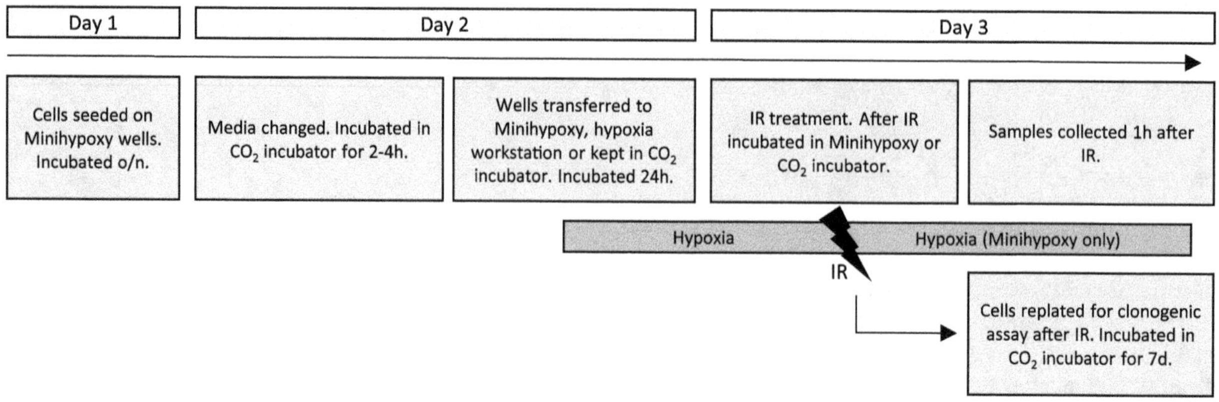

Fig. 3 Work flow chart on in vitro irradiation experiments

irradiation under normoxia and hypoxic preconditioning. The increase in γH2A.X level was irradiation dose-dependent and did not differ between normoxic and preconditioned samples (HW) (Fig. 4a and b). In striking contrast, the response to irradiation was strongly diminished in the Minihypoxy chamber under 1% O_2. To reach the same treatment response in a hypoxic Minihypoxy chamber as in 21% O_2 or preconditioned conditions, the estimated value of radiation dose would need to be approximately three times higher (oxygen enhancement ratio, OER~ 3). The estimation is based on the comparison of the γH2A.X levels in different conditions (Fig. 4b). A similar response was seen in western blot analysis of both HeLa and UT-SCC74 cells. A clear radiation dose-dependent increase in the level of phosphorylated H2A.X seen in normoxic and hypoxia preconditioned (HW) samples was strongly attenuated in hypoxic Minihypoxy chamber (Fig. 4c).

Finally, we determined the clonogenic capacity of the irradiated cells. The cells were irradiated as previously described and plated for clonogenic assay immediately after irradiation (Fig. 3). The clonogenic capacity of the cells decreased rapidly in response to irradiation (Fig. 4d). However, the cells irradiated in the Minihypoxy chambers retained some of their clonogenicity even after 6 Gy dosage, whereas the reference cells grown under normoxia (21% O_2) or preconditioned in the hypoxia workstation (HW) lost their clonogenic potential completely (Fig. 4d). The effect was even more prominent in primary human head and neck carcinoma UT-SCC74 cells (Fig. 4d). Taken together, the data indicate that the Minihypoxy system can mimic the hypoxic microenvironment and maintains hypoxia for prolonged time also when transported and placed inside an irradiator.

Discussion

Hypoxia is one of the major microenvironmental factors affecting carcinogenesis and cancer progression and is characteristic for many pathologies such as inflammation, inflammatory diseases as well as stem cell growth. Moreover, some normal tissues can be considered as permanently hypoxic as the partial oxygen pressure is constantly lower than 5%. Yet, most of the in vitro research on cell cultures is still conducted under partial oxygen pressure up to 21%. There is an obvious need for cost-effective and easy-to-use application for a device with adjustable oxygen concentration. Ideally, all laboratories especially those working on the research fields of cancer, stem cells and inflammation, should have access to the use of a hypoxia incubator.

Here we present a novel device for conducting in vitro experiments in hypoxia. Our results show that experiments in the Minihypoxy system are reproducible and reliable, and results are comparable to studies performed in a hypoxia workstation. Furthermore, the Minihypoxy system maintains hypoxia also when transported to another location as well as when used inside an irradiator. Our results show that performing radiation experiments in the Minihypoxy system markedly reduces the radiosensitivity of carcinoma cells determined as reduced DNA damage and attenuated loss of clonogenic capacity, thus presenting its utility in in vitro radiosensitivity measurements.

There are several advantages of the Minihypoxy system over conventional hypoxia workstations or hypoxia chambers. First, media in the Minihypoxy culture chamber reaches 1% oxygen concentration within 2 h, which is relatively fast as compared to media placed into a hypoxia workstation where it may take up to 24 h for media to reach the set point [41]. The Minihypoxy chambers are made of silicone elastomer which is gas permeable material and therefore enhances the gas exchange inside the chamber. Second, in the Minihypoxy system, the cells are steadily kept on a heat plate, which eliminates the stress effects caused by the temperature changes. Even small temperature changes might affect

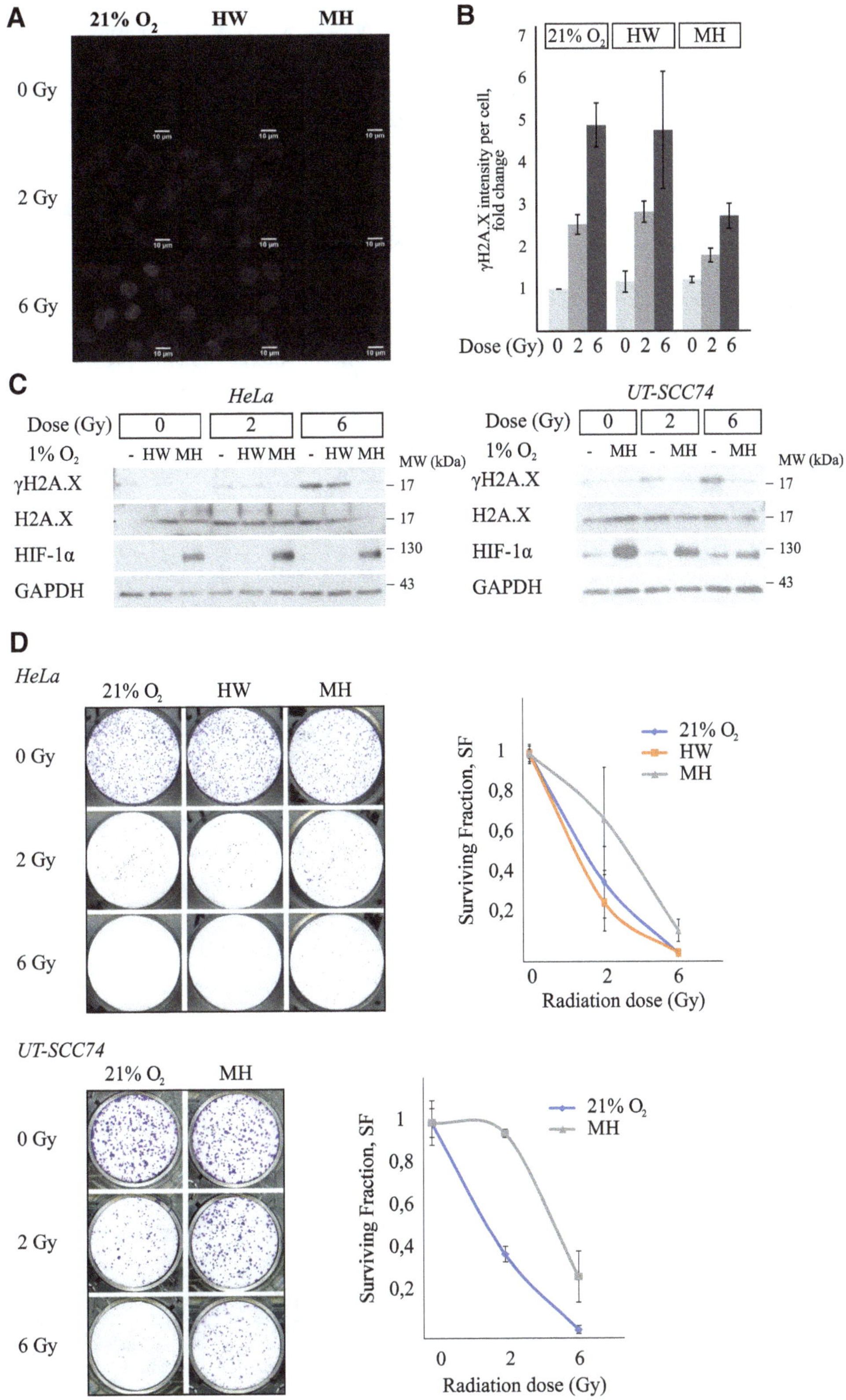

Fig. 4 (See legend on next page.)

(See figure on previous page.)
Fig. 4 The radiosensitivity of cells treated in Minihypoxy chambers is decreased. **a** The phosphorylation of H2A.X histone (γH2A.X) marks the double strand breakages on. The γH2A.X level is gradually increased in HeLa cells with dosage in normoxia (21% O_2) and in hypoxia preconditioned samples (HW) but in Minihypoxy samples (MH) there is significantly less damage. **b** Quantification of three independent biological experiments ($n = 3$). **c** The western blots showing γH2A.X level in HeLa and UT-SCC74 cells. Representative blot is shown. **d** The clonogenicity of the HeLa and UT-SCC74 cells is decreased in all conditions but especially in normoxic (21% O_2) and in hypoxia preconditioned (HW) samples (HeLa only). Quantification of three independent biological experiments ($n = 3$)

significantly the behaviour of cells [42, 43]. Third, the pH changes in the Minihypoxy system are minimized compared to other hypoxia systems as the constant CO_2 supply maintains the buffering capacity of the media. Even inside a standard incubator, the conditions may vary if the incubator is heavily used. In addition, the closed structure of the Minihypoxy culture chamber decreases the evaporation and prevents the concentration of the culture media. Evaporation increases the osmolarity of the cell culture media and has a negative effect on cells [31, 44]. In other words, the optimal composition of the culture media can be maintained in the Minihypoxy system. Fourth, the Minihypoxy system also enables live cell imaging under low oxygen conditions as the chambers are designed with undisrupted optical path (Additional file 1: Figure S1). Everyday monitoring of the cells while in culture can be performed with the adjacent heat plate. Therefore, the cells can also be observed and imaged during the long-term hypoxia culturing. Moreover, high resolution live cell imaging of individual Minihypoxy chambers requires heated microscope chamber to keep the temperature stable during a long-term imaging experiment. Most importantly, the Minihypoxy system is transportable and allows experimental planning with several different independent irradiation treatments and time points at the same time.

The sample collection procedure is similar in hypoxia containers and Minihypoxy culture chambers as opening of the container or the chamber exposes the cells to a short period of reoxygenation stress. A benefit of the Minihypoxy chambers compared to the hypoxia containers is that the Minihypoxy chambers can be handled one chamber at a time while the conditions in the other chambers are not affected. We found no difference in the level of the marker protein HIF-1α between the samples collected using non-preconditioned washing buffer versus samples where preconditioned buffer was used or which were collected inside the hypoxia workstation (Additional file 2: Figure S2). However, as many experimental setups would benefit from a perfusion system, this need has been taken under consideration when developing the next generation Minihypoxy chambers. Taken together, the Minihypoxy system offers many benefits over current methodologies for creating low oxygen atmosphere for cell culture experiments in a compact device. It also provides benefits compared to other hypoxia solutions in regards its mobility and capability of maintaining optimal cell growth conditions during transportation.

Conclusions

The Minihypoxy system provides a transportable easy-to-use platform for controlling oxygen concentration in in vitro cell cultures. In addition to the oxygen level, the Minihypoxy system also maintains the temperature and pH of the culture constant. Here we present the utility of the Minihypoxy system in in vitro irradiation experiments on carcinoma cell cultures under reduced oxygen level. Besides simultaneous hypoxia and irradiation the transportability of the system enables other experimental designs performed under hypoxia.

Additional files

Additional file 1: Figure S1. Live cell images of EGFP expressing prostate cancer cell line LNCaP cells. The images were obtained using 10x and 63x magnifications. (PDF 1137 kb)

Additional file 2: Figure S2. The samples can be collected without performing hypoxic preconditioning on the washing buffer. The cells were washed twice before collecting using either PBS stored in normal 21% oxygen concentration (N) or preconditioned for 24 h in 1% oxygen concentration (pre). As a control there is a sample which is collected inside the hypoxia incubator using preconditioned washing buffer (H). (PDF 207 kb)

Abbreviations

PE: Plating efficiency; ROS: Reactive oxygen species, oxygen radicals; SF: Surviving fraction

Acknowledgements

The Cell Imaging Core in Turku Centre for Biotechnology is acknowledged for the help in imaging the Minihypoxy chambers and image processing.

Funding

This work was supported by the Cancer Society of Finland, Finnish Cultural Foundation Varsinais-Suomi Regional Fund, Finnish Funding Agency for Technology and Innovation (TEKES) (Decision no. 2868/2015), The Sigrid Juselius Foundation and Turku University Hospital (EVO1303).

Authors' contributions

OM and HH carried out the study design and data interpretation. OM performed the protein expression experiments, irradiations and clonogenic assays. PM performed the immunostainings and protein expression experiments. JK and PK provided the Minihypoxy system, and PK also revised the manuscript. JK performed the measurements of oxygen concentration, pH and osmolarity. HH wrote the manuscript with OM, JK and PJ. PJ also participated in designing the study with HH and OM. All authors read and approved the final manuscript.

Competing interests

OM, HH, PM and PMJ declare no competing interest. JK and PK hold a patent application for Minihypoxy.

Author details

[1]Turku Centre for Biotechnology, University of Turku and Åbo Akademi University, Tykistökatu 6, FIN-20520 Turku, Finland. [2]Faculty of Medicine, Institute of Biomedicine, University of Turku, Kiinamyllynkatu 10, FIN-20520 Turku, Finland. [3]BioMediTech, Institute and Faculty of Biosciences and Engineering, Tampere University of Technology, Korkeakoulunkatu 3, FIN-33720 Tampere, Finland. [4]Turku PET Centre, University of Turku and Turku University Hospital, Kiinamyllynkatu 4-8, FIN-20521 Turku, Finland. [5]Helsinki University Hospital Comprehensive Cancer Center and Department of Oncology, University of Helsinki, Haartmaninkatu 4, FIN-00029 HUS Helsinki, Finland.

References

1. Tazzyman S, Murdoch C, Yeomans J, Harrison J, Muthana M. Macrophage-mediated response to hypoxia in disease. Hypoxia (Auckl). 2014;2:185–96.
2. Peers C, Dallas ML, Boycott HE, Scragg JL, Pearson HA, Boyle JP. Hypoxia and neurodegeneration. Ann N Y Acad Sci. 2009;1177:169–77.
3. Vaupel P, Kelleher DK, Hockel M. Oxygen status of malignant tumors: pathogenesis of hypoxia and significance for tumor therapy. Semin Oncol. 2001;28:29–35.
4. Ruan K, Song G, Ouyang G. Role of hypoxia in the hallmarks of human cancer. J Cell Biochem. 2009;107:1053–62.
5. Moeller BJ, Richardson RA, Dewhirst MW. Hypoxia and radiotherapy: opportunities for improved outcomes in cancer treatment. Cancer Metastasis Rev. 2007;26:241–8.
6. Carreau A, El Hafny-Rahbi B, Matejuk A, Grillon C, Kieda C. Why is the partial oxygen pressure of human tissues a crucial parameter? Small molecules and hypoxia. J Cell Mol Med. 2011;15:1239–53.
7. Chen HHW, Kuo MT. Improving radiotherapy in cancer treatment: promises and challenges. Oncotarget. 2017;8:62742–58.
8. Shah MA, Schwartz GK. Cell cycle-mediated drug resistance: an emerging concept in Cancer therapy. Clin Cancer Res. 2001;7:2168–81.
9. Terasima T, Tolmach LJ. Variations in several responses of HeLa cells to x-irradiation during the division cycle. Biophys J. 1963;3:11–33.
10. Zhu Y, Zhao T, Itasaka S, Zeng L, Yeom CJ, Hirota K, Suzuki K, Morinibu A, Shinomiya K, Ou G, et al. Involvement of decreased hypoxia-inducible factor 1 activity and resultant G1-S cell cycle transition in radioresistance of perinecrotic tumor cells. Oncogene. 2013;32:2058–68.
11. Bertout JA, Patel SA, Simon MC. The impact of O2 availability on human cancer. Nat Rev Cancer. 2008;8:967–75.
12. Byrne MB, Leslie MT, Gaskins HR, Kenis PJA. Methods to study the tumor microenvironment under controlled oxygen conditions. Trends Biotechnol. 2014;32:556–63.
13. Pappas D. Single-cell hypoxia: current analytical techniques and future opportunities. In: Encyclopedia of analytical chemistry. Wiley, Wiley Online Library; 2006. https://doi.org/10.1002/9780470027318.a9537.
14. Moeller BJ, Dewhirst MW. HIF-1 and tumour radiosensitivity. Br J Cancer. 2006;95:1–5.
15. Sun Y, Xing X, Liu Q, Wang Z, Xin Y, Zhang P, Hu C, Liu Y. Hypoxia-induced autophagy reduces radiosensitivity by the HIF-1alpha/miR-210/Bcl-2 pathway in colon cancer cells. Int J Oncol. 2015;46:750–6.
16. Hammond EM, Dorie MJ, Giaccia AJ. ATR/ATM targets are phosphorylated by ATR in response to hypoxia and ATM in response to Reoxygenation. J Biol Chem. 2003;278:12207–13.
17. Bussink J, Kaanders JH, Rijken PF, Raleigh JA, Van der Kogel AJ. Changes in blood perfusion and hypoxia after irradiation of a human squamous cell carcinoma xenograft tumor line. Radiat Res. 2000;153:398–404.
18. Milas L, Hunter NR, Mason KA, Milross CG, Saito Y, Peters LJ. Role of reoxygenation in induction of enhancement of tumor radioresponse by paclitaxel. Cancer Res. 1995;55:3564–8.
19. Milas L, Hunter N, Mason KA, Milross C, Peters LJ. Tumor reoxygenation as a mechanism of taxol-induced enhancement of tumor radioresponse. Acta Oncol. 1995;34:409–12.
20. Lagadec C, Dekmezian C, Bauché L, Pajonk F. Oxygen levels do not determine radiation survival of breast Cancer stem cells. PLoS One. 2012;7:e34545.
21. Allen CB, Schneider BK, White CW. Limitations to oxygen diffusion and equilibration in in vitro cell exposure systems in hyperoxia and hypoxia. Am J Physiol Lung Cell Mol Physiol. 2001;281:L1021.
22. Cui H, Qin Q, Yang M, Zhang H, Liu Z, Yang Y, Chen X, Zhu H, Wang D, Meng C, et al. Bortezomib enhances the radiosensitivity of hypoxic cervical cancer cells by inhibiting HIF-1α expression. Int J Clin Exp Pathol. 2015;8:9032–41.
23. Spiro IJ, Rice GC, Durand RE, Stickler R, Ling CC. Cell killing, radiosensitization and cell cycle redistribution induced by chronic hypoxia. Int J Radiat Oncol Biol Phys. 1984;10:1275–80.
24. Sørensen BS, Busk M, Olthof N, Speel EJ, Horsman MR, Alsner J, Overgaard J. Radiosensitivity and effect of hypoxia in HPV positive head and neck cancer cells. Radiother Oncol. 2013;108:500–5.
25. Kato Y, Yashiro M, Fuyuhiro Y, Kashiwagi S, Matsuoka J, Hirakawa T, Noda S, Aomatsu N, Hasegawa T, Matsuzaki T, et al. Effects of acute and chronic hypoxia on the Radiosensitivity of gastric and esophageal Cancer cells. Anticancer Res. 2011;31:3369–75.
26. Ito A, Aoyama T, Yoshizawa M, Nagai M, Tajino J, Yamaguchi S, Iijima H, Zhang X, Kuroki H. The effects of short-term hypoxia on human mesenchymal stem cell proliferation, viability and p16(INK4A) mRNA expression: investigation using a simple hypoxic culture system with a deoxidizing agent. J Stem Cells Regen Med. 2015;11:25–31.
27. Chaachouay H, Fehrenbacher B, Toulany M, Schaller M, Multhoff G, Rodemann HP. AMPK-independent autophagy promotes radioresistance of human tumor cells under clinical relevant hypoxia in vitro. Radiother Oncol. 2015;116:409–16.
28. Wang R, Jin F, Zhong H. A novel experimental hypoxia chamber for cell culture. Am J Cancer Res. 2014;4:53–60.
29. Signorelli S, Jennings P, Leonard MO, Pfaller W. Differential effects of hypoxic stress in alveolar epithelial cells and microvascular endothelial cells. Cell Physiol Biochem. 2010;25:135–44.
30. Mathupala SP, Kiousis S, Szerlip NJ. A lab assembled microcontroller-based sensor module for continuous oxygen measurement in portable hypoxia chambers. PLoS One. 2016;11:e0148923.
31. Blau A, Neumann T, Ziegler C, Benfenati F. Replica-moulded polydimethylsiloxane culture vessel lids attenuate osmotic drift in long-term cell cultures. J Biosci. 2009;34:59–69.
32. Kreutzer J, Ylä-Outinen L, Kärnä P, Kaarela T, Mikkonen J, Skottman H, Narkilahti S, Kallio P. Structured PDMS chambers for enhanced human neuronal cell activity on MEA platforms. J Bionic Eng. 2012;9:1–10.
33. Kreutzer J, Ylä-Outinen L, Mäki AJ, Ristola M, Narkilahti S, Kallio P. Cell culture chamber with gas supply for prolonged recording of human neuronal cells on microelectrode array. J Neurosci Methods. 2017;280:27–35.
34. Välimäki H, Verho J, Kreutzer J, Kattipparambil Rajan D, Ryynänen T, Pekkanen-Mattila M, Ahola A, Tappura K, Kallio P, Lekkala J. Fluorimetric oxygen sensor with an efficient optical read-out for in vitro cell models. Sensors Actuators B Chem. 2017;249:738–46.
35. Franken NA, Rodermond HM, Stap J, Haveman J, van Bree C. Clonogenic assay of cells in vitro. Nat Protoc. 2006;1:2315–9.
36. Ebbesen P, Eckardt KU, Ciampor F, Pettersen EO. Linking measured intercellular oxygen concentration to human cell functions. Acta Oncol. 2004;43:598–600.
37. Wang GL, Jiang BH, Rue EA, Semenza GL. Hypoxia-inducible factor 1 is a basic-helix-loop-helix-PAS heterodimer regulated by cellular O2 tension. PNAS. 1995;92:5510–4.
38. Jewell UR, Kvietikova I, Scheid A, Bauer C, Wenger RH, Gassmann MAX. Induction of HIF-1α in response to hypoxia is instantaneous. FASEB J. 2001;15:1312–4.

39. Salceda S, Caro J. Hypoxia-inducible factor 1α (HIF-1α) protein is rapidly degraded by the ubiquitin-proteasome system under normoxic conditions: its stabilization by hypoxia depends on redox-induced changes. J Biol Chem. 1997;272:22642–7.
40. Foster ER, Downs JA. Histone H2A phosphorylation in DNA double-strand break repair. FEBS J. 2005;272:3231–40.
41. Newby D, Marks L, Lyall F. Dissolved oxygen concentration in culture medium: assumptions and pitfalls. Placenta. 2005;26:353–7.
42. Zhao Y, Boulant JA. Temperature effects on neuronal membrane potentials and inward currents in rat hypothalamic tissue slices. J Physiol. 2005;564:245–57.
43. Das SK, Chung S, Zervantonakis I, Atnafu J, Kamm RD. A microfluidic platform for studying the effects of small temperature gradients in an incubator environment. Biomicrofluidics. 2008;2:34106.
44. Heo YS, Cabrera LM, Song JW, Futai N, Tung YC, Smith GD, Takayama S. Characterization and resolution of evaporation-mediated osmolality shifts that constrain microfluidic cell culture in poly(dimethylsiloxane) devices. Anal Chem. 2007;79:1126–34.

Escalated radiation and prophylactic extended field nodal irradiation are beneficial for FIGO IIIB cervical cancer patients' prognosis

Qingyu Meng†, Weiping Wang†, Xiaoliang Liu, Xiaorong Hou, Xin Lian, Shuai Sun, Junfang Yan, Zhikai Liu, Zheng Miao, Ke Hu* and Fuquan Zhang*

Abstract

Background: Currently, the standard treatment for locally advanced cervical cancer patients is concurrent chemoradiotherapy. Here we aim to evaluate therapeutic efficacy, treatment failure, toxicity and prognostic factors for FIGO IIIB cervical cancer patients.

Methods: A comprehensive retrospective analysis was performed to understand various factors which contribute to IIIB cervical cancer prognosis. In total 223 well defined patients were assigned according to their pathological subtype, age, pre-treatment HGB level, tumor size, pelvic lymph node (LN) metastasis, para-aortic LN metastasis as well as external irradiation technologies, treatment duration, point A EQD2 dose and concurrent chemotherapy cycles. We then performed correlation studies of these factors and OS, DFS, LCR, DMFS using univariate and multivariate analysis respectively.

Results: We managed to achieve 207 (92.8%) complete response (CR) and 16 (7.2%) partial response (PR) with acceptable adverse effects. Notably, the 5 years OS, DFS, LCR, DMFS for these patients were 61.1, 55.2, 83.6 and 66.4% respectively. Importantly, our studies suggest that escalated point A EQD2 can significantly improve OS, DFS and LCR for FIGO IIIB cervical cancer patients, furthermore, patients without para-aortic LN metastasis who received prophylactic extended field irradiation have significant survival advantage for DFS and a tendency to improve OS and DMFS.

Conclusions: Our results suggest that FIGO IIIB cervical cancer patients should receive higher EQD2 ($\geq 98Gy_{10}$) radiotherapy, moreover, patients without para-aortic LN metastasis should receive prophylactic extended field nodal irradiation to improve prognosis.

Keywords: FIGO IIIB, Cervical cancer, EQD2, IMRT, Prophylactic extended field irradiation

Background

Cervical cancer is the fourth most common cancer in women worldwide, with approximately 528,000 newly reported cases and 266,000 death cases every year [1, 2]. Currently, the International Federation of Gynecology and Obstetrics (FIGO, http://www.figo.org/) clinical staging criteria is the standard for cervical cancer classification, according to which local advanced cervical cancer refers to the Ib2-IVa stages. Specifically, FIGO IIIB cervical cancer patients usually exhibit parametrial invasion which has extended to the pelvic wall. Moreover, patients usually display hydronephrosis and impaired renal function [3]. Nearly 25% of local advanced cervical cancers are defined as IIIB cervical cancer [4]. As the determination of IIIB cervical cancer is usually supported by pelvic and/or abdominal aortic lymph node metastasis [5], the prognosis for IIIB cervical cancer patients is generally unfavorable;

* Correspondence: huke8000@163.com; zhangfuquan3@sina.com
†Qingyu Meng and Weiping Wang contributed equally to this work.
Department of radiation oncology, Peking Union Medical College Hospital, Chinese Academy of Medical Sciences and Peking Union Medical College, Beijing, People's Republic of China

previous studies have indicated that the local control failure can be varied from 10.63 to 41% [4–7], which could be as high as 50% for patients with bilateral uterine involvement.

The classical treatment strategy for FIGO IIIB cervical cancer patients is concurrent chemoradiotherapy (CCRT) [5, 6]. Notably, the intensity modulated radiotherapy (IMRT) is now the most widely used clinical radiotherapy technology which can deliver high dose internal irradiation while causing significantly less radiation-related tissue damage, with its unique dosimetric distribution feature, IMRT can reduce the radiation to organs at risks (OARs) without affecting the dose distributed to clinical target volume (CTV) [7]. A combination of radiotherapy with cisplatin-based chemotherapy is recommended by the National Cancer Institute (NCI), which has been used as the standard treatment strategy for cervical cancer for almost two decades. Several studies have been performed to evaluate the clinical efficacy and to define the prognostic factors for local advanced cervical cancer [8–11]. However, such studies focusing on IIIB cervical cancer patients in Chinese populations are still lacking. Here, we retrospectively analyzed therapeutic efficacy, treatment failure, toxicity and prognostic factors for 223 FIGO IIIB cervical cancer patients who were hospitalized in the Peking Union Medical College Hospital (PUMCH) from 2000 to 2014.

Methods

Patient characteristics

In total 223 FIGO IIIB cervical cancer patients were retrospectively analyzed in this study. Patients' age was from 29 to 79 years old, with a median age of 50 years old. The clinical stage was determined by clinical checkup combined with biopsy analysis before the first treatment and supported by CT or PET imaging in some cases. We then divided these patients not only based on their clinical characteristics, but also according to the treatment they received. All detailed information is summarized in Table 1.

Radiation therapy

All patients received both external beam radiation therapy (EBRT) and intracavitary brachytherapy (ICBT) when the patient's health condition was allowed.

The radiation treatment was carried out as previously described [12]. The EBRT technologies included three-dimensional conformal radiotherapy (3D-CRT) and intensity modulated radiation therapy (IMRT). Forty-eight patients received 3D-CRT. Briefly, by using 15MV-X rays, we applied box irradiation technology with a total dose of 36-40Gy_{10} fractioned in 20 times followed by 5 fractions of a total 10Gy_{10} irradiation. The patients' bladders and rectums were protected by a 4 cm central lead block. The other 175 patients received IMRT with a total dose of 45–50.4Gy_{10} fractioned for 25 to 28 times using 6MV-X rays which could cover 95% PTV (1.8Gy_{10}/day, 5 days a week, 5 to 6 weeks). For patients with lymph nodes metastasis, the dosage was increased to 56-60Gy_{10} and an additional dose for proximal uterus area was administrated with a total 10Gy_{10} divided in 5 fractions.

The ICBT usually started 3 weeks after EBRT and was given once or twice a week. The standard protocol for ICBT was a cumulative dose of 36Gy_{10} prescribed to point A in 5 to 7 fractions according to the International Commission on Radiation Units and Measurements (ICRU) report 38. CT imaging was performed to support real-time treatment plans determination after the applicator implantation. The irradiation dose for rectum and bladder was strictly controlled as less than 70% of the point A. For the current study, the range for prescribed point A dose was from 22.5 to 130.4 Gy_{10} (EBRT from 10 to 70.2Gy_{10} and ICBT from 6 to 60Gy_{10}).

Table 1 General patients' information

Character	Group definition	Case	Ratio (%)
Age	≥65	24	10.7
	< 65	199	89.3
Pathology type	Squamous	206	92.3
	Adenocarcinoma, Adeno/squamous Carcinoma	17	7.7
Tumor size	≤4 cm	48	21.5
	> 4 cm	175	78.5
HGB prior treatment	< 110 g/L	69	30.9
	≥110 g/L	149	66.8
	N.A.	5	2.2
Pelvic LN metastasis	w/t	82	25.9
	w/o	141	74.1
Para-aortic LN metastasis	w/t	31	13.9
	w/o	192	86.1
Concurrent chemotherapy	≥4 cycles	155	69.5
	< 4 cycles	45	20.10
	N.A	21	9.4
Radiotherapy	3D-CRT	48	21.5
	IMRT	175	78.5
EQD2 (point A)	22-90Gy_{10}	30	13.4
	90–98 Gy_{10}	54	24.2
	≥98Gy_{10}	139	62.3
Therapy duration	≤63 days	175	78.5
	> 63 days	48	21.5
Prophylactic extended field irradiation	w/t	107	48.0
	w/o	85	38.1

Concurrent chemotherapy

One hundred fifty-five patients received more than 4 cycles of concurrent chemotherapy, 68 patients were treated with less than 4 cycles including 21 patients who didn't receive any chemotherapy due to personal reasons. Patients diagnosed as squamous were treated with a weekly cisplatin-based regimen at a dose of 40 mg/m^2/week for 4 to 6 weeks; for those adenocarcinoma patients, we applied PF regimen in addition which included cisplatin 70 mg/m^2 on day 1 and fluorouracil 1000 mg/m^2 from day 1 to day 4. The PF regimen was given every 3 weeks for a total of 1–2 cycles. When the treatment was finished, the outcome was evaluated according to guidelines proposed previously [13].

Toxicity and adverse effect assessment

All the patients were monitored for toxicities and adverse effects every week during the treatment. The severity of acute complications is classified according to the Common Terminology Criteria for Adverse Events (CTCAE v2.0) (https://ctep.cancer.gov/protocolDevelopment/electronic_applications/docs/ctcv20_4-30-992.pdf). Late complications were graded according to the RTOG/EORTC 1987 toxicity scales [14].

Follow-up

All patients were required to have a review check every 3 months during the first 2 years after the final treatment, and twice a year during the third to fifth year after the treatment, and once a year starting from the 5th year after the last treatment. The review check includes blood biochemistry, SCC Ag, gynecological examination, pelvic MRI, chest and abdomen enhanced CT. The last follow up for the current study was carried out in May 2018.

Statistics analysis

Overall survival (OS) is defined as the time from the start of treatment to the date of death or to the date of censoring. Disease-free survival (DFS) is defined as the time interval between the start of treatment and the detection of recurrence, metastasis or death. Local control rate (LCR) is defined as the percentage of the arrest of cancer growth at the site of origin. Distant metastasis-free survival (DMFS) is defined as the beginning of radiotherapy to the detection of distant metastasis or distant metastasis -related death. OS, DFS, LCR and DMFS were calculated with the Kaplan-Meier method by using SPSS 17.0 statistical software and compared using the log-rank test. Log-rank method was also used to perform univariate analysis, when the factor was found significant ($P < 0.05$), the Cox regression model was used to execute multivariate analysis. P value < 0.05 was considered statistically significant.

Results

Treatment outcome evaluation

For the 223 FIGO IIIB cervical cancer patients included in this study, 207 of them showed complete response (CR) after the therapy (92.8%), and only 16 patients (7.2%) exhibited partial response (PR). Importantly, the 5-year OS, DFS, LCR and DMFS were 61.1, 55.2, 83.6 and 66.4% (Fig. 1a-d), suggesting the standard concurrent chemoradiotherapy was indeed very effective for FIGO IIIB cervical cancer patients.

Treatment failure patterns and toxicity

We observed 36 cases (16.1%) of local recurrence and 73 (32.7%) patients with distant metastasis, the details of which are summarized in Additional file 1: Table S1. Of note, there were 7 patients with both local recurrence and distant metastasis.

One major concern for CCRT treatment is the therapy-related toxicity. We have carefully evaluated both the acute toxicity and delayed toxicity. The most frequent grade 3 or 4 acute toxicity was hematological toxicity, followed by other symptoms such as frequent urination and diarrhea (Table 2). For the delayed toxicity, only few cases of complications in the urinary system and lower digestive tract were observed (Table 2). All these results indicated that CCRT was a safe therapeutic option for FIGO IIIB cervical cancer patients.

Prognostic factors analysis

To comprehensively understand FIGO IIIB cervical cancer prognosis factors, the 223 patients were divided not only based on their clinical appearance but also according to the difference in their treatment (Additional file 1: Table S2). We then performed univariate analysis to determine prognostic factors for OS, DFS, LCR and DMFS respectively. Our data indicated that pre-treatment HGB level, tumor size, pelvic LNM, para-aortic LNM, EQD2 and concurrent chemotherapy significantly correlated with OS (Additional file 1: Figure S1 A-G); pre-treatment HGB level, tumor size, pelvic LNM, para-aortic LNM, treatment duration, EQD2 and concurrent chemotherapy cycles were significantly correlated with DFS (Additional file 1: Figure S2 A-G); moreover, tumor size, para-aortic LNM and EQD2 were highly associated with LCR (Additional file 1: Figure S3 A-C); finally, pelvic LNM, para-aortic LNM, treatment duration and concurrent chemotherapy cycles were prognostic factors for DMFS (Additional file 1: Figure S4 A-D).

Prognostic factors found to be significant ($P < 0.05$) by univariate analysis were then further analyzed using multivariate analysis. Our results suggested that pelvic LNM, para-aortic LNM, EQD2 and concurrent chemotherapy were independent prognostic factors for OS; pre-treatment HGB level, pelvic LNM, para-aortic LNM,

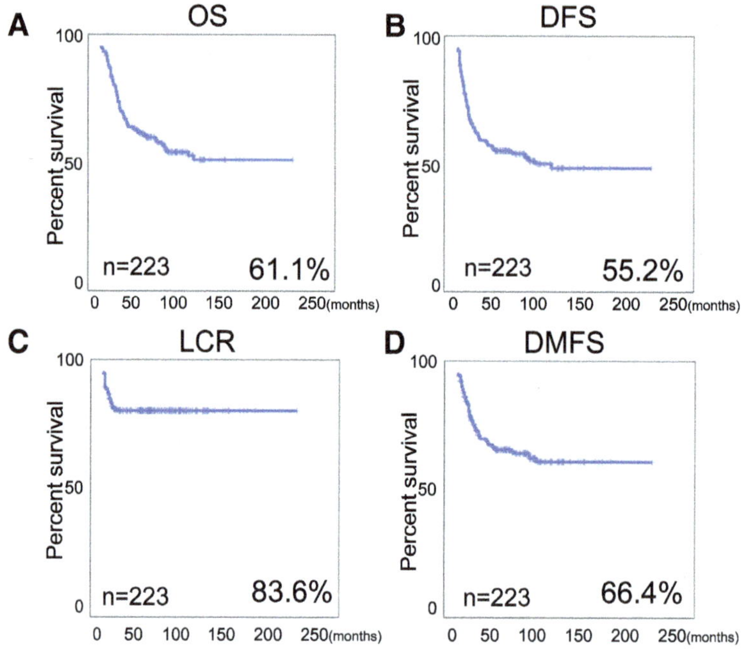

Fig. 1 An overview of 5 years survival of FIGO IIIB cervical cancer patients treated with CCRT. The Kaplan-Meier survival curves for overall survival (OS) (**a**); disease progression-free survival (DFS); (**b**) local control rate (LCR); (**c**) and distant metastasis-free survival (DMFS); (**d**). The detail survival information is indicated separately in each figure, n = 223 patients for all survival analysis

EQD2 and concurrent chemotherapy cycles were independent prognostic factors for DFS; the independent prognostic factors for LCR included tumor size, para-aortic LNM and EQD2; and concurrent chemotherapy cycles was the only independent prognostic factor for DMFS (Table 3).

Higher EQD2(point A) is correlated with better treatment outcome

As our data constantly suggested that EQD2 dosage was a detrimental factor for FIGO IIIB cervical cancer prognosis in various analysis, we further analyzed the correlation between EQD2 level and OS, DFS and LCR by distributing all the patients into high (($\geq$98Gy$_{10}$), medium (90Gy$_{10}$ $\leq$ EQD2 < 98Gy$_{10}$) and low EQD2(22Gy$_{10}$ < EQD2 < 90Gy$_{10}$). As expected, high and medium EQD2 significantly improved patients' OS and DFS compared to low EQD2 (Fig. 2a, b); surprisingly, we observed not only a markedly LCR improvement in patients treated with medium EQD2 compared to low EQD2, but also a significant advantage for LCR in high EQD2 treated patients compared to medium EQD2 treated patients (Fig. 2c). These data further strengthen our finding that higher EQD2 is associated with better prognosis.

Table 2 Acute and delayed toxicity after treatment

	Grade 3	Grade 4
Acute toxicity (CTCEA 2.0)		
Hemoglobin	37 (16.6%)	16 (7.2%)
Leukocyte	86 (38.5%)	12 (5.3%)
Neutrophils	44 (19.7%)	11 (4.9%)
Blood platelet	26 (11.7%)	0 (0)
Frequent urination	9 (4.0%)	0 (0)
Diarrhea	16 (7.2%)	0 (0)
Delayed toxicity (RTOG/EORTC1987)		
Urinary system	7 (3.1%)	4 (1.8%)
Lower digestive tract	10 (4.5%)	5 (2.2%)

Prophylactic extended field irradiation is an important treatment option for patients without para-aortic LN metastasis

Extended field irradiation is widely used for cervical cancer patients with para-aortic LN metastasis in clinical. In our department, for those patients (192 case) who exhibited no para-aortic LN metastasis suggested by CT or PET imaging, but with other aggressive tumor features such as common iliac LN metastasis [15], tumor size> 4 cm, pelvic wall involvement in both sides, we also applied prophylactic extended field irradiation as a supplementary treatment (107 cases). Surprisingly, when compared to those non-para-aortic LN metastases patients who didn't receive such therapies (85 cases), we found a significant survival advantage in DFS and improved OS and DMFS (Fig. 3a-c) in patients with prophylactic extended field irradiation treatment, indicating that prophylactic extended field nodal irradiation is indeed

Table 3 Multivariate analysis for prognostic factors

Subject	HR	CI 95%	*P* value	Reference
OS				
Pelvic LN metastasis	0.558	0.363–0.858	0.008	No pelvic LN metastasis
para-aortic LN metastasis	0.381	0.232–0.624	0.000	No para-aortic LN metastasis
EQD2(point A)	3.168	1.915–5.241	0.000	EQD2 < $90Gy_{10}$
Concurrent chemotherapy	1.867	1.219–2.861	0.004	< 4 cycles
DFS				
Pelvic LN metastasis	0.530	0.352–0.800	0.002	No pelvic LN metastasis
Para- aortic LN metastasis	0.446	0.275–0.722	0.001	No para-aortic LN metastasis
EQD2(point A)	3.416	2.061–5.664	0.000	EQD2 < $90Gy_{10}$
HGB	0.652	0.435–0.979	0.039	*HGB prior treatment < 110 g/L*
Concurrent chemotherapy	1.907	1.266–2.873	0.002	< 4 cycles
LCR				
Tumor size	0.254	0.060–1.069	0.062	Tumor≤4 cm
Para- aortic LN metastasis	0.354	0.172–0.727	0.005	No para-aortic LN metastasis
EQD2(point A)	5.925	3.019–11.630	0.000	EQD2 < $90Gy_{10}$
DMFS				
Concurrent chemotherapy	1.874	1.160–3.028	0.010	< 4 cycles

an important supplement to improve prognosis of none para-aortic LN metastasis FIGO IIIB cervical cancer patients.

Discussion

Most cervical cancer cases can be prevented by routine screening, treatment of precancerous lesions or HPV vaccination, which dramatically decreases cervical cancer incidence and its related mortality [16]. Nevertheless, in many countries and regions which are lacking such procedures, cervical cancer is still a big threat to women as the survival ratio for advanced cervical cancer has not been significantly improved. Sangkittipaiboon et al analyzed 19 cases of stage III cervical cancer patients and revealed that both 5 years OS was 42.1% [17]. Gadducci et al reported a 5-year overall survival of 60% in 61 stage III cervical cancer patients [18], which was similar to our findings specifically in Chinese FIGO IIIB cervical cancer patients.

The treatment failure for cervical cancer therapy is usually defined as distant metastasis or local recurrence. Hong et al analyzed 1292 FIGO I-IV cervical cancer patients and observed that among 410 treatment failure cases, 82% of were reported within 2 years after therapy [19]. Of these

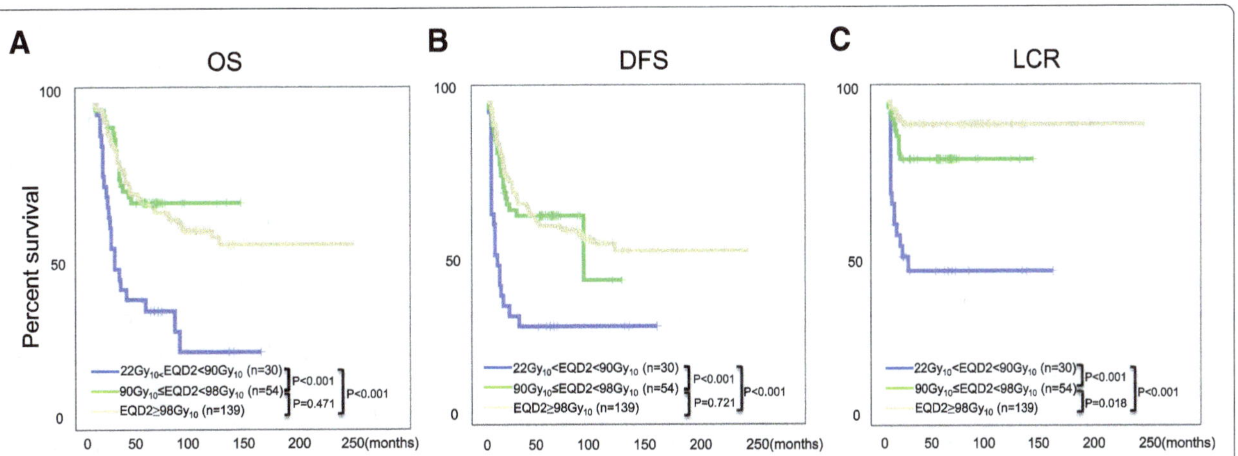

Fig. 2 Higher EQD2 (point A) is correlated with better treatment outcome. All patients were further divided into 3 groups based on the EQD2 (point A), namely low EQD2($22Gy_{10}$<EQD2<$90Gy_{10}$, blue line), medium EQD2 ($90Gy_{10}$≤EQD2<$98Gy_{10}$, green line) and high EQD2(≥$98Gy_{10}$, grey line). The correlation between EQD2 (point A) and OS (**a**), DFS (**b**) and LCR (**c**) are presented. *P* values are indicated separately in the figures. *n* = 223 patients in total

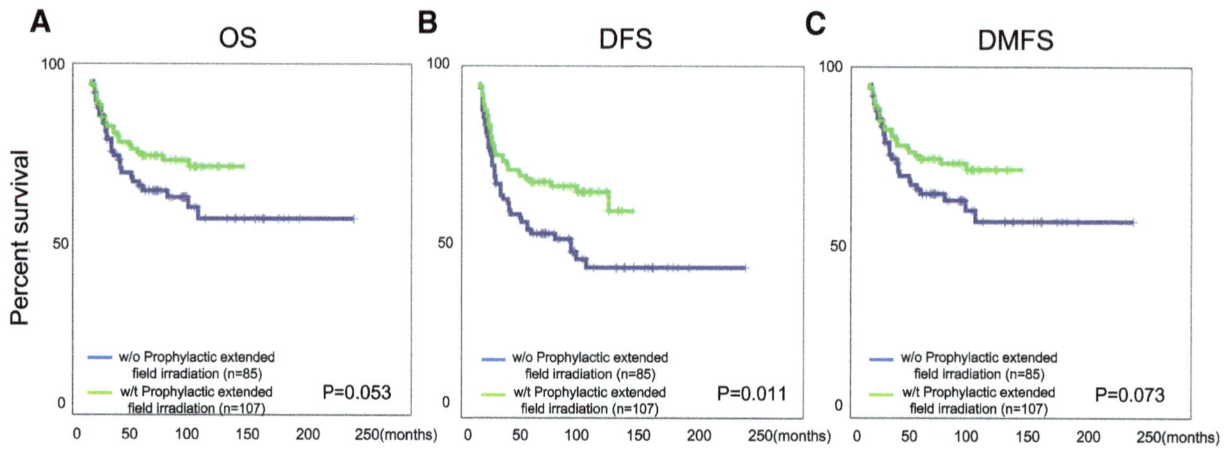

Fig. 3 Prophylactic extended field irradiation can improve prognosis in FIGO IIIB cervical cancer patients without para-aortic LN metastasis. The patients without para-aortic LN metastasis (n = 192) were divided into 2 groups according to whether they were treated with or without prophylactic extended field irradiation. The survival difference in OS (**a**), DFS (**b**) and DMFS (**c**) are presented and P values are indicated in each figure

patients, 213(52%) had distant metastasis, 162(40%) had local recurrence, and 35(8%) had both distant metastasis and local recurrence [19]. Waggoner reported that 90% of cervical cancer recurrence occurred within 3 years after the first treatment [2]. Katanyoo described that pelvic recurrence was one major treatment failure type for FIGO IIIB cervical cancer patients [20]. In our study, 36(16.1%) patients displayed local recurrence, which occurred between 6.5–25.9 months (median time was 13.3 months) after first therapy; while 73 (32.7%) patients had distant metastasis, which occurred within 30 months (median time was 12.2 months). In line with previous studies, lung was the most common metastatic target for FIGO IIIB cervical cancers. Of note, most patients who experienced treatment failure had tumors' diameter > 4 cm, therefore, special or additional treatment are required for these patients.

The major concern for FIGO IIIB cervical cancer patient's treatment is the side effects. Many studies have already shown that IMRT can significantly reduce cervical cancer radiotherapy-related adverse effects compared to 3D-CRT. Chen et al reported that IMRT could induce 36 and 30% digestive and urinary tract acute adverse effects respectively compared to 80 and 60% of such effects induced by 3D-CRT [7]. Similarly, the incidence of IMRT-related digestive and urinary system chronic adverse effects were 6 and 9% compared to 34 and 23% which induced by 3D-CRT [21]. Importantly, we didn't observe any survival difference between IMRT and 3D-CRT treated patients, indicating that IMRT was a safer radiotherapy technology compared to 3D-CRT without compromising any therapeutic efficacy. Importantly, we did notice extended-field irradiation or higher dose escalation were associated with more severe side effects, but the difference were not significant when compared to those patients with only pelvic irradiation or lower dose irradiation treatment.

The radiotherapy for FIGO IIIB cervical cancer patients includes both external beam radiation therapy (EBRT) and intracavitary brachytherapy (ICBT). ICBT, which uses point A as a reference [9] to modulate the equivalent total dose in 2-Gy fractions (EDQ2) in the targeting area, is an essential treatment to cervical cancer radiotherapy. Eifel et al reported that when point A EQD2 was less than 85Gy_{10}, the five-year pelvic recurrence ratio was 33%, in contrast, this ratio was only 16% when point A EQD2 was greater than 85Gy_{10} [6]. Consistently, Schmid et al performed three-dimensional intracavitary radiation therapy and found that when EQD2 for the high-risk CTV (HRCTV) was greater than 87Gy_{10}, the cervical cancer local control ratio was more than 95% [11]. In this study, most patients were treated with IMRT as external radiation therapy, in addition, intracavitary radiation therapy was designed and performed according to real-time CT or PET imaging to reduce radiation-related organ damage. When patients showed no obvious contraindications, 6 fractions of 6Gy_{10} intracavitary radiation was administrated. Thus, the point A EQD_2 for intracavitary radiation was 48Gy_{10}, and the total EQD_2 for both IMRT and intracavitary radiation for point A could reach as high as 98 Gy_{10}. This dose is higher than any other previous reports [22] and we believe this why we could achieve better prognosis. Indeed, the further investigation revealed escalated EQD2(point A) was associated with better survival. However, this strategy also introduced much more acute toxicity compared to a recent reported clinical trial result in India [23], we therefore tried to overcome these complications as previously described [24, 25], for example, we prescribed leucogen or rhG-CSF to control hematological toxicity; live Combined Bifidobacterium, Lactobacillus and Enterococcus Capsules were used to rescue intestinal flora as well as sulfasalazine or mesalazine to alleviate intestinal inflammation; when necessary, we applied levofloxacin to control kidney infection. With these measures, the delayed toxicity percentage in our patients was comparable to the Indian study [23].

Extended field nodal irradiation has been widely used to treat patients with para-aortic LN metastasis and has shown great benefit for such patients [26, 27]. In our study, for those patients without para-aortic LN metastasis but showing aggressive tumor features, we also prescribed them with prophylactic extended field nodal irradiation. Our data suggested that these patients showed marked survival advantage in DFS and improved OS as well as DMFS when compared to none para-aortic LN metastasis patients who didn't receive such treatment. Although the advantage in OS and DMFS was not significant, which might be explained as the limited sample size, the other reason was the patients who received prophylactic extended field irradiation usually showed more aggressive carcinoma features before the treatment. Therefore, albeit further investigation with a larger patient's sample is required, we propose that prophylactic extended field nodal irradiation is beneficial for cervical cancer patients with or without para-aortic LN metastasis.

We admitted that our study also had some limitations, first, this is a single-center retrospective analysis, a multi-centers study included many more patients will be more informative; secondly, the intracavitary brachytherapy used in our study was 2 dimensional, thus we could only evaluate the dosage using EQD2, which might not be so accurate when compared to 3 dimensional intracavitary brachytherapy; thirdly, only 30 patients received less than $90Gy_{10}$ irradiation, this limited numbers might impair the accuracy when interpreting the correlations between higher dosage irradiation and prognosis.

Conclusion

Our retrospective study confirms that concurrent chemoradiotherapy (CCRT) is an efficient and safe treatment for FIGO IIIB cervical cancer patients. We provide systematic understanding of various prognostic factors which contribute to IIIB cervical cancer patients' prognosis in China. Moreover, we propose that FIGO IIIB cervical cancer patients should be treated with higher EQD2 ($\geq 98Gy_{10}$) radiotherapy plus at least 4 rounds of chemotherapy when possible, and patients without para-aortic LN metastasis should be also treated with prophylactic extended field irradiation to improve prognosis.

Additional file

Additional file 1: Figure S1. Univariate analysis of different prognostic factors for overall survival (OS). (A) Pathology type and OS. $P = 0.062$; (B) pre-treatment HGB level and OS. $P = 0.018$; (C) Tumor size and. $P = 0.019$; (D Pelvic LNM and. $P = 0.001$; (E) Para-aortic LNM and OS. $P < 0.001$; (F) EQD2 (Point A) and OS. $P < 0.001$; (G) Concurrent chemotherapy cycles and OS. $P = 0.004$. **Figure S2.** Univariate analysis of different prognostic factors for disease free survival (DFS). (A) pre-treatment HGB level and DFS. $P = 0.022$; (B) Tumor size and DFS. $P = 0.044$; (C) Pelvic LNM and DFS. $P < 0.001$; (D) Para-aortic LNM and DFS. $P < 0.001$; (E) Treatment duration and DFS. $P = 0.04$; (F) EQD2 (Point A) and DFS. $P < 0.001$; (G) Concurrent chemotherapy cycles and DFS. $P = 0.005$. **Figure S3.** Univariate analysis of different prognostic factors for local control rate (LCR). (A) Tumor size and LCR. $P = 0.039$; (B) Para-aortic LNM and LCR. $P < 0.001$; (C) EQD2 (Point A) and LCR. $P < 0.001$; **Figure S4.** Univariate analysis of different prognostic factors for distant metastasis free survival (DMFS). (A) Pelvic LNM and DMFS. $P < 0.001$; (B) Para-aortic LNM and DMFS. $P < 0.001$; (C) Treatment duration and DMFS. $P = 0.018$; (D) Concurrent chemotherapy cycles and DMFS. $P = 0.024$. **Table S1.** Details for treatment failure patterns. **Table S2.** Univariate analysis for prognostic factors. (DOCX 474 kb)

Abbreviations

3D-CRT: Three-dimensional conformal radiotherapy; CCRT: Concurrent chemoradiotherapy; CR: Complete response; CT: Computed tomography; CTV: Clinical target volume; DFS: Disease-free survival; DMFS: Distant metastasis-free survival; EBRT: External beam radiation therapy; EQD2: Equivalent dose in 2 Gy fractions; FIGO: Federation of Gynecology and Obstetrics; HGB: Hemoglobin; ICBT: Intracavitary brachytherapy; ICRU: International Commission on Radiation Units; IMRT: Intensity modulated radiotherapy; LCR: Local control rate; LN: Lymph node; NCI: National Cancer Institute; OARs: Organs at risks; OS: Overall Survival; PET: Positron emission tomography; PR: Partial response

Acknowledgements

We would like to thank all the patients involved in this study for sharing their information during the follow-up period. We are also very grateful to all the members of our department for helpful discussions.

Funding

This project was supported by the Ministry of Science and Technology of the People's Republic of China (grant number 2016YFC0105207).

Authors' contributions

The study was conceived and designed by KH and FZ, QM and WW performed data collection, data analysis and data interpretation; XL, XH, XL, SS, JY, ZL and ZM helped with patient's follow-up and data collection; KH and FZ coordinated the whole study; QM and KH wrote the manuscript and prepared the figures together with help of WW and FZ. All authors read and approved the final manuscript.

Competing interests

The authors declare that they have no competing interests.

References

1. Ferlay J, Soerjomataram I, Dikshit R, Eser S, Mathers C, Rebelo M, et al. Cancer incidence and mortality worldwide: sources, methods and major patterns in GLOBOCAN 2012. Int J Cancer. 2015;136:E359–86.
2. Waggoner S. Cervical cancer. Lancet. 2003;361:2217–25.
3. Patel K, Foster NR, Kumar A, Grudem M, Longenbach S, Bakkum-Gamez J, et al. Hydronephrosis in patients with cervical cancer: an assessment of morbidity and survival. Support Care Cancer. 2015;23:1303–9.
4. Zuliani AC, Cunha Mde O, Esteves SC, Teixeira JC. Brachytherapy for stage IIIB squamous cell carcinoma of the uterine cervix: survival and toxicity. Rev Assoc Med Bras. 2010;56:37–40.
5. Ahmed RS, Kim RY, Duan J, Meleth S, De Los Santos JF, Fiveash JB. IMRT dose escalation for positive para-aortic lymph nodes in patients with locally advanced cervical cancer while reducing dose to bone marrow and other organs at risk. Int J Radiat Oncol Biol Phys. 2004;60:505–12.
6. Eifel PJ, Winter K, Morris M, Levenback C, Grigsby PW, Cooper J, et al. Pelvic irradiation with concurrent chemotherapy versus pelvic and para-aortic irradiation for high-risk cervical cancer: an update of radiation therapy oncology group trial (RTOG) 90-01. J Clin Oncol. 2004;22:872–80.
7. Chen MF, Tseng CJ, Tseng CC, Kuo YC, Yu CY, Chen WC. Clinical outcome in posthysterectomy cervical cancer patients treated with concurrent cisplatin and intensity-modulated pelvic radiotherapy: comparison with conventional radiotherapy. Int J Radiat Oncol Biol Phys. 2007;67:1438–44.
8. Parker K, Gallop-Evans E, Hanna L, Adams M. Five years' experience treating locally advanced cervical cancer with concurrent chemoradiotherapy and high-dose-rate brachytherapy: results from a single institution. Int J Radiat Oncol Biol Phys. 2009;74:140–6.
9. Grigsby PW, Williamson JF, Chao KSC, Perez CA. Cervical tumor control evaluated with ICRU 38 reference volumes and integrated reference air kerma. Radiother Oncol. 2001;58:19–23.
10. Morris M, Eifel PJ, Lu J, Grigsby PW, Levenback C, Stevens RE, et al. Pelvic radiation with concurrent chemotherapy compared with pelvic and para-aortic radiation for high-risk cervical cancer. N Engl J Med. 1999;340:1137–43.
11. Schmid MP, Kirisits C, Nesvacil N, Dimopoulos JC, Berger D, Pötter R. Local recurrences in cervical cancer patients in the setting of image-guided brachytherapy: a comparison of spatial dose distribution within a matched-pair analysis. Radiother Oncol. 2011;100:468–72.
12. Wang W, Meng Q, Hou X, Lian X, Yan J, Sun S, et al. Efficacy and toxicity of image-guided intensity-modulated radiation therapy combined with dose-escalated brachytherapy for stage IIB cervical cancer. Oncotarget. 2017;8: 102965–73.
13. Therasse P, Arbuck SG, Eisenhauer EA, Wanders J, Kaplan RS, Rubinstein L, et al. New guidelines to evaluate the response to treatment in solid tumors. European Organization for Research and Treatment of Cancer, National Cancer Institute of the United States, National Cancer Institute of Canada. J Natl Cancer Inst. 2000;92:205–16.
14. Herrmann T, Knorr A, Dörner K. The RTOG/EORTC classification criteria for early and late radiation reactions. Radiobiol Radiother (Berl). 1987;28:519–28.
15. Huang L, Zheng M, Liu JH, Xiong Y, Ding H, Tang L, et al. Risk factors and prognosis of IB-IIB cervical carcinoma with common iliac lymph node metastasis. Chin J Cancer. 2010;29:431–5.
16. Tota JE, Ramana-Kumar AV, El-Khatib Z, Franco EL. The road ahead for cervical cancer prevention and control. Curr Oncol. 2014;211:255–64.
17. Sangkittipaiboon S. Long-term outcomes of concurrent chemoradiotherapy with weekly carboplatin in locally-advanced carcinoma of the uterine cervix patients. J Med Assoc Thail. 2014;97:12–9.
18. Gadducci A, Fabrini MG, Perrone F, Manfredi B, Fanucchi A, Laliscia C, et al. Pattern of failures and clinical outcome of patients with locally advanced cervical cancer treated with a tailored integrated therapeutic approach. Anticancer Res. 2010;30:3731–6.
19. Hong JH, Tsai CS, Lai CH, Chang TC, Wang CC, Chou HH, et al. Recurrent squamous cell carcinoma of cervix after definitive radiotherapy. Int J Radiat Oncol Biol Phys. 2004;60:249–57.
20. Katanyoo K. Comparing treatment outcomes of stage IIIB cervical cancer patients between those with and without lower third of vaginal invasion. J Gynecol Oncol. 2017;28:e79.
21. Novetsky AP, Einstein MH, Goldberg GL, Hailpern SM, Landau E, Fields AL, et al. Efficacy and toxicity of concomitant cisplatin with external beam pelvic radiotherapy and two high-dose-rate brachytherapy insertions for the treatment of locally advanced cervical cancer. Gynecol Oncol. 2007;105:635–40.
22. Pötter R, Tanderup K, Kirisits C, de Leeuw A, Kirchheiner K, Nout R, et al. The EMBRACE II study: the outcome and prospect of two decades of evolution within the GEC-ESTRO GYN working group and the EMBRACE studies. Clin Transl Radiat Oncol. 2018;9:48–60.
23. Shrivastava S, Mahantshetty U, Engineer R, Chopra S, Hawaldar R, Hande V, et al. Cisplatin chemoradiotherapy vs radiotherapy in FIGO stage IIIB squamous cell carcinoma of the uterine cervix: a randomized clinical trial. JAMA Oncol. 2018;4:506–13.
24. Sturdza A, Potter R, Fokdal LU, Haie-Meder C, Tanj LT, Mazeron R, et al. Image guided brachytherapy in locally advanced cervical cancer: improved pelvic control and survival in RetroEMBRACE, a multicenter cohort study. Radiother Oncol. 2016;120:428–33.
25. Rijkmans EC, Nout RA, Rutten IHHM, Ketelaars M, Neelis KJ, Laman MS, et al. Improved survival of patients with cervical cancer treated with image-guided brachytherapy compared with conventional brachytherapy. Gynecol Oncol. 2014;135:231–8.
26. Rotman M, Pajak TF, Choi K, Clery M, Marcial V, Grigsby PW, et al. Prophylactic extended-field irradiation of para-aortic lymph nodes in stage IIB and bulky IB and IIA cervical carcinomas. JAMA. 1995;274:387–93.
27. Kim JH, Kim JY, Yoon MS, Kim YS, Lee JH, Kim HJ, et al. Prophylactic irradiation of para-aortic lymph nodes for patients with locally advanced cervical cancer with and without CA9 expression (KROG 07-01):a randomized, open-label, multicenter, phase 2 trial. Radiother Oncol. 2016;120:383–9.

Permissions

All chapters in this book were first published in RO, by BioMed Central; hereby published with permission under the Creative Commons Attribution License or equivalent. Every chapter published in this book has been scrutinized by our experts. Their significance has been extensively debated. The topics covered herein carry significant findings which will fuel the growth of the discipline. They may even be implemented as practical applications or may be referred to as a beginning point for another development.

The contributors of this book come from diverse backgrounds, making this book a truly international effort. This book will bring forth new frontiers with its revolutionizing research information and detailed analysis of the nascent developments around the world.

We would like to thank all the contributing authors for lending their expertise to make the book truly unique. They have played a crucial role in the development of this book. Without their invaluable contributions this book wouldn't have been possible. They have made vital efforts to compile up to date information on the varied aspects of this subject to make this book a valuable addition to the collection of many professionals and students.

This book was conceptualized with the vision of imparting up-to-date information and advanced data in this field. To ensure the same, a matchless editorial board was set up. Every individual on the board went through rigorous rounds of assessment to prove their worth. After which they invested a large part of their time researching and compiling the most relevant data for our readers.

The editorial board has been involved in producing this book since its inception. They have spent rigorous hours researching and exploring the diverse topics which have resulted in the successful publishing of this book. They have passed on their knowledge of decades through this book. To expedite this challenging task, the publisher supported the team at every step. A small team of assistant editors was also appointed to further simplify the editing procedure and attain best results for the readers.

Apart from the editorial board, the designing team has also invested a significant amount of their time in understanding the subject and creating the most relevant covers. They scrutinized every image to scout for the most suitable representation of the subject and create an appropriate cover for the book.

The publishing team has been an ardent support to the editorial, designing and production team. Their endless efforts to recruit the best for this project, has resulted in the accomplishment of this book. They are a veteran in the field of academics and their pool of knowledge is as vast as their experience in printing. Their expertise and guidance has proved useful at every step. Their uncompromising quality standards have made this book an exceptional effort. Their encouragement from time to time has been an inspiration for everyone.

The publisher and the editorial board hope that this book will prove to be a valuable piece of knowledge for researchers, students, practitioners and scholars across the globe.

List of Contributors

Heejung Kim
Department of Biomedical Engineering, Seoul National University, Seoul, Korea
Department of Radiation Oncology, Soonchunhyang University Hospital, Seoul, Korea

Ah Ram Chang
Department of Radiation Oncology, Soonchunhyang University Hospital, Seoul, Korea

Sungwoo Cho
Department of Surgery, Soonchunhyang University Hospital, Seoul, Korea

Sung-Joon Ye
Department of Transdisciplinary Studies, Seoul National University, Seoul, Korea
Advanced Institutes of Convergence Technology, Seoul National University, Suwon, Korea
Biomedical Research Institute, Seoul National University Hospital, Seoul, Korea

Nikolaos Koutsouvelis
Radiation Oncology, Geneva University Hospital, CH-1211, 14 Geneva, Switzerland

Thomas Zilli and Raymond Miralbell
Radiation Oncology, Geneva University Hospital, CH-1211, 14 Geneva, Switzerland
Faculty of Medicine, Geneva University, Geneva, Switzerland

Marta Scorsetti
Radiation Oncology, Humanitas University, Rozzano, Milan, Italy
Radiation Oncology, Humanitas Research Hospital and Cancer Center, Rozzano, Milan, Italy

Ciro Franzese and Giuseppe Roberto D'Agostino
Radiation Oncology, Humanitas Research Hospital and Cancer Center, Rozzano, Milan, Italy

Daniel Zwahlen and Michel Zimmermann
Radiation Oncology, Kantonsspital Graubünden, Chur, Switzerland

Robert Förster and Matthias Guckenberger
Radiation Oncology, University Hospital Zürich, Zürich, Switzerland

Niccolò Giaj-Levra
Radiation Oncology, Sacro Cuore Don-Calabria, Negrar, Italy

Filippo Alongi
Radiation Oncology, Sacro Cuore Don-Calabria, Negrar, Italy Faculty of Medecine, University of Brescia, Brescia, Italy

Aurelie Bertaut
Methodology and biostatistic unit, Centre Georges François Leclerc, Dijon, France

Jackson M. May, Mark R. Waddle, Daniel H. Miller, William C. Stross, Tasneem A. Kaleem, Byron C. May, Robert C. Miller, Gerald W. Strong and Daniel M. Trifiletti
Department of Radiation Oncology, Mayo Clinic, 4500 San Pablo Road South, Jacksonville, FL 32224, USA

Jennifer L. Peterson
Department of Radiation Oncology, Mayo Clinic, 4500 San Pablo Road South, Jacksonville, FL 32224, USA
Department of Neurological Surgery, Mayo Clinic, Jacksonville, Florida, USA

Kaisorn L. Chaichana and Ronald Reimer
Department of Neurological Surgery, Mayo Clinic, Jacksonville, Florida, USA

Liuyan Jiang
Department of Pathology and Laboratory Medicine, Mayo Clinic, Jacksonville, Florida, USA

Han W. Tun
Department of Hematology and Medical Oncology, Mayo Clinic, Jacksonville, Florida, USA

Dong-Yun Kim and Hyun-Cheol Kang
Department of Radiation Oncology, Seoul National University College of Medicine, 101 Daehak-ro, Jongno-gu, Seoul 03080, Republic of Korea

Il Han Kim
Department of Radiation Oncology, Seoul National University College of Medicine, 101 Daehak-ro, Jongno-gu, Seoul 03080, Republic of Korea

Seoul National University Cancer Research Institute, 101 Daehak-ro, Jongno-gu, Seoul 110-779, Republic of Korea

Sung-Soo Yoon
Department of Internal Medicine, Seoul National University College of Medicine, 101 Daehak-ro, Jongno-gu, Seoul 03080, Republic of Korea
Seoul National University Cancer Research Institute, 101 Daehak-ro, Jongno-gu, Seoul 110-779, Republic of Korea

Hyoung Jin Kang and Hee Young Shin
Department of Pediatrics, Seoul National University College of Medicine, 101 Daehak-ro, Jongno-gu, Seoul 03080, Republic of Korea
Seoul National University Cancer Research Institute, 101 Daehak-ro, Jongno-gu, Seoul 110-779, Republic of Korea

Hendrik Dapper, Markus Oechsner, Kai Borm, Jan Peeken, Michael Mayinger and Daniel Habermehl
Department of Radiation Oncology, Klinikum rechts der Isar, TU München, Ismaninger Str. 22, 81675 Munich, Germany

Stephanie E. Combs
Department of Radiation Oncology, Klinikum rechts der Isar, TU München, Ismaninger Str. 22, 81675 Munich, Germany
Institute for innovative Radiotherapie (iRT), Helmholtz Zentrum München, Ingolstädter Landstr. 1, Neuherberg, Germany
Deutsches Konsortium für Translationale Krebsforschung (DKTK), Partner Site Munich, Munich, Germany

Stefan Münch
Department of Radiation Oncology, Klinikum rechts der Isar, TU München, Ismaninger Str. 22, 81675 Munich, Germany
Deutsches Konsortium für Translationale Krebsforschung (DKTK), Partner Site Munich, Munich, Germany

Xue Wang
School of Medicine and Life Sciences, University of Jinan-Shandong Academy of Medical Sciences, Jinan, Shandong Province, China
Department of Thoracic Radiation Oncology, Shandong Cancer Hospital affiliated to Shandong University, Shandong Academy of Medical Sciences, No. 440 Jiyan Road, Jinan 250117, Shandong Province, China

Jin-Zhi Wang, Jian-Bin Li, Ying-Jie Zhang, Feng-Xiang Li, Wei Wang, Qian Shao, Min Xu and Xi-Jun Liu
Department of Thoracic Radiation Oncology, Shandong Cancer Hospital affiliated to Shandong University, Shandong Academy of Medical Sciences, No. 440 Jiyan Road, Jinan 250117, Shandong Province, China

Yan-Luan Guo
Department of PET-CT Room, Shandong Cancer Hospital affiliated to Shandong University, Shandong Academy of Medical Sciences, Jinan, Shandong Province, China

Yue Wang
Medical imaging department, Shandong Cancer Hospital affiliated to Shandong University, Shandong Academy of Medical Sciences, Jinan, Shandong Province, China

Jung-in Kim
Department of Radiation Oncology, Seoul National University Hospital, Seoul, South Korea
Institute of Radiation Medicine, Seoul National University Medical Research Center, Seoul, South Korea
Biomedical Research Institute, Seoul National University Hospital, Seoul, South Korea

Jong Min Park
Department of Radiation Oncology, Seoul National University Hospital, Seoul, South Korea
Institute of Radiation Medicine, Seoul National University Medical Research Center, Seoul, South Korea
Biomedical Research Institute, Seoul National University Hospital, Seoul, South Korea
Institute for Smart System, Robotics Research Laboratory for Extreme Environments, Advanced Institutes of Convergence Technology, Suwon, South Korea

So-Yeon Park
Department of Radiation Oncology, Veterans Health Service Medical Center, Seoul, South Korea

Do Hoon Oh
Department of Radiation Oncology, Myongji Hospital, Goyang, South Korea

Sang-Tae Kim
Nuclear Emergency Division, Radiation Protection and Emergency Preparedness Bureau, Nuclear Safety and Security Commission, Seoul, South nKorea

Narges Miri, Kimberley Legge and Kim Colyvas
University of Newcastle, Newcastle, NSW, Australia

Joerg Lehmann and Peter B. Greer
University of Newcastle, Newcastle, NSW, Australia
Calvary Mater Newcastle, Newcastle, NSW, Australia

Philip Vial
Liverpool and Macarthur Cancer Therapy Centres and Ingham Institute, Liverpool, NSW, Australia
University of Sydney, Sydney, NSW, Australia

Alisha Moore and Monica Harris
TROG Cancer Research, Newcastle, NSW, Australia

Howard J. Lee Jr
Duke University School of Medicine, 10 Duke Medicine Circle, Durham, NC 27710, USA

Meghan W. Macomber, Matthew B. Spraker, Stephen R. Bowen, Kenneth J. Russell, George E. Laramore, Ramesh Rengan, Jay Liao, Smith Apisarnthanarax and Jing Zeng
Department of Radiation Oncology, University of Washington School of Medicine, 1959 NE Pacific Street, Campus, Seattle, WA 98195, USA

Daniel S. Hippe
Department of Radiology, University of Washington School of Medicine, 1959 NE Pacific Street, Campus, Seattle, WA 98195, USA

Angela Fung
Seattle Cancer Care Alliance Proton Therapy Center, 1570 N 115th St, Seattle, WA 98115, USA

Yvonne Dzierma, Katharina Mikulla, Patrick Richter, Katharina Bell, Patrick Melchior, Frank Nuesken and Christian Rübe
Department of Radiotherapy and Radiation Oncology, Saarland University Medical Centre, Kirrberger Str. Geb. 6.5, 66421 Homburg, Saar, Germany

Yukiko Hattori and Shingo Hashimoto
Department of Radiation Oncology, Nagoya Proton Therapy Center, Nagoya City West Medical Center, 1-1-1 Hirate-cho, Kita-ku, Nagoya 462-8508, Japan

Koichiro Nakajima, Hiromitsu Iwata and Hiroyuki Ogino
Department of Radiation Oncology, Nagoya Proton Therapy Center, Nagoya City West Medical Center, 1-1-1 Hirate-cho, Kita-ku, Nagoya 462-8508, Japan
Department of Radiology, Nagoya City University Graduate School of Medical Sciences, 1 Kawasumi, Mizuho-cho, Mizuho-ku, Nagoya 467-8601, Japan

Jun-etsu Mizoe
Department of Radiation Oncology, Nagoya Proton Therapy Center, Nagoya City West Medical Center, 1-1-1 Hirate-cho, Kita-ku, Nagoya 462-8508, Japan
Osaka Heavy Ion Therapy Center, 3-1-10 Otemae, Chuo-ku, Osaka 540-0008, Japan

Yuta Shibamoto
Department of Radiology, Nagoya City University Graduate School of Medical Sciences, 1 Kawasumi, Mizuho-cho, Mizuho-ku, Nagoya 467-8601, Japan

Toshiyuki Toshito
Department of Proton Therapy Physics, Nagoya Proton Therapy Center, 1-1-1 Hirate-cho, Kita-ku, Nagoya 462-8508, Japan

Kensuke Hayashi
Department of Proton Therapy Technology, Nagoya Proton Therapy Center, 1-1-1 Hirate-cho, Kita-ku, Nagoya 462-8508, Japan

Kenji Akita
Department of Respiratory Medicine, Thoracic Oncology Center, Nagoya City West Medical Center, 1-1-1 Hirate-cho, Kita-ku, Nagoya 462-8508, Japan

Fumiya Baba
Department of Radiation Therapy, Nagoya City West Medical Center, 1-1-1 Hirate-cho, Kita-ku, Nagoya 462-8508, Japan

Katsumi Nakamae
Department of Thoracic Surgery, Thoracic Oncology Center, Nagoya City West Medical Center, 1-1-1 Hirate-cho, Kita-ku, Nagoya 462-8508, Japan

Yung-Chih Chou
Radiation Oncology, Chang Gung Memorial Hospital at Linkou and Chang Gung University, No. 5, Fuxing St., Guishan Dist, Taoyuan City 33305, Taiwan, Republic of China

Kang-Hsing Fan
Radiation Oncology, Chang Gung Memorial Hospital at Linkou and Chang Gung University, No. 5, Fuxing St., Guishan Dist, Taoyuan City 33305, Taiwan, Republic of China

Head and Neck Oncology Group, Chang Gung Memorial Hospital at Linkou and Chang Gung University, Taoyuan City, Taiwan, Republic of China

Hung-Ming Wang
Medical Oncology, Chang Gung Memorial Hospital at Linkou and Chang Gung University, Taoyuan City, Taiwan, Republic of China
Head and Neck Oncology Group, Chang Gung Memorial Hospital at Linkou and Chang Gung University, Taoyuan City, Taiwan, Republic of China

Chun-Ta Liao
Otorhinolaryngology, Head and Neck Surgery, Chang Gung Memorial Hospital at Linkou and Chang Gung University, Taoyuan City, Taiwan, Republic of China
Head and Neck Oncology Group, Chang Gung Memorial Hospital at Linkou and Chang Gung University, Taoyuan City, Taiwan, Republic of China

Ku-Hao Fang
Otorhinolaryngology, Head and Neck Surgery, Chang Gung Memorial Hospital at Linkou and Chang Gung University, Taoyuan City, Taiwan, Republic of China
Head and Neck Oncology Group, Chang Gung Memorial Hospital at Linkou and Chang Gung University, Taoyuan City, Taiwan, Republic of China
Graduate Institute of Clinical Medical Science, Chang Gung University, Taoyuan City, Taiwan, Republic of China

Christiane Matuschek, Jan Haussmann, Edwin Bölke, Stephan Gripp, Bálint Tamaskovics, Freddy-Joel Djiepmo-Njanang, Klaus Orth and Wilfried Budach
Department of Radiotherapy and Radiooncology, Medical Faculty, Heinrich Heine University, Moorenstr. 5, 40225 Dusseldorf, Germany

Patrick J. Schuler
Department of Oto-Rhino-Laryngology, Head and Neck Surgery, Ulm University Medical Center, Ulm, Germany

Peter Arne Gerber
Department of Dermatology, Medical Faculty Heinrich Heine University Dusseldorf, Dusseldorf, Germany

Kai Kammers
Division of Biostatistics and Bioinformatics, Department of Oncology, The Sidney Kimmel Comprehensive Cancer Center at Johns Hopkins, The Johns Hopkins University School of Medicine, Baltimore, MD, USA

Christian Plettenberg
Department of Oto-Rhino-Laryngology, Head and Neck Surgery, Heinrich Heine University Dusseldorf, Dusseldorf, Germany

Bahar Anooshahr
Vincere Cancer Center, Scottsdale, AZ, USA

Simona Marzi
Medical Physics Laboratory, IRCCS Regina Elena National Cancer Institute, Via Elio Chianesi 53, 00144 Rome, Italy

Alessia Farneti, Laura Marucci, Filomena Spasiano and Giuseppe Sanguineti
Department of Radiotherapy, IRCCS Regina Elena National Cancer Institute, Via Elio Chianesi 53, 00144 Rome, Italy

Antonello Vidiri
Radiology and Diagnostic Imaging Department, IRCCS Regina Elena National Cancer Institute, Via Elio Chianesi 53, 00144 Rome, Italy

Francesca Di Giuliano
Radiology and Diagnostic Imaging Department, IRCCS Regina Elena National Cancer Institute, Via Elio Chianesi 53, 00144 Rome, Italy
Department of Biomedicine and Prevention, University of Rome "Tor Vergata", Viale Oxford 81, 00133 Rome, Italy

Irene Terrenato
Biostatistics-Scientific Direction, IRCCS Regina Elena National Cancer Institute, Via Elio Chianesi 53, 00144 Rome, Italy

Sophie C. Huijskens, Irma W. E. M. van Dijk, Jorrit Visser, Brian V. Balgobind, Coen R. N. Rasch, Tanja Alderliesten and Arjan Bel
Department of Radiation Oncology, Cancer Center Amsterdam, Amsterdam UMC, University of Amsterdam, Office Z1-217, Meibergdreef 9, 1105, AZ, Amsterdam, The Netherlands

Stefania Clemente and Caterina Oliviero
Azienda Ospedaliera Universitaria Federico II, Naples, Italy

Giuseppe Palma, Vittoria D'Avino, Raffaele Liuzzi and Laura Cella
National Research Council, Institute of Biostructures and Bioimaging, Naples, Italy

Manuel Conson and Roberto Pacelli
Department of Advanced Biomedical Sciences, Federico II University School of Medicine, Naples, Italy

Hui Wang and Qianxi Ni
Department of Radiation Oncology, Key Laboratory of Translational Radiation Oncology, Hunan Province. Department of Radiation Oncology, Hunan Cancer Hospital and The Affiliated Cancer Hospital of Xiangya School of Medicine, Central South University, Changsha, Hunan Province, China

Yue Zhou
Department of Radiation Oncology, Key Laboratory of Translational Radiation Oncology, Hunan Province. Department of Radiation Oncology, Hunan Cancer Hospital and The Affiliated Cancer Hospital of Xiangya School of Medicine, Central South University, Changsha, Hunan Province, China
Xiangya School of Medicine, Central South University, Changsha, Hunan Province, China

Shibin Zhan
Department of Head and Neck Surgery, Hunan Cancer Hospital and The Affiliated Cancer Hospital of Xiangya School of Medicine, Changsha, Hunan Province, China

Xiao Zhou
Department of Head and Neck Surgery, Hunan Cancer Hospital and The Affiliated Cancer Hospital of Xiangya School of Medicine, Changsha, Hunan Province, China
Translational Medical Center, Hunan Cancer Hospital and The Affiliated Cancer Hospital of Xiangya School of Medicine, Central South University, Changsha, Hunan Province, China

Feiyan Deng
Department of Head and Neck Surgery, Hunan Cancer Hospital and The Affiliated Cancer Hospital of Xiangya School of Medicine, Changsha, Hunan Province, China
University of South China, Hengyang, Hunan Province, China

Yong Zeng
Translational Medical Center, Hunan Cancer Hospital and The Affiliated Cancer Hospital of Xiangya School of Medicine, Central South University, Changsha, Hunan Province, China

Xiaowu Sheng
Translational Medical Center, Hunan Cancer Hospital and The Affiliated Cancer Hospital of Xiangya School of Medicine, Central South University, Changsha, Hunan Province, China
Central Laboratory, Hunan Cancer Hospital and The Affiliated Cancer Hospital of Xiangya School of Medicine, Central South University, Changsha, Hunan Province, China

Liangfang Shen
Department of Tumor, Xiangya Hospital of Central South University, Changsha, Hunan Province, China

Gracinda Mondlane
Department of Physics - Medical Radiation Physics, Stockholm University, Stockholm, Sweden
Department of Physics, Universidade Eduardo Mondlane, Maputo, Mozambique

Ana Ureba
Department of Oncology and Pathology, Karolinska Institutet, Stockholm, Sweden

P A Lind and Albert Siegbahn
Department of Oncology and Pathology, Karolinska Institutet, Stockholm, Sweden
Department of Oncology, Södersjukhuset, Stockholm, Sweden

Michael Gubanski
Department of Oncology and Pathology, Karolinska University Hospital, Stockholm, Sweden

Xianzhi Zhao, Xiaofei Zhu, Yangsen Cao, Xiaoping Ju and Huojun Zhang
Department of Radiation Oncology, Shanghai Changhai Hospital, the Second Military Medical University, Shanghai 200433, China

Jianfeng Fei
Department of Radiology, Shanghai Changhai Hospital, the Second Military Medical University, Shanghai 200433, China

Haipeng Ren
Department of Oncology, Weifang People's Hospital, Weifang 261041, China

Zhiyong Yuan
Department of Radiation Oncology and CyberKnife Center, Key Laboratory of Cancer Prevention and Therapy, Tianjin's Clinical Research Center for Cancer, Tianjin Medical University Cancer Institute and Hospital, National Clinical Research Center for Cancer, Tianjin 300060, China

Angela Caroli, Francesco Apicella and Lucia Turri
Radiotherapy, University Hospital "Maggiore della Carità", Novara, Italy

Letizia Deantonio and Marco Krengli
Radiotherapy, University Hospital "Maggiore della Carità", Novara, Italy
Department of Translational Medicine, University of "Piemonte Orientale", Novara, Italy

Erinda Puta and Gianmauro Sacchetti
Nuclear Medicine, University Hospital "Maggiore della Carità", Novara, Italy

Daniela Ferrante
Department of Translational Medicine, Unit of Medical Statistics and Cancer Epidemiology, CPO Piemonte and University of "Piemonte Orientale", Novara, Italy

Marco Brambilla
Medical Physics, University Hospital "Maggiore della Carità", Novara, Italy

Manuel Grote
Department of Radiation Oncology, University Hospital, LMU Munich, 81377 Munich, Germany
Department of Orthopaedics, Physical Medicine and Rehabilitation, University Hospital, LMU Munich, 81377 Munich, Germany
Department of Health Promotion/Occupational Health Management, AOK Baden-Württemberg, 70191 Stuttgart, Germany

Cornelius Maihöfer and Claus Belka
Department of Radiation Oncology, University Hospital, LMU Munich, 81377 Munich, Germany
Clinical Cooperation Group 'Personalized Radiotherapy in Head and Neck Cancer' Helmholtz Zentrum München, German Research Center for Environmental Health GmbH, 85764 Neuherberg, Germany

Martin Weigl and Patricia Davies-Knorr
Department of Orthopaedics, Physical Medicine and Rehabilitation, University Hospital, LMU Munich, 81377 Munich, Germany

Sung Jun Ma, Kavitha M. Prezzano, Gregory M. Hermann and Anurag K. Singh
Department of Radiation Medicine, Roswell Park Comprehensive Cancer Center, Elm and Carlton Streets, Buffalo, NY 14263, USA

Olli Metsälä and Petra Miikkulainen
Turku Centre for Biotechnology, University of Turku and Åbo Akademi University, Tykistökatu 6, FIN-20520 Turku, Finland
Faculty of Medicine, Institute of Biomedicine, University of Turku, Kiinamyllynkatu 10, FIN-20520 Turku, Finland

Panu M. Jaakkola
Turku Centre for Biotechnology, University of Turku and Åbo Akademi University, Tykistökatu 6, FIN-20520 Turku, Finland
Faculty of Medicine, Institute of Biomedicine, University of Turku, Kiinamyllynkatu 10, FIN-20520 Turku, Finland
Helsinki University Hospital Comprehensive Cancer Center and Department of Oncology, University of Helsinki, Haartmaninkatu 4, FIN-00029 HUS Helsinki, Finland

Heidi Högel
Turku Centre for Biotechnology, University of Turku and Åbo Akademi University, Tykistökatu 6, FIN-20520 Turku, Finland
Turku PET Centre, University of Turku and Turku University Hospital, Kiinamyllynkatu 4-8, FIN-20521 Turku, Finland

Joose Kreutzer and Pasi Kallio
Bio Medi Tech, Institute and Faculty of Biosciences and Engineering, Tampere University of Technology, Korkeakoulunkatu 3, FIN-33720 Tampere, Finland

Qingyu Meng, Weiping Wang, Xiaoliang Liu, Xiaorong Hou, Xin Lian, Shuai Sun, Junfang Yan, Zhikai Liu, Zheng Miao, Ke Hu and Fuquan Zhang
Department of radiation oncology, Peking Union Medical College Hospital, Chinese Academy of Medical Sciences and Peking Union Medical College, Beijing, People's Republic of China

Index

www.ingramcontent.com/pod-product-compliance
Lightning Source LLC
LaVergne TN
LVHW080921210926
848485LV00004B/704
* 9 7 8 1 6 3 2 4 2 9 4 8 3 *